6th
EDITION

Professional Issues in Nursing

CHALLENGES AND OPPORTUNITIES

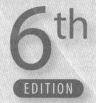

6th EDITION

Professional Issues in Nursing

CHALLENGES AND OPPORTUNITIES

Carol J. Huston, RN, MSN, MPA, DPA, FAAN
Professor Emerita
School of Nursing
California State University
Chico, California

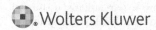 Wolters Kluwer

Philadelphia • Baltimore • New York • London
Buenos Aires • Hong Kong • Sydney • Tokyo

Vice President and Publisher: Julie K. Stegman
Director of Nursing Education and Practice Content: Jamie Blum
Senior Acquisitions Editor: Susan Hartman
Supervisory Development Editor: Staci Wolfson
Editorial Coordinator: Anju Radhakrishnan
Marketing Manager: Brittany Clements
Editorial Assistant: Molly Kennedy
Art Director, Illustration: Jennifer Clement
Senior Production Project Manager: Sadie Buckallew
Manufacturing Coordinator: Margie Orzech-Zeranko
Prepress Vendor: S4Carlisle Publishing Services

Sixth edition

10 9 8 7 6 5 4 3 2

Printed in Mexico

Library of Congress Cataloging-in-Publication Data

ISBN-13: 978-1-975175-61-0
ISBN-10: 1-975175-61-1

Library of Congress Control Number: 2021922502

QUADM0623

I dedicate this book to those nurses who work on the frontlines of the COVID-19 pandemic: doing what you can to improve patient outcomes, despite physical and emotional risks to self. You are the true heroes in the health care system and make such a difference in the lives of patients and families we care for. Thank you for all that you do.

Carol J. Huston

Contributors

Sheila A. Burke, DNP, MSN, MBA, RN, NEA-BC
Vice President of Nursing
Nursing Division
Education Affiliates, Inc.
Baltimore, Maryland
(CHAPTER 25)

Cynthia M. Clark, PhD, RN, ANEF, FAAN
Professor Emeritus; Boise State University
Founder and Consultant; Civility Matters
Boise, Idaho
(CHAPTER 13)

Elizabeth O. Dietz, EdD, RN, CS-NP, CSN, FAAN
Professor Emeritus—San Jose State University
Disability Integration Regional Lead & Disaster Health Services Manager
Northern CA Coastal Region— American Red Cross
The Valley Foundation School of Nursing
San Jose State University
Part-Time District School Nurse, San Jose Unified School District
San Jose, California
(CHAPTER 10)

Cassandra D. Ford, PhD, RN, FAHA, FGSA
Associate Professor
Capstone College of Nursing
The University of Alabama
Tuscaloosa, Alabama
(CHAPTER 5)

Lynn Gallagher-Ford, RN, PhD, DPFNAP, FAAN
Evidence-based Practice (CH)
Chief Operating Officer and Clinical Core Director
Helene Fuld Health Trust National Institute for Evidence-Based Practice in Nursing and Healthcare
College of Nursing
The Ohio State University
Columbus, Ohio
(CHAPTER 3)

Perry M. Gee, PhD, RN, FAAN
System Nurse Scientist & Associate Professor of Research
Intermountain Healthcare
Adjunct Assistant Professor
College of Nursing
University of Utah
Salt Lake City, Utah
(CHAPTER 14)

Barbara Ann Graves, PhD, RN
Professor
Capstone College of Nursing
University of Alabama
Tuscaloosa, Alabama
(CHAPTER 5)

Paul C. Herman, DNP, MSN, RNC
Associate Professor (Retired)
School of Nursing
California State University
Chico, California
(CHAPTER 4)

Erica D. Hooper-Arana, DNP, RN, CNS, CNL, PHN
Kaiser Permanente Regional Program Manager
Academic Relations and Community Health
Northern California Regional Patient Care Services
Oakland, California
(CHAPTER 2)

Carol J. Huston, RN, MSN, MPA, DPA, FAAN
Professor Emerita
School of Nursing
California State University
Chico, California
(CHAPTERS 1, 6, 7, 8, 9, 11, 12, 15, 17, 18, 20, 21, 22, 23, 24)

Holly T. Kralj, DNP, CNM, PHN
Associate Professor
School of Nursing
California State University
Certified Nurse Midwife
Enloe Medical Center
Chico, California
(CHAPTER 4)

Jennifer Lillibridge, PhD, RN
Emeritus Professor
School of Nursing
California State University
Chico, California
(CHAPTER 18)

Michelle L. Litchman, PhD,
    FNP-BC, FAANP, FADCES,
    FAANP
Assistant Professor
College of Nursing
University of Utah
Salt Lake City, Utah
(CHAPTER 14)

Kathy Malloch, PhD, MBA, RN,
    FAAN
Associate Director of Education
    and Evidence-Based Regulation
Clinical Professor
College of Nursing
The Ohio State University
Columbus, Ohio
(CHAPTER 3)

Bernadette Mazurek Melnyk,
    PhD, APRN-CNP, FAANP,
    FNAP, FAAN
Vice President for Health
    Promotion
University Chief Wellness Officer
Dean and Helene Fuld Health Trust
    Professor of Evidence-Based
    Practice, College of Nursing
Professor of Pediatrics &
    Psychiatry, College of Medicine
Executive Director, the Helene Fuld
    Health Trust National Institute
    for EBP
Founder & President, the
    National Consortium for
    Building Healthy Academic
    Communities (BHAC)
Editor, Worldviews on Evidence-
    based Nursing
Columbus, Ohio
(CHAPTER 3)

Donna M. Nickitas, PhD, RN,
    NEA-BC, CNE, FNAP, FAAN
Dean and Professor
Rutgers School of
    Nursing-Camden—Rutgers
    University
Camden, New Jersey
Editor
Nursing Economic$
The Journal for Health Care
    Leaders
Pitman, New Jersey
(CHAPTER 25)

George C. Pittman, RN, CCRN,
    MSN
Associate Professor (Retired)
School of Nursing
California State University
Chico, California
(CHAPTER 19)

Gwen Sherwood, PhD, RN,
    FAAN, ANEF
Professor Emeritus
School of Nursing
University of North Carolina at
    Chapel Hill
Chapel Hill, North Carolina
(CHAPTER 16)

Patricia E. Thompson, EdD
CEO, Retired
Sigma Theta Tau International
Indianapolis, Indiana
(CHAPTER 26)

Cynthia Vlasich, MBA, RN, CEC,
    FAAN
Principal
Cynthia Vlasich & Associates
Indianapolis, Indiana
(CHAPTER 26)

Jonalyn Wallace, DNP, RN, CENP
Regional Director, Scholars
    Academy
Kaiser Permanente Northern
    California Patient Care Services
Oakland, California
(CHAPTER 2)

Nikki West, MPH
Director
Health Care Education
    Management
Patient Care Services
Community Health Kaiser
    Permanente
Oakland, California
(CHAPTER 2)

Preface

As a nursing educator for nearly 40 years, I taught many courses dealing with the significant issues that impact the nursing profession. I often felt frustrated that textbooks that were supposed to be devoted to professional issues in the field instead deviated significantly into other areas, including nursing research and theory. In addition, while many of the existing professional issues books dealt with the enduring issues of the profession, it was difficult to find a book for my students that incorporated those with the "hot topics" of the time. The first five editions of *Professional Issues in Nursing: Challenges and Opportunities* were efforts to address both needs. The sixth edition maintains this precedent with significant content updates, the deletion of one chapter, and the addition of two new chapters.

This book continues, to be first and foremost a professional issues book. Although an effort has been made to integrate research and theory into chapters where it seemed appropriate, these topics in and of themselves are too broad to be fully addressed in a professional issues book. This book is also directed at what my expert nursing colleagues and I have identified as both enduring professional issues and the most pressing contemporary issues facing the profession. It is my hope, then, that this book fills an unmet need in the current professional issues text market. It has an undiluted focus on professional issues in nursing and includes many timely issues not addressed in other professional issues texts. This is an edited book, with 15 chapters contributed by the primary author, 1 chapter coauthored with the primary author, and the remaining 10 chapters by guest contributors with expertise in the specific subject material.

This book has been designed primarily for use at both the baccalaureate and the graduate levels. It is envisioned that it will be used as a primary textbook or as a supplement for a typical two- to three-unit professional issues course. It would also be appropriate for most RN–BSN bridge courses and may be considered by some faculty as a supplemental reader to a leadership/management course that includes professional issues.

The book can be used in both the traditional classroom and online courses because the discussion question format works well for both small and large groups onsite as well as in bulletin board and chat room venues.

ORGANIZATION

The book is divided into five units, representing contemporary and enduring issues in professional nursing including Furthering the Profession, Workforce Issues, Workplace Issues, Legal and Ethical Issues, and Professional Power. Each unit has four to six chapters.

FEATURES

Each chapter begins with **Learning Objectives** and an overview of the professional issue being discussed. Multiple perspectives on each issue are then identified in an effort to reflect the diversity of thought found in the literature as well as espoused by experts in the field and varied professional nursing and health care organizations. **Discussion Points** encourage readers to pause and reflect on specific questions (individually or in groups), and **Consider This** features encourage active learning, critical thinking, and values clarification by the users. In addition, at least one current research study is profiled in every chapter in **Research Fuels the Controversy**, an effort to promote evidence-based analysis of the issue. Each chapter ends with **Conclusions** about the issues discussed, questions **For Additional Discussion**, and a comprehensive and current reference list. Also included in each chapter are multiple displays, boxes, and tables to help the user visualize important concepts.

NEW TO THIS EDITION

- New chapters on disaster planning as well as resilience and self-care in nursing have been added. This content seemed critical given the significant impact of the COVID-19 pandemic on nursing globally. Indeed, the impact of the pandemic is noted in multiple chapters throughout the book including workforce shortages, nurse migration, whistleblowing, academic integrity, and shifting health care policy.

- The chapter on health care reform has been updated to reflect the stated intent of newly elected President Joe Biden to revive and bolster the Affordable Care Act.

- Additional new or updated content has been added throughout the book to reflect cutting-edge trends in health care, including the ongoing demand for quality and safety in the workplace for patients as well as workers; workforce projections and changing population demographics; approaching health care with a global mindset; the need to balance emerging technologies with the human element; the recommendations of the Institute of Medicine put forth in *The Future of Nursing: Leading Change, Advancing Health*; and the challenges and opportunities that accompany the provision of nursing care in an increasingly complex, global, inter-professional, and rapidly changing world.

TEACHING/LEARNING RESOURCES

Professional Issues in Nursing: Challenges and Opportunities, sixth edition, includes additional resources for both instructors and students that are available on the book's companion website at http://thePoint.lww.com/Huston6e.

Instructor Resources

Approved adopting instructors will be given access to the following additional resources:

• Test Generator containing NCLEX-style questions
• PowerPoint Presentations
• Journal Articles

Student Resources

Students who have purchased *Professional Issues in Nursing: Challenges and Opportunities*, sixth edition, have access to the following additional resources:

• Journal Articles
• Journal Articles Critical Thinking Questions
• Internet Resources
• Learning Objectives

In addition, purchasers of the text can access the searchable full text online by going to the Professional Issues in Nursing: Challenges and Opportunities, sixth edition, website at http://thePoint.lww.com/Huston6e. See inside the front cover of this text for more details, including the passcode you will need to gain access to the website.

Carol J. Huston, RN, MSN, MPA, DPA, FAAN

Contents

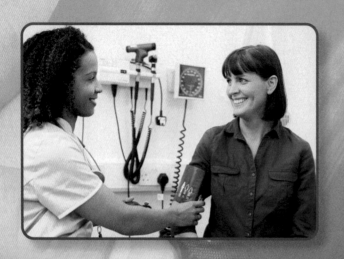

1

FURTHERING THE PROFESSION

Entry Into Practice

Carol J. Huston

ADDITIONAL RESOURCES

Visit the Point for additional helpful resources.
• eBook
• Journal Articles
• Web Links

CHAPTER OUTLINE

LEARNING OBJECTIVES

The learner will be able to:

1. Identify what, if any, progress has been made on increasing the educational entry level for professional registered nursing since publication of the 1965 position paper of the American Nurses Association on entry into practice.

2. Describe basic components of associate degree educational programs as outlined by Mildred Montag and compare those with typical associate degree programs in the 21st century.

3. Identify similarities and differences between contemporary associate and baccalaureate degree nursing programs.

4. Discuss the driving and restraining forces for establishing two levels of National Council Licensure Examination (NCLEX) licensing exams for RNs based on educational entry level.

5. Identify key driving and restraining forces for increasing the educational entry level for professional nursing.

6. Analyze current research that explores the impact of registered nurse educational level on patient outcomes.

7. Explore how shifting health care delivery sites and increasing registered nursing competency requirements are impacting employer preferences for hiring a more educated nursing workforce.

8. Compare the nursing profession's educational entry standards with those of the other health care professions.

9. Consider the potential impacts of raising the educational entry level on the current nursing shortage, workforce diversity, and intraprofessional conflict.

10. Identify positions taken by specific professional organizations, certifying bodies, and employers regarding the appropriate educational level for entry into practice for professional nursing.

11. Explore personal values, beliefs, and feelings regarding whether the educational entry level in nursing should be increased to a baccalaureate or higher degree.

INTRODUCTION

Few issues have been as long-standing or contentious in nursing as the entry-into-practice debate. Although the entry-into-practice debate dates back to the 1940s with the publication of Esther Lucile Brown's classic *Nursing for the Future*, the debate came to the forefront with a 1965 position paper by the American Nurses Association (ANA, 1965a, 1965b). This position paper suggested an orderly transition from hospital-based diploma nursing preparation to nursing education in colleges or universities based on the following premises:

- The education of all those who are licensed to practice nursing should take place in institutions of higher education.
- Minimum preparation for beginning professional nursing practice should be a baccalaureate education in nursing.
- Minimum preparation for beginning technical practice should be an associate degree education in nursing.
- Education for assistants in the health care occupations should be short, intensive, preservice programs in vocational education institutions rather than on-the-job training programs.

In essence, two levels of preparation were suggested for registered nurses (RNs): *technical* and *professional*. Individuals interested in technical practice would enroll in junior or community colleges and earn associate degrees in 2-year programs. Those interested in professional nursing would enroll in 4-year programs in colleges or universities. Hospital-based diploma programs were to be phased out.

The curricula for the two programs were to be different, as were each program's focus. The 2-year technical degree was to result in an associate degree in nursing (ADN). This degree, as proposed by Mildred Montag (Fig. 1.1) in her dissertation in 1952, with direction and support from R. Louise McManus, would prepare a beginning, technical practitioner who would provide care in acute care settings under the supervision of a professional nurse.

In a typical associate degree program, approximately half of the credits would be fulfilled by general education courses such as English, anatomy, physiology, speech, psychology, and sociology and the other half fulfilled by nursing courses. The 4-year degree would result in a Bachelor of Science in nursing (BSN) and would encompass coursework taught in ADN programs as well as more in-depth treatment of the physical and social sciences, nursing research, public and community health, nursing management, and the humanities. The additional coursework in the BSN program was intended to enhance the students' professional development, prepare them for a broader scope of practice, and provide a better understanding of the cultural, political, economic, and social issues affecting patients and health care delivery.

The ANA 1965 position statement was reaffirmed by a resolution at the ANA House of Delegates in 1978, which set forth the requirement that the baccalaureate degree would be the entry level into professional nursing practice by 1985. Associate degree and diploma programs responded strongly to what they viewed as inflammatory terminology and clearly stated that not being considered "professional" was unacceptable. In the end, both ADN and diploma programs refused to compromise title or licensure.

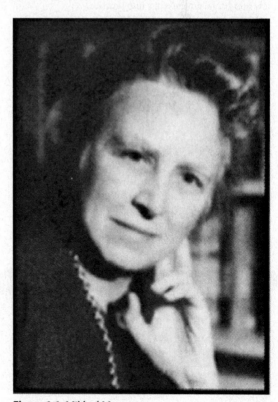

Figure 1.1 Mildred Montag.

Dissension ensued both within and among nursing groups, but little movement occurred to make the position statement a reality.

> *Consider This* Titling (professional versus technical) was and will be an important consideration before consensus can be reached on the entry-into-practice debate.

Finally in 2008, 30 years later, the ANA House of Delegates stepped forth once again to pass a resolution supporting initiatives to require diploma- and associate degree–educated nurses to obtain a BSN within 10 years of license. The responsibility for mandating and implementing this new resolution was passed on to individual states.

However, only one state, North Dakota, became successful in changing its Nurse Practice Act so that baccalaureate education was necessary for initial RN licensure. For 15 years, it was the only state to recognize baccalaureate education as the minimal education for professional nursing despite challenges from opposing groups. However, North Dakota repealed this act in 2003, bowing to pressure from nurses and some health care organizations to once again allow non-baccalaureate entry into practice.

Other states, however, continue to consider increasing educational entry levels. California, for example, requires a BSN for certification as a public health nurse in that state, and multiple states require a BSN to be a school nurse because it is part of public health nursing. In addition, New York signed a "BSN in 10" bill into law on December 19, 2017, making it a leader in recognizing the significance of baccalaureate preparation for RNs. The purpose of the law was to increase the level of education for professional RNs, requiring that newly licensed nurses already have a BSN at the time of entry into practice or achieve a BSN within 10 years after initial licensure. New Jersey's legislature also held hearings in 2020 on a BSN in 10 law but had not enacted anything as of early 2021 (NursingLicensure.org, 2021).

In addition, over the past few years, state nursing associations or other nursing coalitions in California, Rhode Island, and New Jersey have called for initiatives to establish the BSN as the entry level for nursing. Other states are pursuing some type of initiative requiring newly graduated RNs to obtain BSNs within a certain time frame to maintain their licensure.

The result, however, is that more than 57 years after the initial ANA resolution, entry into practice at the baccalaureate level has not been accomplished. Even the strongest supporters of the BSN for entry into practice cannot deny that, despite almost six decades of efforts, RN entry at the baccalaureate level continues to be an elusive goal.

PROLIFERATION OF ADN EDUCATION

It is doubtful that Mildred Montag had any idea in 1952 that ADN programs would someday become the predominant entry level for nursing practice or that this education model would proliferate like it did in the 1960s, just one decade after she completed her doctoral work. While the overwhelming majority of nurses in the early 1960s were educated in diploma schools of nursing, enrollment in baccalaureate programs was increasing and associate degree programs were just beginning. By 2000, diploma education had virtually disappeared, and although BSN education had increased significantly, it was ADN education that represented nearly two-thirds of all nursing school graduates.

Yet, enrollment in baccalaureate nursing programs is on the rise with almost two decades of consecutive enrollment growth. Indeed, with each passing year, the proportion of entry-level National Council Licensure Examination (NCLEX) test takers has moved closer to a 50–50 split between BSN and ADN graduates (Table 1.1). Indeed, just under 50% (49.95%) of first-time United States-educated NCLEX test takers in 2020 were graduates of baccalaureate nursing programs (National Council of State Boards of Nursing, 2020).

LICENSURE AND ENTRY INTO PRACTICE

Critics of BSN as a requirement for entry into practice argue that there is no need to raise entry levels because

TABLE 1.1	2020 NCLEX-RN Passage Rate Per Educational Program Type	
Program Type	**Number of Graduates**	**NCLEX-RN Passage Rate (%)**
Diploma	1,931	87.57
Associate degree	77,508	84.03
Baccalaureate degree	79,320	90.96

Source: Data from National Council of State Boards of Nursing. (2019, October 16). *2017: Number of candidates taking NCLEX examination and percent passing, by type of candidate.* Retrieved September 5, 2020, from https://www.ncsbn.org/Table_of_Pass_Rates_2019.pdf

passing rates for the NCLEX show only small differences between ADN, diploma, and BSN graduates (see Table 1.1). Although some might argue that this suggests similar competencies across the educational spectrum, the more commonly accepted explanation is that the NCLEX is a test that measures minimum technical competencies for safe entry into basic nursing practice and, as such, may not measure performance over time or test for all of the knowledge and skills developed through a BSN program.

Consider This Critics of BSN entry into practice argue that ADN-, diploma-, and BSN-educated nurses all take the same licensing examination and therefore have earned the title of RN. In addition, nurses prepared at all three levels have successfully worked side by side under the same scope of practice for more than five decades.

One must also ask why the nursing profession has not differentiated RN licensure testing (two levels of NCLEX-RN licensing) based on educational preparation for RNs, just as has been done for practical nurses and advanced practice nurses. This would recognize each level of nursing education and help clarify differentiated levels of practice. Complicating the picture, however, is that both ADN and BSN schools preparing graduates for RN licensure meet similar criteria for state board approval and have roughly the same number of nursing coursework units. These factors contribute to confusion about differentiations between ADN- and BSN-prepared nurses and result in an inability to move forward on implementing the BSN as the entry level for professional nursing.

Discussion Point

Should separate licensing examinations be developed for ADN-, diploma-, and BSN-educated nurses?

In addition, many employers state that they are unable to differentiate roles for nurses based on education because both ADN- and BSN-prepared nurses hold the same license. However, state boards of nursing have asserted their inability to develop a different licensure system given the fact that employers have not developed different roles.

Discussion Point

Should licensure be equated with professional status?

EDUCATIONAL LEVELS AND PATIENT OUTCOMES

Perhaps the most common argument against raising the entry level in nursing is an emotional one, with ADN-prepared nurses arguing that "caring does not require a baccalaureate degree." Many ADN-educated nurses argue passionately that patients do not know or care what educational degree is held by their nurses as long as they receive high-quality care from nurses at the bedside. ADN nurses also frequently claim that BSN-prepared nurses are too theoretically oriented and thus are less in touch with real practice. In addition, many ADN nurses suggest that baccalaureate-prepared nurses are deficient in basic skills mastery and conclude that care provided by ADN nurses is at least as good as if not better than that provided by their BSN counterparts.

Discussion Point

Most ADN-prepared nurses argue that significant differences exist between their practice and that of a licensed vocational/practical nurse (LVN/LPN), despite typically only 12 months' difference in the length of educational preparation. Yet, many ADN-educated nurses argue that the additional education that BSN-educated nurses have makes little difference in their practice over that of their ADN counterparts. How can this argument be justified?

An increasing number of studies, however, report differences between the performance levels of ADN- and BSN-prepared nurses as well as patient outcomes. In a landmark study, Aiken et al. (2003) at the University of Pennsylvania identified a clear link between higher levels of nursing education and better patient outcomes (American Association of Colleges of Nursing [AACN], 2019b). This study found that surgical patients have a "substantial survival advantage" if treated in hospitals with higher proportions of nurses educated at the baccalaureate or higher degree level and that a 10% increase in the proportion of nurses holding BSN degrees decreased the risk of patient death and failure to rescue by 5% (AACN, 2019b).

Research by Aiken and colleagues also showed that hospitals with better care environments, the best nurse staffing levels, and the most highly educated nurses had the lowest surgical mortality rates. In fact, the researchers found that every 10% increase in the proportion of BSN nurses on the hospital staff was associated with a 4% decrease in the risk of death (Aiken et al., 2008).

Another study found that a 10-point increase in the percentage of nurses holding a BSN within a hospital was associated with an average reduction of 2.12 deaths for every

1,000 patients—and for a subset of patients with complications, an average reduction of 7.47 deaths per 1,000 patients (AACN, 2019b).

In addition, in a cross-sectional study of 21 University Health System Consortium hospitals, Blegen et al. (2013) analyzed the association between RN education and patient outcomes. The researchers found that hospitals with a higher percentage of RNs with baccalaureate or higher degrees had lower rates of congestive heart failure mortality, decubitus ulcers, failure to rescue, and postoperative deep vein thrombosis or pulmonary embolism as well as shorter lengths of stay (AACN, 2019b).

Another follow-up study by Aiken and colleagues found that a greater proportion of professional nurses at the bedside in adult acute care hospitals in six European nations was associated with better outcomes for patients and nurses. Reducing nursing skill mix by adding assistive personnel without professional nurse qualifications was suggested as a possible contributor to preventable deaths, erosion of care quality, and nurse shortages (AACN, 2019b).

Even more recently, a 2019 study by Djukic and colleagues found that baccalaureate-prepared RNs reported being significantly better prepared than ADNs on 12 out of 16 areas related to quality and safety, including evidence-based practice, data analysis, and project implementation (AACN, 2019b).

Another recent study by Sitzman et al. (2020) affirmed that practice differences occur for RNs who return to school for baccalaureate degrees as well. The most prominent theme voiced by participants was gaining new understanding, focus, and confidence related to the use of research and evidence-based practice to improve clinical practices and patient care. In addition, participants reported enhanced verbal and written communication skills, an improved ability to effectively engage in the nursing process, improved critical thinking skills, and broadened perspectives related to working within increasingly diverse and complex professional situations.

As more outcome research suggesting an empirical link between educational entry level of nurses and patient outcomes becomes available, nursing leaders, professional associations, and employers are increasingly speaking out on the need to raise the profession's entry level as a means of improving quality patient care and patient safety. Yet, Clarke (2017) raises at least some doubt about concluding that these outcomes are clearly due to baccalaureate-educated nurses providing a higher quality of care. He notes it is possible that conditions favoring better patient outcomes, such as an attractive labor market, a range of higher education opportunities, and a better professional practice environment may simply be more common in hospitals where there are more baccalaureate-prepared nurses.

EMPLOYERS' VIEWS AND PREFERENCES

Nursing employers are still somewhat divided on the issue of entry into practice. The academic requirements of associate degree, diploma, and baccalaureate programs vary widely, yet health care settings that employ nursing graduates may make no distinction in the scope of practice among nurses with different levels of preparation. Furthermore, many employers provide little or no incentives for BSN education in terms of pay, recognition, or career mobility and are afraid to do so, fearing they may be unable to fill vacant nursing positions.

The starting rate of pay for ADN- and BSN-prepared nurses historically has not been significantly different, though this appears to be changing. Koivisto (2020) reports that according to the U.S. Bureau of Labor Statistics, the median hourly wage for RNs in the United States in May 2018 was $34.48 with a median annual wage of $71,730. That includes RNs both with bachelor's degrees and with associate degrees. When separated out by degree, on average, ADN nurses earned $28.99 per hour, and BSN nurses earned $45.38 per hour. These figures result in a mean annual wage of $53,760 for ADN-educated nurses and $87,129 for nurses with BSN degrees. Therefore, on average, BSN-educated nurses earned approximately $33,000 more than their ADN counterparts (Koivisto, 2020).

In addition, employers appear to be increasingly aware of purported differences between BSN and ADN graduates, and this is increasingly being reflected in their hiring preferences. One reason is the Magnet Recognition Program's requirement that nurse managers and leaders have at least a baccalaureate in nursing. Magnet hospitals are also required to have a higher percentage of nurses educated at the baccalaureate level. In addition, some employers are now giving preference for clinical placements to students in baccalaureate and higher degree programs over those enrolled in associate degree programs.

Indeed, LaRocco (2014) suggests that

… while state boards of nursing and legislatures fail to act to change the entry requirements for professional nursing, in many areas of the country the baccalaureate is becoming the de facto requirement. Major medical centers in the Boston area no longer hire nurses with associate's degrees. At least one large, for-profit hospital chain has decreed that their nurses must obtain a baccalaureate within a stipulated period of time, typically 3 to 5 years. Nurses with associate's degrees are limited in both their initial employment and their long-term options. (p. 11)

Similarly, NursingLicensure.org (2021) notes that while the ADN has been the benchmark credential for getting a nursing job for 40 years, change is now afoot. A small but growing number of U.S. hospitals are now hiring nurses who have only a BSN or higher and indicators are that many more hospitals will join them in years to come.

Discussion Point

If employers prefer hiring BSN-prepared RNs, why don't more employers offer pay differentials for nurses with BSN degrees?

With its 100,000 nurse corps (VA Celebrates, 2020), the Veterans Administration (VA) is leading the nation in raising the bar for higher educational entry levels in nursing. The VA established the BSN as the minimum education level for new hires and as the minimum preparation its nurses must have for promotion beyond the entry level (AACN, 2019b).

SHIFTING HEALTH CARE DELIVERY SITES AND REQUIRED COMPETENCIES

Although hospitals continue to be the main site of employment for nurses, there is an ongoing shift in health care from acute care settings to the community and integrated health care settings. This shift will clearly require more highly educated nurses who can function autonomously as caregivers, leaders, managers, and change agents. In addition, nurses must now be skilled in evidence-based practice, population health, and quality measurement. These are all skills that are emphasized in a baccalaureate nursing curriculum.

Consider This Baccalaureate and graduate-level skills in research, leadership, management, and community health are increasingly needed in nursing as health care extends beyond the acute care hospital.

In May 2010, the Tri-Council for Nursing, a coalition of four steering organizations for the nursing profession (AACN, ANA, the American Organization of Nurse Executives [AONE], and the National League for Nursing [NLN]), issued a consensus statement calling for all RNs to advance their education in the interest of enhancing quality and safety across health care settings. The statement suggested that a more highly educated nursing workforce will be critical to meeting the nation's nursing needs and delivering safe, effective patient care and that failure to do so will place the nation's health at further risk (AACN, 2019a).

The recommendations of the 2010 Institute of Medicine (IOM) report, *The Future of Nursing*, were even stronger (Campaign for Action, 2013). This landmark report called for increasing the number of baccalaureate-prepared nurses in the workforce from 50% to 80% over the next 10 years and doubling the population of nurses with doctorates to meet the demands of an evolving health care system and changing patient needs.

In addition, in December 2009, Patricia Benner and her team at the Carnegie Foundation for the Advancement of Teaching released a new study titled *Educating Nurses: A Call for Radical Transformation*, which recommended preparing all entry-level RNs at the baccalaureate level and requiring all RNs to earn a master's degree within 10 years of initial licensure (Benner et al., 2010). The authors found that many of today's new nurses are "undereducated" to meet practice demands across settings. Their strong support for high-quality baccalaureate degree programs as the appropriate pathway for RNs entering the profession is consistent with the views of many leading nursing organizations, including the AACN (2019a).

Similarly, the National Advisory Council on Nurse Education and Practice (NACNEP) suggests that nursing's role for the future calls for RNs to manage care along a continuum, to work as peers in interdisciplinary teams, and to integrate clinical expertise with knowledge of community resources. This increased complexity of scope of practice will require the capacity to adapt to change; critical thinking and problem-solving skills; a social foundation in a broad range of basic sciences; knowledge of behavioral, social, and management sciences; and the ability to analyze and communicate data (AACN, 2015). All these are integral components of a BSN education. As a result, the NACNEP has recommended to Congress that at least two-thirds of the nurse workforce hold baccalaureate or higher degrees in nursing (AACN, 2015, 2019b).

The Council on Physician and Nurse Supply also released a statement in 2007 calling for a national effort to substantially expand baccalaureate nursing programs, citing the growing body of evidence that nursing education impacts both the quality and safety of patient care. Consequently, the group is calling on policymakers to shift federal funding priorities in favor of supporting more baccalaureate-level nursing programs (AACN, 2019b). Some nurse leaders have even suggested that a BSN degree may not be an adequate preparation for these expanded roles and that instead, master's or doctoral degrees should be required for entry into practice for registered nursing.

Discussion Point

Would raising the entry level to the master's or doctoral degree eliminate the tension between supporters of ADN and BSN as entry levels into nursing, since both educational preparations would be considered inadequate? Is a graduate degree currently feasible as the entry level for professional nursing? If not, what would it take to make it happen?

ENTRY LEVEL AND PROFESSIONAL STATUS

Nurses, consumers, and allied health care professionals are currently questioning why the entry level into professional nursing is so much lower than that of other health care professions. Does nursing require less skill? Is the knowledge base needed to provide nursing care skill-based instead of knowledge-based? Should nursing be reclassified as a vocational trade and not a profession? The answer to these questions, of course, is no. Yet clearly, nurses have resisted the normal course of occupational development that other health care professions have pursued. As a result, nurses are now the least educated of the health care professionals, with most health care professions now requiring graduate degrees for entry. Indeed, one must question whether nursing is at risk for losing its designation as a profession because of its failure to maintain educational equity.

Discussion Point

Is nursing in danger of losing its designation as a "profession" if it fails to maintain educational entry levels comparable to those of the other health professions?

The primary identity of any professional group is based on the established education entry level. Attorneys, physicians, social workers, engineers, clergy, and physical therapists, to list a few examples, have in common an essential education at the bachelor's level. Nursing is unique among the health care professions in having multiple educational pathways that lead to the same entry-level license to practice. In fact, advanced degrees are required in many professions for entry positions at the professional level. Only nursing continues implying that education is unimportant and does not make a difference. Only nursing allows individuals with no college coursework or with limited college study that lacks a well-rounded global college education to lay claim to the same licensure and identity as that held by nurses who have a baccalaureate education.

Consider This Failure to maintain educational parity with other health care professions also contributes to nursing being viewed as a "second-class citizen" in the health care arena. It is difficult to justify the profession's argument that nursing should be an equal partner in health care decision making when other professions are so much better educated, suggesting that nurses are either undereducated for the roles they assume or that the nursing role lacks complexity.

Indeed, the educational gap between nursing and other health professions continues to grow (Table 1.2). Disciplines such as occupational therapy, physical therapy, speech therapy, and social work all require master's or doctoral degrees. Pharmacy has also raised its educational entry level standards to that of a doctoral degree.

TABLE 1.2 **Entry-Level Degrees for the Health Professions**	
Health Profession	**Entry-Level Degree**
Medicine	Doctorate
Pharmacy	Doctorate
Dentistry	Doctorate
Audiology	Doctorate
Optometry	Doctorate
Physical therapy	Doctorate
Podiatry	Doctorate
Social work	Master's (Required to become a licensed clinical social worker [LCSW])
Speech pathology	Master's (Required for the professional Certificate of Clinical Competence [CCC-SLP] through the American Speech-Language-Hearing Association)
Occupational therapy	Master's (Doctorate as entry-level degree has been proposed but is currently tabled)
Nursing	Associate

THE 2-YEAR ADN PROGRAM

Many ADN-prepared nurses also express frustration when discussing the need to raise the entry level in professional nursing because they feel the ADN degree does not appropriately represent the scope of their education or the time they had to put in to earn what is typically considered to be a 2-year degree. ADN nurses argue that the "2-year" ADN program is a myth. Many ADN students follow nontraditional education paths, and almost all ADN programs currently require three or more years of education, not two, with a minimum of 12 to 24 months of prerequisites and a full 2 years of nursing education. Most associate degrees require approximately 60 semester units or 90 quarter units of coursework, though there is a great deal of variance with some programs now requiring more than 70 semester units and over 100 quarter units.

Indeed, it is almost impossible to graduate from an ADN program in less than 3 years, and often 4 or more years is required to complete the general education, prerequisite, and nursing requirements. Given that most BSN programs require approximately 120 semester units for graduation, the question must be asked whether requiring so many units at the associate degree level without granting the upper division credit that could lead to a BSN degree is an injustice to ADN graduates.

This addition of units and extension of educational time in ADN programs has generally been attributed to the need to respond to a changing job market; that is, the need to

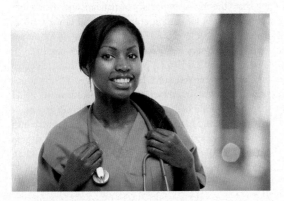

prepare ADNs to work in more diverse environments (non-hospital) and to increasingly assume positions requiring management skills. While Montag clearly intended a differentiation between level of education and level of practice between ADN- and BSN-prepared nurses, many ADN programs have added leadership, management, research, and home health and community health courses to their curricula in the past two decades.

One must ask then, what part of the associate degree curriculum should be cut to add these new experiences? What should the balance be between community and acute care experiences in ADN programs? How much management content do ADN nurses need, and what roles will they be expected to assume? If no content is removed from the ADN programs to accommodate the new content, how can ADN education reasonably be completed within a 2-year framework?

Montag expressed concern that when ADN programs add content inappropriate for technical practice, appropriate content may have to be deleted to maintain the estimated time for completion. The question that follows then is, if ADN education now incorporates much of what was meant to be BSN content, and if the time needed to complete this education is near that of a bachelor's degree, why are ADN graduates being given associate degrees, which reflect expertise in technical practice, rather than BSN degrees, which reflect achievement of these higher-level competencies?

SHORTAGES AND ENTRY-LEVEL REQUIREMENTS

Whenever there are shortages, legislators and workforce experts suggest a need to reexamine or reduce educational requirements. Indeed, Montag's original project to create ADN education was directed at reducing the workforce shortage of nurses that existed at that time by reducing the length of the education process to 2 years. Clearly, the immediate short-term threat of raising the entry level to the bachelor's degree may be to exacerbate predicted nursing shortages.

In addition, raising the entry level may in the long run elevate the public image of nursing and increase recruitment to the field since the best and the brightest may seek professions with greater academic prestige. Raising the entry level may also impact retention rates in nursing. Having more BSN nurses may actually then stabilize the nursing workforce as a result of their higher levels of job satisfaction, a key to nurse retention.

The other reality is that periodic shortages of nursing personnel have persisted despite the proliferation of ADN programs. This negates the argument that any current nursing shortage should be used as an excuse for postponing action to raise educational standards. A nursing shortage existed at the time of the 1965 ANA proposal and has occurred intermittently since then. Clearly, nursing has been swept along by a host of social, economic, and educational circumstances that have little to do with nursing or the patients we serve. Perhaps, then, the decision to raise the entry-to-practice level in nursing should be made because it is the right and necessary thing to do and not as a result of the influence of external communities of interest.

> *Consider This* Nurses, professional health care and nursing organizations, credentialing programs, and employers are divided on the entry-into-practice issue.

Debate over entry into practice is as varied among professional health care and nursing organizations, credentialing programs, and employers as it is among individual nurses. Getting support for the BSN as the entry-level requirement for nursing will be difficult because nearly half of registered nurses are currently ADN-prepared, and there are inadequate workplace incentives to increase entry requirements to the BSN degree.

PROFESSIONAL ORGANIZATIONS, UNIONS, AND ADVISORY BODIES SPEAK UP

Not surprisingly, a 2006 position statement issued by the National Organization for Associate Degree Nursing (NOADN) on entry into practice reaffirmed the role and value of ADN education and practice. The position statement suggested that ADN graduates were essential members of the interdisciplinary health care team, that these nurses were prepared to function in diverse health care settings, and that associate degree education provided a dynamic pathway for entry into professional RN practice. A follow-up position statement issued by the NOADN in 2008 suggested that a BSN should not be required for continued practice beyond initial licensure as an RN and that the choice to pursue further education should remain the choice of each ADN graduate based on their personal preferences and professional career goals.

Similarly, the position of the NLN, the national voice for nurse educators in all types of nursing education programs, was historically that the nursing profession should have multiple entry points. As such, the NLN suggested that instead of investing energy debating entry into the profession, the focus should turn toward opportunities for lifelong learning and progression for those who enter the nursing profession through diploma and associate degree programs.

More recently, however, the NOADN partnered with the American Association of Community Colleges, the Association of Community College Trustees, AACN, and NLN to author a joint statement acknowledging their full support for the academic progression of every nursing student and nurse. This statement was endorsed by the ANA in January 2014 (AACN, 2021). The joint statement suggests that it is only through the collaboration and partnering of organizations that a seamless academic progression of students and nurses will occur.

An increasing number of professional nursing organizations, however, are now supporting the BSN requirement for entry into professional nursing. Indeed, the notion that many more nurses should be BSN-credentialed has gained momentum in national health care policymaking circles, with the IOM and the Robert Wood Johnson Foundation jointly calling for increasing the U.S. nurses holding BSNs to 80% by 2020 (NursingLicensure.org, 2021). In addition, organizations such as the AACN, the National Association of Neonatal Nurses (NANN), the American Nephrology Nurses' Association, the Association of periOperative Registered Nurses (AORN), and the AONE have published position statements supporting BSN entry.

For example, the AACN suggests that the primary pathway for entry into professional-level nursing, as compared to technical-level practice, is a 4-year BSN. In addition, in March 2019, AACN's members endorsed a new position statement titled *Academic Progression in Nursing: Moving Together Toward a Highly Educated Nursing Workforce*, which highlights the need for collaborative solutions that enable all nurses to take the next step in their educational development to better serve the health needs of the nation (AACN, 2019a).

NANN issued its position statement in 2009, arguing that "the increasing acuity of patients and their more complex needs for care in community and home settings demand a higher level of educational preparation for nurses than was necessary in the past" (NANN, 2009, para. 1).

The AORN has also supported the baccalaureate degree for entry into nursing since 1979. The AORN's current position statement on entry into practice reaffirms its belief that there should be one level for entry into nursing practice and that the minimal preparation for future entry into the practice of nursing should be the baccalaureate degree (AORN, 2020). In 2004, the AONE also published guiding principles suggesting that "the educational preparation of the nurse of the future should be at the baccalaureate level."

The NACNEP, which advises the secretary of the U.S. Department of Health and Human Services and the U.S. Congress on policy issues related to nurse workforce supply, education, and practice improvement, in 2017 urged that a minimum of two-thirds of working nurses hold baccalaureate or higher degrees in nursing by 2010 (AACN, 2019b). Yet, federal and state regulation of entry into practice has, for the most part, not occurred. In addition, the Tri-Council for Nursing issued a consensus statement in 2010 calling for all RNs to advance their education in the interest of patient safety and enhanced quality of care across all settings.

Consider This The Tri-Council organizations argue that a more highly educated nursing profession is no longer a preferred future; rather, it is a necessary future in order to meet the nursing needs of the nation and to deliver effective and safe care (AACN, 2019a).

GRANDFATHERING ENTRY LEVELS

Traditionally, when a state licensure law is enacted or when a current law is repealed and a new law enacted, a process called "grandfathering" occurs. Grandfathering allows individuals to continue to practice their profession or occupation despite new qualifications having been enacted into law. Should the entry-level requirement for nursing be raised to a bachelor's or higher degree, debate will undoubtedly occur as to how and when grandfathering should be applied.

Consider This "Grandfathering" current ADN nurses as professional nurses would smooth political tensions between current educational entry levels but threaten the essence of the goal.

Several professional organizations have actively advocated that all RNs should be grandfathered if the entry level is raised. Other professional organizations have argued that it should not occur at all. Still others believe that grandfathering should be conditional. For example, all RNs licensed at the time of the law would be allowed to retain their current title for a certain time but would be required to return to school later to increase their educational preparation if it did not meet the new entry level.

LINKING ADN AND BSN PROGRAMS

Returning to school, unfortunately, is not part of the career path for many nurses, which makes the entry level even more important. Intimidation, costs, impact on family, and lack of clarity about the possible gains from additional education deter many nurses from returning to school. Many RNs feel that furthering their education would provide more career opportunities but are unsure that the benefits will outweigh the costs.

There are cost differences. Koivisto (2020) notes that according to the National Center for Education Statistics, the mean annual tuition costs for a 2-year ADN degree in the United States between 2016 and 2017 was $10,598. The mean annual tuition costs for 4-year bachelor's degree studies was $23,091 (Koivisto, 2020). This means that on average, a bachelor's degree costs $48,000 more than an associate degree.

Indeed, there are many internal and external motivators that encourage or discourage RNs from pursuing higher degrees. RNs identify a desire to achieve personal and job satisfaction, new knowledge, career advancement opportunities, and professional achievement as important motivators for degree completion. Time and money, however, are perceived as significant barriers to pursuing an entry-level baccalaureate degree (Sabio & Petges, 2020). See Research Fuels the Controversy 1.1. Indeed, RN-to-BSN education typically takes 2 to 3 years, though fast-track baccalaureate programs may take as little as 11 to 18 months to complete, including prerequisites (AACN, 2019c). Fast-track master's degree programs generally take about 3 years to complete (AACN, 2019c).

Currently, 777 RN-to-BSN programs nationally build on the education provided in diploma and ADN programs, including more than 600 programs that are offered at least partially online (AACN, 2019d). There are also 219 programs available nationwide to transition RNs with diplomas and associate degrees to the master's degree level (MSN, MS, or Master of Science in Nursing degree; AACN, 2019d). The number of RN-to-MSN programs has more than tripled in the past 20 years from 70 programs in 1994 to 219 programs as of 2019; 24 new RN-to-MSN programs are in the planning stages (AACN, 2019d).

In addition, statewide articulation agreements exist in many states, including Florida, California, Connecticut, Arkansas, Texas, Iowa, Maryland, North Carolina, South Carolina, Idaho, Alabama, and Nevada, to facilitate credit transfer from community colleges to universities with BSN programs. Indeed, adequate numbers of quality RN-to-BSN completion pathways will be essential to raising the educational preparation of the nursing workforce with the aim of improving patient outcomes.

Jeffreys (2020) notes, however, that while improvements have been made in articulation agreements, credit transfers, and concurrent enrollments, meeting the 80% BSN by 2020

Research Fuels the Controversy 1.1

This qualitative study, using a phenomenological approach, conducted focus group interviews of ADN students in community colleges in one Midwestern state. The purpose of the study was to ask ADN students about their education, the influence of their nontraditional attributes, their perceived barriers to baccalaureate nursing education, their opinions about lowering the barriers, and their thoughts about the various proposals for advancing nurses' education.

Source: Sabio, C., & Petges, N. (2020, January). Understanding the barriers to BSN education among ADN students: A qualitative study. *Teaching and Learning in Nursing, 15*(1), 45–52. Retrieved September 7, 2020, from https://www.sciencedirect.com/science/article/pii/S1557308719302112

Study Findings

All participants agreed that because they were self-supporting, cost was the main barrier to entry-level baccalaureate nursing education. In addition, many reported having children, so they expressed a need to achieve the RN degree in as short a time as possible. The geographic location of baccalaureate programs was also a significant barrier, primarily because of the participants' home responsibilities. In addition, participants expressed that because most of their cohorts "have to work and go to school" with "a lot" of them working fulltime, it was more difficult to pursue the baccalaureate route.

In terms of RN-to-BSN completion, only a few were beginning to contemplate the prospect of BSN completion, though they noted that the task of obtaining a baccalaureate degree in nursing after the ADN was perceived as daunting and exhausting. In addition, participants expressed some concerns about the quality of such programs and felt they had received what they needed to know about nursing from their ADN courses.

Given the nontraditional and place-bound characteristics of the participants, making classes more accessible and flexible so they can attend to their obligations was foremost when it came to seeking an entry-level BSN. For the RN-to-BSN program, participants also stressed the importance of accessibility through online classes and the importance of financial support in the form of tuition reimbursement from employers.

However, two participants enrolled in a dual ADN-to-BSN program noted that higher education did lead to a higher level of critical thinking. They also suggested the ADN program focused more on skills attainment and the BSN program more on knowledge and asking "why."

goal fell short because students at key transitional points (such as first- and last-semester students) continue to be faced with numerous academic and career path challenges and opportunities simultaneously, often leaving them overwhelmed and in need of additional support and resources.

In addition, the growth in RN pathways to baccalaureate and graduate degrees has been so rapid in the past decade that some nurse leaders have suggested that this has resulted in a lack of educational standardization and significant variability in expectations and requirements among RN-to-BSN programs. In addition, sometimes there is little integration, standardization, or cooperation between public systems of education. Such integration, standardization, and cooperation will be essential for transition to BSN entry levels. This is why one of the key recommendations in *The Future of Nursing* was that all nursing schools should offer defined academic pathways that promote seamless access for nurses to higher levels of education (IOM, 2010). Transition programs or services for nonbaccalaureate-prepared nurses must be designed to facilitate entry into baccalaureate and advanced education and practice programs. In addition, funding must continue to be increased for colleges and universities sponsoring baccalaureate and advanced practice nursing education programs.

Consider This   A broad new system composed of direct transfer, linkage, and partnership programs is needed between community college and baccalaureate institutions to ensure a smooth transition from ADN to BSN as the entry-level requirement for professional nursing practice. This transition will be costly.

Clearly, barriers for educational reentry must be removed if the educational entry level in nursing is to be raised to a bachelor's or higher degree. Alternative pathways for RN education must be developed to create opportunities for learners who might not otherwise be able to pursue additional nursing education.

ENTRY INTO PRACTICE AS AN INTERNATIONAL ISSUE

The entry-into-practice debate in nursing is not limited to the United States, though several countries have already established the baccalaureate degree as the minimum entry level and grandfathered in all those with licenses before that date. For example, since 1982, all the provincial and territorial nurses associations in Canada have advocated the baccalaureate degree as the education entry-to-practice standard, and most provincial and territorial regulatory bodies have achieved this goal (except Québec). The Canadian Nurses Association (2021) believes that the knowledge, skills, and personal attributes that today's health system demands of its RNs can be gained only through broad-based bachelor's nursing programs.

Similarly, Australia moved toward adoption of a BSN for entry into nursing during the 1980s, initially encountering resistance by both physicians and nurses themselves, who feared university education would minimize needed hands-on training. Registered nursing as a university degree, however, was mandated in the 1990s. *Enrolled nurses* (scope of practice similar to LPNs/LVNs in the United States) continue to be educated in diploma programs and work under the supervision of the RN. Postgraduate diplomas provide further vocational training for specialist areas.

Similarly, in South Africa, nurses who complete a 2-year course of study are called *enrolled nurses* or *staff nurses*, while those who complete 4 years of study attain *professional nurse* or *sister* status. Enrolled nurses can later complete a 2-year bridging program and become *registered general nurses*.

Wales, Scotland, and Northern Ireland also offer only one entry point for nursing, and that is a 3-year university degree. Other one-entry-point countries include Italy, Norway, and Spain (3-year university degree); Ireland (4-year university degree); and Denmark (3.5-year degree at nursing school in university college sector). Many countries, such as Sweden, Portugal, Brazil, Iceland, Korea, Greece, and the Philippines, already require a 4-year undergraduate degree to practice nursing. All new nurses in England were required to hold a degree-level qualification to enter the profession after 2013. The aim was to increase skills and train a medical workforce capable of operating in a more analytical and independent manner.

Consider This A growing list of countries, states, and provinces now require baccalaureate education in nursing.

Thus, international efforts to advance nursing education appear to be gaining momentum. The 2009 World Health Organization's Global Standards for the Initial Education of Professional Nurses and Midwives, written between 2005 and 2007 with participation from Sigma Theta Tau International, called for all nurses to be educated with bachelor's degrees, recognizing that country-specific standards would be necessary due to differing resources, histories, and environments.

CONCLUSIONS

The entry-into-practice debate in the United States continues to be one of the oldest professional issues nurses face as we enter the third decade of the 21st century. Indeed, Krugman and Goode (2018) suggest the issue of educational entry into professional nursing practice is an "old" issue, and that nurse leaders must act now to eliminate the multiple educational levels and require a minimum BSN degree for professional nurse practice. Yet only limited progress has been made since 1965 in creating a consensus to raise the entry level into professional nursing practice.

Complicating the argument to increase nursing's educational entry level is research that suggests that there are differences in the demographics of BSN and ADN graduates with BSN nurses being younger as a cohort than their ADN counterparts. In addition, students who are older, married, and have dependents are more likely to choose the ADN route (Sabio & Petges, 2020). It is also generally believed that ADN graduates represent greater diversity in race, gender, and educational experiences than BSN-prepared nurses. Critics of the BSN requirement for entry into professional nursing suggest that greater diversity is needed in nursing, and this may be lost if entry levels are raised as more disadvantaged minorities may seek lower cost education in community colleges than universities.

There are costs that must be considered as well. University education simply costs more than education at community colleges and significant increases in federal and state funding for baccalaureate and graduate nursing education will need to occur. Given the significant budget deficit currently faced by most states, the likelihood of funding increases for nursing education is directly related to the public and legislative understanding of the complexity of roles nurses assume each day and the educational level they perceive is needed to accomplish these tasks.

In addition, Krugman and Goode (2018) ask why federal money is still being directed to more than 35 diploma schools (embedded as part of graduate medical resident funding) when most state boards of nursing closed these schools 30 years ago and there is no such funding for BSN students. They argue that closure of the remaining diploma schools is overdue and that associated government funds should be reallocated to professional nursing education and nurse residency programs.

Achieving the BSN as the entry degree for professional nursing practice will take the best thinking of our nursing leaders. It will also require courage, as well as a respect for persons not seen in the entry debate, and collaboration of the highest order. It will also require nurses to depersonalize the issue and look at what is best for both the patients they serve and the profession, rather than for them individually.

LaRocco (2014) suggests:

While the leaders of 1965 were visionary in their proposal of baccalaureate education as the entry to professional nursing, they were less effective in creating the change that they proposed. Will our current nursing leaders be successful in completing this unfinished business? (p. 11)

Even the most patient planned-change advocate would agree that nearly 60 years is a long time for implementation of a position. Clearly, the driving forces for such a change have not yet overcome the restraining forces, though movement is apparent. The question seems to come down to whether the nursing profession wants to spend another 60 years debating the issue or whether it wants to proactively take the steps necessary to make the goal a reality.

For Additional Discussion

1. What are the greatest driving and restraining forces for increasing entry into practice to a bachelor's or higher level?

2. Are the terms *professional* and *technical* unnecessarily inflammatory in the entry-into-practice debate? Why do these terms elicit such a "personal" response?

3. Is calling the ADN program a 2-year vocational degree an injustice to its graduates?

4. What is the legitimacy of requiring so many units at the community college level for an ADN degree? Should the current movement by community colleges to award baccalaureate degrees in nursing be encouraged?

5. How does the complexity of nursing roles and responsibilities compare to that of other health professions with higher entry levels?

6. What is the likelihood that nurses and the organizations that represent them will be able to achieve consensus on the entry-into-practice issue?

7. If the entry level is raised, should grandfathering be used? If so, should this grandfathering be conditional?

8. Is the goal of BSN entry a realistic one by 2025? If not, when?

References

Aiken, L. H., Clarke, S. P., Cheung, R. B., Sloane, D. M., & Silber, J. H. (2003). Educational levels of hospital nurses and surgical patient mortality. *JAMA, 290*(12), 1617–1623. https://doi.org/10.1001/jama.290.12.1617

Aiken, L. H., Clarke, S. P., Sloane, D. M., Lake, E. T., & Cheney, T. (2008). Effects of hospital care environment on patient mortality and nurse outcomes. *The Journal of Nursing Administration, 38*(5), 223–229. https://doi.org/10.1097/01 .NNA.0000312773.42352.d7

American Association of Colleges of Nursing. (2015). *Talking points. HRSA report on nursing workforce projections through 2025.* Retrieved September 5, 2020, from http:// www.njccn.org/wp-content/uploads/2015/07/HRSA-Nursing-Workforce-Projections.pdf

American Association of Colleges of Nursing. (2019a). *Fact sheet: Creating a more highly qualified nursing workforce.* Retrieved September 5, 2020, from http://www.aacnnursing .org/News-Information/Fact-Sheets/Nursing-Workforce

American Association of Colleges of Nursing. (2019b). *Fact sheet: The impact of education on nursing practice.* Retrieved September 5, 2020, from https://www.aacnnursing.org/Portals/42/ News/Factsheets/Education-Impact-Fact-Sheet.pdf

American Association of Colleges of Nursing. (2019c). *Accelerated baccalaureate and master's degrees in nursing.* Retrieved September 5, 2020, from http://www.aacnnursing.org/ Nursing-Education-Programs/Accelerated-Programs

American Association of Colleges of Nursing. (2019d). *Degree completion programs for registered nurses: RN to-master's-degree and RN to baccalaureate programs.* Retrieved April 12, 2018, from https://www.aacnnursing.org/News-Information/Fact-Sheets/Degree-Completion-Programs

American Association of Colleges of Nursing. (2021). *Joint statement on academic progression for nursing students and graduates. AACC, ACCT, AACN, NLN, NOADN.* Retrieved January 21, 2021, from http://www.aacnnursing.org/ News-Information/Position-Statements-White-Papers/ Academic-Progression

American Nurses Association. (1965a). *A position paper.* Author.

American Nurses Association. (1965b). *Educational preparation for nurse practitioners and assistants to nurses: A position paper.* Author.

Association of periOperative Registered Nurses. (2020-sunset review). *AORN position statement on entry into practice.* First drafted House of Delegates 1979. https://www.aorn.org/guidelines/clinical-resources/position-statements

Benner, P., Sutphen, M., Leonard, V., & Day, L. (2010). *Educating nurses: A call for radical transformation: Preparation for the professions.* Jossey-Bass/The Carnegie Foundation for the Advancement of Teaching.

Blegen, M. A., Goode, C. J., Park, S. H., Vaughn, T., & Spetz, J. (2013, February). Baccalaureate education in nursing and patient outcomes. *Journal of Nursing Administration, 43*(2), 89–94. https://doi.org/10.1097/NNA.0b013e31827f2028

Campaign for Action. (2013). *The future of nursing: IOM report.* Retrieved September 5, 2020, from https://campaignforaction.org/resource/future-nursing-iom-report/

Canadian Nurses Association. (2021). *Education.* Retrieved September 5, 2020, from https://www.cna-aiic.ca/en/becoming-an-rn/education

Clarke, S. P. (2017). The BSN entry into practice debate. *Nursing Made Incredibly Easy! 15*(1), 6–8. https://doi.org/10.1097/01.NUMA.0000502806.22177.c4

Jeffreys, M. R. (2020, May/June). ADN-to-BSN articulation, academic progression, and transition: A proactive, holistic approach. *Nurse Educator, 45*(3), 155–159. https://doi.org/10.1097/NNE.0000000000000708

Koivisto, I. (2020). *ADN vs BSN salary, competencies, and pros and cons.* Retrieved September 7, 2020, from https://normalnurselife.com/adn-vs-bsn/

Krugman, M., & Goode, C. J. (2018, February). BSN-preparation for RNs: The time is now! *Journal of Nursing Administration, 48*(2), 57–60. https://doi.org/10.1097/NNA.0000000000000572

LaRocco, S. (2014). Where are the visionary nursing leaders of 1965? *American Journal of Nursing, 114*(4), 11. https://doi.org/10.1097/01.NAJ.0000445661.74531.b8

National Association of Neonatal Nurses. (2009). *Educational preparation for nursing practice roles* (Position Statement No. 3048, NANN Board of Directors). Retrieved September 5, 2020, from http://nann.org/uploads/About/Position PDFS/1.4.11_Education%20Preparation%20for%20 Nursing%20Practice%20Roles.pdf

National Council of State Boards of Nursing. (2020, October 16). *2020: Number of candidates taking NCLEX examination and percent passing, by type of candidate.* Retrieved January 22, 2021, from https://www.ncsbn.org/Table_of_Pass_Rates_2020_Q3.pdf

NursingLicensure.org. (2021). *The future of the associate degree in nursing program.* Retrieved January 22, 2021, from https://www.nursinglicensure.org/articles/adn-program-future.html

Sabio, C., & Petges, N. (2020, January). Understanding the barriers to BSN education among ADN students: A qualitative study. *Teaching and Learning in Nursing, 15*(1), 45–52. Retrieved September 7, 2020, from https://www.sciencedirect.com/science/article/pii/S1557308719302112

Sitzman, K., Carpenter, T., & Cherry, K. (2020). Student perceptions related to immediate workplace usefulness of RN-to-BSN program content. *Nurse Educator, 45*(5), 265–268. https://doi.org/10.1097/NNE.0000000000000775

VA celebrates Year of the Nurse by thanking the nurses who serve Veterans. (2020, January 14). VAntage Point. Retrieved September 5, 2020, from https://www.blogs.va.gov/VAntage/70344/va-celebrates-year-nurse-thanking-nurses-serve-veterans/

World Health Organization. (2009). *Global standards for the initial education of professional nurses and midwives.* Retrieved September 5, 2020, from http://www.who.int/hrh/nursing_midwifery/hrh_global_standards_education.pdf

Bridging the Academic–Practice Gap in Nursing

Jonalyn Wallace, Erica D. Hooper-Arana, and Nikki West

ADDITIONAL RESOURCES

Visit thePoint for additional helpful resources.
- eBook
- Journal Articles
- Web Links

CHAPTER OUTLINE

LEARNING OBJECTIVES

The learner will be able to:

1. Define the academic–practice gap in prelicensure nursing.

2. Describe the academic–practice gap's impact on the current and future nursing workforce.

3. Describe changes in the U.S. health care landscape that widen the academic–practice gap.

4. Define nursing practice specialties and care settings that are at risk due to the widening academic–practice gap.

5. Discuss the national spotlight on the academic–practice gap.

6. Describe innovative solutions and effective tactics to address opportunities and challenges in building a robust nursing workforce.

INTRODUCTION

A gap exists between completion of academic programs and entry into employment (also referred to as service or practice) as a registered nurse (RN). This chapter explores how the changing U.S. health care landscape, projected workforce needs, and the evolving role of the RN are making the academic–practice gap more challenging to bridge. It discusses the value of implementing evidence-based interventions to build a thriving and responsive nursing workforce. Innovative approaches are described, including those led by academia, practice, and collaborative partnerships. National attention to the academic–practice gap is presented, as well as current research supporting interventions to meet health care system demands. The chapter concludes with considerations and risks if the gap is not bridged.

Consider This Evidence of an academic–practice gap is well documented. Academic institutions are criticized for not providing curriculum and training experiences that fully prepare nurses to practice in the current health care environment, while practice settings are criticized for having unrealistic expectations of schools of nursing as well as the ability of newly licensed nurses to practice safely (Huston et al., 2018).

THE ACADEMIC–PRACTICE GAP

Negotiating the transition from student to professional nurse can feel daunting. Newly licensed registered nurses (NLRNs) report feeling overwhelmed, unprepared, and shocked by the level of responsibility necessary to navigate the transition from the familiar role of student to the realities of nursing practice. This can result in feelings of anxiety and distress and increase the potential for clinical errors, job dissatisfaction, and NLRN turnover in the first year of practice (Alghamdi & Baker, 2020; Alshahrani et al., 2018; Ankers et al., 2018; Blegan et al., 2017; Huston et al., 2018; Kim & Shin, 2019; Kramer, 1974; Kramer et al., 2013; Powers et al., 2019; Preston et al., 2019).

Complicating the situation are differences in the perceptions of NLRNs' readiness for practice. Nurse researchers have discovered a significant discrepancy between how deans and chief nurse executives view NLRNs' readiness

for practice. Among 400 nursing school deans surveyed, 90% reported that NLRNs were fully prepared to enter clinical practice. In sharp contrast, only 10% of the 5,700 nurse executives responded that new nurses were fully prepared to provide safe and effective care (Berkow et al., 2008; Huston et al., 2018; Powers et al., 2019; Preston et al., 2019). In a study of 352 NLRNs, 51% reported they lacked adequate training in pharmacology and felt unprepared to safely administer medication (Candela & Bowles, 2008; Preston et al., 2019).

In another study, novice nurses expressed a similar viewpoint with more than 50% saying that while their programs prepared them to pass the National Council Licensure Examination (NCLEX), it did not prepare them for "real-world" practice. In addition, more than 76% believed they did not have enough clinical hours in their nursing programs (Berkow et al., 2008, 2009; Preston et al., 2019). Additionally, researchers noted an increase in medication and clinical errors during times when inexperienced NLRNs transitioned into the hospital environment (Duckett & Moran, 2018; Preston et al., 2019; Spector et al., 2015).

Similarly, Kavanagh and Szweda (2017) examined the disconnect between NLRN entry-level competency and NCLEX pass rates. All participants in the study passed the NCLEX. However, the competency assessment tool found that only 23% of new graduates scored in the "safe to practice independently" range. The other 77% were rated as unsafe to practice independently. These competency gaps put patients, NLRNs, and health systems at risk (see Research Fuels the Controversy 2.1).

These challenges are the result of several interconnected issues and are linked to discussions regarding accountability for "fixing" the academic–practice gap. Some researchers suggest that the focus on preparing students to pass the NCLEX limits the scope of education and clinical training that can be accomplished during nursing school. Others suggest that full-time faculty have difficulty staying clinically current and may not present the most relevant or up-to-date material. One survey of nursing students indicated they perceived most of their clinical faculty as lacking the expertise to work in the clinical setting. In addition, poor communication between theory-based and clinical faculty made it hard for them to link what they were learning in class with direct patient care (Dimino et al., 2020; Huston et al., 2018; Preston et al., 2019; Salifu et al., 2019).

Research Fuels the Controversy 2.1

NCLEX Success Versus Real-World Competency

Kavanagh and Szweda (2017) examined the disconnect between NLRN entry-level competency and NCLEX pass rates. In their study, the nurse researchers explored the relationship between successful completion of the NCLEX and the level of clinical competency of recent graduates to work amid the complexity of real-world practice. The study administered a nationally recognized competency assessment tool to more than 5,000 NLRNs over a period of 5 years. Nurses in the study came from more than 140 U.S. nursing programs across 21 states. The assessment tool examines critical thinking learning needs and ability to differentiate urgency and justification for actions, provides insight into the thought processes of the nurse, and assists in the development of an individualized orientation action plan to prepare each nurse for safe clinical practice.

Source: Kavanagh, J., & Szweda, C. (2017). A crisis in competency: The strategic and ethical imperative to assessing new graduate nurses' clinical reasoning. *Nursing Education Perspectives, 38*(2), 57–62. https://doi.org/10.1097/01.NEP.0000000000000112

Study Findings

All participants in the study passed the NCLEX. However, the competency assessment tool found that only 23% of new graduates scored in the "safe to practice independently" range. The other 77% were rated as unsafe to practice independently. To note, there was no significant difference in ratings between baccalaureate and associate degree graduates.

These findings demonstrate the gap between the skills and knowledge required to pass the NCLEX and the competency needed to practice safely as an independent RN. The study authors suggest that the issue belongs to academia and practice alike. Hospital educators must be competent in coaching, guided facilitation, and adult learning theories. Prelicensure academic faculty must respond to the changing landscape of health care as well as the changing learner. This must be achieved while both sides face mounting challenges such as budget cutbacks, aging faculty, lack of trained preceptors, and competition for clinical sites.

More recently, Hensel and Billings (2020) explored the value of incorporating the NCSBN clinical judgment model (CJM) into academic course work. Their study suggests that integrating CJM into nursing curricula is a strategy that prepares students to think through complex clinical problems more effectively and facilitate a safer transition to practice (Hensel & Billings, 2020). Together, undergraduate education and practice partners must prepare nurses beyond the ability to simply pass the NCLEX. Instead, nursing leaders need to look toward knowledge acquisition, clinical application, and critical thinking as desired outcomes for the education of new RNs. The NCLEX is a crucial step in the journey to become a RN. However, many steps must follow initial licensure to obtain the clinical competency necessary for safe and independent RN practice.

Concern exists that the education-to-practice gap is widening. If the academic–practice gap is not addressed through partnership, education redesign, and new teaching strategies, what are the implications for the gap as the U.S. population and health care landscape continue to change?

Discussion Point

Until the 1960s, most nurses were trained in diploma programs associated with hospitals. Diploma programs provided an immersive, clinically focused, and protocol-driven curriculum. During their training, student nurses lived on the hospital grounds, helped staff the hospital, and worked alongside of experienced nurses (Moss et al., 2018).

- What can we learn from the diploma model of nursing?
- Could schools of nursing and clinical settings work together more effectively to bridge the academic–practice gap?
- What would make this model challenging to implement today?

UNDERSTANDING THE ACADEMIC–PRACTICE GAP

Discussed for decades, a recognition of the need to bridge the academic–practice gap gained momentum in 1974 with the release of Kramer's groundbreaking book *Reality Shock: Why Nurses Leave Nursing*. Kramer argued that the idealized versions of nursing promoted by academic faculty contrasted significantly with new nurses' experiences upon entering the workforce. This often led to a shock-like reaction, putting the new graduate nurse at risk for job dissatisfaction and disillusionment with the profession of nursing (Kramer, 1974). The book stimulated the development of programs designed to support newly licensed RNs as they entered professional practice.

Benner's novice-to-expert theory broadened understanding of how NLRNs acquire the skills necessary to expertly care for patients. According to Benner's research, nurses acquire skill over time by engaging in focused educational opportunities and a multitude of clinically relevant experiences. Through these activities, nurses move along a continuum from novice to advanced beginner; competent; proficient; and, finally, expert nurse (Benner, 1984).

The transition shock model (Duchscher, 2009) showed how important supportive relationships are to a NLRN's successful integration into the practice environment (Huston et al., 2018; Kim, 2020). Hickerson and colleagues (2016) identified three themes describing the impact of the academic–practice gap: evidence of a gap is clear; it is costly; and finding solutions will require partnership and collaboration.

TRANSITION-TO-PRACTICE PROGRAMS DEFINED

Transition-to-practice programs (TTPs) are an evidence-based solution designed to support NLRNs as they progress from student to professional nurse. The National Council of State Boards of Nursing (NCSBN, 2015) and the American Association of Colleges of Nursing (AACN, 2007) define TTP as a formal program of active learning that includes a series of facilitated educational sessions and precepted work experiences for NLRNs (Spector et al., 2015). TTPs are structured to address specific needs and have been given various names including "nurse residencies," "nurse fellowships," "externships," and "work–study internships" (Rush et al., 2019; Spector et al., 2015; Wallace, 2016).

THE CHANGING HEALTH CARE LANDSCAPE

The U.S. population is growing older and getting sicker, significant workforce shifts are occurring, and nursing roles are being redefined to meet current and future health care needs as care moves away from acute care settings and toward population health. In addition, unprecedented environmental and medical disasters (i.e., wildfires, hurricanes) and the 2020 novel coronavirus pandemic provide opportunities to further develop skills to meet emerging needs. These factors will impact the transition to practice for NLRNs and could potentially widen the academic–practice gap.

An Aging and Sicker Population

Americans are growing older, generally living longer, and the complexity of patient needs continues to grow. Baby boomers (born between 1946 and 1964) make up the largest generation in history to reach older adulthood. By 2030, all baby boomers will be over 65 years of age, resulting in approximately 20%

of Americans estimated to be of retirement age (Vespa et al., 2020). It is estimated that the U.S. population 85 years and older will double from 6.3 million in 2015 to nearly 13 million by 2035. In addition, the number of U.S. citizens aged 100 years or more will triple between 2017 and 2045 (Buerhaus et al., 2017a; Kirch & Petelle, 2017; Vespa et al., 2020).

Despite medical and technologic advances, lower rates of smoking, decreased incidence of emphysema, and access to healthier lifestyles, the prevalence of chronic disease is increasing among aging U.S. adults. Adding burden to an already taxed system, the need for Medicare, the health insurance plan available to U.S. citizens aged 65 years and older, people with specific disabilities, and/or people with end-stage renal failure, is anticipated to rise to 92.5 million people by 2050 (Dickman et al., 2017). The growth in Medicare is directly related to the surge in U.S. population from the early 1940s through the early 1960s—the baby boomer generation. By 2030, 40% of baby boomers are expected to be diagnosed with diabetes, 43% will have heart disease, and 25% will have received a diagnosis of cancer (Buerhaus et al., 2017b). The aging population, coupled with an increasing prevalence of chronic disease, increases the complexity of patient care exponentially for both the newly licensed and experienced RNs (Buerhaus et al., 2017b; Gaudette et al., 2015; Goldman & Gaudette, 2015).

Nursing has an opportunity to help mitigate issues related to chronic condition care through preventative measures and a focus on social determinants of health (SDOH) and population health. The U.S. Department of Health and Human Services (USDHHS, 2020) defines SDOH as the conditions in environments where people are born, live, learn, work, play, worship, and age that affect a wide range of health, functioning, and quality-of-life outcomes and risks. SDOH are being considered important contributors to health, with factors outside of direct care significantly impacting well-being (USDHHS, 2020). There is growing focus on understanding the communities in which people live and work and how this affects access to care and health care utilization as well as outcomes (Centers for Medicare and Medicaid Services (CMS), 2021).

Health Care Reform

The United States has the world's costliest health care: in 2018, U.S. spending on health care grew 4.6% to $3.6 trillion, or $11,172 per person. These costs account for 17.7% of the gross domestic product (GDP). Rising costs are threatening the health of the American economy. The nation's total annual health care spending is projected to reach $6.2 trillion by 2028 (CMS, 2020).

Significant reform was instituted in 2010 with the Affordable Care Act (ACA). The law passed with the goals of making affordable health insurance available to more people, expanding Medicaid, and supporting innovative medical care delivery methods designed to lower the costs of health care (CMS, 2020).

There is ongoing debate of the effectiveness of the ACA and its implementation, and health care reform remains a much-discussed topic from a political and social perspective. Health care delivery remains in a predominantly fee-for-service model that can favor more (rather than better) services, treatments, and tests. One approach to tackling rising health care costs and improving quality is value-based payment models. Value-based models shift financial incentives toward reduced costs, efficiencies, and better health outcomes. These models focus on preventive care and management of diseases and conditions with fewer complications. The CMS is taking steps in this direction (Lyford & Lash, 2019–2020).

Health care reform and the concept of value-based payments present an opportunity for both academia and practice to evaluate and prepare nurses to deliver high-quality care that is also cost-effective. Nurses have an opportunity to be recognized as high-value contributors. To do this, nurses must look at costs and their use of resources, thinking about how they can improve quality and use resources more wisely. Many nurses do not understand how their actions impact costs (Kerfoot, 2020).

Workforce Changes

Demands on the health care workforce are shifting. The number of nurses and other health professionals needed as well as the skills and competencies they require are changing and will continue to evolve.

Nurses

RNs play a key role in the delivery of health care. It is estimated that nurses from the baby boomer generation are leaving practice at the rate of more than 70,000 annually, with 1 million nurses anticipated to retire between 2015 and 2030 (Buerhaus et al., 2017a). Shortages of nurses by 2030 are projected to be most acute in California (193,100), Florida (128,364), and Texas (109,779) (Juraschek et al., 2019). Offsetting this loss are national initiatives like the Johnson & Johnson Campaign for Nursing's Future (2002) and the Institute of Medicine's (IOM) *The Future of Nursing* report (2011) that sparked engagement and action across the profession (Fig. 2.1). Together, these initiatives and others have resulted in an increase of over 1 million fulltime-equivalent nurses between 2001 and 2015 and are predicted to expand the profession by another 1 million by 2030 (Buerhaus et al., 2017c).

Another benefit of the initiative is increased educational levels for the current and future nursing workforce. Academia may experience challenges as health systems adjust

and pivot to function in a dynamic health care environment, including educational pipeline interruption, cancellation of clinical rotations, regulatory and licensure changes, and adjustments to reimbursement (AAMC, 2020). Overall, however, the age composition is rapidly shifting, with growing numbers of RNs aged 35 and younger joining the workforce as older nurses retire and leave the profession (Buerhaus et al., 2017c). These achievements are significant and position nurses to embrace current and future challenges.

Meanwhile, demand for access to high-quality affordable care is growing exponentially as the U.S. population grows older and sicker. The impact of nurse retirements and integration of younger nurses into a complex health care system is significant and multifaceted. Not only must nurse leaders fill vacant positions in hard-to-fill clinical specialties, they must also account for the loss of accumulated nursing knowledge, expertise, and wisdom as experienced nurses leave practice. Buerhaus et al. (2010) quantified the impact of this loss; calculations show that the loss of "experience years" during this transition is significant and will impact nurse leaders as they address health system challenges with less experienced teams.

Physicians

Anticipated changes in the physician workforce will impact health care delivery as well. Over the next two decades, significant numbers of physicians will retire or leave their medical practices. Total numbers vary as do estimates of anticipated shortages that could result. The Association of American Medical Colleges (AAMC, 2020) predicts physician demand will grow faster than supply, leading to a projected total shortage of between 54,100 and 139,000 physicians and specifically a primary care physician shortage of between 21,400 and 55,200 by 2033.

Currently, rural America has fewer physicians, averaging 60 primary care physicians per 100,000 residents compared to urban areas that have 80 primary care providers per 100,000 residents. Researchers anticipate that the uneven distribution of physicians across the United States will worsen in the future. People seeking care may notice significant wait times and difficulty accessing necessary care (AAMC, 2020; Kirch & Petelle, 2017).

Nurses may be able to help address the growing physician gap in innovative ways, including broadening the use of nurse practitioners to meet primary care needs. Patients in primary care settings are receiving care from an array of providers, not just physicians. Advanced practice nurses, which include nurse practitioners, clinical nurse specialists, certified RN anesthetists, and certified nurse midwives, may be filling a growing shortage of physicians with the scope of services they can provide (AAMC, 2020).

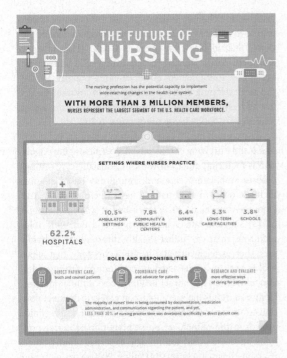

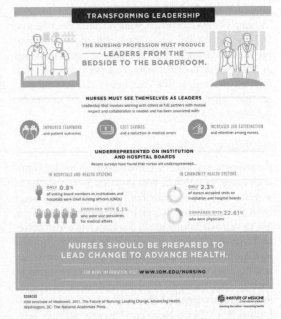

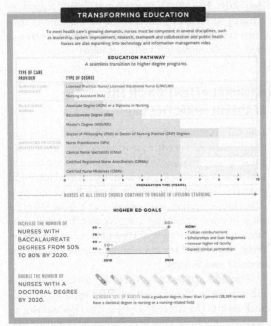

Figure 2.1 Infographic—The IOM's *Future of Nursing*. (Infographic based on Institute of Medicine. (2011). *The future of nursing: Leading change, advancing health.* National Academies Press. https://doi.org/10.17226/12956. Reprinted with permission from the National Academy of Sciences, Courtesy of the National Academies Press, Washington, DC.)

Discussion Point

Upon completion of medical school, newly licensed physicians typically attend a 1-year internship followed by a multiyear residency in a designated specialty. How does this compare to the pathway of a newly licensed nurse?

Behavioral Health Workforce

The demand for behavioral health care is growing. According to the National Institute of Mental Health (NIMH), nearly one in five U.S. adults live with a mental illness (51.5 million in 2019) (NIMH, 2020). As demand remains high, mental health workforce supply is unlikely to meet needs. Estimates suggest that only half of people with mental illnesses receive treatment.

According to the Health Resources and Services Administration (HRSA) health workforce data, psychiatrists and addiction counselors are anticipated to experience shortages by 2030.

The supply of psychiatrists is projected to decline as retirements exceed new entrants. Rapid growth in supply of psychiatric nurse practitioners and psychiatric physician assistants may help but not fully offset this. In 2030, the supply of psychiatrists, psychiatric nurse practitioners, and psychiatric physician assistants will not be enough to provide any higher level of care than the national average in 2017, which does not fully meet need (HRSA, n.d.). Focused on whole-person care, nurses can help fill gaps related to identifying behavioral health issues, an area for consideration in academia.

New Roles for Nurses

For nurses to help meet the current needs of the U.S. health care system, they must be both prepared for and willing to step into new and nontraditional roles. Given that Gallup has reported nurses as the most trusted professionals for the last 18 years (Reinhart, 2020), it is imperative that nurses are prepared to continue to cultivate this trust by providing high-quality and comprehensive holistic care. Nurses are now expected to take on nontraditional roles in a variety of settings across the care continuum while using an innovative, inclusive, technologically savvy, and preventative care-focused lens (Carson-Newman University Online, 2020; Demiris et al., 2019; Knoff, 2019; Lopez et al., 2019; Moore, 2018; Nursing School Hub, 2020).

Furthermore, nursing education must prepare nurses beyond the bedside to understand broader concepts like population health, health equity, global citizenship, social justice, and SDOH in order to produce nurses able to contribute to national efforts such as attaining the United Nations' Sustainable Development Goals (Hassmiller & Kuehnert, 2020). Nursing leaders with a solid understanding of how to implement evidence-based practice are crucial to developing and supporting the innovation needed for addressing shortfalls within the health care system (Noles et al., 2019; Shelby & Wermers, 2020).

The current health care landscape with hospital downsizing and a growing chronically ill, complex, aging population is requiring nurses to work in nonacute care settings, such as ambulatory care and community-based environments in order to meet patient needs (Demiris et al., 2019; Hooper-Arana et al., 2019; Jones-Bell et al., 2020). Pittman (2019) suggests nurses take on new and emerging roles, requiring them to utilize health information technologies, such as telehealth and health technology, that allows health care to be delivered in community settings while also addressing the unmet health needs of the population. Common trends include a focus on geriatric nursing, positions working as nursing faculty and in retail health clinics, growth in the number of nurse practitioners, nurse positions on boards, and technologic expertise among nurses (Carson-Newman University Online, 2020; Nursing School Hub, 2020; Ross, 2018). Demiris et al. (2019) support leveraging nurses as innovators and leaders to deliver value-based care to an older population in need of services to meet complex social and health care needs.

NATIONAL ATTENTION ON THE ACADEMIC–PRACTICE GAP

National recommendations have been put forth to help narrow the academic–practice gap by supporting nurses in being adequately prepared to meet the health care system and workforce needs. These recommendations are highlighted in several significant documents identifying specific areas of nursing education and practice that require strengthening of nurse knowledge, competencies, and skills. The following discussion reviews some of those documents reflecting national efforts and recommendations to close the academic–practice gap.

Recommendations to develop the nursing profession and improve health outcomes are stated in the IOM's landmark report, *The Future of Nursing* (2011); it includes an emphasis on six focal areas (e.g., transforming nursing education) and four key strategies (e.g., nurses should practice to the full extent of their education and training) for helping nurses overcome barriers for effectively practicing in a rapidly changing health care environment. As a result of this report, the Robert Wood Johnson Foundation (RWJF) and the American Association of Retired Persons (AARP) collaborated to create the Future of Nursing Campaign for Action to use the power of the largest group of health professionals to help transform health and health care (RWJF & AARP, 2020). An expert committee is now undertaking the task of extending the IOM 2011 report and the Future of Nursing Campaign for Action in the Future of Nursing 2020–2030 to establish further recommendations to take nurses into the next decade with the ability to meet health care system challenges and needs (National Academy of Medicine, 2020). There are various areas to be considered in this initiative, including the preparation of nurses to ensure the ability to work in areas outside of acute care settings and to attain health equity.

At the national level, population health has been identified as an important area that all current and future nurses must understand. The RWJF conducted a project to review nursing education and practice models designed to support population health improvement (RWJF & AARP, 2019). Out of this project came a report articulating how nursing education can support improving population health. Key recommendations include having a core population health course for all nursing students while also weaving population health concepts throughout all nursing curriculum. Noted as relevant population health content to address within nursing curriculum are SDOH, interprofessional team building and skills, and health equity.

Nationally recognized as another area for further development to help close the academic–practice gap is the preparation of nurses to work outside the acute care setting. The Josiah Macy Jr. Foundation held its annual conference in 2016 for enhanced nursing roles in primary care. Six conference recommendations were developed:

1. Changing the cultures of both nursing schools and practices to place greater value on primary care and the role of nurses in it
2. Redesigning practices to make full use of the expertise of nurses
3. Rebalancing nursing education to elevate primary care content
4. Promoting the career development of nurses in primary care
5. Developing primary care expertise in nursing school faculty
6. Increasing opportunities for interprofessional education and teamwork development in both education and practice (Bodenheimer & Mason, 2016)

Primary care nursing roles were highlighted including coordinating the care of chronically ill patients between the primary care home and the surrounding health care neighborhood and promoting population health, including working with communities to create healthier spaces for people to live, work, learn, and play.

The AACN has recently updated its *AACN Essentials* (2021) to provide a framework for entry-level and advanced-level professional nursing education. The competency areas for education recommended to best prepare nurses to meet the needs of the current health care system include:

1. Knowledge for nursing practice
2. Person-centered care
3. Population health
4. Scholarship for the nursing discipline
5. Quality and safety
6. Interprofessional partnerships
7. Systems-based practice
8. Informatics and health care technologies
9. Professionalism
10. Personal, professional, and leadership development

The AACN has highlighted various key content areas that should be threaded throughout all nursing curricula, such as SDOH.

All these national recommendations demonstrate trends in support of closing the academic–practice gap. These trends indicate a need for placing high importance on continually monitoring the health care landscape to appropriately revise nursing curricula to allow new graduates to meet ever-changing health care system demands. It is of importance to continue reviewing nursing education and care delivery outcomes to determine if nurses are adequately prepared with the necessary knowledge and experiences to smoothly transition from academia to practice.

STRATEGIES AND INNOVATIONS TO BRIDGE THE GAP

Both academia and practice partners have developed and implemented programs to help assimilate NLRNs into the profession through experiences that help develop improved critical thinking, clinical skills, and professional confidence. Programs are of value to health systems, mitigating concerns for patient safety, recruitment, retention, and turnover costs during the initial year of a nurse's career (Blegan et al., 2017; Dimino et al., 2020; Huston et al., 2018; Powers et al., 2019).

Huston et al. (2018) identified several strategies that successfully address the education-to-practice gap, organized into three categories: educational, practice, and collaborative strategies. These evidence-based concepts provide guidance for academic and practice partners who want to work together to more effectively manage this critical issue (Huston et al., 2018).

Educational Strategies

Simulation

Simulation is an evidence-based, adaptable methodology to address faculty and student needs. Simulation facilitates discussion and problem solving, exposes curriculum gaps, and shapes learning experiences. A multifaceted longitudinal study conducted by the NCSBN considered the impact on student outcomes when simulation was substituted for clinical practicum hours (Hayden et al., 2014). Positive results were reported in both the control group (students who received 25% of their clinical practicum hours in the simulation lab) and the research group (students who received 50% of their clinical practicum hours via simulation). These findings suggest learning is enhanced when simulation and debriefing are conducted in a safe, nonthreatening manner. Additionally, simulation is customizable; thus, specific gaps in knowledge can be addressed in "real time" with a student rather than waiting until the next patient interaction.

The 2020 novel coronavirus pandemic presented an opportunity to increase the use of clinical simulation. Practice partners faced myriad challenges during pandemic surges, resulting in many cases in a curtailment of clinical training placements. Schools were required to quickly adjust to this new reality, and many did so by more fully integrating simulation into their programs. Despite the disadvantages of missing face-to-face interactions with patients, use of simulation and debriefing sessions offered students a way to continue to improve both their clinical judgment and critical thinking skills. While not a replacement for interaction with patients and staff, simulation provides a proven solution to enhance clinical training experiences (Hayden et al., 2014; Huston et al., 2018; Waxman et al., 2019).

Active Learning

In active learning, instruction shifts from reliance on lecture and slide decks and focuses on activities that promote critical thinking and development of clinical judgment (Huston et al., 2018). Faculty may present questions or use case studies, scenarios, and experiences to give students an opportunity to reason through a patient care problem and work together to solve it. The flipped classroom is another approach in which students are assigned to read and learn content prior to class time and apply the learning during remote or face-to-face class sessions. This strategy requires students to use higher-level skills as opposed to memorization, and improves the transfer of knowledge (Hessler, 2017; Huston et al., 2018).

Competency-Based Education

In this learner-centric solution, educators structure learning and provide students with specific ways to demonstrate competency for both "soft" and technical skills necessary for safe nursing practice (AACN, 2021; Huston et al., 2018).

Practice Strategies

Practice partners typically provide transition experiences to address workforce needs, giving newly licensed and hired RNs an opportunity to prepare for their new role.

Nurse Residency Programs

There is growing evidence that nurse residency programs (NRPs) are a gold-standard solution to successful transition to practice. The structure and length of NRPs vary by region, health system, and budget. Programs are structured to provide a multitude of experiences to participants including online modules, didactic sessions, simulation, and direct patient care under the supervision of an experienced nurse preceptor. Numerous solutions have been implemented by health systems and academia and through academic–practice partnerships and other collaborative efforts (AACN, 2007; Barr et al., 2019; Benner et al., 2010; Brook et al., 2019; Chant & Westendorf, 2019; Goode et al., 2018).

Differences in program design, definitions, and standardized outcome measures have hampered efforts to identify essential elements and best practices of successful programs. That said, empirical data suggest that NRPs lasting between 6 and 12 months with a focus on both clinical competence and integration into the organization's culture result in positive outcomes including improved confidence, competence, critical thinking, professional engagement, and retention (Goode et al., 2018). Chant and Westendorf (2019) link structured NRPs with clearly defined outcomes promoting clinical competency, quality, safety, and professional leadership skills to satisfaction and retention. Finally, a key factor of successful programs relates to the quality of relationships in the care environment. Prioritizing positive professional relationships between experienced RNs and NLRNs as resources, precepts, and mentor factors strongly in successful program outcomes (AACN, 2007; Barr et al., 2019; Benner et al., 2010; Brook et al., 2019; Chant &

Westendorf, 2019; Frogeli et al., 2018; Goode et al., 2018; Kaihlanen et al., 2020; Murry et al., 2019; Spector, 2015; Oblea et al., 2019; Rush et al., 2019; Tyndall et al., 2019; Warren et al., 2018).

Health systems may either purchase a commercially developed program or develop their own program in-house. Commercial programs provide content, data analysis, and proprietary tools as a framework for the residency team. In-house or homegrown programs developed by hospital system staff are also widely used. Tailored to the specific needs of a health system, homegrown programs offer another avenue for safely and effectively transitioning NLRNs into practice.

Of note, data show that whether the program is homegrown or commercially purchased, a key element to success is the quality of relationships; strong clinical and leadership support for NLRNs correlates with job satisfaction and retention (Alghamdi & Baker, 2020; Cline et al., 2017).

Collaborative Strategies

Academia and practice have come together in effective, creative ways to prepare NLRNs and bridge the gap. Multiple examples of collaborative solutions and strategies follow.

Academic–Practice Partnership: Transition to Practice

A 12-week TTP was developed in the San Francisco Bay area to address difficulties caused by the 2008 recession (2017). Few health systems were hiring new graduate nurses, and many NLRNs were unable to find jobs, losing clinical skills and confidence in the interim. The partnership included several practice partners and both public and private schools of nursing. A structured curriculum was developed using Quality and Safety Education for Nurses (QSEN) competencies as a framework, student skills were assessed, and the team worked with participants to develop a robust learning plan. NLRNs were placed in clinical sites across northern California. The standardized curriculum and support resulted in positive outcomes including improved competence, confidence, employment, and retention. The program was adopted for use in acute care, home health, hospice, and public health settings (Jones & West, 2017).

Student Work–Study Internships/ Externships

Work–study programs provide senior-level nursing students with paid clinical immersion experience, exposing interns to the realities of clinical practice and allowing them to hone skills they've learned in nursing school. Students work in a variety of settings including hospital units, procedural suites, clinical education, quality and risk teams, and infection prevention departments. Programs are structured as clinical courses with syllabi, faculty of record, and malpractice coverage by the academic partner. Programs may include both clinical and didactic sessions depending on the setting and usually take place in the summer semester when students have fewer school-related obligations. Interns show increased confidence and competence as a result of these programs (Wallace, 2016).

Specialty-Specific Clinical Immersion

Academic–practice partnerships that provide structured clinical immersion experiences for nursing students in specialty areas anticipating critical workforce shortages (i.e., perioperative nursing, maternal–child health) are another example of collaboration. The immersion experience is structured as a clinical practicum course in which the school and clinical site collaborate to develop curriculum, select students, and create evaluation tools. In this model, tuition may be paid by the student, covered by the practice partner, or covered through other means, such as grant funding. Students are exposed to the clinical environment, gain proficiency in basic nursing skills, and have an opportunity to integrate theory into practice.

Dedicated Education Unit

Dedicated education units (DEUs) are student-centered care units where nursing students learn theory and direct patient care. In this model, staff nurses are key partners in the students' education and professional role development. An added benefit to DEUs is that they require sharing of resources and a willingness to work collaboratively to solve operational issues, the foundation of a true partnership. Positive outcomes include better clinical and professional preparation, confidence communicating within the interprofessional team, and a sense of engagement with the unit team when compared to students not participating in DEUs (Dimino et al., 2020).

Formal Academic–Practice Partnerships

A formal academic–practice partnership moves beyond transactional tasks to embrace a true partnership bound by clearly defined expectations, alignment of vision and values, establishment of mutual trust and respect, the sharing of knowledge, and a commitment to creating programs, projects, structure, and processes to address issues and meet identified goals. Through partnership, organizations can move beyond traditional roles and rethink nursing education, evidence-informed practice, and nursing research. This provides an opportunity to design and implement more effective strategies to address the education-to-practice gap (AACN, 2021).

> ## Discussion Point
> What ideas do you have for better alignment of academia to emerging practice needs?

THINKING BIGGER: CURRICULUM REDESIGN

The academic and practice strategies shared previously are built on traditional models of nursing education. The changing health care landscape provides the nursing profession with an opportunity to disrupt current thinking and fundamentally rethink how to prepare a future nursing workforce. Through partnership, academia and practice can redesign curricula that prepare students to pass their board exams and safely and effectively provide patient care. What might a new model look like? How might education and practice partners collaborate to create an innovative approach to nursing education? It can be difficult to envision innovative approaches that bridge the academic–practice gap. Fortunately, examples do exist and can be used to illustrate this idea.

Redesign Example from the Past: Kaiser Foundation School of Nursing

The Kaiser Foundation School of Nursing (KFSN) opened in 1947 as a 3-year diploma program based in Oakland, California. The school was designed to meet a growing need for nurses after World War II and to prepare a nursing workforce with the ability to care for patients in the new and disruptively innovative Kaiser Health System. The school was led by a doctorally prepared nurse with expert faculty made up of both nurses and physicians. Together, they developed and taught a curriculum that included scientific and social theory, disease prevention and wellness, and traditional medical knowledge. Students often accompanied physicians during patient rounds. The integrated curriculum aligned with Kaiser Permanente's model of care and focused on prevention and wellness rather than a traditional sick care or disease-focused model of care. In a departure from other diploma schools, the students were not onsite to staff the hospital; rather, their clinical practicums aligned with coursework and included both typical hospital rotations as well as rehabilitation, home care,

ambulatory clinics, and occupational health. The accredited Permanente School of Nursing graduated its first class in 1950 and offered tuition-free education and training for its first 7 years. In 1953, the name of the school was changed to KFSN and it became an independent institution. The last class graduated in 1976.

KFSN focused on developing nurses to have a solid understanding of preventative care, interdisciplinary collaboration, accountability, self-care, patient-centered care, leadership, and professionalism (Moss et al., 2018).

Jones and D'Alfonso (2020) state that:

> *Innovations in nursing education and lasting legacies of the school of nursing were formed. … Many of these legacies shape the professional practice of nursing today: the values of preventive care, diversity and antidiscrimination, encouraging continuing education, a flourishing sense of community among students that built a culture of caring and team-work, an emphasis on self-care, and life-balancing cultural and social development. (p. 65)*

Nursing students were strictly instructed to represent KFSN and honor the rich traditions of the nursing profession with the utmost integrity, values, excellence, and professionalism. KFSN consistently raised the bar in nursing education by surpassing regulatory expectations and standard practice to promote nursing excellence and influence innovation. Students were taught to value team-based care and continuing education as well as interprofessionalism; they were educated both in the classroom and practice setting by physicians and specialists in addition to nurses. To promote the resilience of nurses, encouragement was provided to students to develop a wellness lifestyle promoting self-care both inside and outside of school. The KFSN model of nursing education paved the way for caring for oneself and others as well as creatively envisioning the future of the nursing that continues to exist within the current nursing practice at Kaiser Permanente (Moss et al., 2018).

Modern Redesign Example: California Nursing Schools Pilot Project

In 2018, a cross-sector team assembled to support four nursing schools in a pilot program focused on revising curricula with the goal of better preparing nurses for evolving roles in rapidly changing practice environments. A unique feature of the redesign project was the team, which included:

- Leaders from a large regional employer with experience and interest in nursing workforce needs, who provided grant funding
- Two faculty from an academic health sciences university that had recently successfully revised its curriculum;

the faculty had advised and led faculty and administrators of the four pilot schools through a process

- The state's nursing workforce center and action coalition that served as the convener and subject matter expert in developing the workforce to be consistent with health care trends

- Nursing education consultants from the state's licensing and regulatory board who were active participants in helping schools of nursing understand the statutes and regulations in support of curriculum redesign

With this collaborative approach, the schools were supported and led through a process of discovery and exploration for how to best bridge the academic–practice gap.

Two associate degree–awarding schools and two bachelor degree–awarding schools were selected for the pilot. They worked both independently with their own school faculty and together as a multischool learning community to create four unique curricula, one designed for each school, that best met evolving health care environmental needs and the needs of their specific local populations. An important aspect of their redesign process was identifying and increasing engagement with clinical partners, both traditional and nontraditional, who gave input to how they could best utilize nurses. Nontraditional clinical input was obtained from county health departments, health centers, and nonprofit organizations providing care transitions for special populations. Each school integrated this input and developed its own revised curriculum based around critical thinking skills, flexibility, and care across a continuum of settings from inpatient through community. These schools are now more intentionally focusing on SDOH, health equity, and access (Swan et al., 2020).

Discussion Point

Have your prelicensure clinical experiences prepared you to work in settings outside of the hospital? How much experience are you gaining outside the hospital?

WHAT CAN WE DO TO BRIDGE THE GAP? WHAT IS HOLDING US BACK?

Despite data validating the risks of not addressing the academic–practice gap, many organizations continue to resist change. Change can be complex. Schools and clinical sites may be open to new ways of thinking and working, yet they might lack the understanding of or experience with how to successfully manage organizational change and the

inevitable disruptions that accompany innovation. Strategies such as redesigning relationships between academic and practice partners, providing opportunities for employees to work as clinical faculty, and creating DEUs require collaboration, clear communication, patience, persistence, and resources to conceive and adopt. It is a challenge and a skill to address nursing workforce competencies for evolving health care trends while simultaneously addressing the current demand to graduate nurses and treat a population with chronic disease and illness. In other words, the need and finite resources with which to address immediate issues and challenges can compete with the longer-term investment of time, effort, and funds to create the type of nurse anticipated to be in increasing demand.

Academia faces pressure to meet current educational and regulatory requirements established by accrediting agencies and state boards of nursing. Universities and colleges may be steeped in tradition and committed to adhere to long-established policies, procedures, and approaches to academic learning. The school's business model may be reliant on traditional ways of providing nursing education. Recommendations for fundamentally redesigning curricula and shifting how knowledge is transferred may challenge both the academic and business sides of universities and colleges. Moving beyond the traditional prelicensure models focused on inpatient medical-surgical nursing represents a dramatic change in paradigm, which may be challenging to overcome.

CONCLUSION

Despite numerous data points, health care trends and recommendations from national sources, schools, and practice settings have yet to uniformly adopt solutions to address the academic–practice gap. The U.S. population is growing older, and the need to manage chronic health conditions continues to expand. This is occurring simultaneously with health care reform and significant changes in the clinical workforce. With the right education, nursing can support changing care needs through the emergence of new roles and care delivery models. If academia and practice do not address these trends in American health care, then the academic–practice gap is likely to grow wider.

Much of prelicensure nursing education continues to focus on tasks and memorization. This curriculum was designed for a role that does not match expectations of a contemporary RN. As evidence shows, focusing on NCLEX pass rates does not adequately measure the NLRN's ability to meet the demands of real-world clinical practice. Unlike the physician education model, nursing lacks a standardized approach to role acquisition through robust TTPs. This places both NLRNs and the providers they work for at risk.

Physician residency is not required following initial licensure as a medical doctor. However, it is the standard of practice in most communities across the country. Newly licensed physicians seek placements in competitive multiyear residency programs that help bridge the gap between medical school and safe independent practice. As RN roles and the overall health care system become more complex, standardization of RN TTPs becomes an increasingly important consideration. Facing a multitude of conflicting priorities, providers have yet to recognize the importance of requiring the same rigor of education for NLRNs. Lack of adequate preparation for practice may result in clinical errors, reality shock, job dissatisfaction, and ultimately nurse attrition.

Regulatory and accrediting bodies, such as state boards of nursing and the NCSBN, must critically evaluate prelicensure and postlicensure standards. Revisions to state-mandated prelicensure curriculum outlines may be necessary. Further, TTPs should become the standard of practice to ensure quality and consistency across health systems. Federal regulatory bodies like the CMS should also take an interest in supporting TTPs for NLRNs. Improving initial RN competency could help close the quality and affordability gap that is draining the national economy.

In the current environment, there are opportunities for academia and practice to find creative ways to create the nurse of the future. Examples exist for how academia and practice have aligned to prepare nurses for the modern needs of clinical practice. These examples of schools and practice sites working collaboratively have been possible through openness to innovation. Stronger collaborative relationships need to be developed between regulatory bodies, academia, and practice partners to advance new models of prelicensure and postlicensure nursing education.

Risks are high if nursing maintains the status quo; the health of the U.S. population and the value of the profession are on the line. Can we afford not to change?

For Additional Discussion

1. In the future, should all practice settings be required to offer NRPs to all NLRNs? What role might academia play in these programs? What role might the CMS or other public funders play?

2. Do you feel your nursing program has prepared you to fill nursing roles in the community? Have you learned about population-based care and SDOH?

3. Which specialty areas have you been exposed to (e.g., emergency department, operating room, catheterization lab, labor and delivery)? Did the exposure provide enough experience for you to work as a competent nurse in that field?

4. How many of your faculty members are still active in clinical practice? Do you think this makes a difference in your education as a future RN?

5. What learning experiences should be offered in the future to help better prepare prelicensure RNs for real-world nursing practice? What gaps do you see?

References

Alghamdi, M. S., & Baker, O. G. (2020). Identifying the experiences of new graduate nurses during the transition period to practice as a professional nurse. *Journal of Clinical Nursing, 29*, 3082–3088. https://doi.org/10.1111/jocn.15344

Alshahrani, Y., Cusack, L., & Rasmussen, P. (2018). Undergraduate nursing students' strategies for coping with their first clinical placement descriptive survey study. *Nurse Education Today, 69*, 104–108. https://doi.org/10.1016/j.nedt.2018.07.005

American Association of Colleges of Nursing. (2007, February). *White paper on the education and role of the clinical nurse leader.* https://nursing.uiowa.edu/sites/default/files/documents/academic-programs/graduate/msn-cnl/CNL_White_Paper.pdf

American Association of Colleges of Nursing. (2021, April). *The essentials: Core competencies for professional nursing education.* https://www.aacnnursing.org/Portals/42/AcademicNursing/pdf/Essentials-2021.pdf

Ankers, M. D., Barton, C. A., & Parry, Y. K. (2018). A phenomenological exploration of graduate nurse transition to professional practice within a transition to practice program. *Collegian, 25*(3), 319–325. https://doi.org/10.1016/j.colegn.2017.09.002

Association of American Medical Colleges. (2020, June). *The complexities of physician supply and demand: Projections from 2018 to 2033.* https://www.aamc.org/system/files/2020-06/stratcomm-aamc-physician-workforce-projections-june-2020.pdf

Barr, S., Ferro, A., & Prion, S. (2019). An innovative academic-practice partnership to enhance the development and training of military nurses. *Journal of Professional Nursing, 35*(5), 369–378. https://doi.org/10.1016/j.profnurs.2019.04.008

Benner, P. (1984). *From novice to expert: Excellence and power in clinical nursing practice.* Addison-Wesley Publishing Company.

Benner, P., Sutphen, M., Leonard, V., & Day, L. (2010). *Educating nurses: A call for radical transformation.* Jossey-Bass.

Berkow, S., Virkstis, K., Stewart, J., & Conway, L. (2008). Assessing new graduate nurse performance. *Journal of Nursing Administration, 38*(11), 468–474. https://doi.org/10.1097/01.NNA.0000339477.50219.06

Berkow, S., Virkstis, K., Stewart, J., & Conway, L. (2009). Assessing new graduate nurse performance. *Nurse Educator, 34*(1), 17–22. https://doi.org/10.1097/01.NNE.0000343405.90362.15

Blegan, M. A., Spector, N., Lynn, M. R., Barnsteiner, J., & Ulrich, B. (2017, October). Newly licensed RN retention: Hospital and nurse characteristics. *Journal of Nursing Administration, 47*(10), 508–514. https://doi.org/10.1097/NNA.0000000000000523

Bodenheimer, T., & Mason, D. (2016, June). *Registered nurses: Partners in transforming primary care.* Proceedings of a Conference on Preparing Registered Nurses for Enhanced Roles in Primary Care, Atlanta, GA. Josiah Macy Jr. Foundation.

Brook, J., Aitken, L., Webb, R., MacLaren, J., & Salmon, D. (2019). Characteristics of successful interventions to reduce turnover and increase retention of early career nurses: A systematic review. *Journal of Nursing Students, 91*, 47–59. https://doi.org/10.1016/j.ijnurstu.2018.11.003

Buerhaus, P. (2010). Dr. Peter Buerhaus' perspective on the short- and long-term outlook for registered nurses in the US. *New Jersey Nurse, 40*(4),7.

Buerhaus, P., Auerbach, D., & Staiger, D. (2017a). How should we prepare for the wave of retiring baby boomer nurses? *Health Affairs Blog.* https://www.healthaffairs.org/do/10.1377/hblog20170503.059894/full/

Buerhaus, P., Skinner, L. E., Auerbach, D. I., & Staiger, D. O. (2017b). Four challenges facing the nursing workforce in the United States. *Journal of Nursing Regulation, 8*(2), 40–46. https://doi.org/10.1016/S2155-8256(17)30097-2

Buerhaus, P., Skinner, L. E., Auerbach, D. I., & Staiger, D. O. (2017c). State of the registered nurse workforce as a new era of health reform emerges. *Journal of Nursing Economics, 35*(5), 229–237. http://healthworkforce studies.com/news/state_of_the_nursing_workforce_paper.pdf

Candela, L., & Bowles, C. (2008). Recent RN graduate perceptions of educational preparation. *Nursing Education Perspectives (National League for Nursing), 29*(5),266–271. https://search.ebscohost.com/login.aspx?direct=true&db=c8h&AN=105700684&site=ehost-live

Carson-Newman University Online. (2020). *25 Nursing trends we expect to see in 2020.* https://onlinenursing.cn.edu/news/nursing-trends

Centers for Medicare and Medicaid Services. (2020, March). *National Health Expenditure (NHE) fact sheet.* https://www.cms.gov/Research-Statistics-Data-and-Systems/Statistics-Trends-and-Reports/NationalHealthExpendData/NHE-Fact-Sheet

Centers for Medicare and Medicaid Services. (2021, January). *SHO# 21-001 RE: Opportunities in Medicaid and CHIP to address Social Determinants of Health (SDOH).* https://www.medicaid.gov/federal-policy-guidance/downloads/sho21001.pdf

Chant, K. J., & Westendorf, D. S. (2019). Nurse residency programs: Key components for sustainability. *Journal of Nursing Professional Development, 35*(4), 185–192. https://doi.org/10.1097/NND.0000000000000560

Cline, D., La Frentz, K., Fellman, B., Summers, B., & Brassil, K. (2017). Longitudinal outcomes of an institutionally developed nurse residency program. *Journal of Nursing Administration, 47*(7/8), 384–390. https://doi.org/10.1097/NNA.0000000000000500

Demiris, G., Hodgson, N. A., Sefcik, J. S., Travers, J. L., McPhillips, M. V., & Naylor, M. D. (2019). High-value care for older adults with complex care needs: Leveraging nurses as innovators. *Nursing Outlook, 68*(1), 26–32. https://doi.org/10.1016/j.outlook.2019.06.019

Dickman, L., Himmelstein, D. U., & Woolhandler, S. (2017). Inequality and the health-care system in the USA. *The Lancet, 389*(10077), 1431–1441. https://doi.org/10.1016/S0140-6736(17)30398-7

Dimino, K., Kem, L., Banks, J., & Mahon, E. (2020). Exploring the impact of a dedicated education unit on new graduate nurses' transition to practice. *Journal for Nurses in Professional Development, 36*(3), 121–128. https://doi.org/10.1097/NND.0000000000000622

Duchscher, J. E. (2009). Transition shock: The initial stage of role adaptation for newly graduated registered nurses. *Journal of Advanced Nursing, 65*(5), 1103–1113. https://doi.org/10.1111/j.1365-2648.2008.04898.x

Duckett, S., & Moran, G. (2018). *Why you should avoid hospitals in January.* http://theconversation.com/why-you-should-avoid-hospitals-in-January-89857

Frogeli, E., Rudman, A., Ljotsson, B., & Gustavsson, P. (2018). Preventing stress-related ill health among newly registered nurses by supporting engagement in proactive behaviors: Development and feasibility testing of a behavior change intervention. *Pilot Feasibility Studies, 4*, 28. https://doi.org/10.1186/s40814-017-0219-7

Gaudette, E., Tysinger, B., Cassil, A., & Goldman, D. P. (2015). Health and health care of Medicare beneficiaries in 2030. *Forum Health Econ Policy, 12*(2), 75–96. https://doi.org/10.1515/fhep-2015-0037

Goldman, D., & Gaudette, É. (2015). Strengthening Medicare for 2030. *Brookings Institute.* https://www.brookings.edu/wp

Goode, C. J., Glassman, K. S., Reid Ponte, P., Krugman, M., & Peterman, T. (2018). Requiring a nurse residency for newly licensed registered nurses. *Nursing Outlook, 66*(3), 329–332. https://doi.org/10.1016/j.outlook.2018.04.004

Hassmiller, S. B., & Kuehnert, P. (2020). Building a culture of health to attain the sustainable development goals. *Nursing*

Outlook, 68(2), 129–133. https://doi.org/10.1016/j.outlook
.2019.12.005

Hayden, J. K., Smiley, R. A., Alexander, M. A., Kardongedgren,
S., & Jeffries, P. R. (2014). The NCSBN National Simulation
Study: A longitudinal, randomized, controlled study replac-
ing clinical hours with simulation in prelicensure nursing
education. *Journal of Nursing Regulation, 5*(2 suppl):
S3–S40. https://doi.org/10.1016/S2155-8256(15)30062-4

Health Resources and Services Administration. (n.d.). *Behavioral Health Workforce Projections, 2017-2030.* https://bhw
.hrsa.gov/sites/default/files/bhw/nchwa/projections/bh-
workforce-projections-fact-sheet.pdf

Hensel, D., & Billings, D. M. (2020). Strategies to teach the
National Council of State Boards of Nursing Clinical Judgment Model. *Nurse Educator, 45*(3), 128–132. https://doi
.org/10.1097/NNE.0000000000000773

Hessler, K. L. (2017). *Flipping the nursing classroom.* Jones &
Bartlett Learning.

Hickerson, K. A., Taylor, L. A., & Terhaar, M. F. (2016).
The preparation-practice gap: An integrative literature
review. *The Journal of Continuing Education in Nursing,
47*(1), 17–23. https://doi.org/10.3928/00220124-
20151230-06

Hooper-Arana, E. D., Li, J. N., Borges, W. J., & Bodenheimer,
T. (2019). Clinical training innovation for prelicensure
graduate nursing students to expand roles in primary care.
Nurse Educator, 45(1), 25–29. https://doi.org/10.1097/
NNE.0000000000000664

Huston, C. L., Phillips, B., Jeffries, P., Todero, C., Rich, J.,
Knecht, P., & Lewis, M. P. (2018). The academic-practice
gap: Strategies for an enduring problem. *Nursing Forum,
53*(1), 27–34. https://doi.org/10.1111/nuf.12216

Institute of Medicine. (2011). *The future of nursing: Leading
change, advancing health.* The National Academies Press.
https://doi.org1.17226/12956

Jones, D., & D'Alfonso, J. (Eds.). (2020). *Kaiser Foundation
School of Nursing: A legacy of disruptive innovation,
1947-1976.* Moss Communications.

Jones, D., & West, N. (2017). New graduate RN transition
to practice programs. In C. J. Huston (Ed.), *Professional
issues in nursing: Challenges and opportunities* (4th ed.,
pp. 233–249). Wolters Kluwer.

Jones-Bell, J., Parker, N. W., Donnelly, M. K., Hooper-Arana, E. D.,
Schiff, S., & Ziehm, S. (2020). Using innovative models in
transition to practice and master's entry programs to teach
ambulatory and primary care nursing. *Journal of Professional Nursing, 37*(2), 435–440. https://doi.org/10.1016/j
.profnurs.2020.04.017

Juraschek, S. P., Zhang, X., & Ranganathan, V. (2019). United
States Registered Nurse Workforce report card and shortage forecast. *American Journal of Medical Quality, 34*(5),
473–481. https://doi.org/10.1177/1062860619873217

Kaihlanen, A. M., Elovainio, M., Haavisto, E., Salminen, L.,
& Sinervo, T. (2020). The associations between the final
clinical practicum elements and the transition experience
of early career nurses: A cross-sectional study. *Nurse Education in Practice, 42.* https://doi.org/10.1016/j.nepr.2019
.102680

Kavanagh, J. M., & Szweda, C. (2017). A crisis in competency:
The strategic and ethical imperative to assessing new graduate nurses' clinical reasoning. *Nursing Education Perspectives, 38*(2), 57–62. https://doi.org/10.1097/01.NEP
.0000000000000112

Kerfoot, K. M. (2020). The international year of the nurse: An
interview with Peter Buerhaus. *Nursing Economics, 38*(5),
238–243. https://www.proquest.com/docview/2452331725

Kim, J. S. (2020). Relationships between reality shock, professional self-concept, and nursing students' perceived trust
from nursing educators: A cross-sectional study. *Nurse Education Today, 88,* 104369. http://doi.org/10.1016/j.nedt
.2020.104369

Kim, S. Y., & Shin, Y. S. (2019). Validity and reliability of the
transition shock scale for undergraduate nursing students. *Journal of Korean Academic Society of Nursing Education, 25*(1), 17–26. https://doi.org/10.5977/jkasne
.2019.25.1.17

Kirch, D. G., & Petelle, K. (2017). Addressing the physician
shortage: The peril of ignoring demography. *JAMA, 317*(19),
1947–1948. https://doi.org/10.1001/jama.2017.2714

Knoff, C. R. (2019). A call for nurses to embrace their innovative spirit. *The Online Journal of Issues in Nursing, 24*(1).
https://doi.org/10.3912/OJIN.Vol24No01PPT48

Kramer, M. (1974). *Reality shock: Why nurses leave nursing.* CV
Mosby.

Kramer, M., Brewer, B. B., & Maguire, P. (2013). Impact of
healthy work environments on new graduate nurses'
environmental reality shock. *Western Journal of Nursing
Research, 35*(3), 348–383. https://doi.org/10.1177/
0193945911403939

Lopez, E., Cordo, J. A., Fitzpatrick, T. A., Gonzalez, J. L., &
Janvier-Anglade, M. (2019). EntrepreNurses: Nursing's
evolving role in innovation strategy. *Nursing Economics,
37*(3), 159–163. https://www.proquest.com/docview/
2452331725

Lyford, S., & Lash, T. A. (2019–2020, Winter). America's
healthcare cost crisis. *Journal of the American Association
on Aging,* 7–12. https://online.flippingbook.com/view/
115850/8/

Moore, E. (2018). Emerging trends in nursing. *American Nurse
Today, 13*(9), 1. https://www.myamericannurse.com/wp-
content/uploads/2018/09/ant9-ANA-Leadership-822.pdf

Moss, T., D'Alfonso, J., & Jones, D. (2018). Kaiser's School of
Nursing: A 70-year legacy of disruptive innovation. *Nursing
Administration Quarterly, 42*(1), 35–42. https://doi.org/
10.1097/NAQ.0000000000000262

Murray, M., Sundin, D., & Cope, V. (2019). New graduate
nurses' understanding and attitudes about patient safety
upon transition to practice. *Journal of Clinical Nursing,
28*(10):2543-2552. https://doi.org/10.1111/jocn.14839

National Academy of Medicine. (2020, July 30). *The future of
nursing 2020-2030: A consensus study from the National
Academy of Medicine.* https://nam.edu/publications/the-
future-of-nursing-2020-2030/

National Institute of Mental Health. (2020). *Mental health
information.* https://www.nimh.nih.gov/health/statistics/
mental-illness.shtml

Noles, K., Barber, R., James, D., & Wingo, N. (2019). Driving innovation in health care: Clinical nursing leader role. *Journal of Nursing Care Quality, 34*(4), 307–311. https://doi .org/10.1097/NCQ.0000000000000394

Nursing School Hub. (2020). *30 big trends in the field of nursing.* https://www.nursingschoolhub.com/nursing-trends/

Oblea, P. N., Berry-Caban, C., Dumayas, J. Y., Adams, A. R., & Beltran, T. A. (2019). Evaluation of clinic nurse transition program at US army hospitals. *Military Medicine, 184*(11/12), 914–921. https://doi.org/10.1093/milmed/usz108

Patient Protection and Affordable Care Act, 42 U.S.C. § 18001 (2010).

Pittman, P. (2019, March). *Activating nursing to address the unmet needs of the 21st century.* Robert Wood Johnson Foundation.

Powers, K., Herron, E. K., & Pagel, J. (2019). Nurse preceptor role in new graduate nurses' transition to practice. *Dimensions of Critical Care Nursing, 38*(3), 131–136. https:// doi.org/10.1097/DCC.0000000000000354

Preston, P., Leone-Sheehan, D., & Keys, B. (2019). Nursing student perceptions of pharmacology education and safe medication administration: A qualitative research study. *Nurse Education Today, 74*, 76–81. https://doi.org/10.1016/j .nedt.2018.12.006

Reinhart, R. J. (2020). *Nurses continue to rate highest in honesty, ethics.* Gallup, Inc. https://news.gallup.com/poll/274673/ nurses-continue-rate-highest-honesty-ethics.aspx

Robert Wood Johnson Foundation and AARP Foundation. (2019, March). *Nursing education and the path to population health improvement.* https://campaignforaction.org/wp-content/uploads/2019/03/NursingEducationPathto HealthImprovement.pdf

Robert Wood Johnson Foundation and AARP Foundation. (2020). *Campaign for action: Our story and timeline.* https:// campaignforaction.org/about/our-story/

Ross, S. (2018). Emerging trends in nursing. *American Nurse Today, 13*(9), 1. https://www.myamericannurse.com/ wp-content/uploads/2018/09/ant9-ANA-Leadership-822.pdf

Rush, K. L., Janke, R., Duchsher, J. E., Phillips, R., & Kaur, S. (2019). Best practice of formal new graduate transition programs: An integrative review. *International Journal of Nursing, 94*, 139–158. https://doi.org/10.1016/j.ijnurstu .2019.02.010

Salifu, D. A., Gross, J., Salifu, M. A., & Ninnoni, J. P. K. (2019). Experiences and perceptions of the theory-practice-gap in nursing in a resource-constrained setting: A qualitative

description study. *Nursing Open, 6*(1), 72–83. https://doi .org/10.1002/nop2.188

Shelby, M., & Wermers, R. (2020). Complexity science fosters professional advanced nurse practitioner role emergence. *Nursing Administration Quarterly, 44*(2), 149–158. https:// doi.org/10.1097/NAQ.0000000000000413

Spector, N. (2015). The National Council of State Boards of Nursing's Transition to Practice Study: Implications for Educators. *Journal of Nursing Education, 54*(3),119–120.

Spector, N., Blegen, M. A., Silvestre, J., Barnsteiner, J., Lynn, M. R., Ulrich, B., & Alexander, M. (2015). Transition to practice study in hospital settings. *Journal of Nursing Regulation, 5*(4), 24–38. https://doi.org/10.1016/S2155-8256(15)30031-4

Swan, B. A., Hilden, P., West, N., Chan, G., Shaffer, K., Berg, J., Dickow, M., & Jones, D. (2020). Redesigning nursing education to build healthier communities: An innovative cross-sector collaboration. *Nursing Education Perspectives, z41*(5), 301–303. https://doi.org/10.1097/01.NEP.0000000000000711

Tyndall, D. E., Scott, E. S., Jones, L. R., & Cook, K. J. (2019). Changing new graduate nurse profiles and retention recommendations for nurse leaders. *The Journal of Nursing Administration, 49*(2), 93–98. https://doi.org/10.1097/ NNA.0000000000000716

U.S. Centers for Medicare and Medicaid Services. (2020, November). *Healthcare.gov, Affordable Care Act.* https:// www.healthcare.gov/glossary/affordable-care-act/

U.S. Department of Health and Human Services. (2020, November). *Healthy People 2030: Social determinants of health.* https://health.gov/healthypeople/objectives-and-data/social-determinants-health

Vespa, J., Armstrong, D. M., & Medina, L. (2020). *Demographic turning points for the United States: Population projections for 2020 to 2060.* US Census Bureau. https://www.census .gov/library/publications/2020/demo/p25-1144.html

Wallace, J. (2016). Nursing student work-study internship program: An academic partnership. *Journal of Nursing Education, 55*(6), 357–359. https://doi.org/10.3928/ 01484834-20160516-11

Warren, J. I., Perkins, S., & Greene, M. A. (2018). Advancing new nurse graduate education through Implementation of statewide standardized nurse residency programs. *Journal of Nursing Regulation, 8*(4), 14–21. https://doi.org/10.1016/ S2155-8256(17)30177-1

Waxman, K. T., Bowler, F., Forneris, S. G., Kardong-Edgren, S., & Rizzolo, M. A. (2019). Simulation as a nursing education disrupter. *Nursing Administration Quarterly, 43*(4), 300–305. https://doi.org/10.1097/NAQ.0000000000000369

Developing Effective Leaders to Meet Today's Health Care Challenges

Bernadette Mazurek Melnyk, Kathy Malloch, and Lynn Gallagher-Ford

ADDITIONAL RESOURCES

Visit the Point for additional helpful resources.
- eBook
- Journal Articles
- Web Links

CHAPTER OUTLINE

LEARNING OBJECTIVES

The learner will be able to:

1. Describe factors that are driving the need for innovative and transformational leaders in health care for the 21st century.

2. Identify nine health care leadership challenges of the 21st century.

3. Delineate effective strategies to promote and sustain an evidence-based practice organizational culture.

4. Explain why effective leaders in the 21st century must engage in mentoring young leaders and succession planning.

5. Discuss the importance of teamwork, effective communication, and transdisciplinary/de-siloed work as they relate to health care outcomes.

6. Describe the characteristics required of leaders in order to effectively promote innovation and change.

7. List 13 essential characteristics of effective leaders.

8. Recognize the areas of change that have occurred as a result of advances in technology.

9. Discuss the strengths and weaknesses of three leadership models: transactional, transformational, and complexity.

10. Distinguish the unique leadership components required in the complexity leadership model.

TODAY'S HEALTH CARE: IN CRITICAL CONDITION

The American health care system is in critical condition. Preventable medical errors are the third leading cause of death, with up to 250,000 unintended patient deaths every year (Anderson & Abrahamson, 2017; Makary & Daniel, 2016). Half of the hospitals in the United States are functioning in deficit. The United States ranks number one in health care spending, yet ranks 34th in life expectancy outcomes (OECD, 2020; World Health Organization, 2021) when compared to 38 industrialized nations across the globe. Furthermore, we are living in an era in which patients do not consistently receive evidence-based care (Melnyk & Fineout-Overholt, 2019). Americans' health care needs also are increasing, with one out of every two Americans living with a chronic condition (e.g., overweight/obesity, hypertension, diabetes, mental health disorder) (Boersma et al., 2020).

Over 50% of clinicians in the United States are currently suffering from burnout, depression, and compassion fatigue, compromising the quality and safety of health care (Dzau et al., 2018; Melnyk, Orsolini, Tan et al., 2018; Melnyk, Tan, Hsieh, & Gallagher-Ford, 2021; Shanafelt et al., 2017). The health care system is also facing the most severe shortage of health professionals, including physicians and nurses, ever encountered (Juraschek et al., 2019; Zhang et al., 2020). The changing nature of morbidities in the United States, the current condition of the health care system, and the severe shortage of health care professionals call for transformational and innovative leaders. These leaders will be charged with creating health care systems that empower transdisciplinary teams to create new models of high-quality, reliable, evidence-based care and healthy work environments that support clinician health and well-being.

This chapter presents nine critical leadership challenges for nurse leaders in the 21st century as well as 13 competencies needed to overcome these challenges. The chapter concludes with a discussion of leadership models for the 21st century and suggests that the complexity leadership model offers a new perspective for leadership and potential to support improved organizational performance.

TODAY'S LEADERSHIP CHALLENGES

Today's health care issues provide challenges or "character-builders" to nursing and health care leaders. These challenges are listed in Box 3.1. Individual nurse leaders have the opportunity to leverage the challenges of these times or be overwhelmed by them. Old models of autocratic, hierarchic leadership are inadequate to handle the fast-paced, complex health care environment of the future. Leaders of today need to be evidence based, innovative, flexible, engaging, courageous, relationship based, and dynamic.

Leadership is not a "solo act"; it is embedded in relationships, effective communication, shared ownership, and coaching and motivating others. Leadership must move from an autocratic, transactional model to innovative complexity leadership. Leaders who are steeped in traditional

Nine 21st Century Leadership Challenges

- Meeting expectations for increased productivity within budgetary constraints
- Advancing evidence-based practice
- Planning for succession and mentoring young nurse leaders
- Facilitating and enhancing teamwork and effective communication
- Embracing and supporting transdisciplinary health care
- Positioning nursing to influence decision making in organizational and health policies
- Promoting workplace wellness
- Striking a balance between technology and interpersonal relationships to deliver best care
- Creating cultures of innovation and change

leadership styles and unwilling to grow and change their own practices are particularly challenged by the dynamics of the current health care environment. Leaders who are proactive and embrace new approaches are better suited for chaotic times and will be in the best position to navigate future challenges.

Meeting Expectations for Increased Productivity Within Rigorous Budgetary Constraints

Even in an era of major federal, state, and organizational budget reductions, leaders are expected to be highly productive. In the theater of nursing, what exactly does "productive" encompass? Productivity includes both resource stewardship and delivery of the nursing "product" of safe, evidence-based, quality care. A major challenge for nurse leaders is to advocate for, attain, and maintain a balance between these two key factors. Nurse leaders need to use strategies in which "caring management and financial constraints can coexist while promoting quality patient care" (Cara et al., 2011).

Nurse leaders also need to understand and clearly articulate the connectedness of nurse engagement, productivity, and retention with caring and quality outcomes, which ultimately drive satisfaction and the financial well-being of the organization. Therefore, nurse leaders must be evidence based, innovative, and resourceful in garnering new resources and strategizing to maintain the core nursing value of caring to drive quality outcomes.

Advancing Evidence-Based Practice When Care Often Remains Steeped and Mired in Tradition

Consider This   A large number of medical errors occur because clinicians do not practice evidence-based health care.

The Institute of Medicine (IOM) named evidence-based practice (EBP) as a core competency for health care professionals in a landmark document (Greiner & Knebel, 2003). Shortly thereafter, the National Institutes of Health roadmap initiative prioritized the acceleration of the transfer of knowledge from research into practice (Zerhouni, 2005) (see Research Fuels the Controversy 3.1). Today, health care systems are striving to meet the quadruple aim in health care, which includes enhancing the experience of care (e.g., quality and safety); improving population health; decreasing costs; and enhancing clinician well-being and joy in work (Melnyk & Fineout-Overholt, 2019). Studies indicate that EBP positively impacts each of these outcomes and therefore is essential for health care systems to integrate EBP to reach the quadruple aim. Yet, EBP is not the standard of practice in many health care organizations (Harding et al., 2014; Melnyk & Fineout-Overholt, 2019; Melnyk, Gallagher-Ford, Zellefrow et al., 2018) despite the fact that specific research-derived competencies for EBP have been developed and can easily be integrated into clinical organizations (Melnyk et al., 2014, 2015).

Findings from a survey of over 1,000 nurses randomly sampled from the American Nurses Association indicated that only one-third of the nurses reported that their colleagues consistently implemented EBP, and only one-third said they had EBP mentors. Further, the older the nurse, the less they were interested in gaining more knowledge and skills in EBP (Melnyk et al., 2012). Top barriers to EBP included time, organizational culture, and politics; lack of EBP knowledge and education; lack of access to evidence and information; and leader/manager resistance. Identification of leaders as a major barrier to EBP prompted another survey of over 270 chief nurse executives across the United States. The study revealed that although they reported that their top priorities were health care quality and safety, EBP was a low priority. These findings revealed a major disconnect in that many chief nurses do not see EBP as a direct pathway to quality and safety. Other recent studies have reinforced these findings. Välimaki et al. (2018) identified that the most common barriers to EBP were nursing leadership and organizational characteristics, and Pittman and

Research Fuels the Controversy 3.1

The Establishment of Evidence-Based Practice Competencies for Practicing Registered Nurses and Advanced Practice Nurses in Real-World Clinical Settings: Proficiencies to Improve Health Care Quality, Reliability, Patient Outcomes, and Costs

In 2014, the first set of evidence-based practice (EBP) competencies for practicing nurses and advanced practice nurses was created. Consensus among a national panel of seven EBP experts was the first step in establishing the competencies followed by two rounds of a Delphi survey with 80 EBP mentors across the United States who validated them.

Source: Melnyk, B. M., Gallagher-Ford, L., Long, L. E., & Fineout-Overholt, E. (2014). The establishment of evidence-based practice competencies for practicing registered nurses and advanced practice nurses in real-*world* clinical settings: Proficiencies to improve health care quality, reliability, patient outcomes, and costs. *Worldviews on Evidence-Based Nursing, 11*(1), 5–15. https://doi.org/10.1111/wvn.12021

Study Findings

Two rounds of a Delphi survey with the 80 mentors resulted in a final set of 13 EBP competencies for practicing registered nurses and 11 additional competencies for advanced practice nurses. Leaders must create cultures and environments that support the implementation and sustainability of EBP. Integration of these competencies into health care system expectations, orientations, job descriptions, performance appraisals, and clinical ladder promotion processes will enhance health care quality, safety, and consistency of health care interventions as well as reduce costs.

---

team (2019) found that nursing leadership was a key influence on organizational context and enhancing a culture of EBP within organizations.

Leaders must have the knowledge and skills to create cultures of EBP that ignite a spirit of inquiry throughout the organization and cultivate an environment where EBP is the standard of care, not the exception. They also need to implement system-wide models that have been demonstrated through research to enhance EBP implementation. One such model is the *Advancing Research and Clinical Practice Through Close Collaboration* (ARCC) model. In the ARCC model, the key strategy used to enhance and sustain EBP is a critical mass of EBP mentors, typically advanced practice clinicians competent in EBP, who work with clinicians at the point of care to improve patient care and outcomes (Melnyk, 2012; Melnyk & Fineout-Overholt, 2019; Melnyk et al., 2017; Melnyk, Tan, Hsieh et al., 2021).

Unfortunately, although leaders report they believe in the value of EBP, their own implementation of it is low (Melnyk et al., 2016). It will be critical for nurse leaders to integrate evidence into their individual professional practices to deliver best leadership practice as well as to serve as EBP role models, which will influence their staff's EBP beliefs and implementation of evidence-based care. Recently developed tools, such as the new EBP competencies for practicing nurses and advanced practice nurses (Melnyk et al., 2014) and shortened EBP Scales (Melnyk, Hsieh et al., 2021), are examples of resources to support and assess the state of EBP. The Helene Fuld Health Trust National Institute for

Evidence-based Practice in Nursing and Healthcare at The Ohio State University College of Nursing also has excellent resources to support EBP, including a new EBP implementation toolkit (Helene Fuld Health Trust National Institute for Evidence-based Practice in Nursing and Healthcare, 2007–2021).

Discussion Point

As a new nurse leader, you may be faced with an organization of nurses who, in large part, do not believe in or have the skills to deliver evidence-based care. What strategies would you embark upon early in your new role to begin to change that paradigm?

Planning for Leadership Succession and Mentoring Young Nurse Leaders

Continuity is a vital aspect of effective organizations; it is critical to strategic and operational goals. Disruption in an organization's continuity can have dire consequences. Disruption is particularly challenging in health care organizations because of the potential damage to confidence from the community and employees, the cost of unfinished business and negative impact on financing, and the harm to the organization's image and history (Bowen, 2014). In 2018, Phillips and colleagues noted that by the year 2020, an estimated 75% of nurse managers would leave the workforce and that less than 7% of health care organizations had formal leadership succession planning programs in place. Hughes-Warden et al. (2021) offered equally distressing predictions in their 2021 findings that over 50% of nurses in formal leadership positions planned to leave their jobs within the next 5 years, with half of those planning to leave within 2 years. Of those planning to leave, just over 30% were planning to retire, making succession planning critical.

Succession planning is the cure for this as the process is intended to create a leadership pipeline that identifies internal candidates to be promoted. It is a proactive approach used to identify and prepare high-potential intellectual talent for future leadership roles. It allows an organization to develop a pool of qualified, prepared, and promotable leaders and ensures leadership continuity within an organization (McCallin et al., 2009; Titzer et al., 2013). These internal candidates require less time and effort to become oriented and are likely to be successful in the new position. This, in turn, allows organizations to accomplish at least two major goals during times of transition and turnover: (1) effective resource stewardship and (2) ongoing focus on accomplishing the strategic mission.

Succession planning can also be a positive experience for developing leaders in an organization. As individuals in the organization are given expanded opportunities, planned support, intentional mentorship, and effective and meaningful rewards and recognition, they develop their leadership portfolio and are less likely to leave the organization (Blouin et al., 2006).

Discussion Point

Succession planning requires ... planning! Have you thought about who will follow you and how you can influence their success?

One critical aspect of effective succession planning is mentoring. Studies indicate that nurses and physicians who have mentors tend to be more successful and satisfied with their careers (Beecroft et al., 2006; Sambunjak et al., 2006). Creating a mentoring and coaching work environment that facilitates positive relationships is necessary for succession planning to be successful (Phillips, 2020). Mentoring can range from informal in-the-moment coaching to formal, planned meetings. "Giving talented future leaders the time, energy, advice, and experiences to gain new competencies and learn how to begin to prepare for future roles and responsibilities becomes the 'gift' a current leader can bestow upon a future leader" (Blouin et al., 2006, p. 328). Evidence supports that mentoring programs decrease nursing turnover rates (Zucker et al., 2000).

Despite the associated positive benefits, there has not been enough mentoring and empowering of young nurse leaders by more seasoned leaders in the nursing profession (Huston, 2020; Titzer et al., 2013). As a result, the profession is highly vulnerable as large numbers of established nurse leaders are retiring; the resulting talent gap may cause nursing to lose much of the ground gained in health care in recent years. Intentional as well as informal mentoring of young leaders and strategic succession planning is an imperative for current nurse leaders to sustain the positive changes and significant outcomes cultivated during their tenures.

Facilitating and Enhancing Teamwork and Effective Communication

Communication has always been an important skill for all clinicians and teams. Effective communication among team members has been identified by the IOM as one of the markers of safe and highly reliable care (Kohn et al., 2000). Communication is not simply an exchange of information; it is a complex social process in which each party involved brings history, assumptions, and expectations to the interaction (Lyndon et al., 2011). Each member of the team enters into communication with different values, fears, confidence, and an assumed place within the hierarchy. "Effective (clinical) communication is clear, direct, explicit, and respectful" and "requires excellent listening skills, superb administrative support, and a collective commitment to move past traditional hierarchy and professional stereotyping" (p. 93). Communication, whether effective or ineffective, is jointly owned by all members of a team, and each member is equally capable of engaging in positive or negative communication tactics.

Discussion Point

Communication is a personal attribute and a learned skill. Do you understand your personal communication style? How do you communicate or how do you like people to communicate with you? There are many tools available that you can use to gain a better understanding of your style, how you interact with other individuals and teams, and how you can modify your style to be more effective.

Leaders can significantly impact the success of teams and communication efforts in their organizations in a wide variety of ways. First, leaders must be effective communicators themselves and role model excellent communication skills. In addition, leaders are responsible for establishing and upholding administrative structures that support effective teamwork and communication. Finally, leaders must have the skills to effectively confront and manage conflicts that arise out of poor communication.

Embracing and Supporting Transdisciplinary Health Care

The complex and multidimensional nature of health care and health problems requires an approach different from the traditional, segregated, discipline-siloed approach to patient care that has often been the standard in health care for decades. Transdisciplinary care has received a great deal of attention lately and is emerging as an essential requirement in health care. This approach includes true interprofessional decision making and trust among a variety of health care clinicians (Clark & Greenwald, 2013; Légaré et al., 2008; Regan et al., 2015). Transdisciplinary care assumes that merging the specialized knowledge from different health care disciplines together to act on the same situation results in better and faster results (Vyt, 2008). Interprofessional collaboration, a key component of transdisciplinary care, improves care effectiveness for patients with chronic diseases as well as work satisfaction among health care workers.

The challenge for leaders is to see the dynamics of health care through a contemporary lens, recognize its complexities, and acknowledge that care must be evidence based and patient centered, both of which require a transdisciplinary, de-siloed approach. Leaders need to be well versed in the tenets of this approach, able to model it in their leadership roles, and diligent in creating organizational settings and cultural milieus where this approach can thrive.

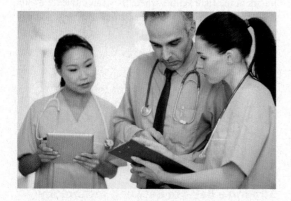

Creating Wellness Cultures and Promoting Well-Being in Clinicians

Wellness includes physical, intellectual, mental, emotional, social, occupational, financial, environmental, and spiritual dimensions (Melnyk & Neale, 2018). Therefore, promoting workplace wellness in nurses and all clinicians is critical, whether they are new hires or long-term employees. This not only promotes the health and well-being of nurses directly but also enhances productivity and decreases absences and high turnover rates, which are costly to the health care system. To address this important problem, health care systems have been appointing chief wellness officers to spearhead the building of wellness cultures and enhance the population health and well-being of clinicians (Kishore et al., 2018; Melnyk, 2019). Investing in wellness of clinicians not only improves return on investment for a health care system but also on value of investment by improving job satisfaction, engagement, and morale (Melnyk, 2019).

Stress, burnout, depression, suicide, and turnover continue to plague the nursing and health professions and are now considered a public health epidemic, which is why the National Academy of Medicine launched the *Action Collaborative on Clinician Well-Being and Resilience* in 2017 (Dzau et al., 2018). This initiative is working to raise visibility on this public health problem and develop evidence-based solutions to improve it.

The COVID-19 pandemic beginning in early 2020 also substantially impacted nurse wellness. More than 50% of nurses are now screening positive for burnout in relation to providing care during the pandemic (Prasad et al., 2021). Inadequate staffing, increased workloads, equipment shortages, fear of disease exposure, and being the primary support person to dying patients are system failures that have created a mental health pandemic inside of the COVID-19 pandemic (Einboden, 2020; Pappa et al., 2020; Prasad et al., 2021; Shechter et al., 2020). Nurses with workplaces supportive of their wellness have fared better than nurses without the same level of support. Amid the COVID-19 pandemic, nurses with workplaces supportive of wellness were three to nine times as likely to have better mental and physical health, no to little stress, no burnout, and higher quality of life when compared to nurses with little to no wellness support (Melnyk et al., in press).

New graduate nurses are particularly affected by stress, resulting in burnout and turnover in their first year of employment (Cho et al., 2006). In the first 12 to 24 months of employment, nursing turnover can be 30% to 60% for new graduate nurses, nearly double the national average of 10% to 15% for experienced nurses (Parker et al., 2014; Unruh & Zhang, 2014). In a study of new graduate nurses, Melnyk et al. (2013) found that higher levels of workplace stress were associated with higher levels of depression and anxiety as well as lower levels of resiliency, job satisfaction, and healthy lifestyle beliefs.

Although nurses are typically effective caregivers of others, they are often lacking in self-care. A 2012 Gallup survey found that nurses had higher rates of smoking, obesity, hypertension, diabetes, and depression than physicians. In a recent national study of 1,790 nurses from 19 U.S. health care systems, Melnyk and colleagues (2018) found that more than 50% of the nurses reported suboptimal physical and mental health. Approximately one-third reported depression, the leading cause of self-reported medical errors. The health and well-being of nurses not only affects the population health of the nurses themselves but it also impacts the safety and quality of the care they deliver. In a study with 771 critical care nurses, 60.9% of nurses reported having made a medical error in the past 5 years (Melnyk, Tan, Hsieh et al., 2021). When compared to nurses in good mental and physical health, medical error occurrence was significantly higher in nurses with poor mental and physical health. Therefore, it is critical to fix system issues and build workplace cultures of wellness for nurses and other health care professionals along with integrating evidence-based strategies and interventions that improve health and well-being outcomes. In a recent systematic review of evidence, Melnyk and colleagues (2020) reported that the following interventions improved the health and well-being as well as healthy lifestyle behaviors and physical health of nurses and physicians: mindfulness, cognitive–behavioral therapy/skills building, health coaches, visual triggers and pedometers, deep abdominal breathing, and gratitude.

All clinicians should be offered the opportunity to participate in screening for depression and suicide, such as that offered by the University of California at San Diego's evidence-based *Healer Education Assessment and Referral* (HEAR) program. The HEAR program provides free anonymous referrals to mental health services for those who screen high for depression and suicidal ideation. Thus, the program successfully identifies and provides care to health care workers struggling with suicidal thoughts, substance use, and other mental health conditions. Another successful evidence-based program that can be delivered by nurses or other nonpsychiatric mental health providers is the MINDBODYSTRONG program, which provides a seven-session manualized cognitive behavioral therapy–based skills building program to nurses and other clinicians. This program was adapted from the evidence-based Creating Opportunities for Personal Empowerment (COPE) program that has been shown to be effective in reducing depression, anxiety, and suicidal ideation as well as improving healthy lifestyle behaviors in children, teens, and young adults (Hart Abney et al., 2019; Hoying & Melnyk, 2016; Hoying et al., 2016). A randomized controlled trial with new nurse residents showed that nurses who completed the MINDBODYSTRONG program as part of orientation had less depression, anxiety, and stress in addition to higher job satisfaction and healthy lifestyle behaviors than did nurses in the control program up to 6 months after completing

the program (Sampson et al., 2019, 2020). Another study found that new graduate nurses who participated in a 2-day energy management workshop entitled "Nurse Athlete," which included healthy nutrition, physical activity, and stress reduction, decreased their weight, body mass index, and depressive symptoms at 6 months following completion of the workshop (Hrabe et al., 2017).

What single action could you take to make your workplace healthier? When can you initiate that action? How healthy are you? What are you doing to promote *your* well-being? What single action could you take to make yourself healthier? When can you initiate that action?

Discussion Point

How healthy is your workplace culture, physically and emotionally? How healthy are you personally? Are you role modeling and supporting healthy behaviors as a leader?

Positioning Nursing to Influence Decision Making in Organizational and Health Policy

Nurse leaders must be present in all health care and health policy venues and be active contributors to key discussions and decision-making forums that influence the science and delivery of health care. In addition, they must proactively ensure that nurse experts are positioned at organizational and health policy tables where the topics of their expertise are being addressed. These nurse leader actions will place nurses in the right venues where they can influence major decisions that influence health care quality, safety, and patient outcomes.

Discussion Point

Nurses are the largest sector of health care professionals, yet they rarely participate in health care policy decisions. Why does this dilemma persist? Individually and as a united group, what can nurses do to change this?

Striking a Balance Between Technology and Interpersonal Relationships to Deliver Best Care

The impact of technology on health care in the past few decades has been startling and will persist into the future. The challenge for leaders as the future unfolds will be in shifting from the current trend of technology driving work to value-based health care quality and relationships driving work with technology supporting those drivers. To this end, technology users (i.e., patients and providers) will need to be engaged and valued throughout the design and development work on the technology that lies ahead.

Health care systems are facing constant and evolving challenges including aging demographics, heightened patient expectations, patients with multiple and complex chronic diseases, and outbreaks of new infectious diseases. The demands brought on by these challenges are occurring while health care budgets are strained and sometimes shrinking. This dynamic threatens an organization's capacity to support the technologies needed to deliver care and further compromises access to technologies that will be needed in the future. Masterful understanding of the value of technology is a leadership imperative, and acumen in balancing technology costs *as well as* non-technology costs (e.g., human resources, equipment, and space) will be critical. Leaders will need to leverage the powerful tool of technology to empower both clinicians and patients and recognize how technology "offers them their best chance of system sustainability" (Barker & Donnelly, 2017, p. 28).

Whether it is a smartphone that puts critical information at a clinician's fingertips in real time, a medication library embedded in an infusion pump to prevent medication errors, an electronic medical record that trends patient progress and issues alerts, or motion sensors that track patient movement to prevent falls, all these technologies are becoming essential to achieving best practice and outcomes.

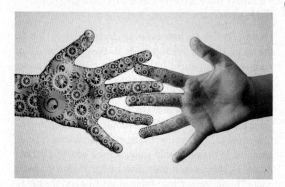

Creating Cultures of Innovation and Change

Innovation is the development and implementation of products, services, or solutions that create new value to an organization, and, as such, innovation is more than an idea; it is an idea that comes to fruition and sustains itself over time (Melnyk & Raderstorf, 2019). Although leaders may say that innovation is important, they often do not model it themselves nor provide opportunities that foster innovation in

others. For an innovation to be sustainable, it is not enough to simply create awareness about the change needed; instead, leaders must have the skills and capacity to manage the dynamics and processes associated with innovation as a lived experience (Porter-O'Grady & Malloch, 2010).

When leaders actively acknowledge, embrace, and model innovation and change in their own practice, a culture of innovation and change is enhanced. However, when leaders do not do so, they become a barrier to creating and sustaining the innovative environment needed for positive change to continually occur (Melnyk & Davidson, 2009).

> ***Consider This*** Many people find change stressful. In addition, many people instinctively resist change. Embracing change and innovation is a challenge for many traditional managers and leaders.

ESSENTIAL CHARACTERISTICS OF EFFECTIVE LEADERS

Many characteristics are essential for transformational and innovative leaders; 13 are detailed in Box 3.2. It is important to remember that titles do not produce effective leaders; leadership is derived from the combination of an individual's personal characteristics and how they mindfully act and

---

BOX 3.2 ### Characteristics of Transformational and Innovative Leaders

- Vision and the ability to inspire a team vision/dream
- Passion for patient care and making a difference
- Transparency, honesty, integrity, and trust
- Effective communication skills
- The ability to lead and not micromanage
- Team-oriented, not "I"-oriented
- Risk taking
- High level of execution
- Positive future orientation
- Innovative and entrepreneurial spirit
- Dedicated to coaching and mentoring
- Committed to motivating and empowering others to act, encouraging the heart
- Passion and persistence through character-building experiences

Conflict Disclosure: Bernadette Melnyk has a company entitled COPE2Thrive, LLC that disseminates the COPE cognitive behavioral therapy–based programs for children, teens, and young adults.

interact with others. Informal leaders without titles who possess these characteristics are often far more respected and influential than formal leaders with titles who do not possess these qualities.

Vision and the Ability to Inspire a Team Vision/Dream

There is nothing more important to achieving success than a potent dream/vision and an ability to inspire that vision in the team. A motivational vision/dream will keep the energy of the leader and the team going when barriers, challenges, or fears are slowing or preventing outcomes from being achieved. Change efforts of many leaders fail because they focus too much on process and not enough on an exciting vision. It is important to recognize that even a great vision without execution will deter success. Effective leaders are those who can set a vision, guide others toward it, acknowledge progress along the way, and celebrate success relentlessly.

When patient care and experience are the focus of the leader's efforts, all of the challenges of the day take on a new perspective. As long as the first question is "what is the best thing to do for this patient?" a plan can be constructed. With the patient as the focus, leaders and staff connect through their passion for serving others and a shared commitment to a set of beliefs about the way patients will be cared for, how families will be treated, how leadership will support that vision, and how staff will help each other. As health care becomes more complex, consumers become more educated, and expectations continue to escalate, a clear vision that drives the work will help nurse leaders be effective and valued.

Transparency, Honesty, Integrity, and Trust

Transparency, honesty, and integrity are critical elements for establishing trust. Over the past several decades and across many disciplines, much has been written about the importance of trust. It is considered by many to be the foundation or the basic building block of healthy relationships and effective functional teams. Leaders who are wise know that trust is critical to their success, and they work continuously to attain and sustain it. Trust is a "two-way street" and to reap its full benefits, leaders must be trusted by team members *and* team members must be trusted by the leader as well. When words and actions match, when one is perceived as authentic, and when humility and reflection are common actions, trust will flourish. The benefits and rewards of relationships forged from trust are immeasurable, and it is in every nurse leader's best interest to cultivate this attribute.

Passion for Patient Care and Making a Difference

Historically, nurses have been perceived as *the* person on the health care team that "represents the patient" and "advocates for the patient." Placing the patient at the center of nursing work is not a stretch for nurses; it is a part of nursing practice and feels natural to nurses. However, in the chaos and pace of modern health care, this basic core value can be lost at times. This simple idea must be reprioritized as the core of nursing from wherever care is being rendered to the leadership suite. Beyond how this defines nurses as clinicians, it must also be translated effectively related to *the value nurses bring* to patients and the health care delivery milieu. As value-based care is the future of reimbursement and therefore of health care survival, it is essential that nurse leaders articulate the value of nurses to an organization and its mission.

Effective Communication Skills

Effective communication is critical to the safety of patients and the wellness of the workforce. By role modeling effective communication skills at all times, leaders can significantly influence the success of teams and organizations. An early lesson in most nursing curricula is paying attention to verbal and nonverbal communication and whether they are congruent within interactions. This lesson resonates whether one is caring for a patient or presenting a strategic proposal at an executive board meeting. Words, tone, and nonverbal cues, including body language, are all critically meaningful parts of communication. Effective leaders say what they mean, share as much information as they possibly can, and fully engage in their interpersonal interactions.

Within the scope of effective communication skills, the ability to listen cannot be emphasized enough. True listening is an incredibly powerful interaction; the listener obtains a tremendous amount of valuable information but also begins, builds, and enhances their relationship with the other person.

Leaders must have the capacity and courage to use communication skills effectively in the challenging times ahead in health care to confront and manage the conflicts, dilemmas, and conundrums of the coming decades. Finally, in addition to being good communicators, leaders are responsible for establishing and upholding administrative structures that ensure effective communication and teamwork in their organizations.

The Ability to Lead and Not Micromanage

As a leader, it is critical to lead and sometimes to manage, but it is important to never micromanage. When you hire qualified people, you must give them the freedom to do their work. Micromanagement is destructive at all levels and in every direction, both vertical (manager to subordinate) as well as horizontal (peer to peer). When employees are micromanaged, they believe the leader does not trust their work or judgment. This often leads to disengagement from their work, resulting in investment of time but not effort or creativity. The resulting dysfunctional work environment is characterized by employees feeling suffocated or abandoned, both of which breeds contempt and distrust. These feelings are dangerous to individuals, teams, organizations, and in health care to patients.

> **Consider This** If you tell people where to go, but not how to get there, you'll be amazed at the results.
> —General Patton

Effective leaders understand and recognize the differences between managing and leading, and they choose to lead whenever possible. Managing people is a skill, whereas leading people is an art and an investment. It requires commitment, relationships, emotional intelligence, critical thinking, finesse, and time. The rewards and joys of effective leading compared to the dangers and burdens of micromanaging make the effort to lead worthwhile every time.

> **Consider This** Informal leaders without a title can be more effective and influential than leaders with a formal title.

Team-Oriented, Not "I"-Oriented

Teamwork is characterized by a set of interrelated activities accomplished by more than one person to achieve a common objective. Teamwork allows for engagement of many, and the distribution of workload enables each person to be more focused and efficient. Being on a team builds bonds among team members (being part of the team is being part of the solution), spawns creativity, and often generates a more robust outcome than could be achieved by a single individual. With all of this in mind, leaders must embrace the opportunity to work with and build effective teams.

Successful leaders understand the nature of teams and their role on a particular team. When working on a team, the effective leader understands that their goal is for the *team* to be successful. The effective leader knows that achieving success requires each person to relinquish their own agenda for personal success and embrace the opportunity to share success with the team. Effective leaders understand that teams need different things from the leader at different stages of development. A young team needs more direction, while a mature team needs more autonomy and freedom. The effective leader guides, motivates, listens to, critiques, cheerleads, and, in the end, earns the unique opportunity to celebrate successes as part of the team.

Risk Taking

Many of the most successful people in life are the greatest risk takers (Melnyk & Raderstorf, 2019). A definition of a risk taker is "a visionary change leader who can cope with the uncertainty that comes with change at the same time promoting innovation" (McGowan, 2007, p. 106). Risk taking is often related to "challenging the status quo." It requires a rigorous spirit of inquiry, relentless curiosity about the possibilities, and the courage to engage in both.

Risk taking is a complex undertaking that includes weighing risks against rewards and moving into a process or project with a clear vision of the benefits overshadowing the doubts. At the same time, successful risk takers proactively recognize the vulnerabilities of moving forward and develop backup plans to address any events that unfold.

> *Consider This*   Progress always involves risk; you can't steal second base and keep your foot on first.
>
> —Frederick Wilcox

Leaders of the future will necessarily have to be comfortable with taking risks because the health care environment in the coming decades is bound to be chaotic, unpredictable, messy, and frenetic. Every day in health care will be peppered with opportunities to be risk averse or risk engaging, and those leaders who embrace and leverage risk effectively will be the success stories, looking at the others in their "rearview mirrors."

Innovative and Entrepreneurial Spirit

The current health care climate calls for leaders who are innovative and entrepreneurial. Resources are dwindling in most health care organizations, which require leaders to be more resourceful and creative in launching initiatives that will lead to enhanced efficiency, revenue generation, and reduced costs. Leaders who create cultures of innovation and entrepreneurship will reap the benefits of an organization that thrives through uncertain times with budget constraints. According to Balik and Gilbert (2010), highly successful leaders in health care should "embrace a spirit of innovation, lead bold change, and find ways to lead from inside and outside health care—not only techniques, but changes in mind-set" and "learn to be prepared to lead an interdependent, agile organization with a non-hierarchic mentality that works as a team, with leaders defined by their actions, not by their title" (p. 256).

Dedication to Coaching and Mentoring

Coaching and mentoring young leaders is an imperative for nurse leaders in order to sustain the positive changes and significant outcomes cultivated during their tenures. The ability and desire to find and cultivate what is good in others is a hallmark of an effective leader. When you ask people, "have you ever been mentored by someone?" they are immediately able to tell you who their mentor was and what that mentor did for them that was so life-changing. Mentors are often described as someone who "saw potential in me that I never saw in myself," "pushed me to do more," "believed in me," and "stood at my side when I was facing a new challenge and encouraged me." Mentoring is a deep and powerful experience that enriches both the mentee and the mentor. Effective leaders understand the potential power to help others grow and engage in mentoring

relationships in order to build effective leaders and, ultimately, better organizations.

> ## Discussion Point
>
> Think of someone who mentored you in your life. What were the characteristics of your mentors? What were the things they did for you? How did you know you were being mentored? Is there someone in your work environment who you could or should be mentoring now? What can you do to begin that process?

High Level of Execution

Effective leaders understand that vision without execution will not lead to success, and so they begin their work with end points in mind and in their plans. They continuously think about outcomes, the bottom line, and/or the product to be delivered, but the critical difference is that great leaders think and plan with the outcome in mind while paying attention to the process and the people involved. They never work without the end result in mind.

> *Consider This*   We are judged by what we finish, not by what we start.
>
> —Unknown

Positive Future Orientation

Transformational leaders aim high, have a positive future orientation, and "live comfortably in the gap between reality and the organization's vision" (Balik & Gilbert, 2010, p. 14). They are never satisfied, and they are energized by dissatisfaction as opposed to being distressed by it. They convey a positive spirit in their organization as they look to the challenges ahead of them as opportunities, not obstacles (Balik & Gilbert, 2010). Leaders in the chaotic health care environment of the future who embody this type of spirit and energy will be more likely to survive and thrive. The key to this attribute is choice; every individual chooses how they will face their day, and those leaders who choose a positive future orientation in their work will be more effective *and* more likely to have a positive future.

Committed to Motivating and Empowering Others to Act, Encouraging the Heart

The ability to motivate and empower others is a skill effective leaders must possess. The wise and effective leader knows that this aspect of leadership can only be fulfilled with pure and real intention or the results will be disastrous. Approaches for connecting with others to motivate them, grow them, and empower them, such as Kouzes and Posner's "encourage the heart," can serve leaders well in developing these attributes (2007). These authors stress that leaders must make sure people believe that what they do matters in their hearts. The practice of encouraging the heart is aligned with two commitments: (1) recognizing contributions by showing appreciation for individual excellence and (2) celebrating the values and victories by creating a spirit of community.

Sharing stories can be an incredibly powerful tool for motivating and empowering others. Hearing about and relating to what others have lived, learned, or survived has helped others for decades. Parents who have suffered the loss of a child and shared their stories with other parents or with clinicians in training have demonstrated the power of storytelling. This type of exchange is emerging as a powerful tool for leaders to add to their toolkits (Melnyk & Fineout-Overholt, 2019).

Passion and Persistence Through Character-Building Experiences

Passion is so critical, especially to avoid burnout and to keep going when life gets tough. Leaders need to know what their passion is and be able to access it and focus on it when the environment intensifies. Persistence, defined as enduring tenaciously, can be expressed quietly or loudly, but either way, it is a key characteristic for effective health care leadership. Persistence is deeply connected to passion in that what one is passionate about they are also likely to be persistent in pursuing. Nurse leaders must learn the power of passion and persistence and leverage both wisely to attain their vision and goals.

> ***Consider This*** Many of life's failures are people who had not realized how close they were to success when they gave up.
>
> —Thomas A. Edison

MODELS OF LEADERSHIP FOR THE 21ST CENTURY

Over the last 30 years, different types and styles of leadership have been used by nurse leaders. Both transactional and transformational models are commonplace in varying degrees in health care organizations. Despite many successes with these models, nurse leaders continue to struggle with patient quality, financial limitations, time management, knowledge access, information sharing, and effective communication. Not surprisingly, leaders are continually

searching for the holy grail of leadership, that ultimate, ideal model that effectively guides success in their respective organizations. It is the work of leaders to continually search for the best leadership model that meets the needs of the current environment. Effective leaders are always searching for better approaches to envisioning the future, engaging people, serving customers, and evaluating outcomes. Ineffective leaders continually work to reinforce current models of leadership that focused on the style, communication, and expectations of the past. For example, command and control leadership behaviors are no longer suitable in the highly technologic, worldwide collaboration with rapid communication that occurs among all individuals on the organizational chart of an organization. Consider the impact of the digital world on how work occurs.

Specifically, the digital world has changed when we work, where work takes place, and the media for information transfer. This digital revolution results in changes in clinical work processes, including relationships between and among employees, patients, and the community, as well as the speed at which information is processed, available, and shared. These changes challenge the best of traditional leadership models and render them ineffectual in many situations and settings. Understanding the dynamics of these changes is the first step in determining optimal leadership models that will be effective moving forward.

Scharmer and Käufer (2000) identified four areas of change as a result of the electronic world: media, time, space, and structure. *Media* is the first area of change and refers to the form in which information is documented, shared, and transmitted. In the information age, the internet has revolutionized how information is transmitted. Cloud-based systems are becoming the norm for data storage. The digitization of information has dramatically reduced the size and format of information. Less physical space is required for papers and files. In many cases, information is virtual, requiring only electronic storage space. It is now possible for information to be sent to nearly anyone at any time anywhere in the world. The majority of documents can be digitized and thus provide for increased consistency and quality of information. For leaders, the written or typed modality is no longer the most reliable; digitized documentation of information is now the more effective and efficient media for information.

With ready access to the internet, *time* for work is now widened as well. Access to information at any time of the day or night increases the emphasis on speed and efficiency. However, this reality can blur the work–personal time boundaries, creating more challenges. Leaders are sometimes now required to shift the emphasis on specific times for work based on a traditional 8-hour day, 5-day week in which an individual is present in the workplace to more flexible models. In health care, different models for work time necessarily exist for those providing patient care. The blurring of boundaries for work time creates two significant challenges: being physically present when there is value in presence, and in assuring separation of work and personal time for a healthy work–life balance.

As time and media conceptualizations have evolved, the *space* required for work has also changed. While single offices are still commonplace, the actual time spent by individuals in offices is decreasing. The portability of media and ready access to the internet allows for work to be completed in many locations rather than in the traditional office. It is now possible for many industries to perform work wherever the information is accessible. The trend is to increase flexible spaces for individual and group meetings while decreasing physical office spaces. Even when the COVID-19 pandemic is "over," aspects of what came to be "business as usual" during this time will continue. This is a rare moment when leaders will have an opportunity to demonstrate many of the attributes described here and excel or not.

The final major change is organizational *structure*. Given these realities of information and communication exchange, the underlying structure for how work is organized is now open and free-flowing. The traditional levels of authority diagrams, communication pathways, and span of control are now secondary guides for the organization rather than the primary expectations for communication and permissions. In the digital age, any employee or patient or community members can now communicate with anyone in the organization using email.

In the next section, an overview of the strengths and weaknesses of transactional and transformational leadership models followed by the emerging complexity leadership model is presented. Table 3.1 presents a comparison of the three model characteristics. This information is designed to assist leaders in understanding leadership models from a historic perspective and also to determine the role of leaders and leadership for the future.

Transactional/Instrumental Leadership

Transactional or *instrumental* leadership is the most common and well-known leadership style used in health care. In this model, the focus is on task orientation, leader direction, and follower participation, with the expectation of rewards, threats, or disciplinary action from the leader (Bass & Bass, 2008; see Table 3.1). Examples of trait theories that focus on the behaviors of the leader include:

- "Great man" theory: Throughout history, revered men such as Abraham Lincoln, John Kennedy, and Bill Gates emerged as leaders. The assumption is that strong people emerge as leaders in certain situations.
- Biologic-genetic theories: Some individuals were born to lead, considered natural leaders. The assumption is that leadership cannot be learned; rather one is born a leader.
- Traits of individuals specific to qualities: Intelligence, scholarship, dependability, situation, age, emotional competence, physique, fluency of speech, self-sufficiency, socioeconomic status, social activity, tact, popularity, and so on are largely common to leaders.

The limitations of transactional leadership include focus on a single individual as the source of knowledge and power; the role of the follower is to follow directions and support the vision of the leader. Creativity, self-actualization, and empowerment of followers are perceived as secondary or unimportant in this model.

TABLE 3.1	**Characteristics of Three Leadership Models**		
	Transactional	**Transformational**	**Complexity**
Focus	Planned work	Planned work	Emerging and transitional work
Locus of Power	Individual leader-centric/position; formal	Individual leader-centric/position; formal	Team/group/relationship-centric network focus; informal
Work	Defined/prescribed; rule driven	Defined/prescribed; rule- and principle driven	Emergent; principle driven
Communication direction	Top-down; authoritarian	Top-down; authoritarian	Multiple directions
Competencies	Plan, organize, direct, reward, punish	Plan, organize, direct, reward, punish, empower, collaborate	Facilitate, coach, collaborate
Organizational boundaries	Defined	Defined	Overlapping, informal

Inspirational/Transformational Leadership

The second most common leadership model is *inspirational* or *transformational* and emphasizes the emotional and ideologic appeals using exemplary behavior, confidence, symbolism, and intrinsic motivation (Bass & Bass, 2008). In a transformational leadership model, the work of managing meaning, infusing ideologic values, and co-creation of goals is recognized as processes of empowerment for both the leader and the follower. The exchange between the leader and the follower is elevated to include the value of personal growth for the follower.

Most recently, the concepts of leader authenticity and mindfulness have gained attention (Table 3.2; Mindful Staff, 2020). Models and descriptions of these concepts focus on leadership traits and their relationships to engagement with others in the organization and community as well as a deeper sense of the positive aspects of leadership engagement. The trait of mindfulness from a transactional perspective and authenticity as a transformational approach to self-actualization further defines these basic leadership theories.

These leadership characteristics reflect the complexity of interactions and the limitless potential of other characteristics yet to be identified to guide leaders in recognizing the most contemporary strategies to lead effectively.

Despite the advancements in the transformational leadership model, the ability of the organization to optimize the knowledge and competencies of all members of the organization in a fluid and timely manner is still limited. Continuing to rely on bureaucratic, top-down processes is counterproductive in the presence of the critical dynamics of the digital media, time, space, and structure advancements. The addition of appreciative leadership behaviors and strategies may indeed mediate these challenges of transformational leadership.

Complexity Leadership

Congruency between the leadership model, namely, how work occurs, and the underlying assumptions, values, and artifacts of the organization are positively correlated and impact organizational efficiency and effectiveness (Casida & Pinto-Zipp, 2008). The *complexity leadership model* offers a futuristic perspective for leadership and potential to support improved organizational performance.

Complexity leadership models are based on complexity leadership theory (CLT) and provide a new lens for leadership to increase effectiveness and efficiency (Uhl-Bien & Marion, 2008).

The assumptions in a complexity leadership model are:

- Positional and informal leaders fulfill diverse functions in the organization.

- Positional leaders carry authority focused on managing organizational dynamics and enabling informal initiatives rather than directing or mandating behaviors.

- Informal leaders emerge based on relationships and do not require a formal title to lead.

- Control is difficult if not impossible; uncertainty is the norm.

- System boundaries cannot be defined as all interactions are human and interconnected. Boundaries are artificial at best and used to focus on specific projects.

- Principles increase the effectiveness of the organization and policies are decreased to allow for application of principles by those accountable for the work.

- Leadership is the accountability of every individual in the organization specific to the assigned role. Rather than one "great man," everyone has the potential to lead.

- Power does not rest solely with one individual; power is distributed among the members of the organization and is located within relationships.

- High degrees of individual interactions are the norm. Communication is critical; transparency about both positive and negative events is essential.

Within the CLT model, three types of leadership functions are identified—*administrative, adaptive,* and *enabling.* The CLT model provides a more robust and congruent model for leadership. The *administrative* leadership component is somewhat similar to the transactional model. This work is about coordinating and planning organizational activities with less hierarchy and formality, thereby sustaining the framework of the organization. The *adaptive* aspect of the model is about the emergence of optimal outcomes from interrelationships and interactions. The *enabling* role is the new dimension and serves to foster and optimize adaptive work processes and mediate the tensions that occur between administrative and adaptive functions. This brief description of CLT serves as the foundation for reframing the contemporary leadership model into a trimodal model to better meet the needs of today's challenges (Malloch, 2010).

Appreciative Leadership

As the complexity of organizations continues to increase, there is a need for leadership that is less hierarchic and more pervasive across networks, cultures, and teams. There is a need for leadership practices that are sensitive to adaptability at the point of service, sensitive to the local environment, and a need for leadership at the intersection of every human system (Miller, 2015).

TABLE 3.2   Appreciative Leadership and Mindfulness

Appreciative Leadership	Mindfulness
Description	
A process that mobilizes creative potential and unleashes positive power. Five relational strategies—inquiry, inclusion, inspiration, integrity and illumination—are the focus on appreciative leadership (Whitney et al., 2010).	Mindfulness is the basic human ability to be fully present, aware of where we are and what we're doing, and not overly reactive or overwhelmed by what's going on around us.
Key Points	
• A leadership strategy to identify and mobilize creative potential for the individual and the organization • Positive power means bringing your best forward. • Recognizing creative potential • Enhancing individual and collective capacity • Opportunities, rather than problems, are the focus.	• The goal is to observe what one is thinking, feeling, and sensing. • Develop a spirit of openness and kindness to oneself and others. • Move from automatic processing of information to a high level of presence and engagement in the moment to gain a greater understanding of events.
Selected References	
• Dewar and Cook (2014) • Keefe and Pesut (2004) • Whitney et al. (2010)	• Black (2011) • Boyatzis and McKee (2005) • Cullen (2011) • Pipe (2008)

Leadership from multiple nodes and networks in a complex system requires behaviors and values that rely less on hierarchical, directive, or controlling competencies and move beyond transformational or servant leadership focused on solving existing problems to appreciative leadership that recognizes the leadership capabilities of every individual in an organization (Malloch & Porter-O'Grady, 2020). In the appreciative leadership model, leadership is emergent from interactions and exchange of new information. The emergent leader is a person who steps up in situations or circumstances in which their expertise, understanding, skill, or particular insight provides guidance at particular moments in time.

Appreciative leadership can be defined as "The capacity to engage others in discovering, magnifying, and connecting all that is good and healthy in people and the world around them—in such a way that deepens relatedness, inspires transformational conversations, and mobilizes cooperative action toward life-affirming social innovations" (Whitney et al., 2010, p. 12). Based on a unique and local position, the appreciative leader has the perspective to lead the implementation of evidence-based interventions. In an appreciative leadership model, each individual's skills are based on the belief that all people in the enterprise have a specific and defined role in relationship to the purposes and practices of the organization and clearly, specifically,

and intentionally contribute to the work done there (Porter-O'Grady & Malloch, 2015).

There are particular leader behaviors that reflect appreciation of the fundamental contribution and value of every role and participant providing service. Three guiding principles are actualized with the five behaviors of inquiry, illumination, inclusion, inspiration, and integrity (Whitney et al., 2010). The application of these appreciative practices and patterns of behavior serve to change the mental model of a culture to be a positive, proactive, and dynamic frame for action (Malloch & Porter-O'Grady, 2020). The guiding principles are:

1. Acting as the role of agent for the system and network, the appreciative leader recognizes the definitive and essential contribution of every individual in the system.

2. Appreciative leaders in complex systems and networks manage movement, not people.

3. The appreciative leader recognizes that the skill sets associated with leading collaterally and representing complex adaptive values and behaviors are unique and differentiated from those historically present in the characteristics of the person of the leader.

Five principles guide the actualization of these three principles through role behaviors (Whitney et al., 2010):

1. Inquiry: The appreciative leader lets people know they and their contributions are valued by routinely asking for input. When the leader asks people to share their thoughts and feelings as well as their stories of success or ideas for the future and sincerely listens to what they say, the leader is telling them, "I value you and your thinking."

2. Illumination: Appreciative leaders help people understand how they can best contribute. Through illumination, the appreciative leader helps people learn about their own strengths and the strengths of others, giving them confidence and encouragement to express themselves, take risks, and support others.

3. Inclusion: Appreciative leaders routinely provide people with a sense of belonging. Inclusion means opening the door for collaboration and co-creation. This in turn creates an environment in which everyone feels they are a part of something larger. When they feel they are part of something, they care for it.

4. Inspiration: The appreciative leader provides people with a sense of direction and excitement. By forging a vision and path forward, the leader gives people hope and unleashes their energy. These are the foundations for transformation, innovation, and sustainable high performance.

5. Integrity: The appreciative leader lets people know they are expected to give their best for the greater good and that they can trust others to do the same. When the leader leads with integrity, people know they can depend on the leader to connect them to the whole.

The opportunities to implement appreciative leadership abound for organizations today. The knowledge, capacity, and expression of each individual leader in their geographic-specific circumstances was called into action to focus intentionally on management and eradication of the novel COVID-19 virus beginning in 2020. Leader actions to address the pandemic provided examples and strategies to address health care differently. Examining leader actions through the lens of appreciation illuminates different and likely more effective leader actions. Following the pandemic will be an ideal time to employ a positivity approach, seek synergistic processes and outcomes, and recognize and enhance the role of a catalyst as new behaviors transformed leadership.

Multiple Leadership Perspectives

Given that the most appropriate leadership model necessarily emerges from the time, place, and circumstances in which the organization exists, the leader often must rely on multiple leadership perspectives to achieve desired goals. For example, a transactional approach is appropriate when there are regulations to enforce; discussion about whether to comply is not appropriate or helpful unless the intent is to propose new regulation. Transformational behaviors—within a complexity leadership model—are appropriate when the focus is on individuals (Malloch, 2014). A complexity approach is often most appropriate for the realities of today's health care world. For example, health care reform requirements, namely, the emphasis on population health, coordination of care across the life span, and the delivery of value to health care users, are ideally supported by an open and networked approach that aligns leadership behaviors and beliefs with the nature of this complex and uncertain work.

CONCLUSION

To be successful, leaders must possess important characteristics to overcome the major challenges ahead of health care in the 21st century. Major challenges facing today's leaders include dwindling resources, organizations and practices steeped in tradition, and intense pressures to achieve high-value, high-reliability organizations. Leaders must possess numerous essential characteristics, such as an ability to inspire a team vision, effective communication skills, integrity, and an ability to mentor and encourage their team to excel among others, in order to be effective.

For Additional Discussion

1. How do traditional attributes associated with the nursing profession (caring, advocacy, service, etc.) promote effective leadership in the 21st century? How might these traditional attributes hinder effective leadership in the 21st century?

2. How could traditional nursing attributes be proactively and thoughtfully leveraged to influence health care decisions in the 21st century?

3. Are health care leaders role modeling EBP by integrating evidence into their daily management decision making? How can this leadership paradigm shift be enhanced?

4. How could formal leadership training for nurse managers and leaders impact hospitals in terms of saving money related to recruitment, nursing satisfaction, nurse wellness, and retention?

5. Compare and contrast three of the leadership models identified. How does each model facilitate patient safety? How can each model be a barrier to patient safety?

6. Is there a model of leadership that better supports leadership at the point of service? Why? Why not?

References

Anderson, J. G., Abrahamson, K. (2017). Your health care may kill you: Medical errors. *Stud Health Technol Inform,234*: 13-17. PMID: 28186008.

Balik, M. B., & Gilbert, J. A. (2010). *The heart of leadership: Inspiration and practical guidance for transforming your health care organization.* AHA Press.

Barker, R., & Donnelly, T. (2017). Transforming healthcare through technology. *HealthcarePapers, 16*(3), 27–33. https://doi.org/10.12927/hcpap.2017.25083

Bass, B. M., & Bass, R. (2008). *Handbook of leadership: Theory, research, and management* (4th ed.). Free Press.

Beecroft, P. C., Santner, S., Lacy, M. L., Kunzman, L., & Dorey, F. (2006). New graduate nurses' perceptions of mentoring: Six-year program evaluation. *Journal of Advanced Nursing, 55*(6), 736–747. https://doi.org/10.1111/j.1365-2648.2006.03964.x

Black, D. S. (2011). A brief definition of mindfulness. *Mindfulness Research Guide.* http://citeseerx.ist.psu.edu/viewdoc/download?doi=10.1.1.362.6829&rep=rep1&type=pdf

Blouin, A. S., McDonagh, K. J., Neistadt, A. M., & Helfand, B. (2006). Leading tomorrow's healthcare organizations: Strategies and tactics for effective succession planning. *The Journal of Nursing Administration, 36*(6), 325–330. https://doi.org/10.1097/00005110-200606000-00009

Boersma, P., Black, L. I., & Ward, B. W. (2020). Prevalence of multiple chronic conditions among US adults, 2018. *Preventing Chronic Disease, 17,* E106. https://doi.org/10.5888/pcd17.200130

Bowen, D. J. (2014). The growing importance of succession planning. *Healthcare Executive, 29*(4), 8.

Boyatzis, R., & McKee, A. (2005). *Resonant leadership: Renewing yourself and connecting with others through mindfulness, hope and compassion.* Harvard Business Press.

Cara, C. M., Nyberg, J. J., & Brousseau, S. (2011). Fostering the coexistence of caring philosophy and economics in today's health care system. *Nursing Administration Quarterly, 35*(1), 6–14. https://doi.org/10.1097/NAQ.0b013e3182048c10

Casida, J., & Pinto-Zipp, G. (2008). Leadership–organizational culture relationships in nursing units of acute care hospitals. *Nursing Economics, 26*(1), 7–15. https://pubmed.ncbi.nlm.nih.gov/18389837/

Cho, J., Laschinger, H. K., & Wong, C. (2006). Workplace empowerment, work engagement and organizational commitment of new graduate nurses. *Nursing Leadership, 19*(3), 43–60. https://doi.org/10.12927/cjnl.2006.18368

Clark, R. C., & Greenwald, M. (2013). Nurse–physician leadership: Insights into interprofessional collaboration. *The Journal of Nursing Administration, 43*(12), 653–659. https://doi.org/10.1097/NNA.0000000000000007

Cullen, M. (2011). Mindfulness-based interventions: An emerging phenomenon. *Mindfulness, 2*(3), 186–193. https://doi.org/10.1007/s12671-011-0058-1

Dewar, B., & Cook, F. (2014). Developing compassion through a relationship centered appreciative leadership programme. *Nurse Education Today, 34*(9), 1258–1264. https://doi.org/10.1016/j.nedt.2013.12.012

Dzau, V. J., Kirch, D. G., & Nasca, T. J. (2018). To care is human—Collectively confronting the clinician-burnout crisis. *New England Journal of Medicine, 378*(4), 312–314. https://doi.org/10.1056/NEJMp1715127

Einboden, R. (2020). SuperNurse? Troubling the hero discourse in COVID times. *Health, 24*(4), 343–347. https://doi.org/10.1177/1363459320934280

Gallup. (2012). *U.S. physicians set good health example.* http://www.gallup.com/poll/157859/physicians-set-good-health-example.aspx

Greiner, A. C., & Knebel, E. (Eds.). (2003). *Health professions education: A bridge to quality*. The National Academies Press.

Harding, K. E., Porter, J., Horne-Thompson, A., Donley, E., & Taylor, N. F. (2014). Not enough time or a low priority? Barriers to evidence-based practice for allied health clinicians. *The Journal of Continuing Education in the Health Professions, 34*(4), 224–231. https://doi.org/10.1002/chp.21255

Hart Abney, B. G., Lusk, P., Hovermale, R., & Melnyk, B. M. (2019). Decreasing depression and anxiety in college youth using the Creating Opportunities for Personal Empowerment Program (COPE*). Journal of the American Psychiatric Nurses Association, 25*(2), 89–98. https://doi.org/10.1177/1078390318779205

Helene Fuld Health Trust National Institute for Evidence-based Practice in Nursing and Healthcare. (2007–2021). *Home/News/EBP implementation and sustainability toolkit released to EBP HQ members*. The Ohio State University College of Nursing. Retrieved September 17, 2021, from https://fuld.nursing.osu.edu/news/ebp-implementation-and-sustainability-toolkit-released-ebp-hq-members

Hoying, J., & Melnyk, B. M. (2016). COPE: A pilot study with urban-dwelling minority sixth grade youth to improve physical activity and mental health outcomes. *Journal of School Nursing, 32*(5), 347–356. https://doi.org/10.1177/1059840516635713

Hoying, J., Melnyk, B. M., & Arcoleo, K. (2016). Effects of the COPE Cognitive Behavioral Skills Building TEEN Program on the healthy lifestyle behaviors and mental health of Appalachian early adolescents. *Journal of Pediatric Health Care, 30*(1), 65–72. https://doi.org/10.1016/j.pedhc.2015.02.005

Hrabe, D. P., Melnyk, B. M., Buck, J., & Sinnott, L. (2017). Effects of the nurse athlete program on the healthy lifestyle behaviors, physical health, and mental well-being of new graduate nurses. *Nursing Administration Quarterly, 41*(4), 353–359. https://doi.org/10.1097/NAQ.0000000000000258

Hughes-Warden, D., Hughes, R. G., Probst, J. C., Warden, D. N., & Adams, S. A. (2021, June 18). Current turnover intention among nurse managers, directors, and executives. *Nursing Outlook*. In Press. Corrected Proof. Retrieved September 17, 2021, from https://www.sciencedirect.com/science/article/abs/pii/S0029655421001044

Huston, C. J. (Eds.) (2020). Professional issues in nursing: Challenges and opportunities. In *The nursing profession's historic struggle to increase its power base (Chapter 22,* 5th ed., pp. 318–333). Wolters Kluwer.

Juraschek, S. P., Zhang, X., Ranganathan, V., & Lin, V. W. (2019). United States registered nurse workforce report card and shortage forecast. *American Journal of Medical Quality, 34*(5), 473–481. https://doi.org/10.1177/1062860619873217

Keefe, M. R., & Pesut, D. (2004). Appreciative inquiry and leadership transitions. *Journal of Professional Nursing, 20*(2), 103–109. https://doi.org/10.1016/j.profnurs.2004.02.006

Kishore, S., Ripp, J., Shanafelt, T., Melnyk, B., Rodgers, D., Brigham, T., Busis, N., Charney, D., Cipriano, P., Minor, L., Rothman, P., Spisso, J., Kirch, D. G., Nasca, T., & Dzau, V. (2018, October 26). Making the case for the chief wellness officer in America's health systems: A call to action. *Health Affairs Blog*. https://doi.org/10.1377/hblog20181025.308059. Retrieved September 17, 2021, from https://www.healthaffairs.org/do/10.1377/hblog20181025.308059/full/

Kohn, L. T., Corrigan, J. M., & Donaldson, M. (Eds.). (2000). *To err is human: Building a safer health system*. Institute of Medicine.

Kouzes, J. M., & Posner, B. Z. (2007). *The leadership challenge* (4th ed.). Jossey-Bass.

Légaré, F., Ratté, S., Gravel, K., & Graham, I. D. (2008). Barriers and facilitators to implementing shared decision-making in clinical practice: Update of a systematic review of health professionals' perceptions. *Patient Education and Counseling, 73*(3), 526–535. https://doi.org/10.1016/j.pec.2008.07.018

Lyndon, A., Zlatnik, M. G., & Wachter, R. M. (2011). Effective physician–nurse communication: A patient safety essential for labor and delivery. *American Journal of Obstetrics & Gynecology, 205*(2), 91–96. https://doi.org/10.1016/j.ajog.2011.04.021

Makary, M. A., & Daniel, M. (2016). Medical error-the third leading cause of death in the U.S. *BMJ, 353*, i2139. Retrieved September 17, 2021, from https://www.bmj.com/content/353/bmj.i2139/

Malloch, K. (2010). Innovation leadership: New perspectives for new work. *The Nursing Clinics of North America, 45*(1), 1–10. https://doi.org/10.1016/j.cnur.2009.10.001

Malloch, K. (2014). Beyond transformational leadership to greater engagement: Inspiring innovation in complex organizations. *Nurse Leader, 12*(2); 60-63.

Malloch, K., & Porter-O'Grady, T. (2020). *Appreciative leadership: Building sustainable partnerships for health*. Jones and Bartlett Learning.

McCallin, A., Bamford-Wade, A., & Frankson, C. (2009). Leadership succession planning: A key issue for the nursing profession. *Nurse Leader, 7*(6), 40–44. https://doi.org/10.1016/j.mnl.2009.07.008

McGowan, J. J. (2007). Swimming with the sharks: Perspectives on professional risk taking. *Journal of the Medical Library Association, 95*(1), 104–113. https://www.ncbi.nlm.nih.gov/pmc/articles/PMC1773030/

Melnyk, B. M. (2012). Achieving a high reliability organization through implementation of the ARCC model for system-wide sustainability of evidence-based practice. *Nursing Administration Quarterly, 36*(2), 127–135. https://doi.org/10.1097/NAQ.0b013e318249fb6a

Melnyk, B. M. (2019). Making an evidence-based case for urgent action to address clinician burnout. *American Journal of Accountable Care, 7*(2), 12–14. https://www.ajmc.com/publications/ajac/2019-vol7-n2

Melnyk, B. M., & Davidson, S. (2009). Creating a culture of innovation in nursing education through shared vision, leadership, interdisciplinary partnerships, and positive deviance. *Nursing Administration Quarterly, 33*(4), 1–8. https://doi.org/10.1097/NAQ.0b013e3181b9dcf8

Melnyk, B. M., & Fineout-Overholt, E. (2019). *Evidence-based practice in nursing & healthcare: A guide to best practice* (4th ed.). Wolters Kluwer.

Melnyk, B. M., Fineout-Overholt, E., Gallagher-Ford, L., & Kaplan, L. (2012). The state of evidence-based practice in US nurses: Critical implications for nurse leaders and educators. *The Journal of Nursing Administration, 42*(9), 410–417. https://doi.org/10.1097/NNA.0b013e3182664e0a

Melnyk, B. M., Fineout-Overholt, E., Giggle, M., & Choy, K. (2017). A test of the ARCC© model improves implementation of evidence-based practice, healthcare culture, and patient outcomes. *Worldviews on Evidence-Based Nursing, 14*(1), 5–9. https://doi.org/10.1111/wvn.12189

Melnyk, B. M., Gallagher-Ford, L., & Fineout-Overholt, E. (2015). *Implementing the evidence-based practice competencies: A practical guide for improving quality, safety and outcomes.* Sigma Theta Tau International.

Melnyk, B. M., Gallagher-Ford, L., Koshy, B., Troseth, M., Wyngarden, K., & Szalacha, L. (2016). A study of chief nurse executives indicates low prioritization of evidence-based practice and shortcomings in hospital performance metrics across the United States. *Worldviews on Evidence-based Nursing, 13*(1), 6–14. https://doi.org/10.1111/wvn.12133

Melnyk, B. M., Gallagher-Ford, L., Long, L. E., & Fineout-Overholt, E. (2014). The establishment of evidence-based practice competencies for practicing registered nurses and advanced practice nurses in real-world clinical settings: Proficiencies to improve healthcare quality, reliability, patient outcomes, and costs. *Worldviews on Evidence-Based Nursing, 11*(1), 5–15. https://doi.org/10.1111/wvn.12021

Melnyk, B. M., Gallagher-Ford, L., Zellefrow, C., Tucker, S., Thomas, B., Sinnott, L. T., & Tan, A. (2018). The first U.S. study on nurses' evidence-based practice competencies indicates major deficits that threaten healthcare quality, safety, and patient outcomes. *Worldviews on Evidence-Based Nursing, 15*(1), 16–25. https://doi.org/10.1111/wvn.12269

Melnyk, B. M., Hrabe, D. P., & Szalacha, L. A. (2013). Relationships among work stress, job satisfaction, mental health, and healthy lifestyle behaviors in new graduate nurses attending the Nurse Athlete program: A call to action for nursing leaders. *Nursing Administration Quarterly, 37*(4), 278–285. https://doi.org/10.1097/NAQ.0b013e3182a2f963

Melnyk, B. M., Hsieh, A. P., Gallagher-Ford, L., Thomas, B., Guo, J., Tan, A., & Buck, J. (2021). Psychometric properties of the short versions of the EBP Beliefs Scale, the EBP Implementation Scale, and the EBP Organizational Culture and Readiness Scale. *Worldviews on Evidence-Based Nursing, 18*(4), 243–250. https://doi.org/10.1111/wvn.12525

Melnyk, B. M., Hsieh, A. P., Tan, A., Teall, A. M., Weberg, D., Jun, J., Gawlik, K., & Hoying, J. (in press). Associations among nurses' mental/physical health, lifestyle behaviors, shift length and workplace wellness support during COVID-19: Important implications for healthcare systems. *Nursing Administration Quarterly*.

Melnyk, B. M., Kelly, S. A., Stephens, J., Dhakal, K., McGovern, C., Tucker, S., Hoying, J., McRae, K., Ault, S., Spurlock, E., &

Bird, S. B. (2020). Interventions to improve mental health, well-being, physical health, and lifestyle behaviors in physicians and nurses: A systematic review. *American Journal of Health Promotion, 34*(8), 929–941. https://doi.org/10.1177/0890117120920451

Melnyk, B. M., & Neale, S. (2018). *9 Dimensions of wellness: Evidence-based tactics for optimizing your health and well-being.* The Ohio State University.

Melnyk, B. M., Orsolini, L., Tan, A., Arslanian-Engoren, C., Melkus, G. D., Dunbar-Jacob, J., Rice, V. H., Millan, A., Dunbar, S. B., Braun, L. T., Wilbur, J., Chyun, D. A., Gawlik, K., & Lewis, L. M. (2018). A national study links nurses' physical and mental health to medical errors and perceived worksite wellness. *Journal of Occupational & Environmental Medicine, 60*(2), 126–131. https://doi.org/10.1097/JOM.0000000000001198

Melnyk, B. M., & Raderstorf, T. (2019). *Evidence-based leadership, innovation, and entrepreneurship in nursing and healthcare: A practical guide for success.* Springer Publishing Company.

Melnyk, B. M., Tan, A., Hsieh, A. P., & Gallagher-Ford, L. (2021). Evidence-based practice culture and mentorship predict EBP implementation, nurse job satisfaction, and intent to stay: Support for the ARCC© Model. *Worldviews on Evidence-Based Nursing, 18*(4), 272–281. https://doi.org/10.1111/wvn.12524

Melnyk, B. M., Tan, A., Hsieh, A. P., Gawlik, K., Arslanian-Engoren, C., Braun, L. T., Dunbar, S., Dunbar-Jacob, J., Lewis, L. M., Millan, A., Orsolini, L., Robbins, L. B., Russell, C. L., Tucker, S., & Wilbur, J. (2021). Critical care nurses' physical and mental health, worksite wellness support, and medical errors. *American Journal of Critical Care, 30*(3), 176–184. https://doi.org/10.4037/ajcc2021301

Miller, J. (2015). *A crude look at the whole: The science of complex systems in business, life, and society.* Basic Books.

Mindful Staff. (2020, July 8). What is mindfulness? *Mindful: Healthy Mind, Healthy Life.* https://www.mindful.org/what-is-mindfulness/

OECD. (2020). *Health spending (indicator).* https://doi.org/10.1787/8643de7e-en

Pappa, S., Ntella, V., Giannakas, T., Giannakoulis, V. G., Papoutsi, E., & Katsaounou, P. (2020). Prevalence of depression, anxiety, and insomnia among healthcare workers during the COVID-19 pandemic: A systematic review and meta-analysis. *Brain, Behavior, and Immunity, 88*, 901–907. https://doi.org/10.1016/j.bbi.2020.05.026

Parker, V., Giles, M., Lantry, G., & McMillan, M. (2014). New graduate nurses' experiences in their first year of practice. *Nurse Education Today, 34*, 150–156. https://doi.org/10.1016/j.nedt.2012.07.003

Phillips, L. K. (2020, July). Concept analysis: Succession planning. *Nursing Forum, 55*(4), 730–736. https://doi.org/10.1111/nuf.12490

Phillips, T., Evans, J. L., Tooley, S., & Shirey, M. R. (2018). Nurse manager succession planning: A cost–benefit analysis. *Journal of Nursing Management, 26*(2), 238–243. https://doi.org/10.1111/jonm.12512

Pipe, T. B. (2008). Illuminating the inner leadership journey by engaging intention and mindfulness as guided by caring theory. *Nursing Administration Quarterly, 32*(2), 117–125. https://doi.org/10.1097/01.NAQ.0000314540.21618.c1

Pittman, J., Cohee, A., Storey, S., LaMothe, J., Gilbert, J., Bakoyanns, G., Ofner, S., & Newhouse, R. (2019). A multi-site health system survey to assess organizational context to support evidence-based practice. *Worldviews on Evidence Based Nursing, 16*(4), 271–280. https://doi.org/10.1111/wvn.12375

Porter-O'Grady, T., & Malloch, K. (2010). Innovation: Driving the green culture in healthcare. *Nursing Administration Quarterly, 34*(4), E1–E5. https://doi.org/10.1097/NAQ.0b013e3181fb48d3

Porter-O'Grady, T., & Malloch, K. (2015). *Innovation leadership: Creating the landscape of health care.* Jones & Bartlett.

Prasad, K., McLoughlin, C., Stillman, M., Poplau, S., Goelz, E., Taylor, S., Nankivil, N., Brown, R., Linzer, M., Cappelucci, K., Barbouche, M., & Sinsky, C. A. (2021). Prevalence and correlates of stress and burnout among U.S. healthcare workers during the COVID-19 pandemic: A national cross-sectional survey study. *EClinicalMedicine, 35*, 100879. https://doi.org/10.1016/j.eclinm.2021.100879

Regan, S., Laschinger, H. K., & Wong, C. A. (2015). The influence of empowerment, authentic leadership, and professional practice environments on nurses' perceived interprofessional collaboration. *Journal of Nursing Management, 24*(1), E54–E61. https://doi.org/10.1111/jonm.12288

Sambunjak, D., Straus, S. E., & Marušić, A. (2006). Mentoring in academic medicine: A systematic review. *The Journal of the American Medical Association, 296*(9), 1103–1115. https://doi.org/10.1001/jama.296.9.1103

Sampson, M., Melnyk, B. M., & Hoying, J. (2019). Intervention effects of the MINDBODYSTRONG cognitive behavioral skills building program on newly licensed registered nurses' mental health, healthy lifestyle behaviors, and job satisfaction. *Journal of Nursing Administration, 49*(10), 487–495. https://doi.org/10.1097/NNA.0000000000000792

Sampson, M., Melnyk, B. M., & Hoying, J. (2020). The MINDBODYSTRONG intervention for new nurse residents: 6 month effects on mental health outcomes, healthy lifestyle behaviors and job satisfaction. *Worldviews on Evidence-Based Nursing, 17*(1), 16–23. https://doi.org/10.1111/wvn.12411

Scharmer, C. O., & Käufer, K. (2000). *Universities as the birthplace for the entrepreneuring human being.* Retrieved August 14, 2011, from https://urldefense.com/v3/__https://presencingcom.sharepoint.com/:b:/s/PresencingInstituteInc/EYIoF_QiKGdOr08ysJ7_rl8Bnar-YSHhVFYCXPa50qkUPw?e=qn7YJR__;!!KGKeukY!n8D0NFrntcs5bZcP4eqjPD-SsYO7PUVJ32jwlrU4SFunuBZOzoAVTFhw_EPejIlfOg$

Shanafelt, T., Goh, J., & Sinsky C. (2017). The business case for investing in physician well-being. *JAMA Internal Medicine, 177*(12), 1826–1832. https://doi.org/10.1001/jamainternmed.2017.4340

Shechter, A., Diaz, F., Moise, N., Anstey, D. E., Ye, S., Agarwal, S., Birk, J. L., Brodie, D., Cannone, D. E., Chang, B., Claassen, J., Cornelius, T., Derby, L., Dong, M., Givens, R. C., Hochman, B., Homma, S., Kronish, I. M., Lee, S., … Abdalla, M. (2020). Psychological distress, coping behaviors, and preferences for support among New York healthcare workers during the COVID-19 pandemic. *General Hospital Psychiatry, 66*, 1–8. https://doi.org/10.1016/j.genhosppsych.2020.06.007

Titzer, J., Phillips, T., Tooley, S., Hall, N., & Shirey, M. (2013). Nurse manager succession planning: Synthesis of the evidence. *Journal of Nursing Management, 21*(7), 971–979. https://doi.org/10.1111/jonm.12179

Uhl-Bien, M., & Marion, R. (Eds.). (2008). *Complexity leadership, Part I: Conceptual foundations.* Information Age.

Unruh, L., & Zhang, N. J. (2014, November/December). The hospital work environment and job satisfaction of newly licensed registered nurses. *Nursing Economics, 32*(6). https://pubmed.ncbi.nlm.nih.gov/26267960/

Välimaki, T., Partanen, P., & Häggman-Laitila, A. (2018). An integrated review of interventions for enhancing leadership in the implementation of evidence-based nursing. *Worldviews on Evidence-Based Nursing, 15*(6), 424–431. https://doi.org/10.1111/wvn.12331

Vyt, A. (2008). Interprofessional and transdisciplinary teamwork in healthcare. *Diabetes/Metabolism Research and Reviews, 24*(Suppl. 1), S106–S109. https://doi.org/10.1002/dmrr.835

Whitney, D., Trosten-Bloom, A., & Rader, K. (2010). *Appreciative leadership: Focus on what works to drive-winning performance and build a thriving organization (Business Skills and Development).* McGraw Hill.

World Health Organization. (2021, September 17). *Global health expenditure database.* Retrieved September 17, 2021, from http://apps.who.int/nha/database

Zerhouni, E. (2005). US biomedical research: Basic, translational, and clinical sciences. *JAMA, 294*(11), 1352–1358. https://doi.org/10.1001/jama.294.11.1352

Zhang, X., Lin, D., Pforsich, H., & Lin, V. W. (2020). Physician workforce in the United States of America: Forecasting nationwide shortages. *Human Resources for Health, 18*(1), 8. https://doi.org/10.1186/s12960-020-0448-3

Zucker, B., Goss, C., Williams, D., Bloodworth, L., Lynn, M., Denker, A., & Gibbs, J. D. (2006). Nursing retention in the era of a nursing shortage: Norton Navigators. *Journal for Nurses in Staff Development, 22*(6), 302–306. https://doi.org/10.1097/00124645-200611000-00006

Advanced Practice Nursing: Evolving Roles and Striving for Autonomy

Holly T. Kralj and Paul C. Herman

ADDITIONAL RESOURCES

Visit the Point for additional helpful resources.
- eBook
- Journal Articles
- Web Links

CHAPTER OUTLINE

LEARNING OBJECTIVES

The learner will be able to:

1. Understand the historic and current roles and impact of advanced practice nursing.

2. Describe the challenges of variations in practice and autonomy across the United States.

3. Discuss the rationale for the National Council of State Boards of Nursing's APRN Campaign for Consensus.

4. Describe the driving and restraining forces for increasing the entry educational level for advanced practice nursing to that of a practice doctorate.

5. Discuss the impetus for and controversies associated with the Doctor of Nursing Practice degree.

INTRODUCTION

In the past few decades, the U.S. health care system has experienced an increased focus on cost efficiency and allocation of resources. Primary and preventative care play an increasingly important role in the overall goal of maintaining health of the U.S. populace (Schober et al., 2016). With the passage of the Affordable Care Act in 2010, coverage was expanded to millions of previously uninsured

Americans, which stressed an already insufficient network of primary care physicians. As a result, many health care policy research organizations including the Robert Wood Johnson Foundation, the Pew Health Commission, and the Institute of Medicine (IOM) recommended the increased utilization of advanced practice registered nurses (APRNs) and other nonphysician primary care providers to fill the gap (Institute of Medicine of the National Academies [IOM], 2010, 2011; Xue & Intrator, 2016).

In 2020, the COVID-19 pandemic stressed the U.S. health care system and threatened to overwhelm regions where the disease burden was high and resources were low (Stucky et al., 2020). In addition, the pandemic exposed major flaws and weaknesses in the U.S. health care system, including severe shortages of providers to meet anticipated patient surges. As a result, emergency regulatory and policy changes were put in place to expand the scope of practice of many APRNs to bolster the pandemic response (Stucky et al., 2020). Indeed, Stucky and colleagues (2020) suggest that the pandemic provided a watershed moment for APRNs to redesign U.S. health care in a sustainable and resilient manner, educate others about the merit of their role, and advocate for permanent and national full practice authority.

ADVANCED PRACTICE REGISTERED NURSING ROLES

Although there are many advanced roles and skills in nursing, only four categories are considered APRNs: nurse practitioners (NPs), clinical nurse specialists (CNSs), certified nurse-midwives (CNMs), and certified registered nurse anesthetists (CRNAs). Each of these designated roles requires graduation from a nationally accredited APRN program, licensure and regulation by a state board of registered nursing, and competency certification from specific national governing bodies (National Council of State Boards of Nursing [NCSBN], 2020a). All advanced practice roles require additional education and training in advanced pathophysiology, advanced pharmacology, and advanced health assessment; however, APRN roles typically have a specific population-based focus.

While CRNAs provide anesthesia services across all age ranges, NP and CNS programs focus on specific population-based competencies including family, neonatal, pediatric (both acute and primary care), adult/gerontology (both acute and primary care), women's health/gender-related, and psychiatric/mental health (NCSBN, 2017). CNMs focus on the primary care and reproductive health care of women from puberty to beyond menopause with a special focus on pregnancy and childbirth. CNMs

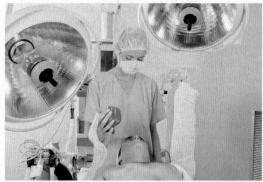

(Tyler Olson/Shutterstock)

can also care for newborns in the first 30 days of life as well as treat sexually transmitted infections in the partners of their patients (American College of Nurse-Midwives [ACNM], 2020b).

In 2008, the APRN Consensus Work Group & NCSBN APRN Advisory Committee (revised 2018) offered the following definition of an APRN:

1. A nurse who has completed an accredited graduate-level education program, preparing them for one of the four recognized APRN roles

2. A nurse who has passed a national certification examination that measures APRN and role- and population-focused competencies and who maintains continued competence as evidenced by recertification in the role and population through the national certification program

3. A nurse who has acquired advanced clinical knowledge and skills preparing them to provide direct care to patients as well as a component of indirect care; however, the defining factor for *all* APRNs is that a significant component of the education and practice focuses on direct care of individuals

4. A nurse whose practice builds on the competencies of registered nurses (RNs) by demonstrating a greater depth and breadth of knowledge, a greater synthesis of data, increased complexity of skills and interventions, and greater role autonomy

5. A nurse who is educationally prepared to assume responsibility and accountability for health promotion and/or maintenance as well as the assessment, diagnosis, and management of patient problems, including the use and prescription of pharmacologic and nonpharmacologic interventions

6. A nurse who has clinical experience of sufficient depth and breadth to reflect the intended license

7. A nurse who has obtained a license to practice as an APRN in one of the four APRN roles (pp. 2–3)

Certification for each APRN role is managed by different certifying organizations with differing educational and competency requirements. For CNMs, certification is governed by the American Midwifery Certification Board (AMCB), while CRNAs are governed by the National Board of Certification and Recertification for Nurse Anesthetists (NBCRNA). Certification for a CNS can occur either through the American Nurses Credentialing Center (ANCC) or through the Clinical Nurse Specialist American Association of Critical-Care Nurses (AACN) Certification Corporation. For NPs, there are five different certifying bodies to choose from depending on area of specialization and provider preference. The four APRN roles, their respective certifying organizations, and specific certifications offered within each category are detailed in Table 4.1.

According to the National Nursing Database, there are over 3 million RNs working in the United States, and of those, more than 350,000 are APRNs (NCSBN, 2020a). According to the American Association of Nurse Practitioners (AANP, 2020), over 290,000 APRNs in the United States are NPs. The National Association of Clinical Nurse Specialists

TABLE 4.1   APRN Role, Certifying Organizations, and Type of Certification

APRN Role	Certifying Organizations	Type of Certification
Certified nurse-midwife	American Midwifery Certification Board (AMCB)	• Certified nurse-midwife (CNM)
Certified registered nurse anesthetist	National Board of Certification and Recertification for Nurse Anesthetists (NBCRNA)	• Certified registered nurse anesthetist (CRNA)
Clinical nurse specialist	Clinical Nurse Specialist American Association of Critical-Care Nurses (AACN) Certification Corporation	• Adult-gerontology CNS (ACCNSAG) • Pediatric CNS (ACCNS-P) • Neonatal CNS (ACCNS-N)
	American Nurses Credentialing Center (ANCC)	• Adult-gerontology CNS (AGCNS-BC)
Nurse practitioner	American Academy of Nurse Practitioners Certification Board (AANPCB)	• Family nurse practitioner (FNP) • Adult-gerontology primary care nurse practitioner (AGPCNP) • Emergency care NP (FNP with emergency department focus)
	American Nurses Credentialing Center (ANCC)	• Adult-gerontology acute care nurse practitioner (AGACNP-BC) • Adult-gerontology primary care nurse practitioner (AGPCNP-BC) • Family nurse practitioner (FNP-BC) • Pediatric primary care nurse practitioner (PPCNP-BC) • Psychiatric mental health nurse practitioner (PMHNP-BC) • Emergency nurse practitioner (ENP-BC)
	American Association of Critical-Care Nurses (AACN) Certification Corporation	• Acute care nurse practitioner: adult-gerontology (ACNPC-AG)
	Pediatric Nursing Certification Board (PNCB)	• Pediatric nurse practitioner primary care (CPNP-PC) • Pediatric nurse practitioner acute care (CPNP-AC)
	National Certification Corporation (NCC)	• Neonatal nurse practitioner (NNP-BC) • Women's health care nurse practitioner (WHNP-BC)

Sources: American Nurses Credentialing Center. (2017). ANCC Certification Center. https://www.nursingworld.org/our-certifications/; Pediatric Nursing Certification Board. (2020). Steps to CPNP-PC certification. https://www.pncb.org/cpnp-pc-certification-steps

(NACNS, 2020a and 2020b) reports that there are more than 72,000 CNSs. The ACNM (2019) reports there are over 12,000 CNMs, and the American Association of Nurse Anesthetists (AANA, 2019) confirms there are more than 54,000 CRNAs in the United States. APRNs constitute nearly 10% of the RN workforce in the United States (U.S. Department of Labor: Bureau of Labor, 2020), and numbers are expected to continue to grow.

As the national populace ages and health care reform continues to evolve, there is a call to provide better care at a lower cost. To achieve this goal, APRNs will likely take an integral role. According to the hallmark IOM (2011) report, "The Future of Nursing: Leading Change, Advancing Health,"

> *The nursing profession has the potential capacity to implement wide-reaching changes in the health care system…. By virtue of their regular, close proximity to patients and their scientific understandings of care processes across the continuum of care, nurses have a considerable opportunity to act as full partners with other health care professionals and to lead in the improvement and redesign of the health care system and its practice environment. (p. 23)*

Yet challenges persist for APRNs regarding acceptance and the ability "to practice to the full extent of their education and training" (IOM, 2010, 2011, p. 29).

History of Advanced Practice Nursing Roles

Historically, nurses have stepped in and filled advanced roles as needed. Nurses administered chloroform to soldiers on the front lines of the Civil War (AANA, 2019), and they cared for impoverished and vulnerable individuals when few would. Some of the first recognized nurse "specialists" were psychiatric nurses who tended to the mentally ill in the late 1800s hoping to create more humane treatments. The first psychiatric nurse specialty program dates to 1882 in McLean Hospital in Massachusetts (McLean Hospital, 2017). Many other advanced nursing roles can be traced to public health nursing at the turn of the 20th century when care was typically delivered in the home or community clinics, especially to pregnant and postpartum women and children living in poverty. Lillian Wald founded the Henry Street Settlement in New York in 1895 and is credited with starting the U.S. public health movement. Mary Breckinridge founded the first U.S. nurse-midwifery service in the Appalachian mountains of Kentucky in the 1920s, servicing people living in poverty and in rural areas with exceptional results (Declercq, 2018).

The formal development and recognition of APRNs in the United States is often attributed to Loretta Ford and Henry Silva who started the first NP program at the University of Rochester Hospital in 1965 (Parker & Hill, 2017). Initially, it was a hospital-based training program, but it soon expanded to include master's and post-master's degrees as well as preparation for national certification. The program expanded on preexisting public health competencies of disease prevention and health promotion and focused heavily on primary preventative care. In addition, APRN programs flourished in the 1970s and 1980s, and along with increased numbers came increased recognition of the need for professional consistency, regulation, and advocacy.

Discussion Point

How might increasing popularity of the APRN degree strain the profession? What benefits might there be to increasing the number of APRNs?

Variations in Role Recognition and Licensing

One challenge APRNs face is the lack of consistency within states regarding APRN education, role recognition, and licensing agencies. Currently all states require a graduate degree or postgraduate certification for APRNs except South Dakota and Indiana (which require only a certificate and board certification), but recognition and regulation of specific APRN roles can vary widely. For example, in Indiana and Mississippi, CNSs are not recognized as APRNs, and in New York and Pennsylvania, only NPs and CNSs are recognized as APRNs (while CNMs are licensed by the state board of medicine, not nursing). In Virginia, CNSs are not recognized, and the other three APRN roles are recognized but are jointly regulated by both the boards of nursing and medicine (NCSBN, 2017). Obviously, the lack of consistency across state lines can make it difficult for APRNs to practice in states other than their home state of licensure. Additionally, this irregularity in role recognition can decrease access to care for underserved populations by creating additional barriers to practice for APRNs who traditionally serve more vulnerable populations (Xue & Intrator, 2016).

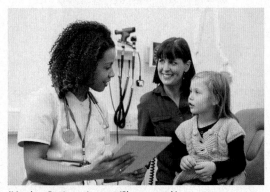

(Monkey Business Images/Shutterstock)

Levels of Independence in Practice

Across the United States, there is also a wide variety of APRN practice environments regarding required physician involvement, prescriptive authority, and the ability to bill third-party payers for services rendered. Not only are there discrepancies in the level of physician involvement in APRN practice across state lines but there are also differing levels of independent practice even between APRN roles within individual states.

The IOM, the Robert Wood Johnson Foundation and the NCSBN all recommend independent practice for APRNs as numerous studies have shown positive patient outcomes, reduced costs, and no compromise on patient safety when APRNs can practice to the full extent of their education and training (AANP, 2019).

Collaborative care has been held up as a best practice for patient outcomes (IOM, 2010, 2011), and great headway has been made legislatively across the United States regarding full practice authority for NPs. As of October 2020, 28 states granted NPs full independent practice with prescriptive authority (Fig. 4.1), but 14 states required a collaborative agreement with a physician or have other limiting elements of NP practice, and 11 states require physician supervision (the most restrictive practice model) (AANP, 2020).

Of the four APRN roles, CNSs have perhaps the greatest variation in practice recognition and requirements. In some states, the role is not recognized at all, or it is recognized as a nonadvanced practice role, like that of a nurse educator. In other states, CNSs are allowed independent practice

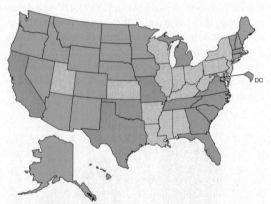

Figure 4.1 Practice models for nurse practitioners: variance by state. States in *blue* grant nurse practitioners (NPs) full independent practice with prescriptive authority. States in *gray* require some type of collaborative agreement or oversight by a physician. States in *orange* require physician supervision, the most restrictive practice model. (*Source:* Data from American Association of Nurse Practitioners. (2020). *NP fact sheet.* http://www.aanp.org/all-about-nps/np-fact-sheet)

to diagnose, treat, and manage patient care in specific patient populations (NACNS, 2020a and 2020b). As of late July 2020, CNSs could practice independently in 28 states and prescribe independently in 19 (CNS Scope of Practice, 2020). Thirteen others recognized CNSs as APRNs but required them to have collaborative practice agreements with physicians. In addition, 19 states required CNSs to have agreements with physicians to prescribe drugs and durable medical equipment (CNS Scope of Practice, 2020).

As of 2020, CNMs had independent practice in 28 states, some type of collaborative agreement required in 17 states, and physician supervision (the most restrictive practice type) in three states: Nebraska, North Carolina, and Georgia. Four states were in "hybrid models" moving toward independent practice: California, Kansas, Virginia, and Florida (ACNM, 2020a).

In California, certified midwives, who lack the nursing education and backgrounds of their CNM counterparts, were granted independent practice in 2013 with the passage of Assembly Bill 1308, no longer requiring physician supervision for non-nurse-certified midwives (California Legislative Information, 2013). In essence, the legislators deemed a hospital or home birth with a CNM in greater need of physician supervision than a homebirth with a non-nurse-midwife.

This speaks of a lack of understanding of key health care issues by many legislators and reinforces the need for strong lobbying in shaping health policy. Finally, in September 2020, Senate Bill 1237 was signed into law granting CNMs independent practice starting in January 2021, nearly 8 years later than their non-nurse-certified midwife counterparts (CNMA, 2020). Again, this illustrates the importance of political competence and engagement on the part of APRNs (Research Fuels the Controversy 4.1).

CRNAs practice almost entirely in inpatient or outpatient surgical suites. As of early 2020, CRNAs had independent practice in 30 states, required some type of physician or dentist agreement or oversight in 13 states, and required physician supervision in 7 states (NCSBN, 2020b).

Impact of the COVID-19 Pandemic on Independence of Practice for CRNAs and NPs

In response to the COVID-19 pandemic, beginning in March 2020, the Centers for Medicare & Medicaid Services (CMS) announced emergency (temporary) waivers allowing CRNAs to practice without physician supervision (CMS, 2020). Because of the surge in patients on ventilators as well as a potential shortage of anesthesiologists available during the pandemic, CRNAs stepped into critical care roles in record numbers. According to the AANA chief executive officer (CEO), "They're intubating patients, they're

Research Fuels the Controversy 4.1

Impact of Education on Professional Involvement for Student Registered Nurse Anesthetists' (SRNAs') Political Activism: Does Education Play a Role?

It is well recognized that political issues strongly impact scope of practice and reimbursement regulations for APRNs, but ways to increase APRN advocacy engagement in legislative advocacy has not been well studied. Poole et al. (2019) explored the impact of specific advocacy education on students' professional involvement in legislative activism.

Noting that registered nurse anesthetist (RNA) programs are required to include 45 hours of professional issue education without specification of the content, the authors set out to investigate the current educational curriculum and its impact on Pennsylvania nurse anesthetist programs. Their objectives were threefold:

- To investigate the extent to which Pennsylvania RNA programs addressed political engagement and advocacy in their curriculum
- To determine whether SRNAs felt they had received advocacy education within their graduate programs
- What correlation, if any, was seen between advocacy education and student advocacy activities

Source: Poole, J., Borza, J., & Cook, L. A. (2019). Impact of education on professional involvement for student registered nurse anesthetists' political activism: Does education play a role? *AANA Journal, 87*(2), 138–143.

Study Findings

The study's literature review suggested that nurses who received education on health policy and advocacy were more likely to engage in efforts to inform legislators on issues important to clinical practice. However, the literature also suggested a lack of standardized or consistent curriculum, leading the researchers to conclude that this "may lead to a lack of policy knowledge resulting in weak political skills and reduced political interest" (p. 138). The authors hypothesized that a shortage of nurse advocacy mentors and limited education on advocacy issues in APRN programs might contribute to a lack of readiness for APRNs to assume critical roles in the health policy arena.

Anonymous surveys were distributed to the 12 RNA programs in Pennsylvania, one directed toward program administrators and one toward senior nurse anesthetist students who had completed at least 1 year of study within the program. Data were analyzed using Pearson r calculations to determine correlations between survey variables. The results showed a strong positive correlation between advocacy education in RNA educational programs and the professional advocacy activities of students ($r = 0.481, p = 0.001$).

The Standards for Accreditation of Nurse Anesthesia Programs Practice Doctorate have since incorporated advocacy education and professional development as a professional role standard for CRNA programs. With CRNA programs set to embrace the DNP as the standard entry to practice in the near future, this research helps inform curricular standards in order to enhance CRNAs to assume crucial health policy advocacy to advance the profession as well as ensure best outcomes for patients.

---

managing ventilators, they're taking care of patients' critical care needs. And this is everywhere" (Terry, 2020, p. 2).

This change, however, caused pushback from physician anesthesiologists. The American Society of Anesthesiologists (ASA) issued a strongly worded statement to "protect older patients and those with disabilities…(we are) asking the Center of Medicare & Medicaid Services (CMS) to rescind the temporary policy that lowers the standard of care and risks patients' lives" (Terry, 2020). The AANA responded, pointing out that in many states as well as the military and Department of Veterans Affairs, CRNAs practice safely without physician supervision and have been doing so for years.

AANA's CEO Randall Moore, DNP, MBA, CRNA, stated in response to the ASA statement:

Their tactic is to stoke fear and obfuscation to try to prevent the modernization of anesthesia care. I say to them, "show up the evidence." Because we have a *mountain of evidence that shows otherwise. Nurse anesthetists have been providing care in this country for over 100 years…the vast majority of anesthesia care in rural, underserved areas is provided by nurse anesthetists without the presence of an anesthesiologist. (Terry, 2020, p. 1)*

Indeed, as far back as 2001, CMS allowed individual states to voluntarily opt out of physician supervision requirements for CRNAs, and as of 2020, 18 of the 45 states with supervision requirements had done so. However, the ASA contends in its position statement that while CRNAs provide excellent technical care in routine cases, when complications arise, having a physician anesthesiologist "can mean the difference between life and death." As of March 2021, 42 states have modified or lifted physician supervision to some degree; 19 of these states opted out of physician supervision entirely.

In addition, to address pandemic-induced workforce shortfalls, the CMS issued waivers in 2020 that enabled hospitals to use NPs to their fullest extent under state emergency preparedness plans (Stucky et al., 2020). One change from the Coronavirus Aid, Relief, and Economic Security Act or the "CARES Act" (H.R. 748) permanently authorized NPs to order and provide care for Medicare-eligible home health patients. Additionally, all but seven states limiting APRN practice have partially or fully waived collaborative practice agreement requirements. While these federal and state regulatory orders were meant to be temporary, permanent policy changes may occur (Stucky et al., 2020).

A MOVEMENT TOWARD AUTONOMY

The IOM's landmark report, *The Future of Nursing* (2010), called for APRNs to be allowed to practice to "the full extent of their education and training" (p. 29). Removing arbitrary, restrictive practice barriers was seen as a key intervention to expand high-quality, cost-effective care to the additional 30 million individuals who received expanded health coverage under the Affordable Care Act (AANP, 2019). Decreasing restrictive practice requirements for NPs has been shown to increase access to quality health care for patients (Kurtzman et al., 2017). Of the recommendations laid out by the IOM, those most impacting APRN practice included "removing scope of practice barriers, expanding opportunities for nurses to lead and diffuse collaborative improvement efforts, doubling the number of nurses with a doctorate by 2020, and preparing and enabling nurses to lead change to advance health" (IOM, 2010, pp. 1–7). However, these milestones have not yet been achieved.

Scope-of-practice restrictions for APRNs vary widely across the United States. According to Mary Chesney, former president and current fellow of the National Association of Pediatric Nurse Practitioners, "The national environmental landscape for APRN practice is at best disparate and fragmented and at worst illogical and highly restrictive. Practice laws vary significantly from state to state without evidence-based explanation" (Chesney, 2015, p. 219).

It has even been suggested that restrictive scope-of-practice legislation without evidence-based justification is a restriction of trade based on economic and political factors, not on best practice or the well-being of Americans. Studies have shown that requiring physician supervision of NPs increases cost of care and physician wages, decreases NP wages, and has no benefit to patient outcomes (Kleiner et al., 2016; Perloff et al., 2016). The IOM report (2011) went so far as to call for an investigation by the Federal Trade Commission (FTC) regarding state policies that restrict APRN practice, since they reduce the well-being of the public through anticompetitive barriers to fair-trade health care practices.

According to the Robert Wood Johnson Foundation (RWJF, 2017), restrictive practice legislation for APRNs unnecessarily decreases access to high-quality, affordable care for some of the most vulnerable Americans. APRNs have historically cared for more underserved patients than have physicians, such as patients in rural or remote areas, those with disabilities, or those living in poverty (RWJF, 2017).

States that require supervising physicians for APRNs or restrict the ability of APRNs to prescribe medications, order tests or medical equipment, and admit patients to hospitals delay crucial care for patients. Some APRNs have to pay collaborating physicians, and some insurance companies are unwilling to reimburse APRNs or they pay them at lower rates than their physician counterparts for the same services rendered (RWJF, 2017). Also, supervisory requirements can take time away from patient care for unnecessary administrative tasks. Most concerning, they can keep APRNs from providing necessary care in rural or remote areas where a supervising physician is unavailable (Kleiner et al., 2016; Kurtzman et al., 2017; Martsolf et al., 2015; RWJF, 2017). Restrictive practice legislation poses economic barriers to practice for APRNs, but, more importantly, it decreases access to care for citizens in need.

Discussion Point

What role could insurance companies play in increasing access to APRNs?

A number of studies have examined the theoretical impact of removing restrictive scope-of-practice barriers for APRNs and standardizing independent practice legislation across the United States. Perloff et al. (2016) conducted a study looking at the cost of primary care for Medicare recipients delivered by NPs versus physicians. After controlling for variables, their results showed no decrease in quality measures but significant cost savings in the NP group. These findings reinforce other research that suggests independent practice for APRNs increases access to care for patients and decreases health care costs with no compromise of patient safety or health outcomes (Fauteux et al., 2017; Kleiner et al., 2016; Kurtzman et al., 2017; Martsolf et al., 2015; Perloff et al., 2016; RWJF, 2017).

NCSBN'S APRN Campaign for Consensus

Inconsistencies in state requirements regarding APRN education and regulations pose barriers for APRNs to work in states other than those of their home licensure. It may also undermine the credibility of the APRN profession among other health care professionals (APRN Consensus Work Group & NCSBN APRN Advisory Committee, 2008). After extensive research, collaboration, and compromise, the APRN Consensus Work Group and the NCSBN APRN Advisory Committee issued a document intended to unify nursing regulations for advanced practice nursing across the country in the areas of licensing, accreditation, credentialing, and education (LACE) (APRN Consensus Work Group & NCSBN APRN Advisory Committee, 2008). The document, *Consensus Model for APRN Regulation: Licensure, Accreditation, Certification, and Education* (2008, 2018), put forth a uniform model of regulation intended to protect the public and create consistency for APRN recognition nationally. The Consensus Model recommended that APRNs within the four designated roles be granted independent practice (APRN Consensus Work Group & NCSBN APRN Advisory Committee, 2008). Licensure would only be granted to graduates or accredited or preaccredited programs, ensuring that the content and core competencies of the program met the national standards in both broad and population-based foci. Professional certification would still be conducted by the national certifying organizations.

Advanced practice registered nurses are licensed independent practitioners who are expected to practice within standards established or recognized by a licensing body. Each APRN is accountable to patients, the nursing profession, and the licensing board to comply with the requirements of the state nurse practice act and the quality of advanced nursing care rendered; for recognizing limits of knowledge and experience, planning for the management of situations beyond the APRNs expertise; and for consulting with or referring patients to other health care providers as appropriate. (APRN Consensus Work Group & NCSBN Committee, 2008, p. 7)

The NCBN's APRN Campaign for Consensus was overwhelmingly endorsed by the vast majority of major nursing organizations, including the AANP, the AACN, the AANA, the ACNM, the American College of Nurse Practitioners (ACNP), and the American Nurses Association (ANA). State boards of nursing would still have the responsibility of licensing APRNs, but the consistency in education and regulation would give APRNs the ability to practice in all states adopting the APRN Consensus Model. This would increase access to care for underserved populations. The goal for adoption in all states was 2015 (APRN Consensus Work Group & NCSBN APRN Advisory Committee, 2008). Unfortunately, legislative issues and lobbying against independent practice for APRNs in certain states have prevented full adoption nationally, but progress has been made.

Legislative sessions from 2017 to 2020 were exceedingly active in enacting or amending laws and regulations pertaining to APRN practice authority, reimbursements, and prescriptive authority in 25 states. Major emphasis was placed on the national opioid crisis. APRNs participated in local state prescription drug monitoring programs, improving access to safe and effective care for patients with chronic pain. Twelve states enacted legislation pertaining to APRN practice authority, including collaborative practice agreements, scope-of-practice improvements, and specification of credentialing, privileging, and educational requirements. Two additional states reported improvement in reimbursement policies for health care services provided by APRNs (Phillips, 2019).

In addition to legislative and regulatory updates to practice authority and reimbursement, states introduced legislation addressing telehealth policy adoption, home health challenges, transition-to-practice struggles, and laws pertaining to tax incentives for APRN preceptors. Five states adopted telehealth service policies, improving access to vital health care services for their residents. Four states proposed tax credit legislation for clinical preceptors; however, only one state was successful in enacting such policy. In 2019, South Carolina's Act No. 45 authorized income tax credit for each clinical rotation provided by an APRN, physician, or physician assistant preceptor. These new statutes clearly define hourly requirements in the practice-payer mix percentage and are limited to family medicine, internal medicine, pediatrics, obstetrics/gynecology, emergency medicine, psychiatry, and general surgery (Phillips, 2019).

The Nurse Practitioner journal puts out a comprehensive annual legislative update that details recent legislative and regulatory changes to practice, reimbursement, and prescriptive authority that have the most impact on NPs and other APRNs across the country. The full legislative update can be found online at https://doi.org/10.1097/01 .NPR.0000615560.11798.5f.

Discussion Point

How might states work together to achieve consensus regarding licensing, accreditation, certification, and education? What stakeholders might pose the greatest roadblocks?

CONTROVERSIES AND ISSUES IN ADVANCED PRACTICE NURSING

APRNs have been on the frontlines of expanding access to health care for some of the most vulnerable individuals for decades, yet controversy still exists regarding scope of practice and acceptance. Discrepancies regarding level of education required for APRN roles exist, and organizations have debated the merits and challenges of moving the educational requirement for all APRNs to the doctoral level, some claiming such a move discourages diversity within APRN roles. For APRNs who have achieved the Doctor of Nursing Practice (DNP) degree, challenges exist within academe regarding the acceptance of the DNP versus the PhD in terms of tenured faculty positions. Finally, ongoing issues exist regarding scope of practice, levels of independence from physician supervision, and relationships and collaboration between physicians and APRNs.

The DNP as the Standard for APRNs?

A lack of doctorally prepared nurses reduces the likelihood of achieving the goal of a patient-centered, cost-effective, and safe health care system. Although APRNs are skilled clinical practitioners, many lack the training and expertise needed to address the persistent professional issues that arise in the health care system. In 2004, the AACN initiated multiple task forces to assess these, comparing various educational models and making future recommendations as to the type of leadership needed to move nursing forward. Ultimately, the board of the AACN proposed that the DNP degree be developed to bring advanced practice nursing to the doctoral level, on par with other clinical health care professionals such as physical therapists and pharmacists (AACN, 2004).

In addition, the *Future of Nursing* report (IOM, 2011) recognized the need for more nurses who have higher degrees and recommended that the number of nurses who hold doctorates be doubled by 2020. According to the most recent data available from the RWJF (2013), of the over 4 million RNs in the United States, fewer than 30,000 obtain a doctoral degree. The AACN (2020) updated fact sheet indicates that as of October 2020, there are over 357 DNP programs in the United States. Enrollment is up from 32,678 in 2018 to 36,061 in 2019, with graduations up from 7,039 to 7,944.

Based on the work of the 2004 task force, the AACN endorsed the *Position Statement on the Practice Doctorate in Nursing* recommending that all advanced practice nursing education change from graduating APRNs with master's degrees to doctoral degrees by 2015. However, this goal was not achieved. In 2020, AACN continued its work in this area and approved a document titled *The Essentials of Doctoral Education for Advanced Practice Nursing*. These *Essentials* are similar in focus to the *Essentials of Baccalaureate Education for Professional Nursing Practice* (AACN, 2020). This *DNP Essentials* document provided schools of nursing with the key content areas that should be included in the DNP curriculum (Box 4.1).

Some of the APRN organizations were quick to respond to the recommendation to adopt the DNP degree as the entry into practice for APRNs by 2015. The National Organization of Nurse Practitioner Faculties (NONPF) began work on the practice doctorate in 2001. In April 2011 and amended in 2012, it released its final document on the core competencies for NP education and practice at the doctoral level. In the end, the NONPF decided that it could not support the 2015 deadline for NP programs to prepare graduates at the doctoral level. In 2017, NONPF redefined the NP core competencies and acknowledged that the DNP is a worthwhile goal for NP programs to attain, recommending that programs transition at a pace that would continue to ensure quality (NONPF, 2017).

The other three advanced practice specialties (CNS, CNM, and CRNA) have taken a more conservative approach to the DNP recommendation. Their representative associations have published position statements that offer different views on the topic. Initially, the NACNS decided to remain neutral about the recommendation and requested

---

BOX 4.1   Essentials of Doctoral Education for Advanced Practice Nursing

1. Scientific underpinnings for practice
2. Organizational and systems leadership for quality improvement and systems thinking
3. Clinical scholarship and analytical methods for evidence-based practice
4. Information systems/technology and patient care technology for the improvement and transformation of health care policy for advocacy in health care
5. Interprofessional collaboration for improving patient and population health outcomes
6. Clinical prevention and population health for improving the nation's health
7. Advanced nursing practice

Source: Data from American Association of Colleges of Nursing. (2006). *The essentials for doctoral education for advanced practice nursing.* http://www.aacn.nche.edu/DNP/pdf/Essentials.pdf

ongoing dialogue in an effort to tackle lingering concerns, voicing support for both MSN and doctoral programs for CNS practice (NACNS, 2020a).

However, in 2015, the organization changed its position, calling for all CNS programs to have a practice doctorate as the entry level to practice by 2030 (NACNS, 2015).

While acknowledging the value of the DNP, the ACNM decided not to require it for entry to practice for CNMs or certified midwives, stating that midwives, "regardless of terminal degree, are safe, cost-effective providers of maternity and women's health care" (ACNM, 2019, para. 3). At last count, 4.8% of CNMs held doctoral degrees (ACNM, 2019). The AANA commissioned a task force in 2007 that extensively studied the issues and advocated for mandating the DNP but decided that the timeline should be extended to 2025 based on concerns about feasibility (AANA, 2007). The ANA has taken the stance that it "supports both master's and doctoral level of preparation as entry into APRN practice through a period of transition" (AACN, 2015, p. 9).

Discussion Point

Does the mandate to make doctoral education the entry level for advanced practice nursing create barriers for students from marginalized backgrounds to pursue advanced practice? If so, what measures can be taken to improve equity in advanced practice nursing while supporting the DNP?

Although the movement to standardize the doctoral degree as the required education for APRNs has not been met, schools have adopted the recommendations with more enthusiasm than previously seen in nursing education. DNP programs saw a 259% enrollment increase from 2018 to 2019, and as of 2020, the goal of doubling the number of doctorally prepared nurses was realized (Campaign for Action, 2020).

There continues, however, to be concern about the lack of doctorally prepared APRNs needed to train incoming students as well as lack of clinical sites and the availability of clinical preceptors (AACN, 2015). Some concern has also been raised that DNP graduates, though doctorally prepared and eligible to fill faculty gaps in nursing programs, may not be able to obtain tenure and equal status with PhDs in academia. Research has suggested that the role ambiguity in research, academia, and academic leadership tends to obscure the distinctness and individuality of the DNP degree, further impacting role identity (Udlis & Mancuso, 2015).

Though discussions continue, nursing schools are adopting the DNP at record speed and nurses are flocking to these programs to obtain practice doctorates (Fang et al., 2017). These doctorally prepared nurses are moving into leadership roles as well as serving as nursing faculty and are helping shape health care practice. It is the hope that DNPs will continue to gain respect and acceptance within academia for the unique perspective they bring to nursing education as well as for their clinical expertise in educating the next generation of nursing professionals.

Increasing Diversity in Advanced Practice Nursing

Healthy People 2020 defines health equity as "attainment of the highest level of health for all people" (ODPHP, n.d., para. 5), yet marginalized groups in the United States continue to experience less access to health care and lower quality than their majority counterparts (Agency for Healthcare Research and Quality, 2019). The National Advisory Council on Nurse Education and Practice (NACNEP) compiled a report to the Secretary of the Department of Health and Human Services and Congress titled *Achieving Health Equity through Nursing Workforce Diversity*. In this report, the authors established the goal of creating a nursing workforce that better mirrors the diversity of the U.S. population. Studies have demonstrated better health outcomes when the language and culture of the patient more closely matches that of the provider, a concept called "concordance." The report also notes that APRNs are more likely to practice in rural and underserved areas than their physician counterparts (NACNEP, 2020).

One concern raised by several APRN organizations regarding mandating the DNP as the entry level for APRNs is the concern that students from disadvantaged backgrounds may have fewer resources and less support for doctoral studies. In the NACNEP Congressional report, the authors presented policy strategies to encourage diversity in the nursing workforce, faculty, and advanced practice. Specifically, they encouraged pipeline (kindergarten through 12th grade) programs to direct underrepresented students into science, technology, engineering, and math (STEM) programs, specifically health care and nursing. Additionally, the report called for continued Health Resources and Services Administration Nursing Workforce Diversity Grants to be funded through the Public Health Service Act. These grants provide financial support to minority students as well as encourage schools of nursing and hospitals to promote diversity in the workplace. Formal programs facilitating financial and mentoring support can help enhance diversity in the nursing workforce, which translates to increased access and quality of care in underserved populations (NACNEP, 2020).

Differences Between DNP/ND and PhD/DNS

There remains some confusion regarding the differences between a research doctorate (PhD or Doctor of Nursing Science [DNS/DNSc]) and a practice doctorate (DNP). The key focus of PhD programs is the development of research, and the primary focus of DNP graduates is to utilize the research work of the PhD or DNS nurse to effect change and improve care through clinical implementation and systems change.

In 2006, the AACN provided a detailed explanation in its introduction to the *DNP Essentials* document: This has been revised and republished as the *DNP Fact Sheet* (AACN, 2020):

> Doctoral programs in nursing fall into two principal types: research-focused and practice-focused. Most research-focused programs grant the Doctor of Philosophy degree (PhD), while a small percentage offers the Doctor of Nursing Science degree (DNS, DSN, or DNSc). Designed to prepare nurse scientists and scholars, these programs focus heavily on scientific content and research methodology, and all require an original research project and the completion and defense of a dissertation or linked research papers. Practice-focused doctoral programs are designed to prepare experts in specialized advanced nursing practice. They focus heavily on practice that is innovative and evidence-based, reflecting the application of credible research findings. The two types of doctoral programs differ in their goals and the competencies of their graduates. They represent complementary, alternative approaches to the highest level of educational preparation in nursing. (p. 3)

For some time, there has been controversy in the literature regarding the value and scope of the DNP degree, and part of the issue arises from differing PhD and DNP pedagogy. The curricula for many DNP programs were initially developed and instructed by PhD faculty. These PhD-prepared faculty, therefore, may not understand the difference between evidence-based practice and translational research from the DNP perspective. Instead of having DNP students conduct rigorous research, which was not the original intent of the DNP degree, faculty need to help DNP students understand how to use best evidence to improve

health care systems and patient outcomes (Melnyk, 2016). The two disciplines are complementary in their scopes and focuses with the overarching goal of safe, effective health care delivery.

Physicians and Advanced Practice Nursing

As APRNs have become more visible and utilized within health care delivery systems, they have experienced some pushback from their physician counterparts. Some physician groups, including the American Medical Association (AMA) and American Academy of Family Physicians (AAFP), have opposed the IOM recommendations for removal of barriers to practice from APRNs, claiming patient safety concerns, though this is not evident in the research (Fauteux et al., 2017; Kleiner et al., 2016; Kurtzman et al., 2017; Martsolf et al., 2015; Perloff et al., 2016; RWJF, 2017). Others have suggested that NPs do not spend an equivalent amount of time in their education and therefore cannot function as well as physicians regarding complex patient decision making (Sarzynski & Barry, 2019).

While it is true that APRNs generally focus on primary care, NPs generally spend 4 years in baccalaureate nursing education plus 2 to 3 additional years obtaining a master's degree and/or 2 to 4 years obtaining a DNP. Most NP programs require applicants to have at least 1 year of clinical experience as an RN before applying to the NP program, and applicants must hold at least a bachelor's degree in nursing. However, many NP students have significantly more years of clinical experience prior to starting their advanced practice programs. It is not unusual for an NP to have 7 to 9 or more years of education and many more years of practice as an RN before taking on the APRN role.

The question must be asked whether APRNs need additional years of education and advanced clinical training to perform the role. Since APRNs have been providing patient care for nearly 50 years with exceptional outcomes in safety, cost-effectiveness, and patient satisfaction (Parker & Hill, 2017), it is clear the level of education for these health care providers is adequate and responsive to changing roles and requirements as illustrated by increasing movement toward acceptance of the DNP.

Most concerns over the quality of care provided by APRNs have been unsupported by multiple studies (Fauteux et al., 2017; Kleiner et al., 2016; Kurtzman et al., 2017; Martsolf et al., 2015; Newhouse et al., 2011; Perloff et al., 2016; RWJF, 2017; Swan et al., 2015). An extensive study by Newhouse and team (2011) reviewed two decades of literature on care provided by APRNs in comparison with physician care. The results indicated that APRNs provide cost-effective, high-quality patient care and have an important role in improving the quality of health care in the United States. More recent reviews have confirmed the quality and efficacy of APRN care (Parker & Hill, 2017). In addition to achieving primary care health outcomes equal to or greater than those of their physician counterparts, APRNs have been shown to reduce costs with no decrease in patient satisfaction (Spetz et al., 2016). This abundance of data should eliminate concerns about whether care provided by APRNs can safely augment the physician supply to support reform efforts aimed at expanding access to care.

It should be clarified, however, that NPs and physicians do not strive to practice identically. Physicians practice from a medical model while APRNs practice from the nursing model, which emphasizes health promotion and disease prevention. This key component of NP practice is one that many patients value. It is also supported by *Healthy People 2030*. It is of note that in recent years, medical schools have increased education about the importance of health promotion and disease prevention, partially in response to this quality and safety movement.

The IOM report, *Health Professions Education: A Bridge to Quality* (2003), notes that health care professionals must "work in interdisciplinary teams—cooperate, collaborate, communicate, and integrate care in teams to ensure that care is continuous and reliable" (p. 45). NPs have always advocated for all health care providers, including physicians, NPs, physical therapists, pharmacists, and respiratory therapists, among others, to work together to provide the highest quality of care. Shared leadership with a patient-centered focus provides an opportunity for all disciplines to bring their expertise with the goal of best outcomes. However, the paradigm is shifting from physician-led care to collaborative care, and doctorally prepared APRNs are poised to bring their knowledge and expertise to the table.

LOOKING TOWARD THE FUTURE

The controversy over the clinical practice doctorate in nursing will likely continue for many years, but advanced practice nursing must continue to self-evaluate the level of education needed to provide top-quality care to patients in today's health care system. Of equal importance, APRNs must develop the advocacy skills needed to survive as a vital constituent of the current evolving health care system. There is no question that advanced practice nursing makes valuable contributions to the health care system. The movement toward the DNP is a crucial part of that process. Continued advocacy and policy support for advanced practice nursing will be critical for APRNs to most significantly impact the health of patients. The nursing profession must continue to be vigilant about attempts to encroach on its right to practice.

> *The integration of APNs into the workforce is a dynamic change in the provision of healthcare services requiring a mind shift by policy makers and healthcare professionals... The development of policy to support this new nursing role to its full potential was found to be essential. (Schober et al., 2016, p. 1322)*

More than a decade ago, the IOM (2010, 2011) recommended that all levels of nursing be allowed and encouraged to perform to the full scope of their practice. Nurses must be strong advocates for the profession by joining and being actively involved in professional associations that focus on monitoring practice issues and voting for legislators who will support advanced practice nursing roles. Legislators must be kept informed of nursing practice as well as provided with documentation of the outstanding patient outcomes from APRN care. The protection of nursing's freedom to practice without undue restrictions and barriers must be ensured, not just for the profession but more importantly for the health and wellness of the patients served. In collaboration, all members of the health care team must strive to enhance the health of the U.S. population, especially its most vulnerable members.

For Additional Discussion

1. Compare and contrast the skill sets of PhD- and DNP-trained nurses bring to nursing education and curriculum development. How can both doctoral degrees work together to impact the profession?

2. Give examples of barriers and facilitators for increasing diversity in advanced practice nursing. Why are diversity and inclusion important?

3. Should physicians be reimbursed more than APRNs for the same services rendered? Why or why not?

4. Would you consider pursuing an advanced practice nursing degree? If not, why? If so, which of the four roles most interests you and why? Provide examples of personality traits you feel are beneficial for the different roles.

5. Do you support the NCSBN Consensus Model for APRNs? What benefits does the model provide for APRNs and consumers? Are there any benefits for physicians? What do you see as potential disadvantages of the Consensus Model?

References

Agency for Healthcare Research and Quality. (2012, updated 2019). *National Healthcare Disparities Report*. U.S. Department of Health and Human Services. https://www.ahrq.gov/research/findings/nhqrdr/index.html

American Association of Colleges of Nursing. (2004). AACN position statement on the practice doctorate in nursing. Washington, D.C.: Author. https://www.aacnnursing.org/Portals/42/News/Position-Statements/DNP.pdf

American Association of Colleges of Nursing. (2015). *White paper: Re-envisioning the clinical education of advanced practice nurses*. https://www.aacnnursing.org/Portals/42/News/White-Papers/APRN-Clinical-Education.pdf

American Association of Colleges of Nursing. (2020, October). *Fact sheet: The Doctor of Nursing Practice (DNP)*. http://www.aacnnursing.org/News-Information/Fact-Sheets/DNP-Fact-Sheet

American Association of Nurse Practitioners. (2019). *State practice environment*. https://www.aanp.org/advocacy/state/state-practice-environment

American Association of Nurse Practitioners. (2020). *NP fact sheet*. http://www.aanp.org/all-about-nps/np-fact-sheet

American College of Nurse-Midwives. (2019). *Midwifery education and the Doctor of Nursing Practice (DNP)*. http://www.midwife.org/ACNM/files/ACNMLibraryData/UPLOADFILENAME/000000000079/Midwifery%20Ed%20and%20DNP%20Position%20Statement%20June%202012.pdf

American Nurses Credentialing Center. (2017). *ANCC Certification Center*. https://www.nursingworld.org/our-certifications/

APRN Consensus Work Group & National Council of State Boards of Nursing APRN Advisory Committee. (2008). *Consensus model for APRN regulation: Licensure, accreditation, certification and education*. https://www.ncsbn.org/Consensus_Model_for_APRN_Regulation_July_2008.pdf

California Legislative Information. (2013). *AB 1308 midwifery*. http://leginfo.legislature.ca.gov/faces/billVotesClient.xhtml?bill_id=201320140AB1308

California Nurse Midwives Association. (2020). *Updated state practice environment map: California isn't red anymore!* https://www.cnma.org/post/decemebr-2020-newsletter

Campaign for Action. (2020). *Transforming nursing education*. https://campaignforaction.org/issue/transforming-nursing-education/

Centers for Medicare & Medicaid Services. (2020). Trump administration makes sweeping regulatory changes to help U.S. healthcare system address COVID-19 patient surge. *CMS Newsroom Press Release*. https://www.cms.gov/newsroom/press-releases/trump-administration-makes-sweeping-regulatory-changes-help-us-healthcare-system-address-covid-19

Chesney, M. L. (2015). Increasing families' health care access and choice through full practice authority. *Journal of Pediatric Health Care, 29*(3), 219–221. https://doi.org/10.1016/j.pedhc.2015.02.001

Declercq, E. (2018). Introduction to a special issue: Childbirth history is everyone's history. *Journal of the History of Medicine and Allied Sciences, 73*(1), 1–6. https://doi.org/10.1093/jhmas/jrx057

Doctors of Nursing Practice. (2015). *DNP scholarly projects*. http://www.doctorsofnursingpractice.org/resources/dnp-scholarly-projects/

Fang, D., Li, Y., Kennedy, K. A., & Trautman, D. E. (2017). *2016-2017 Enrollment and graduations in baccalaureate and graduate programs in nursing*. AACN.

Fauteux, N., Brand, R., Fink, J. L. W., Frelick, M., & Werrlien, D. (2017). *The case for removing barriers to APRN practice*. https://www.rwjf.org/en/library/research/2017/03/the-case-for-removing-barriers-to-aprn-practice.html

Institute of Medicine of the National Academies. (2003). *Health professions education: A bridge to quality*. National

Academies Press. http://books.nap.edu/openbook
.php?record_id=10681&page=45

Institute of Medicine of the National Academies. (2010). *The future of nursing: Leading change, advancing health—Report recommendations.* https://doi.org/10.17226/12956

Institute of Medicine. (2011). *The future of nursing: Leading change, advancing health.* The National Academies Press.

Kleiner, M. M., Marier, A., Park, K. W., & Wing, C. (2016). Relaxing occupational licensing requirements: Analyzing wages and prices for a medical service. *The Journal of Law and Economics, 59*(2), 1–53. https://doi.org/10.1086/688093

Kurtzman, E. T., Barnow, B. S., Johnson, J. E., Simmens, S. J., Infeld, D. L., & Mullan, F. (2017). Does the regulatory environment affect nurse practitioners' patterns of practice or quality of care in health centers? *Health Services Research, 52*(S1), 437–458. https://doi.org/10.1111/1475-6773.12643

Martsolf, G. R., Auerbach, D. I., & Arifkhanova, A. (2015). *The impact of full practice authority for Nurse Practitioners and other Advanced Practice Registered Nurses in Ohio.* RAND Corporation. https://www.rand.org/content/dam/rand/pubs/research_reports/RR800/RR848/RAND_RR848.pdf

McLean Hospital. (2017). *History and progress.* https://www.mcleanhospital.org/about/history-progress

Melnyk, B. M. (2016). An urgent call to action for nurse leaders to establish sustainable evidence-based practice cultures and implement evidence-based interventions to improve healthcare quality. *Worldviews on Evidence-Based Nursing, 13*(1), 3–5. https://doi.org/10.1111/wvn.12150

National Advisory Council on Nurse Education and Practice. (2020). *Annual Report: Meeting of the National Advisory Council on Nurse Education and Practice.* https://www.hrsa.gov/advisory-committees/nursing/about.html

National Association of Clinical Nurse Specialists. (2015). *Position statement on the nursing practice doctorate.* http://www.nacns.org/docs/DNP-Statement1507.pdf

National Association of Clinical Nurse Specialists. (2020a). *CNS scope of practice and prescriptive authority as of 7.31.2020.* Retrieved June 11, 2021, from https://nacns.org/wp-content/uploads/2020/08/PractPrescAuthority7.31.2020.pdf

National Association of Clinical Nurse Specialists. (2020b). *Who are clinical nurse specialists?* https://www.webmd.com/a-to-z-guides/what-is-a-clinical-nurse-specialist

National Council of State Boards of Nursing. (2020a). *National nursing data base.* https://www.ncsbn.org/national-nursing-database.htm

National Council of State Boards of Nursing. (2020b). *APRN consensus model by state.* https://www.ncsbn.org/APRN

National Organization of Nurse Practitioner Faculties. (2017). *Nurse practitioner core competencies.* https://cdn.ymaws.com/www.nonpf.org/resource/resmgr/competencies/20170516_NPCoreCompsContentF.pdf

Newhouse, R. P., Stanik-Hutt, J., White, K. M., Johantgen, M., Bass, E. B., Zangaro, G., Wilson, R. F., Fountain, L., Steinwachs, D. M., Heindel, L., & Weiner, J. P. (2011). Advanced practice nurse outcomes 1990-2008: A systematic review. *Nurse Economics, 29*(5), 230–250. https://pubmed.ncbi.nlm.nih.gov/22372080/

Office of Disease Prevention and Health Promotion. (n.d.). *Healthy People 2020—Disparities.* https://www.healthypeople.gov/2020/about/foundation-health-measures/Disparities

Parker, J. M., & Hill, M. N. (2017). A review of advanced practice nursing in the United States, Canada, Australia and Hong Kong Special Administrative Region (SAR), China. *International Journal of Nursing Sciences, 4*(2), 196–204. https://doi.org/10.1016/j.ijnss.2017.01.002

Pediatric Nursing Certification Board. (2020). *Steps to CPNP-PC certification.* https://www.pncb.org/cpnp-pc-certification-steps

Perloff, J., DesRoches, C. M., & Buerhaus, P. (2016). Comparing the cost of care provided to Medicare beneficiaries assigned to primary care nurse practitioners and physicians. *Health Services Research, 51*(4), 1407–1423. https://doi.org/10.1111/1475-6773.12425

Phillips, S. J. (2019). 31st Annual APRN Legislative Update: Improving state practice authority and access to care. *The Nurse Practitioner, 44*(1), 27–55. https://doi.org/10.1097/01.NPR.0000550248.81655.30

Poole, J., Borza, J., & Cook, L. A. (2019). Impact of education on professional involvement for student registered nurse anesthetists' political activism: Does education play a role? *AANA Journal, 87*(2), 138–143. https://pubmed.ncbi.nlm.nih.gov/31587727/

Robert Wood Johnson Foundation. (2013). *Robert Wood Johnson Foundation announces $20 million grant to support nurse PhD scientists.* https://www.rwjf.org/en/library/articles-and-news/2013/06/a-new-generation-of-nurse-scientists--educators--and-transformat.html

Robert Wood Johnson Foundation. (2017). *Charting nursing future: The case for removing barriers to APRN practice.* http://campaignforaction.org/wp-content/uploads/2017/03/CNF30-online-brief.pdf

Sarzynski, E., & Barry, H. (2019). Current evidence and controversies: Advanced practice providers in healthcare. *American Journal of Managed Care, 25*(8), 366–368. https://www.ajmc.com

Schober, M., Gerrish, K., & McDonnell, A. (2016). Development of a conceptual policy framework for advanced practice nursing: An ethnographic study. *Journal of Advanced Nursing, 72*(6), 1313–1324. https://doi.org/10.1111/jan.12915

Spetz, J., Skillman, S. M., Holly, C., & Andrilla, A. (2016). *Nurse practitioner autonomy and satisfaction in rural settings.* https://healthforce.ucsf.edu/publications/nurse-practitioner-autonomy-and-satisfaction-rural-settings

Stucky, C. H., Brown, W. J., & Stucky, M. G. (2020, October 12). COVID 19: An unprecedented opportunity for nurse practitioners to reform healthcare and advocate for permanent full practice authority. *Nursing Forum.* https://doi.org/10.1111/nuf.12515

Swan, M., Ferguson, S., Chang, A., Larson, E., & Smaldone, A. (2015). Quality of primary care by advanced practice nurses: A systematic review. *International Journal for Quality in Health Care, 27*(5), 396–404. https://doi.org/10.1093/intqhc/mzv054

Terry, K. (2020). Anesthesiologists try to stop CRNAs from practicing independently. *Medscape Medical News.* https://www.medscape.com/viewarticle/942272

Udlis, K. A., & Mancuso, J. M. (2015). Perceptions of the role of the Doctor of Nursing Practice-prepared nurse: Clarity or confusion. *Journal of Professional Nursing, 31*(4), 274–283. https://doi.org/10.1016/j.profnurs.2015.01.004

U.S. Department of Labor: Bureau of Labor. (2020, July 6). *Occupational employment and wage statistics. Occupational employment and wages, May 2019 29-1171 Nurse Practitioners.* Retrieved January 1, 2021, from https://www.bls.gov/oes/current/oes291171.htm

Xue, Y., & Intrator, O. (2016). Cultivating the role of nurse practitioners in providing primary care to vulnerable populations in an era of health care reform. *Policy, Politics, and Nursing Practice, 17*(1), 24–31. https://doi.org/10.1177/1527154416645539

Evidence-Based Practice

Cassandra D. Ford and Barbara Ann Graves

ADDITIONAL RESOURCES

Visit the Point for additional helpful resources.

- eBook
- Journal Articles
- Web Links

CHAPTER OUTLINE

LEARNING OBJECTIVES

The learner will be able to:

1. Differentiate between evidence-based practice and best practices.

2. Explain why the identification and implementation of evidence-based practice are important both for ensuring quality of care and in advancing the development of nursing science.

3. Recognize the need to ask critical questions in the spirit of looking for opportunities to improve nursing practice and patient outcomes.

4. Delineate research and nonresearch sources of evidence for answering clinical questions.

5. Compare the efficacy of randomized controlled trials, integrative reviews, and meta-analyses as reference sources to answer clinical research questions.

6. Describe the types of knowledge and education that nurses need to prepare them for conducting research and leading best practice initiatives.

7. Identify personal, professional, and administrative strategies as well as support systems that promote the identification and implementation of evidence-based practice.

8. Specify institutions, units, teams, or individuals that could be considered regional or national benchmark leaders in the provision of a specialized type of medical or nursing care.

INTRODUCTION

Nurses and other health care providers constantly strive to provide the best care for their patients. As new medications and health care innovations emerge, determining the best options can be challenging. This process becomes more difficult as health care administrators, insurance companies, and other payers, accrediting agencies, and consumers demand the latest and greatest health care interventions. Nurses and physicians are expected to select health care interventions that are supported by research and other credible forms of evidence. They may also be expected to provide evidence to demonstrate that the care they deliver is not only clinically effective but also cost-effective and satisfying to patients. In light of these challenges, the term *evidence-based practice* has emerged as a descriptor of the preferred approach to health care delivery.

This chapter begins by defining the concept of evidence-based practice. Examples of when and where nurses are using evidence-based practice are provided, as are strategies for determining and applying these practices. In addition, the *who* of evidence-based practice is addressed regarding how nurses in various roles can support this approach to care. Finally, future implications are discussed.

WHAT IS EVIDENCE-BASED PRACTICE?

The term "evidence-based practice" is part of the daily discourse among health care providers in progressive clinical environments. Evidence-based practice has a variety of definitions and interpretations. The term "evidence-based practice" evolved in the mid-1990s when discussions of evidence-based medicine were expanded to apply to an interdisciplinary audience, including nurses. David Sackett, one of the original leaders of the movement, defined evidence-based medicine as "the conscientious and judicious use of current best evidence from clinical care research in the management of individual patients" (Sackett et al., 1996, p. 71). The Honor Society of Nursing, Sigma Theta Tau International (STTI, 2005) expanded this definition to address a broad nursing context with the following definition of evidence-based nursing practice: "An integration of the best evidence available, nursing expertise, and the values and preferences of the individuals, families, and communities who are served" (p. 1).

Historically, various industries in health care and beyond have used the term *best practice* to describe the strategies or methods that work most efficiently or achieve the best results. This concept is often associated with the process of *benchmarking*, which involves identifying the most successful companies or institutions in a particular sector of an industry, examining their methods of doing business, using their approach as the goal or gold standard, and then replicating and refining their methods. Today, benchmarking data is one of the less scientific forms of evidence that is used, along with the results of formal research studies, to identify evidence-based nursing practices.

> *Consider This* Today, most nurse experts agree that the best practices in nursing care are also evidence-based practices.

Although this process of identifying the best evidence-based practices has become more scientific, the ultimate goal remains to provide optimal patient care with the goal of enhancing nursing practice and in turn improving patient or system outcomes.

Discussion Point

Are there any situations in which an evidence-based practice might not be considered the best practice?

WHY, WHEN, AND WHERE IS EVIDENCE-BASED PRACTICE USED?

Each week, new developments and innovations occur and are reported in health care—not only in research publications but also in the public media. Contemporary health care consumers are knowledgeable and demanding. They expect the most current, effective, and efficient interventions.

Why Is Evidence-Based Practice Important?

In their quest to provide the highest quality care for their patients, nurses are challenged to stay abreast of new developments in health care, even within the limits of their areas of specialization. Simultaneous with the growth of health care knowledge, health care costs have increased and patient satisfaction has taken on greater importance. Administrators expect health care providers to satisfy their customers and to do it in the most clinically effective and cost-effective manner.

Control of health care costs was one of the early drivers of the evidence-based practice movement. As contracted and discounted reimbursement systems decreased revenue to hospitals and providers, it became increasingly apparent that some providers were capable of providing high-quality care in a more efficient and cost-effective manner than their peers. The practices of these industry leaders were quickly identified and emulated. Within the current litigious and cost-conscious health care environment, there remains a sense of urgency to select and implement the most effective and efficient interventions as quickly as possible.

Nurses are increasingly accepted as essential members, and often leaders, of interdisciplinary health care teams. To effectively participate and lead a health care team, nurses must have knowledge of the most effective and reliable evidence-based approaches to care, and as nurses increase their expertise in critiquing research, they are expected to apply the evidence of their findings to select optimal interventions for their patients.

The processes and tools of evidence-based practice can help nurses respond to these challenges. This approach to care is based on the latest research and other forms of evidence, as well as clinical expertise and patient preferences. All of these factors contribute to providing quality care that is clinically effective, cost-effective, and satisfying to health care consumers.

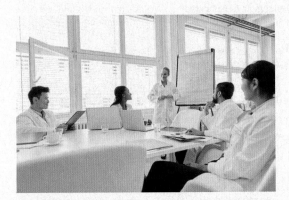

Discussion Point

What type of knowledge and education do nurses need to prepare them for leading evidence-based practice initiatives as described?

When and Where Is Evidence-Based Practice Used?

Over the past two decades, programs and initiatives to advance evidence-based practice have been identified as a priority in nursing. The implementation of evidence-based practice has been positively associated with improved health outcomes and quality care. Historically, evidence-based practice methods have been used to improve outcomes, such as decreasing catheter-associated urinary tract infections, preventing ventilator-associated pneumonia, reducing length of stay and readmission rates in heart failure patients, improving venous leg ulcers, and many others.

A review of current literature yields a plethora of evidence-based practice research studies, projects, and recommendations across both nursing specialties and nursing roles (Table 5.1). Moore et al. (2019) demonstrated improved sepsis outcomes in the emergency department using an evidence-based sepsis bundle. In a research study using evidence-based practice methods, Davis et al. (2020) designed and tested a telehealth intervention for rural populations. Lukes et al. (2019) were able to improve antibiotic administration times for pediatric patients using an evidence-based practice nursing order set.

Central to the future of evidence-based nursing practice will be the ability to enhance nurses' skills and achievement of evidence-based practice competencies (Melnyk et al., 2018). It will be important to continue to provide support systems and resources to help nurses to understand and implement evidence-based practice. Equally important will be the ability of nursing academic programs to refine nursing curricula to ensure evidence-based practice competencies are instilled in students before they enter practice as clinicians (Palese et al., 2018).

Evidence-Based Practice Around the World

A commitment to evidence-based practice is not limited to the United States. A few countries—in particular, Australia, Canada, and the United Kingdom—adopted this approach to care several years before it became popular in the United States. The Joanna Briggs Institute, which started at the University of Adelaide, Australia, in 1996, now has over 75 centers collaborating to provide evidence-based resources to health care providers around the world. The Registered Nurses Association of Ontario has been developing and distributing evidence-based nursing practice guidelines for more than a decade. Nursing Knowledge International, a subsidiary of STTI, also serves as an international clearinghouse and facilitator to promote international nursing communication, collaboration, and sharing of resources in support of evidence-based practice.

Consider This In the past decade, the concept of evidence-based practice has evolved and been embraced by nurses in nearly every clinical specialty, across a variety of roles and positions, and in locations around the globe.

TABLE 5.1   Evidence-Based Practice Across Nursing Specialties

Area of Specialization	Author/Year/Location	Title or Theme	Type of Report
Administration	Lavenberg et al., 2019, United States	Impact of EBP centers on hospital nursing policy/practice	Quality improvement with quantitative analysis
Critical care	Hellyar et al., 2019, United States	Decreased burnout, improving teamwork, nurse satisfaction, and patient safety	Case study investigation
Staff development	Sichieri et al., 2018, Brazil	Improving nursing knowledge and compliance using EBP related to central venous catheter maintenance	Implementation project
Gerontology	Scheepmans et al., 2020, Belgium	Reducing physical restraints for older adults in home care	Development of EBP guidelines
Medical–surgical	Ren et al., 2019, China	Assessment and management of pain during dressing change in patients with diabetic foot injuries	EBP implementation project
Mental health	Davis et al., 2020, United States	Designing a multifaceted telehealth intervention for a rural population	Research study using EBP intervention
Oncology	Reams et al., 2020, United Kingdom	Effectiveness of telephone-delivered interventions for reducing symptoms associated with cancer and its treatment	Systematic review
Pediatrics	Lukes et al., 2019, United States	Improved antibiotic administration times for pediatric patients with therapy-induced neutropenia and fever	Implementation of a nursing-based order set
Urgent care	Moore et al., 2019, United States	Improving 3-hr sepsis bundled care outcomes in the emergency department	Implementation of a nurse-driven sepsis protocol
Women's health	Davies et al., 2019, Ireland	Management of menopausal symptoms in breast cancer survivors	Developing clinical guidelines; process evaluation

EBP, evidence-based practice.

How Do Nurses Determine Evidence-Based Practices?

Evidence-based practice begins with questions that arise in practice settings. Nurses must be empowered to ask critical questions in the spirit of looking for opportunities to improve nursing practice and patient outcomes. In any specialty or role, nurses can regard their work as a continuous series of questions and decisions.

In a given day, a staff nurse may ask and answer questions such as: Should I give the analgesic only when the patient requests it, or should I encourage them to take it every 4 hours? Will aggressive ambulation expedite this patient's recovery, or will it consume too much energy? Will open family visitation help the patient feel supported, or will it interrupt their rest?

A nurse manager or administrator might ask questions like: Who is the most qualified care provider for our sickest patient today? What is the optimal nurse-to-patient ratio for a specific unit? Do complication rates and sentinel events increase with less educated staff? Do longer shifts result in greater staff fatigue and medication errors? Will higher-quality and more expensive mattresses decrease the incidence of pressure injuries? What benefits promote nurse retention? How does the use of supplemental (or agency) staffing affect the morale of existing staff? Can this population be treated on an outpatient, rather than an inpatient, basis? What is the optimal length of time for a comprehensive home care assessment? How many patients can a nurse practitioner see in 8 hours?

Likewise, a nurse educator may ask questions like: Is it more effective to teach a procedure in the simulation laboratory rather than on an actual patient? What are the most efficient methods of documenting continued competency? Do students learning remotely perform as well on standardized tests as students in traditional classrooms?

Each type of question can lead to important decisions that affect outcomes, such as patient recovery, organizational effectiveness, and nursing competency. The best answers and consequently the best decisions come from informed, evidence-based analysis of each situation. See Box 5.1 for a list of questions to assist the nurse in the process of evidence-based decision making for various nursing scenarios.

FINDING EVIDENCE TO ANSWER NURSING QUESTIONS

Nurses rely on various sources to answer clinical questions such as those cited previously. A practicing staff nurse might consult a nurse with more experience, more education, or a higher level of authority to get help in answering such questions. Institutional standards or policy and procedure manuals are also a common reference source for nurses in practice. Nursing coworkers or other health care providers, such as physicians, pharmacists, or therapists, might also be consulted. Although all of these approaches are extremely common, they are more likely to yield clinical answers that are *tradition-based* rather than *evidence-based*.

If evidence-based practice is truly based on best evidence, nursing expertise, and the values and preferences of patients, then local expertise and tradition is not sufficient. However, the optimal source of best evidence is often a matter of controversy.

Discussion Point

In your preferred area of nursing specialization, what are some key questions and decisions that nurses address on a daily basis? What are the best sources of evidence for answering clinical questions?

Research is generally considered a more reliable source of evidence than traditions or the clinical expertise of individuals. However, many experts argue that some types of research are better or stronger forms of evidence than others. In medicine and pharmacology, the *randomized controlled trial* (RCT) has been considered the gold standard of clinical evidence. RCTs yield the strongest statistical evidence regarding the effectiveness of an intervention in comparison with other interventions or a placebo. For many clinical questions in medicine and pharmacy, there may be multiple RCTs in the literature addressing a single question, such as the effectiveness of a particular drug. In such situations, an even stronger form of evidence is an *integrative review* or *meta-analysis* wherein the results of several similar research studies are combined or synthesized to provide the most comprehensive answer to the question.

In nursing literature, RCTs, meta-analyses, and integrative reviews are significantly less common than in medical or pharmaceutical literature. For many clinical questions in nursing, RCTs may not exist or they may not even be appropriate. For example, if a nurse is considering how best to prepare a patient for endotracheal suctioning, it would be helpful to inform the patient what suctioning feels like. This

BOX 5.1   **Key Questions to Ask When Considering Evidence-Based Practices**

- Why have we always done it this way?
- Do we have an evidence-based rationale? Or is this practice merely based on tradition?
- Is there a better (more effective, faster, safer, less expensive, more comfortable) method?
- What approach does the patient (or the target group) prefer?
- What do experts in this specialty recommend?
- What methods are used by leading, or benchmark, organizations?
- Do the findings of recent research suggest an alternative method?
- Is there a review of the research on this topic?
- Are there nationally recognized standards of care, practice guidelines, or protocols that apply?
- Are organizational barriers inhibiting the application of evidence-based practice in this situation?

type of question does not lend itself to an RCT but rather to descriptive or qualitative research. In general, qualitative, descriptive, or quasi-experimental studies are much more common methods of inquiry in nursing research than RCTs or meta-analyses. Furthermore, the body of nursing research overall is newer and less developed than that of some other health disciplines. Thus, for many clinical nursing questions, research studies may not exist.

Although research results are usually considered the optimal form of evidence, many other data sources have been used to support the identification of optimal interventions for nursing and other health care disciplines. Some additional sources are:

- Benchmarking data
- Clinical expertise
- Cost-effectiveness analyses
- Infection control data
- Medical record review data
- National standards of care
- Pathophysiologic data
- Quality improvement data
- Patient and family preferences

Another dilemma for the practicing nurse is the time, access, and expertise needed to search and analyze the research literature to answer clinical questions. Few practicing nurses have the luxury of leaving their patients to conduct a literature search. Many staff nurses practicing in clinical settings have less education than a baccalaureate degree; therefore, many have not been exposed to a formal research course. Findings from research studies are typically technical, difficult to understand, and even more difficult to translate into applications. Searching, finding, critiquing, and summarizing research findings for applications in practice are high-level skills that require substantial education and practice.

Discussion Point

If a practicing nurse has no formal education or experience related to research, what strategies should they use to find evidence that answers clinical questions and supports evidence-based practice?

SUPPORTING EVIDENCE-BASED PRACTICE

In light of the challenges of providing or implementing evidence-based practice, nurses must consider some

BOX 5.2 Mechanisms to Promote Evidence-Based Practice

- Garner administrative support.
- Collaborate with a research mentor.
- Seek assistance from professional librarians.
- Search for sources that have already been reviewed or the research summarized.
- Access resources from professional organizations.
- Benchmark with high-performing teams, units, or institutions.

alternative support mechanisms when searching for the best evidence to support their practice. Recommended mechanisms of support are summarized in Box 5.2.

Garner Administrative Support

The first strategy is to garner administrative support. The implementation of evidence-based practice should not be an individual, staff nurse–level pursuit. Administrative support is needed to access the resources, provide the support personnel, and sanction the necessary changes in policies, procedures, and practices. Recently, nursing administrators have had increased incentives to support evidence-based practice because this approach to care has become recognized as the standard expectation of organizations, such as The Joint Commission (formerly Joint Commission on Accreditation of Healthcare Organizations), which accredits hospitals and other health care institutions. Evidence-based practice is also one of the expectations associated with the highly regarded Magnet Hospital Recognition program. Most nursing administrators who want their institutions to be recognized for providing high-quality care will understand the value of evidence-based practice and should therefore be willing to provide resources to support it.

Collaborate With a Research Mentor

One way nurse administrators can support the use of evidence-based practice is through the provision of nurse experts who can function as research mentors. Advanced practice nurses, nurse researchers, and nursing faculty are examples of nurses who may provide consultation and collaboration to support the process of searching, reviewing, and critiquing research literature and databases to answer clinical questions and identify best practices. Most staff nurses do not have the educational background, research expertise, or time to effectively review and critique extensive research literature in search of the evidence to support

Strategies for the New Nurse to Promote Evidence-Based Practice

- Keep abreast of the evidence; subscribe to professional journals and read widely.
- Use and encourage multiple sources of evidence.
- Find established sources of evidence in your specialty.
- Implement and evaluate nationally sanctioned clinical practice guidelines.
- Question and challenge nursing traditions, and promote a spirit of risk-taking.
- Dispel myths and traditions not supported by evidence.
- Collaborate with other nurses locally and globally.
- Interact with other disciplines to bring nursing evidence to the table.

evidence-based practice. Research mentors can assist with these processes, whereas staff nurses can often provide the best insight on clinical needs and patient preferences. Box 5.3 includes a list of strategies for the new graduate nurse to promote evidence-based practice.

Seek Assistance From Professional Librarians

Another valuable type of support that is available in academic medical centers and in some smaller institutions is consultation with medical librarians. A skilled librarian can save nurses a tremendous amount of time by providing guidance in the most comprehensive and efficient approaches to search the health care literature to find research studies and other resources to support the implementation of evidence-based practice.

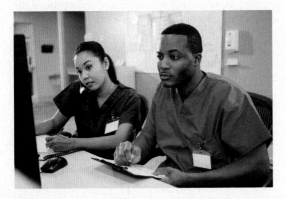

Search Already-Reviewed or Summarized Research

A strategy nurses can use to expedite the search for evidence-based practice is to specifically seek references that have already been reviewed or summarized in the research literature. For example, some journals, such as *Evidence-Based Nursing* and *Worldviews on Evidence-Based Nursing*, specifically focus on providing summaries, critiques, and practice implications of existing nursing research studies. For example, recent issues of *Worldviews on Evidence-Based Nursing* included reviews and summaries on topics like:

- Empowering clinicians during the COVID-19 pandemic
- Preventing surgical site infections
- Transforming organizational culture
- Stress management programs for nurses and nurse assistants

When conducting a literature search, use of keywords, such as "research review" or "meta-analysis," can assist the nurse in identifying published research review articles on the topic of interest.

The *Cochrane Collaboration* is a large international organization composed of several interdisciplinary teams of research scholars that are continuously conducting reviews of research on a wide variety of clinical topics. The Cochrane Collaboration promotes the use of evidence-based practice around the world. Cochrane reviews tend to focus heavily on evaluating the effectiveness of medical interventions, for example, comparing the effects of different medications for specific conditions. Therefore, many of the Cochrane review summaries are more useful for primary care providers, such as physicians and nurse practitioners, than for staff nurse clinicians. Some of the Cochrane projects of interest to nurses in direct care positions include their reviews of products designed to prevent pressure injuries, nursing interventions for smoking cessation, interventions to help patients follow medication regimens, and interventions to promote collaboration between nurses and physicians.

Access Resources From Professional Organizations

Professional nursing organizations can also provide a wealth of resources to support evidence-based practice. For example, the American Association of Critical-Care Nurses (AACN) publishes several "practice alerts" that are relevant to nursing care in critical care units. These documents are based on extensive literature reviews conducted by national panels of nurse researchers and advanced practice nurses. They provide concise recommendations focused on areas where current common practices should change on the basis of the latest research. Some of the topics covered in these alerts include pain assessment in the critically ill adult, ST-segment monitoring, and oral care for critically ill patients.

The Association of Women's Health, Obstetric and Neonatal Nurses (AWHONN, 2020) also provides resources to support evidence-based practice. For example, AWHONN produces evidence-based practice briefs, which include quick reference guides that should be incorporated into clinical practice, including the rationale for these practice changes.

The Association of periOperative Registered Nurses (AORN), the Oncology Nursing Society (ONS), and STTI provide web-based resources to facilitate implementation of evidence-based practice as well. AORN has published *Guidelines for Perioperative Practice*, the ONS published *ONS Guidelines*, and STTI provides web-based continuing education programs and several supportive publications, including *Worldviews on Evidence-Based Nursing*.

Benchmark With High-Performing Teams, Units, or Institutions

Finally, nurses can use benchmarking strategies to poll nurse experts from high-performing teams, units, or institutions to learn more about their practices for specific clinical problems or patient populations. Leaders of professional nursing organizations, such as STTI or the National Association of Clinical Nurse Specialists, can help nurses locate and contact established nurse experts in various areas of specialization. Accrediting organizations, such as The Joint Commission, can assist in identifying institutions that are known as national leaders in providing specific types of care. The University of Iowa, Ohio State University, and McMaster University of Ontario are three North American institutions that have established reputations as leaders in evidence-based nursing practice.

Discussion Point

What institutions, units, teams, or individuals can you identify in your region that would be considered regional or national benchmark leaders in the provision of a specialized type of medical or nursing care?

CHALLENGES AND OPPORTUNITIES: STRATEGIES FOR CHANGING PRACTICE

Nurses use several mechanisms for incorporating new research into current practice in the pursuit of promoting evidence-based practice. Perhaps the most common mechanism is through the development and refinement of research-based policies and procedures. Fortunately, The Joint Commission has mandated that health care institutions must implement formal processes for reviewing the latest research and ensuring that institutional policies and procedures are consistently revised in keeping with current research findings.

Protocols, algorithms, decision trees, standards of care, critical pathways, care maps, and institutional clinical practice guidelines are additional mechanisms used to incorporate new evidence into clinical practice. Each of these formats is used by health care teams to guide clinical decision making and clinical interventions. Although nurses often take the lead in developing or revising these standards and the related procedures, participation and buy-in from the interdisciplinary health care team are essential to achieve successful implementation and consistent changes in practice.

Discussion Point

When the investigation reveals a need for an evidence-based change in practice, what strategies are useful for implementing change?

In addition to consensus from the interdisciplinary team, support from patients and their families is important. This element of the evidence-based practice process is frequently overlooked or not thoroughly considered. As previously mentioned, evidence-based nursing practice involves "an integration of the best evidence available, nursing expertise, and the values and preferences of the individuals, families and communities who are served" (STTI, 2005, p. 1).

If the review of evidence leads the health care team to recommend an intervention that is inconsistent with the patient's values and preferences (such as a specific dietary modification or transfusion of blood products), the recommendation may lead to poor adherence or total disregard by the patient. This situation can also result in loss of the patient's trust and confidence in the health care team.

Discussion Point

Can you think of situations in which the latest research may be inconsistent with the values of an individual or group of patients?

Discussion Point

What obstacles would limit your involvement in pursuing evidence-based practice?

Challenges to Implementing Evidence-Based Practice

Although evidence-based practice is promoted by nurses around the world, several obstacles continue to inhibit the movement. Funk et al. (1991) originally studied this problem in 1991 and developed a survey instrument to quantify those barriers. Spiva et al. (2017) used this instrument in their implementation of a mentoring program to promote evidence-based practice. Practicing nurses often feel overwhelmed by the volume of research on their topics of interest, and they often lack the time and experience to be able to efficiently read and synthesize that literature. They also struggle with the political challenges of attempting to change long-standing policies and procedures in their clinical settings. Still other nurses are not aware that evidence-based practice tools like clinical practice guidelines even exist (Weller et al., 2019). See Research Fuels the Controversy 5.1. Other researchers have investigated the barriers to implementing evidence-based practices and guidelines with similar findings. Advanced practice nurses, such as clinical nurse specialists, nurse practitioners, and clinical nurse leaders, can help to educate, empower, and support staff nurses through this process.

CONCLUSIONS

Many nurses are experiencing success in promoting evidence-based practice. Organizations such as the Cochrane Collaboration provide support to help clinicians overcome some barriers, such as difficulties in obtaining and understanding research reports and the lack of time to synthesize research findings into recommended practices. The many agencies that support teams of research experts to collect, critique, and summarize the research and other forms of evidence pave the way for frontline clinicians to find and adopt evidence-based practices.

Yet challenges continue. Too few nurses understand what evidence-based practice is about. Organizational cultures may not support the nurse who seeks out and uses research to change long-standing practices rooted in tradition rather than science. In addition, a stronger connection is needed between researchers and academics who study evidence-based nursing practice and staff nurses who must translate those findings into the art of nursing practice. Nursing cannot afford to value the art of nursing over the science. Both are critical to making sure that patients receive the highest quality of care possible.

Research Fuels the Controversy 5.1

Barriers and Enablers to the Use of Venous Leg Ulcer Clinical Practice Guidelines in Australian Primary Care: A Qualitative Study Using the Theoretical Domains Framework

The prevalence and cost of venous leg ulcers represent a common problem in primary care. Despite the problem, an evidence-based practice gap exists. While research studies support that clinical practice guidelines (CPGs) for the management of venous leg ulcers can significantly improve outcomes and reduce associated costs, barriers continue to exist in the use of these guidelines in primary care. These CPGs highlight: (1) skilled assessment, examination, and compression treatment; (2) need to exclude arterial insufficiency prior to compression application by measuring the ankle-brachial pressure index or referral to a specialist to exclude arterial insufficiency; and (3) following diagnosis, treatment is below-knee multicomponent compression therapy. The authors conducted a qualitative study using semistructured, face-to-face and telephone interviews with primary care providers.

Source: Weller, C. D., Richards, C., Turnour, L., Patey, A. M., Russell, G., & Teama, V. (2019). Barriers and enablers to the use of venous leg ulcer clinical practice guidelines in Australian primary care: A qualitative study using the theoretical domains framework. *International Journal of Nursing Studies*, 103503. https://doi.org/10.1016/j.ijnurstu.2019.103503

Study Findings

Both barriers and the lack of enablers to the use of venous leg ulcer CPGs in primary care were identified. The most important barrier was that primary care health providers were not aware of the CPG.

For Additional Discussion

1. Can decision support tools such as algorithms, decision trees, clinical pathways, and standardized clinical guidelines ever replace clinical judgment?

2. What causes the disconnection between nurse researchers or faculty studying evidence-based practice and the nurses who seek to implement such research into their practice? Is the problem a lack of communication?

3. Do most nurses have access to evidence-based nursing research findings?

4. Are evidence-based practice findings consistent over time? Can you identify an evidence-based practice that was later found to be ineffective or inappropriate?

5. Should evidence-based practices be institution-specific or should they be more generalizable across different settings?

6. Is evidence-based nursing research grounded more in quantitative or qualitative research? Are both needed?

7. What can be done to increase the research knowledge base of practicing registered nurses given that a significant proportion of those nurses have been educated at the associate degree level?

References

Association of Women's Health, Obstetric and Neonatal Nursing. (2020). *Practice briefs*. Retrieved November 1, 2020, from https://awhonn.org/practice-briefs/

Davies, C., Summers, E., Clarke, V., Mooney, G., Maher, K., Twohig, M., Sharkey, P., Lavern, M., & Furlong, E. (2019). Developing clinical guidelines for the management of menopausal symptoms in breast cancer survivors: Process evaluation. *International Journal of Integrated Care, 19*(4), 229. https://doi.org/10.5334/ijic.s3229

Davis, M. D., Jones, A., Jaynes, M. E., Woodrum, K. N., Canaday, M., Allen, L., & Mallow, J. A. (2020). Designing a multifaceted telehealth intervention for a rural population using a model for developing complex interventions in nursing. *BMC Nursing, 19*(9). https://doi.org/10.1186/s12912-020-0400-9

Funk, S. G., Champagne, M. T., Wiese, R. A., & Tornquist, E. M. (1991). Barriers to using research findings in practice: The clinician's perspective. *Applied Nursing Research, 4*(2), 90–95. https://doi.org/10.1016/S0897-1897(05)80062-X

Hellyar, M., Madani, C., Yeaman, S., O'Connor, K., Kerr, K. M., & Davidson, J. E. (2019). Case study investigation decreases burnout while improving interprofessional teamwork, nurse satisfaction, and patient safety. *Critical Care Nursing Quarterly, 42*(1), 96–105. https://doi.org/10.1097/CNQ.0000000000000243

Lavenberg, J. G., Cacchione, P. Z., Jayakumar, K. L., Leas, B. F., Mitchell, M. D., Mull, N. K., & Umscheid, C. A. (2019). Impact of a hospital evidence-based practice center (EPC) on nursing policy and practice. *Worldviews on Evidence-Based Nursing, 16*(1), 4–11. https://doi.org/10.1111/wvn.12346

Lukes, T., Schjodt, K., & Struwe, L. (2019). Implementation of a nursing-based order set: Improved antibiotic administration

times for pediatric ED patients with therapy-induced neutropenia and fever. *Journal of Pediatric Nursing, 46*, 78–82. https://doi.org/10.1016/j.pedn.2019.02.028 0882-5963/

Melnyk, B. M., & Fineout-Overholt, E. (2019). *Evidence-based practice in nursing & healthcare: A guide to best practice* (4th ed.). Wolters Kluwer Health.

Melnyk, B. M., Gallagher-Ford, L., Zellefrow, C., Tucker, S., Thomas, B., Sinnott, L. T., & Tan, A. (2018). The first U.S. study on nurses' evidence-based practice competencies indicates major deficits that threaten healthcare quality, safety, and patient outcomes. *Worldviews on Evidence-Based Nursing, 15*(1), 16–25. https://doi.org/10.1111/wvn.12269

Moore, W. R., Vermuelen, A., Taylor, R., Kihara, D., & Wahome, E. (2019). Improving 3-hour sepsis bundled care outcomes: Implementation of a nurse-driven sepsis protocol in the emergency department. *Journal of Emergency Nursing, 45*(6), 690–698. https://doi.org/10.1016/j.jen.2019.05.005

Palese, A., Gonella, S., Grassetti, L., Destrebecq, A., Mansutti, I., Terzoni, S., Lucia Zannini, L., Altini, P., Bevilacqua, A., Brugnolli, A., Ponte, A., De Biasio, L., Fascì, A., Grosso, S., Mantovan, F., Marognolli, O., Nicotera, R., Randon, G., Tollini, M., … Dimonte, V. (2018). Multilevel national analysis of nursing students' perceived opportunity to access evidence-based tools during their clinical learning experience. *Worldviews on Evidence-Based Nursing, 15*(6), 480–490. https://doi.org/10.1111/wvn.12328

Ream, E., Hughes, A. E., Cox, A., Skarparis, K., Richardson, A., Pedersen, V. H., Wiseman, T., Forbes, A., & Bryant, A. (2020). Telephone interventions for symptom management in adults with cancer. *Cochrane Database of Systematic Reviews*, (6), CD007568. 10.1002/14651858.CD007568.pub2

Ren, Y., Luo, X., Xie, C., Zhang, P., Meng, M., & Song, H. (2019). Assessment and management of pain during dressing change in patients with diabetic foot ulcers: A best practice implementation project. *JBI Database of Systematic Reviews and Implementation Reports, 17*(10), 2193–2201. https://doi.org/10.11124/JBISRIR-2018-004039

Sackett, D. L., Rosenberg, W. M., Gray, J. A., Haynes, R. B., & Richardson, W. S. (1996). Evidence based medicine: What it is and what it isn't. *British Medical Journal, 312*(7023), 71–72. https://doi.org/10.1136/bmj.312.7023.71

Scheepmans, K., Dierckx de Casterlé, B., Paquay, L., Gansbeke, H. V., & Milisen, K. (2020). Reducing physical restraints by older adults in home care: Development of an evidence-based guideline. *BMC Geriatrics, 20*(169). https://doi.org/10.1186/s12877-020-1499-y

Sichieri, K., Iida, L. I. S., Menezes, I. R. S. C., Garcia, P. C., Santos, T. R. S., Peres, E., Shimoda, G. T., Maia, F. O. M., & Secoli, S. R., & Puschel, V. A. A. (2018). Central line bundle maintenance among adults in a university hospital intensive care unit in São Paulo, Brazil: A best practice implementation project. *JBI Database of Systematic Reviews and Implementation Reports, 16*(6), 1454–1473. https://doi.org/10.11124/JBISRIR-2017-003561

Sigma Theta Tau International. (2005). *Evidence-based nursing position statement*. Retrieved December 10, 2017, from http://www.sigmanursing.org/why-sigma/about-sigma/position-statements-and-resource-papers/evidence-based-nursing-position-statement

Spiva, L., Hart, P. L., Patrick, S., Waggoner, J., Jackson, C., & Threatt, J. L. (2017). Effectiveness of an evidence-based practice nurse mentor training program. *Worldviews on Evidence-Based Nursing, 14*(3), 183–191. https://doi.org/10.1111/wvn.12219

Weller, C. D., Richards, C., Turnour, L., Patey, A. M., Russell, G., & Teama, V. (2019). Barriers and enablers to the use of venous leg ulcer clinical practice guidelines in Australian primary care: A qualitative study using the theoretical domains framework. *International Journal of Nursing Studies,* 103503. https://doi.org/10.1016/j.ijnurstu.2019.103503

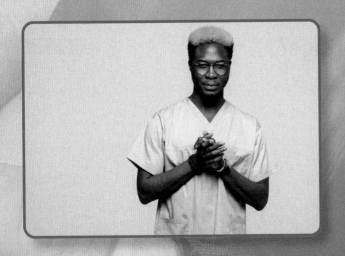

2

WORKFORCE
ISSUES

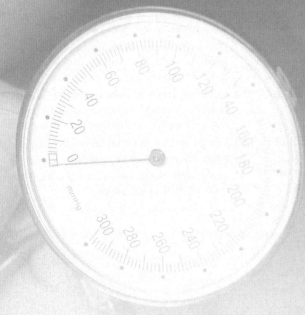

Is There a Nursing Shortage?

Carol J. Huston

LEARNING OBJECTIVES

The learner will be able to:

1. Explore factors affecting the current supply of registered nurses (RNs) in the United States as well as the current and projected demand through 2030.

2. Identify the relationship between nursing shortages and the state of the national economy.

3. Compare regional differences in the supply and demand for RNs in the United States.

4. Address the educational challenges inherent in solving projected nursing shortages given unfilled faculty positions, resignations, projected retirements, low faculty pay schedules, and the shortage of students being prepared for the faculty role.

5. Differentiate between and provide examples of both short- and long-term solutions to nursing shortages.

6. Analyze the impact of salary as an incentive for resolving nursing shortages.

7. Discuss consequences of nursing shortages on quality of health care, working conditions for RNs, and RN retention rates.

8. Outline strategies directed at both supply and demand factors that have been proposed to reduce nursing shortages and analyze the efficacy of each.

9. Identify specific strategies being used to recruit and retain older nurses in the workforce.

10. Reflect upon the personal commitment of RNs to a career in professional nursing.

INTRODUCTION

As government and private insurer reimbursement declined in the 1990s and managed care costs soared, many health care organizations, hospitals in particular, began downsizing to achieve cost containment by eliminating registered nursing jobs or by replacing registered nurses (RNs) with unlicensed assistive personnel. Even hospitals that did not downsize during this period often did little to recruit qualified RNs.

This downsizing and shortsightedness regarding recruitment and retention contributed to the beginning of an acute shortage of RNs in many health care settings by the late 1990s. The health care quality and safety movement also exacerbated this shortage in the late 1990s as research emerged to demonstrate that having more RNs in the staffing mix and smaller RN-to-patient ratios improved patient outcomes. In addition, the public became aware of how important an adequately sized workforce was to patient safety. Unlike earlier nursing shortages, which typically lasted only a few years, this shortage was longer and more severe than earlier nursing shortages. Indeed, even as late as 2010, most states in the United States reported nursing shortages.

When the economy soured, however, late in the first decade of this century, new graduate nurses began struggling to find jobs, and vacancy rates fell at most hospitals across the country. This occurred, at least in part, because many part-time nurses sought fulltime employment and some nurses delayed cutting back on their work hours or seeking retirement. Thus, the economic crisis of a decade ago both eased the nursing shortage and obscured its depth and breadth. As the economy improved, however, fears of a shortage began emerging again though many experts felt that increases in supply due to increasing nursing school enrollments would likely keep up with the increases in the projected retirement of baby boomer (those born between 1946 and 1964) nurses (Caruso, 2020).

New concerns emerged again, however, with the onset of the COVID-19 pandemic in 2020, due to a wave of earlier-than-planned retirements (Arends, 2020). Indeed, fears grew that the virus could diminish the supply of new nurses at the exact time the workforce needed to be growing. In addition, as hospitals began seeing an influx of patients with COVID-19, the older experienced nurses who were desperately needed to help lead their younger colleagues through the crisis were the ones at a higher risk for severe outcomes from COVID-19, increasing the likelihood they would be unable to care for patients or lead younger staff (Caruso, 2020).

Indeed, the World Health Organization (WHO) noted that while nurses are on the front line fighting COVID-19, there is "an alarming failure" in the global supply of protective clothing and new coronavirus tests. Together with "unprecedented" overwork, this is leading to increased global staffing shortages (Narain, 2020). This suggests a vulnerability in nursing workforce numbers that may obscure the more stable workforce projections made just a few months before the emergence of the pandemic.

> **Consider This** The economic crisis late in the first decade of this century both eased and obscured any nursing shortage. The emergence of COVID-19 in 2020 also further obscured and may have increased shortage numbers.

To accurately assess the depth or significance of any current nursing shortage, data must be examined regarding both the demand for RNs and the supply. Assessing the demand for RNs is in many ways more complicated than assessing the supply. However, from an economic perspective, more recent nursing shortages have been driven more by the supply side of the supply/demand equation than the demand side. Supply shortages are more difficult to solve than demand-induced shortages because they require longer-term solutions.

This chapter will explore whether a nursing shortage exists or is likely to occur by examining the present and projected demand for RNs, as well as the supply. In addition, the potential consequences of an unaddressed shortage will be examined with strategies needed to keep the shortage from increasing.

THE DEMAND FOR NURSES

Demand is defined by *Merriam-Webster* (2021a) as the quantity of a commodity or service wanted at a specified price and time. In the case of nursing, demand is the amount of RNs (the good or service) that an employer (the consumer) would be willing to acquire at a given price. A shortage occurs when employers want more employees at the current market wages than they can get. Demand then is derived from the health status of a population and the use of health services.

The demand for professional nurses in both the short- and long-term future appears to be high. In fact, in 2019, nursing was ranked as the third highest in-demand job of any profession in the United States, and this trend shows no signs of slowing down (Nurse Journal, 2020). Indeed, according to the Bureau of Labor Statistics' Employment Projections 2016–2026, registered nursing is listed among the top occupations in terms of job growth through 2026 (American Association of Colleges of Nursing [AACN],

2021a). Indeed, the RN workforce is expected to grow from 2.9 million in 2016 to 3.4 million in 2026, an increase of 438,100 or 15%. In addition, the Bureau also projects the need for an additional 203,700 new RNs each year through 2026 to fill newly created positions and to replace retiring nurses (AACN, 2021a). Similarly, in a 2017 report, the National Center for Health Workforce Analysis projected that by 2030, the number of RNs needed in the United States would skyrocket by 28.4% from 2.8 million to 3.6 million ("The States with the Largest Nursing Shortages," 2020).

While most states are projected to keep up with demand, some states are expected to have significant shortages in RNs. The National Center for Health Workforce Analysis report noted that California is expected to have the greatest shortage of RNs (45,500), while Alaska is projected to have the most job vacancies (22.7%). Texas, New Jersey, South Carolina, Georgia, and South Dakota are expected to experience shortages as well. Florida will have the most extra nurses (53,700), along with Ohio, Virginia, and New York. Wyoming will have the biggest overage of RNs (50.9%) followed by New Mexico and Ohio ("The States with the Largest Nursing Shortages," 2020).

> *Consider This* While the number of nurses employed is expected to grow by 7% between 2019 and 2029 (Bureau of Labor Statistics, 2020b), at least 500,000 nurses are expected to retire by the year 2022 (American Nurses Association, n.d.). As a result, the U.S. Bureau of Labor Statistics projects the need for 1.1 million new RNs for expansion and replacement of retirees and to avoid a nursing shortage.

CAUSES OF INCREASED DEMAND

There are multiple factors driving the demand for RNs, including a growing population, medical advances that increase the need for adequately educated nurses, and the increased acuity of hospitalized patients. Other factors driving demand are the technologic advances in patient care and an increasing emphasis on health care prevention.

In addition, a growing older adult population with extended longevity and more chronic health conditions requires more nursing care. As life expectancy in the United States increases, more nurses will be needed to assist the individuals who are surviving serious illnesses and living longer with chronic diseases. The American Association of Colleges of Nursing (AACN, 2021a) concurs, suggesting that as baby boomers enter their retirement years, their demand for care will escalate. As a result, the demand for health care is expected to steadily increase in the next few decades, and the numbers of nurses to care for these patients will lag.

In addition, Spurlock (2020) notes that continuing spikes in COVID-19 infections due to premature ending of social distancing will continue to stress and overwhelm hospitals and health systems, locally and regionally, as outbreaks move from place to place within the country until effective treatments or vaccines become widespread. For example, Oklahoma has experienced a nursing shortage for decades, but the pandemic further exacerbated the problem (Sweeney, 2020).

THE SUPPLY OF NURSES

Supply refers to the quantity of goods or services that are ready for use or purchase (*Merriam-Webster*, 2021b). As of September 2020, hospitals employed about 60% of working nurses. Of these, 18% worked in ambulatory care services, 7% in nursing and residential care facilities, 5% in government, and 3% in educational services (Bureau of Labor Statistics, 2020c).

To evaluate the supply of RNs in the United States, it is necessary to look at both RNs who are currently working and those who are eligible to work but do not. In addition, the current and potential student pool must be part of the supply discussion.

As of April 2020, the United States had 3,059,800 RNs filling just under 3 million jobs (Bureau of Labor Statistics, 2020a). Despite declining vacancy rates, particularly at hospitals, the RN population does not appear to be large enough to meet either short- or long-term needs in hospitals or other health care settings. This is because the supply of RNs is expected to grow in the coming decade, but large numbers of nurses are also expected to retire.

In fact, the American Nurses Association (ANA) estimates that 23% or 187,200 RNs plan to retire in the next 2 to 3 years, and an additional 81,900 will switch to part-time status. Faller (2020) suggests that this tsunami of retirements among baby boomer nurses will create a particular drain on clinical expertise and institutional knowledge, which are critical to quality patient care and organizational success for health care providers.

Actual turnover in acute care hospitals for bedside nurses in 2020 was 19.5%, up 1.7% from 2019 (Nursing Solutions Inc., 2021). Voluntary terminations accounted for 93.9% of all hospital separations (Nursing Solutions Inc., 2021). Career advancement, relocation, and retirement were the top drivers for turnover in 2020, with retirement moving from 5th place in 2019 to 3rd place in 2020 (Nursing Solutions Inc., 2020). As the U.S. population ages, however, health care organizations should expect retirement to increase even further, a driving force for future separations.

High turnover is also expensive. Nursing Solutions Inc. (2021) suggests that while only 57% of hospitals track the actual cost of turnover, the average cost of turnover for a bedside nurse in 2020 was $40,038, with a range of $28,400 to $51,700 resulting in the average hospital losing $5.1 million dollars per year. Each percent change in RN turnover costs will cost/save the average hospital $270,800 (Nursing Solutions Inc., 2021). In addition, the average time to fill an RN vacancy in 2020 ranged from 66 to 126 days, depending on specialty (Nursing Solutions Inc., 2021).

In addition, with the risks and impacts of COVID-19 on RNs already in the workforce becoming apparent in 2020, especially for older nurses (Buerhaus et al., 2020), the extent to which nurses leaving the workforce—and perhaps the profession—earlier than planned due to psychological trauma and possibly physical disability will only exacerbate any current nursing shortages (Spurlock, 2020).

> **Consider This** Supply shortages are more difficult to solve than demand-induced shortages because they require longer-term solutions.

Nursing as a "Graying" Population

One factor impacting supply is the aging nursing workforce. Indeed, nursing is a "graying" population—even more so than the population at large. The median age of U.S. nurses is 46 years, and older nurses make up the largest age group in the nursing profession at around 25% ("What Is the Average Age," 2021). An online nursing forum noted that most nurses expect to retire in their 50s ("What Is the Average Age," 2021). This means that the nursing workforce will be retiring at a rate faster than it can be replaced.

Given the demographics of the nursing workforce, an aging pattern is expected to continue over the next decade. Indeed, the average age of the working nurse has been increasing for some time, reflecting a two- to three-decade-long trend toward older students entering nursing education programs. According to a 2017 study by Dr. Peter Buerhaus and colleagues, 1 million RNs will retire by 2030, and "the departure of such a large cohort of experienced RNs means that patient care settings and other organizations that depend on RNs will face a significant loss of nursing knowledge and expertise that will be felt for years to come" (AACN, 2021b, para. 3).

> ### Discussion Point
> Why is there so little discussion about the "expertise gap" that will occur as a result of impending nursing retirements? What factors have led to the "graying" of the nursing workforce? Does there appear to be any short-term resolution of these factors?

In addition, nursing faculty are even older than the nursing population at large. The average age of nursing faculty members continues to increase, narrowing the number of productive years nurse educators can teach. The AACN (2021b) notes in their *2019–2020 Salaries of Instructional and Administrative Nursing Faculty* that the average ages of doctorally prepared nurse faculty holding the ranks of professor, associate professor, and assistant professor were 62.6, 56.9, and 50.9 years, respectively. For master's degree–prepared nurse faculty, the average ages for professors, associate professors, and assistant professors were 57.1, 56.0, and 49.6 years, respectively. The AACN concludes that a wave of faculty retirements is expected across the United States over the next decade.

According to a *Special Survey on Vacant Faculty Positions* released by AACN in October 2018, a total of 1,567 faculty vacancies were identified in a survey of 821 nursing schools with baccalaureate and/or graduate programs across the country (85.7% response rate). Besides the vacancies, schools cited the need to create an additional 133 faculty positions to accommodate student demand. The data show a national nurse faculty vacancy rate of 7.9%. Most of the vacancies (92.8%) were faculty positions requiring or preferring a doctoral degree.

One must question where the faculty will come from to teach the new nurses needed to solve the current shortage. In addition, given the lag time required to educate master's prepared or doctorally prepared faculty, the faculty shortage may end up being the greatest obstacle to solving any short-term nursing shortages. A concerted effort must be made immediately to encourage nurses to return to school for advanced degrees and to provide scholarship support for students interested in teaching careers.

> **Consider This** Even if enough students can be recruited to become nurses, there will likely not be enough faculty to teach them.

Enrollment in Nursing Schools

The number of students enrolled or projected to enroll in nursing programs is also an important factor in getting the full picture of the RN supply. Unfortunately, some schools have closed nursing programs because of funding cuts or to reduce program size. Still others have been forced to turn away potential students because of a lack of faculty. Despite this, enrollment in nursing schools has steadily increased almost every year for the past decade (Table 6.1). These increases, however, are not predicted to be adequate to replace those nurses who will be lost to retirement in the coming decade or to meet the increasing demand for more nurse faculty, researchers, and primary care providers (AACN, 2021b).

TABLE 6.1	Number of Candidates Taking the National Council Licensure Examination for Registered Nurses: First-Time, U.S.-Educated Candidates Only					
Program	**2015**	**2016**	**2017**	**2018**	**2019**	**2020**
Diploma	2,607	2,745	2,222	1,968	1,921	1,931
Baccalaureate	70,857	72,637	75,944	79,235	76,496	79,320
Associate	84,379	81,653	79,511	82,000	76,973	77,508
Total	157,882	157,053	157,720	163,238	214,443	158,797

Sources: National Council of State Boards of Nursing. (2020, October 16). *2020: Number of candidates taking NCLEX examination and percent passing, by type of candidate.* Retrieved January 20, 2020, from https://www.ncsbn.org/Table_of_Pass_Rates_2020_Q3.pdf; National Council of State Boards of Nursing. (2019, October 16). *2019: Number of candidates taking NCLEX examination and percent passing, by type of candidate.* Retrieved September 1, 2020, from https://www.ncsbn.org/table_of_pass_rates_2019.pdf; National Council of State Boards of Nursing. (2019, January 16). *2018: Number of candidates taking NCLEX examination and percent passing, by type of candidate.* Retrieved September 1, 2020, from https://floridasnursing.gov/forms/Table_of_Pass_Rates_2018.pdf; National Council of State Boards of Nursing. (2018, January 19). *2017: Number of candidates taking NCLEX examination and percent passing, by type of candidate.* Retrieved September 1, 2020, from https://www.ncsbn.org/Table_of_Pass_Rates_2017.pdf; National Council of State Boards of Nursing. (2017, January 23). *2016: Number of candidates taking NCLEX examination and percent passing, by type of candidate.* Retrieved September 1, 2020, from https://ncsbn.org/Table_of_Pass_Rates_2016.pdf; National Council of State Boards of Nursing. (2016, January 21). *2015: Number of candidates taking NCLEX examination and percent passing, by type of candidate.* Retrieved September 1, 2020, from https://ncsbn.org/Table_of_Pass_Rates_2015_(3).pdf

Unfortunately, nursing program enrollment increases are not possible without a significant boost in federal and state funding to prepare new faculty, enhance teaching resources, and upgrade nursing school infrastructure. More money is needed in the form of nursing scholarships and loans to encourage young people to enter nursing. In addition, individual nurses and professional organizations must support legislation to improve financial access to nursing education. The Tri-Council for Nursing (comprising the AACN, the ANA, the American Organization for Nursing Leadership, the National Council of State Boards of Nursing, and the National League for Nursing [NLN]) has urged nurses to advocate for increased nursing education funding under Title VIII of the Public Health Service Act, as well as other publicly funded initiatives, so that there will be the necessary capacity and resources to educate future nurses.

There have been increases in federal money for nursing education over the last decade. The passage of legislation such as the 2002 Nurse Reinvestment Act encouraged more students to choose nursing as a career and helped students financially to complete their education. It also encouraged graduate students to complete their studies and assume teaching positions in nursing schools. In addition, many states introduced or passed legislation designed to improve working conditions and attract more nurses.

In addition, some hospitals have joined forces with local schools of nursing to offer scholarships in exchange for a student's willingness to work in that institution after graduation. Hospitals are also lending master's prepared and doctorally prepared nurses such as nurse practitioners, clinical nurse specialists, and clinical nurse leaders to supplement faculty positions.

Private foundations have also stepped up to offer funding for nursing education. For example, in 2008, the Robert Wood Johnson Foundation (RWJF, 2016) joined with the AACN to create the RWJF New Careers in Nursing. Through grants to schools of nursing, the program has provided scholarships of $10,000 each annually to more than 3,500 scholars. Similarly, foundations set up by nursing organizations such as the Association of periOperative Registered Nurses, the National Student Nurses' Association, and the ANA provide scholarships and financial assistance to students and RNs pursuing degrees in nursing.

Recruitment efforts into the nursing profession in the last decade have been successful, and the problem is no longer a lack of nursing school applicants. Indeed, enrollment in nursing programs of education has increased steadily since 2001. The problem is that there are inadequate resources to provide nursing education to those interested in pursuing nursing as a career, including an insufficient number of clinical sites, classroom space, nursing faculty, and clinical preceptors. As a result, qualified applicants are turned away despite the current shortage of nurses.

Indeed, the AACN (2021b) reported that U.S. nursing schools turned away 75,029 qualified applicants from baccalaureate and graduate nursing programs in 2018 because of an insufficient number of faculty, clinical sites, classroom space, clinical preceptors, and budget constraints. Most nursing schools responding to the survey pointed to faculty shortages as a reason for not accepting all qualified applicants into baccalaureate programs. Robert Rosseter, spokesman for the AACN, called it a "catch 22 situation," noting a tremendous demand from hospitals and clinics to hire more nurses as well as a tremendous demand from students who want to enter nursing programs. Yet schools cannot accommodate either demand (Kavilanz, 2018).

Educational costs are also a deterrent to increasing nursing school enrollment. Nursing is often called an "expensive major" given relatively low faculty-to-student ratios in clinical courses and the need for financially strapped states to subsidize the cost of education at state universities.

Discussion Point

Should the increased cost of nursing education be passed on to students? Would students enrolled in public universities be willing to pay more for their education than students in other majors?

The greatest challenge, however, to increasing nursing school enrollment is an inadequate number of nursing faculty to teach students interested in pursuing nursing as a career. According to an October 2018 *Special Survey on Vacant Faculty Positions* released by the AACN (2021b), a total of 1,715 faculty vacancies were identified in a survey of 872 nursing schools with baccalaureate and/or graduate programs across the country (85.8% response rate). Besides the vacancies, schools cited the need to create an additional 138 faculty positions to accommodate student demand. The data show a national nurse faculty vacancy rate of 7.9%. Most of the vacancies (90.7%) were faculty positions requiring or preferring a doctoral degree. Most schools identify difficulty finding doctorally prepared faculty and noncompetitive salaries as roots of the problem (AACN, 2021b).

Research conducted by the NLN (n.d.) and the Carnegie Foundation Preparation for the Professions Program supports AACN's assertions. This research found aging, overworked faculty earning far less than nurses entering clinical practice. In fact, this study reported that nurse faculty earned less than faculty in other academic disciplines and that they earned far less than their RN counterparts in clinical practice. This lack of competitive pay for nurse educators is a significant obstacle to recruiting new nursing faculty.

At the professor rank, nurse educators suffered the largest deficit, with salaries averaging 45% lower than those of their non-nurse colleagues. Associate and assistant nursing professors were also at a disadvantage, earning 19% and 15% less than similarly ranked faculty in other fields. Those employed as nursing instructors experienced the only advantage, with salaries averaging 8% higher than those of non-nurses (NLN, n.d., para. 2).

Increasing the number of nursing students in the pipeline as a strategy for addressing the current nursing shortage depends on having enough qualified faculty to teach them. Clearly, the same energy that was directed at recruiting young people for nursing must now be directed at recruiting nursing faculty.

In response, programs have been created both to encourage nurses to consider careers in nursing education and to support them in that role. For example, the Division of Labor Workforce Investment Act has created a Faculty Loan Repayment Program for nurses willing to serve in faculty roles after graduation. Furthermore, the National Institute of Nursing Research, the Agency for Health Care Research and Quality, Department of Veterans Affairs, and some private foundations have funds available to enhance nursing education and faculty development.

In addition, AACN and the Johnson & Johnson Campaign for Nursing's Future announced the creation of a Minority Nurse Faculty Scholars program in 2008 (AACN, 2021b). This program seeks to address the nursing faculty shortage and diversity of the faculty population by providing financial support to graduate nursing students from minority backgrounds who agree to teach in a school of nursing after graduation. In late 2012, the Jonas Nurse Leaders Scholar Program expanded nationally and now provides funding and support to 198 doctoral nursing students in 87 schools across the United States, making it one of the largest programs addressing the nation's dire shortage of doctorally prepared nursing faculty (AACN, 2021b).

Other long-term strategies for addressing the nursing faculty shortage are shown in Box 6.1.

Consider This   Unfilled faculty positions, resignations, and projected retirements continue to pose a threat to the nursing education workforce.

Using Foreign-Born Nurses to Relieve the Shortage

Nursing shortages have been alleviated at least in part by bringing in RNs from foreign markets, and widespread, transnational nursing migration was expected to continue for some time given the success hospitals have had with foreign recruitment and the time required to strengthen the domestic nurse supply pipeline. The emergence of COVID-19 in 2020 may, however, reduce the availability of foreign-born nurses to relieve nursing shortages in the

---

BOX 6.1   **Long-Term Strategies for Addressing the Nursing Faculty Shortage**

1. Recruitment
   - Provide a positive image for a career in nursing education.
   - Provide incentives for part-time and adjunct faculty to return to school to earn doctoral degrees.
   - Provide fellowships or tuition forgiveness in exchange for teaching service.
   - Develop mentoring and support programs for new academics.
2. Retention
   - Provide salaries and benefits for nursing faculty similar to those of nonacademic settings.
   - Establish positive work environments and reasonable teaching assignments.
   - Recognize and reward teaching excellence.
   - Create academic environments that foster innovation.
   - Fund faculty development and mentorship programs.
3. Collaboration
   - Partner with health care stakeholders to create support for higher education in nursing.

---

short-term future (Narain, 2020). Although two major suppliers of nursing staff globally—the Philippines and India—train more health professionals than they need, in the knowledge that many will work abroad, the two countries are now encountering potentially significant "emerging shortages" within their own national health services.

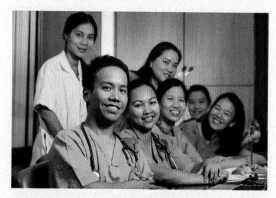

In addition, using foreign-born labor has complex international implications, creating a drain on some countries' health care systems while shoring up the economies of countries that purposefully export their workers through remittance income. Because hiring foreign-born nurses has such complex ramifications, Chapter 7 is devoted to this discussion.

ROOTS OF NURSING SHORTAGE

Many factors contribute to the current nursing shortage in acute care settings, including an aging workforce, high turnover because of worker dissatisfaction, inadequate long-term pay incentives, and an increasing recognition by

nurses that they can make more money and act more autonomously as free agents than as fulltime employees of a health care organization. These factors and others (Box 6.2) will be discussed in this section.

The Free Agent Nurse

An increase in the number of free agent nurses is another aspect that must be examined in assessing supply and demand factors of the current nursing shortage. Fulltime employment of nurses is decreasing. Instead, nurses are increasingly assuming the role of free agent, and this contributes to an RN shortage in acute care agencies. A *free agent* nurse is often an independent contractor who contracts their services with an employer with the condition that they maintain control over the number of hours they are willing to work and their working conditions.

Per diem and *traveling nurses* are two types of free agents. The relationship between the free agent and their employing organization is based on a free and open exchange, more of a partnership than an unequal dependency relationship. Typically, the free agent nurse makes a higher hourly wage than other fulltime or part-time employees in a health care organization in exchange for not receiving health care and retirement benefits. Such nurses also have greater control over if and when they want to work.

Historically, health care organizations sought to employ fulltime workers (employees) so that they could better control the availability of needed human resources. However, the free agent model of nursing is gaining momentum in health care organizations as they recognize that they need to supplement their fulltime employee pool with these skilled workers and that significant benefit costs can be saved from using free agent or temporary workers.

Causes of the Current Nursing Shortage

- Increasing older adult population (more individuals who have chronic illnesses)
- Increased acuity in acute care settings, requiring higher-level nursing skills
- Downsizing and restructuring of the late 1990s, which eliminated many RN positions
- A relatively healthy economy in the late 1990s and early 2000s, which encouraged some nurses to change from full-time employment to part-time or to quit
- An aging RN workforce
- Workplace dissatisfaction
- Women choosing fields other than nursing for a career
- Aging faculty for RN programs
- Inadequate nursing programs to accommodate interested applicants
- Low ceiling on wages for RNs without advanced degrees
- Future educator pool for RNs more limited than demand
- COVID-19 pandemic inducing stress, trauma, and retirement

Critics of the increased use of free agent nurses, particularly traveling nurses, suggest that this practice may negatively affect the quality of care related to inconsistency of caregivers and a reduced ability to determine the competencies of each specific free agent nurse. More research is needed, however, on the effect of the free agent nurse on the current nursing shortage.

Workplace Dissatisfaction

Perhaps one of the most significant yet least addressed factors leading to RN shortages is workplace dissatisfaction, resulting in high turnover levels and nurses leaving the profession entirely. Long shifts, low autonomy, mandatory overtime, a lack of leadership, and being forced to work during weekends, nights, and holidays prompt many nurses to look for other jobs. In addition, many nurses feel they are underpaid for the work they do.

Inadequate staffing also continues to demoralize nurses. Hood (2020) notes that a recent poll conducted by the ANA showed that 68% of nurses fear working when shifts are understaffed. The inability or unwillingness of hospitals to ensure that each shift has a reasonable nurse-to-patient ratio is directly linked to increased risk of nurses experiencing exhaustion, mental illness, and/or posttraumatic stress disorder. This has only worsened with the COVID-19 pandemic during which staff reported relentless work hours under extremely stressful conditions.

As a result, many highly trained, employable nurses are voluntarily leaving the profession. So too are early career registered nurses (ECRNs), those in the first 5 years of their practice. Indeed, ECRNs are at increased risk of leaving the profession due to burnout and role strain (Douglas et al., 2020).

Research by Douglas et al. (2020) reported that ECRNs experienced disorienting dilemmas, unfamiliar situations, and uncertainty in their new role as an RN. The "overnight transition from nursing student to RN" and the unexpected levels of RN responsibility were difficult, and many ECRNs experienced unprofessional bullying or humiliating behavior from senior colleagues, supervisors, and managers. Thus, the experience of being an RN was different from what they had imagined it would be (Research Fuels the Controversy 6.1).

Douglas et al. (2020) concluded that issues impacting but beyond the control of the ECRN must be addressed by nursing leaders to create and preserve workplaces that promote learning, growth, and retention of these novice nurses. In addition, supportive relationships must be provided to help ECRNs navigate these disorienting dilemmas, particularly those involving difficult interactions with colleagues and managers. This will discourage these nurses from leaving both their current employment as well as their chosen profession.

It is important to remember though that some organizational turnover is normal and in fact desirable because it infuses the organization with fresh ideas. It also reduces the probability of *groupthink*, in which everyone shares similar thought processes, values, and goals (Marquis & Huston, 2021). However, excessive or unnecessary turnover is disruptive to organizational functioning and threatens the quality of patient care. Thus, retention becomes a critical goal when workforce shortages exist and the achievement of desired outcomes is critical to organizational success.

Consider This Retention of precious nurse resources must be a real part of the solution to the nursing shortage; health care institutions must make a commitment to improving working conditions for nurses.

Research Fuels the Controversy 6.1

Factors Influencing Early Career Registered Nurse Retention

A purposive sample of 13 Australian early career registered nurses (ECRNs) working in a variety of clinical settings participated in face-to-face, semistructured interviews to explore factors that cause them to stay or leave the nursing profession.

Source: Douglas, J. A., Bourgeois, S., & Moxham, L. (2020, August). Early career registered nurses: How they stay. *Collegian, 27*(4), 437–442. https://doi.org/10.1016/j.colegn.2020.01.004

Study Findings

Participants spoke of two specific and significant disorienting dilemmas as ECRNs. The first resulted from the "overnight transition from nursing student to RN" and the unexpected levels of RN responsibility. The second was "difficult" and "unexpected workplace relationships" involving unprofessional behavior from senior colleagues, supervisors, and managers. ECRNs suggested that the experience of being an RN was very different from what they had imagined it to be.

In addition, balancing the desire to fit in with new colleagues against the need to work effectively as an RN was a challenge shared by most participants. Many described situations of exclusion and isolation in the workplace, where their abilities to work as RNs were questioned because they were university educated, alongside their feelings of needing to prove themselves constantly. Many study participants also described being humiliated in front of other staff, both as students and then as ECRNs.

The researchers concluded that how these dilemmas are approached and managed is significant to whether ECRNs choose to continue working as nurses. Professional, educational, and government bodies with responsibility for the education, regulation, and employment of ECRNs must acknowledge the shared accountability for helping develop, structure, and implement processes to support ECRNs in lifelong and relational learning. In addition, safe learner-centric workplaces must be created that employ zero tolerance for uncivil and bullying behavior.

In addition, not all health care organizations have high turnover rates. Organizations perceived to be employers of choice, such as magnet hospitals, retain their employees and are more capable of replacing losses than less-sought-after employers. Therefore, having a healthy work environment provides an advantage in the competition for scarce nursing resources. Clearly, organizations that pay attention to the employee market and understand what people are looking for in the work environment have a better chance to recruit and retain top talent.

Consider This Nursing shortages cannot be resolved until we address the underlying issues of worker dissatisfaction that caused them in the first place.

Is Pay an Issue?

Salaries also provide mixed incentives for young people to become nurses and for nurse retention. The economy at the end of the 20th century was fairly strong, with low unemployment and rising consumer confidence. This resulted in some RNs, who were often the second income provider in the family unit, reducing their work hours or leaving the workplace entirely. Many of these same RNs, however, returned to work in the past decade because of declining stock market values, a rising recession, and lower levels of consumer confidence.

Wages for RNs have, however, increased with rising demand and threatened shortages. The mean annual wage of RNs as of January 2021 was $65,452 (PayScale, 2021a). As of January 2021, late career nurses, on average, earn more than those at entry level, with $72,922 median annual salary as compared to $56,785, respectively (PayScale, 2021a).

In addition, current average base salaries for U.S. nurse practitioners range from $79,000 to $122,000, with bonuses and profit sharing often adding up to $20,000 additional wages annually (PayScale, 2021b). The average salary of a nurse practitioner across settings and specialties was $97,518 in January 2021 (PayScale, 2021b).

Discussion Point

Historically, nursing has been considered an altruistic profession. How critical do you think pay is as a motivator for people who want to become nurses today?

In contrast to the findings for nurse practitioners, salary is a deterrent for nursing faculty. PayScale (2021c) reported that the median salary in January 2021 for a nurse educator was $76,480. One reason that nursing faculty salaries are poorer comparatively than nurses with graduate degrees in advanced practice roles is that nursing education has never had the same federal funding support as medical education. In addition, securing advanced academic degrees is costly. Indeed, many graduate students who may have become educators in the past are now opting instead for better-paying positions in clinical and private practice. Clearly, increasing faculty salaries and providing tuition support for graduate students considering a career as a nursing faculty will be an essential part of addressing the increasing faculty shortage.

Discussion Point

What incentives should be offered to nurses who earn a master's or doctoral degree to become nursing faculty members rather than advanced practice nurses engaged in clinical practice?

CONSEQUENCES OF NURSING SHORTAGES

What are the consequences of a nursing shortage? To answer this question, it is critical first to recognize that patient outcomes are sensitive to nursing interventions and that as a result, nurse staffing (total hours of care as well as staffing mix) affects patient outcomes. This supposition is certainly supported by a review of the literature, which increasingly suggests that RN staffing affects patient outcomes such as inpatient mortality and other measures of quality of hospital care. Indeed, numerous studies have been conducted to describe the relationship between nurse staffing levels and clinical outcomes of patients at both the hospital and unit levels. These studies are summarized in Chapter 11.

ADDITIONAL STRATEGIES FOR SOLVING NURSING SHORTAGE

Just as the issues that caused nursing shortages are complex, so too must be the solutions. Only some of the solutions that have been presented to address the current nursing shortage are included here, including increasing the number of nursing students in the pipeline, increasing the nursing faculty pool, hiring foreign nurses, redesigning the workplace, and improving nursing's image.

Redesigning the Workplace for an Older Workforce

The age of the current nursing workforce is an important factor in the current nursing shortage because nursing can be both physically and mentally taxing, even to those who are young. Some experts have suggested that more attention should be given to retaining older workers or bringing retired nurses back into the workforce because these employees are generally more productive, more reliable, and highly experienced. Indeed, Nursing Solutions Inc. (2021) notes that while most hospitals have strategies in place to retain new hires, only 52.6% have a strategy for retaining older workers. With retirement a major driver of turnover, the retention of the existing older workforce should be a priority.

In addition, experienced nurses possess intellectual capital and institutional memory. If large numbers of this experienced workforce retire all at once, both tacit knowledge and institutional wisdom will be lost (Fackler, 2019). In addition, there will be insufficient mentors for the large numbers of newly licensed nurses entering the workforce (Fackler, 2019).

Some adaptations of the working environment may be needed, however, to meet the needs and limitations of an aging workforce such as flexible work shift options and job sharing. Indeed, recent research by Fackler (2019) found that older nurses want to practice in ways that were still patient focused but to have more options for shorter or fewer hours and less physical demands.

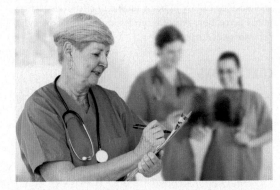

In addition, these older RNs must be made to feel valued, and relationships reflecting collegiality and collaboration should be fostered. In addition, environments of shared governance should be created in which these experienced nurses actively participate in all decision making related to patient care. This need for organizations to foster an environment where older nurses feel respected and heard and where personal and professional needs are addressed was found to be the primary strategy for retaining older workers in an integrative literature review completed by Markowski et al. (2020). The study also found that supervisors must provide support for the aging nurse's professional and personal needs, including flexibility in work schedules, support in retirement preparation, and specific professional development. Additional strategies for retaining older workers are outlined in Box 6.3.

Strategies for Retaining Older Workers

- Flexible shift options with more options for shorter shifts
- Job sharing
- Work redesign to limit physical energy expenditure
- Use of lift teams, special beds, and equipment to reduce work-related injuries and strain
- Benefit packages that recognize the needs of mature workers
- Recognition and use of experienced workers as mentors and preceptors
- Job design that emphasizes autonomy and empowered decision making

Changing Nursing's Image

In addition, inaccurate and negative stereotypes continue to plague the nursing profession. This may discourage the best and brightest students from pursuing nursing as a career. Changing nursing's public image will not be an easy task, given the historic roots of nursing stereotypes and the profession's long history of being unable to effectively change public perceptions regarding professional nursing roles and behaviors (see Chapter 24).

CONCLUSIONS

Many factors led to a significant professional nursing shortage in the early 21st century and a mitigation of that shortage early in the second decade. This shortage is again recurring as demand increases, an aging workforce retires, and a global pandemic consumes nursing resources. Health care providers, the public, and legislators are beginning to recognize that both the problem and the potential consequences could be severe. One would be hard-pressed to find a congressperson or senator who would not identify health care workforce shortages as one of the most serious issues affecting health care today.

Yet, efforts to proactively address the coming shortage have to date been few and far between. Short-term solutions to the shortage have been attempted, including hiring foreign-born nurses and increasing federal money for nursing education. The passage of current legislation has encouraged more students to choose nursing as a career and has helped students financially to complete their education. It has also encouraged graduate students to complete their studies and assume teaching positions in nursing schools. Long-term planning and aggressive intervention, however, will be needed for some time at the national and regional levels to ensure that an adequate, highly qualified nursing workforce will be available in the future to meet health care needs in the United States.

More must be done to address the projected nursing shortage to come, and it is increasingly clear that multiple solutions to the shortage will be needed. These solutions will require expert thinking and will likely reshape fundamental core underpinnings that have been a part of the nursing work world for decades, if not centuries.

For Additional Discussion

1. In what ways do other professions do a better job of attracting younger workers?
2. Are salaries a significant driver in the current nursing shortage? At what level would salaries not be a factor?
3. How would increasing the educational level for entry into practice affect the current nursing shortage?
4. Will the demand for RNs in the future be affected by growing technologic developments?
5. Why has the nursing workforce historically suffered some degree of a shortage every 10 to 15 years?
6. If magnet hospital criteria (increased number of BSN-educated nurses on staff) become the baseline for organizational structure and performance, would nursing shortages exist?
7. Why are starting salaries for nurses with master's and doctoral degrees in academia so low?
8. Why do many health care organizations choose to expend more money on recruitment than on retention strategies? Which is more effective in the short term and in the long term?
9. Is implementation of mandatory minimum staffing ratios in acute care hospitals likely to reduce the nursing shortage in California?

References

American Association of Colleges of Nursing. (2021a). *Fact sheets: Nursing shortage.* Retrieved September 1, 2020, from http://www.aacnnursing.org/News-Information/Fact-Sheets/Nursing-Shortage

American Association of Colleges of Nursing. (2021b). *Fact sheets: Nursing faculty shortage.* Retrieved September 1, 2020, from http://www.aacnnursing.org/News-Information/Fact-Sheets/Nursing-Faculty-Shortage

American Nurses Association. (n.d.). *Workforce.* Retrieved September 3, 2020, from https://www.nursingworld.org/practice-policy/workforce/

Arends, B. (2020, May 2). *Opinion: COVID-19 crisis sparks 'early retirement' wave.* Retrieved September 3, 2020, from https://www.marketwatch.com/story/covid-19-crisis-sparks-early-retirement-wave-2020-04-30

Buerhaus, P. I., Auerbach, D. I., & Staiger, D. O. (2020). Older clinicians and the surge in novel coronavirus disease 2019 (COVID-19). *JAMA, 323*(18), 1777–1778. https://doi.org/10.1001/jama.2020.4978

Bureau of Labor Statistics, U.S. Department of Labor. (2020a). *Occupational outlook handbook—Registered nurses. Summary.* Retrieved September 1, 2020, from http://www.bls.gov/ooh/Healthcare/Registered-nurses.htm

Bureau of Labor Statistics, U.S. Department of Labor. (2020b). *Occupational outlook handbook—Registered nurses. Job outlook.* Retrieved September 1, 2020, from https://www.bls.gov/ooh/healthcare/registered-nurses.htm#tab-6

Bureau of Labor Statistics, U.S. Department of Labor. (2020c). *Occupational outlook handbook—Registered nurses. Work environment.* Retrieved September 1, 2020, from https://www.bls.gov/ooh/healthcare/registered-nurses.htm#tab-3

Caruso, M. (2020, April 13). *Outlook for nurse supply and demand shifting amid COVID-19. Modern Healthcare, 50*(15), 14.

Douglas, J. A., Bourgeois, S., & Moxham, L. (2020, August). Early career registered nurses: How they stay. *Collegian, 27*(4), 437–442. https://doi.org/10.1016/j.colegn.2020.01.004

Fackler, C. A. (2019). Retaining older hospital nurses: Experienced hospital nurses' perceptions of new roles. *Journal of Nursing Management, 27*(6), 1325–1331. https://doi.org/10.1111/jonm.12814

Faller, M. (2020). *Retirement wave hits: Nursing shortages may worsen.* The Staffing Stream. Retrieved September 1, 2020, from http://www.thestaffingstream.com/2018/01/09/retirement-wave-hits-nursing-shortages-may-worsen/

Hood, S. R. (2020, August 30). *The national nursing shortage has serious ramifications.* Retrieved September 1, 2020, from https://www.mcgowanhood.com/2020/08/31/the-national-nursing-shortage-has-serious-ramifications/

Kavilanz, P. (2018, April 30). *Nursing schools are rejecting thousands of applicants—In the middle of a nursing shortage.* CNN Money. Retrieved September 1, 2020, from http://money.cnn.com/2018/04/30/news/economy/nursing-school-rejections/index.html

Markowski, M., Cleaver, K., & Weldon, S. M. (2020, September). An integrative review of the factors influencing older nurses' timing of retirement. *Journal of Advanced Nursing, 76*(9), 2266–2285. https://doi.org/10.1111/jan.14442

Marquis, B., & Huston, C. (2021). *Leadership roles and management functions in nursing* (10th ed.). Wolters Kluwer.

Merriam-Webster. (2021a). *Demand (definition).* Retrieved January 20, 2021, from https://www.merriam-webster.com/dictionary/demand

Merriam-Webster. (2021b). *Supply (definition).* Retrieved January 21, 2021, from https://www.merriam-webster.com/dictionary/supply

Narain, A. (2020, April 7). *COVID-19 highlights nurses' vulnerability as backbone to health services worldwide.* Retrieved September 3, 2020, from https://news.un.org/en/story/2020/04/1061232

National League for Nursing. (n.d.). *NLN nurse educator shortage fact sheet.* Retrieved September 1, 2020, from http://www.nln.org/docs/default-source/advocacy-public-policy/nurse-faculty-shortage-fact-sheet-pdf.pdf?sfvrsn=0

Nurse Journal. (2020, June 3). *The U.S. nursing shortage: A state-by-state breakdown.* Retrieved September 1, 2020, from https://nursejournal.org/community/the-us-nursing-shortage-state-by-state-breakdown/

Nursing Solutions Inc. (2021). *2020 NSI national health care retention & RN staffing report.* Retrieved September 1, 2020, from https://www.nsinursingsolutions.com/Documents/Library/NSI_National_Health_Care_Retention_Report.pdf

PayScale. (2021a). *Average registered nurse (RN) hourly pay.* Retrieved January 20, 2021, from http://www.payscale.com/research/US/Job=Registered_Nurse_(RN)/Hourly_Rate

PayScale. (2021b). *Average nurse practitioner (NP) salary.* Retrieved January 20, 2021, from http://www.payscale.com/research/US/Job=Nurse_Practitioner_(NP)/Salary

PayScale. (2021c). *Average nurse educator salary.* Retrieved January 20, 2021, from http://www.payscale.com/research/US/Job=Nurse_Educator/Salary

Robert Wood Johnson Foundation. (2016). *New careers in nursing. About.* Retrieved September 1, 2020, from http://www.newcareersinnursing.org/about-ncin.html

Spurlock, D. (2020). The nursing shortage and the future of nursing education is in our hands. *Journal of Nursing Education, 59*(6), 303–304. https://doi.org/10.3928/01484834-20200520-01

Sweeney, C. (2020, August 21). *COVID-19 exacerbates Oklahoma's decades-old nursing shortage.* Retrieved September 3, 2020, from https://stateimpact.npr.org/oklahoma/2020/08/21/covid-19-exacerbates-oklahomas-decades-old-nursing-shortage/

The states with the largest nursing shortages. (2020, October 30). Retrieved January 20, 2021, from https://www.registerednursing.org/largest-nursing-shortages/

What is the average age of retirement for nurses in the United States? (2021). Retrieved January 20, 2021, from https://www.bestmasterofscienceinnursing.com/faq/what-is-the-average-age-of-retirement-for-nurses-in-the-united-states/

Foreign Nurse Migration

Carol J. Huston

CHAPTER OUTLINE

Introduction

Global Migration of Nurses: "Push" and "Pull" Factors

Effects of Global Migration on Developing Countries
    Remittance Income
    Brain Drain

Global Nurse Recruitment and Migration as an Ethical Issue

Professional Organizations Respond

The International Council of Nurses

The International Centre on Nurse Migration

Voluntary Code of Ethical Conduct for International Nurse Recruitment

The World Health Organization

The Mistreatment of Foreign Nurses

Assimilating the Foreign Nurse Through Socialization

The International Community Addresses the Problem
    Some Governments Respond
    U.S. Immigration Policy

Ensuring Competency of Foreign Nurses: Commission on Graduates of Foreign Nursing Schools and the NCLEX-RN Examination

Conclusions

LEARNING OBJECTIVES

The learner will be able to:

1. Examine how the scope of global nurse migration has changed over the last decade.

2. Identify primary donor and recipient countries of migrating nurses.

3. Analyze "push" and "pull" factors that encourage nurses to migrate internationally.

4. Explore potential negative effects of international migration on donor countries, including "brain drain" in donor countries.

5. Apply the ethical principles of autonomy, utility, and justice in arguing for or against global nurse recruitment and migration.

6. Explore the ethical dimensions of nurse migration.

7. Outline common key components of position statements on nurse migration adopted by professional associations such as the International Council of Nurses, the International Centre on Nurse Migration, Academy Health, and the World Health Organization.

8. Explore national and international efforts to develop best practices or regulatory oversight of international nurse recruitment and migration.

9. Discuss the need for ongoing cultural, professional, and psychological support for foreign nurses after

their arrival in a new country to assist them in successful socialization.

10. Differentiate between the types of work visas foreign nurses use to gain entry for employment in the United States.

11. Outline the certification process required by the Commission on Graduates of Foreign Nursing

Schools for migratory nurses to be able to take the National Council Licensure Examination (NCLEX) examination and obtain visas for work in the United States.

12. Reflect on personal beliefs and values regarding the use of widespread international recruitment and nurse migration to address nursing shortages.

INTRODUCTION

Many countries experience cyclic shortages of nurses. Indeed, currently, half of the world does not have an adequate number of nurses. According to the World Health Organization (WHO)'s *State of the World's Nursing 2020* report, there is a projected shortfall of 5.7 million nurses in the global nursing workforce in the coming decade unless nations increase funding to educate and employ more nurses (Stringer, 2020). In addition, even though more than 4 million nurses have been added to the global nursing workforce since 2013, the vast majority are working in countries that account for only half of the world's population. That leaves some countries in the African, Southeast Asian, Eastern Mediterranean, and Latin American regions with severe shortages.

One means of alleviating these shortages, particularly in developed countries, has been to recruit foreign workers. International recruitment and *nurse migration*—moving from one country to another in search of employment—has been viewed as a relatively inexpensive, "quick-fix" solution to health care worker shortages. For example, due to the shortage of qualified health care workers, immigrants held 1% of all registered nursing positions in the United States in 2020 (Narea, 2020). Indeed, developed nations have seen a 60% increase in the number of foreign-educated health care professionals within their borders since 2010 (Zolot, 2019).

Developed countries, such as Australia, the United Kingdom, the United States, Norway, Australia, Ireland, and Saudi Arabia, are the primary destinations of most migrant nurses, and developing nations are primarily the donors. Some developed countries are both a source and a recipient for migrating nurses.

Unfortunately, however, unlike 20 to 30 years ago when nurse migration was mostly based on individual motivation and typically followed previous colonial ties, now there is more active planning of large-scale international nurse recruitment, often from developing countries that can least afford to lose their most highly educated health care workers.

This has significant local and regional implications. For example, nurse migration from developing countries has occurred at the same time that international resources are finally available to address human immunodeficiency virus and acquired immunodeficiency syndrome (HIV/AIDS) and improve immunization coverage around the world. This undermines efforts to address those problems in the donor countries.

Another example is apparent in China, which has increasing numbers of elderly people accompanied by a severe nursing shortage. The result is that the wait time for a slot at a nursing home in Beijing amounted to 100 years in 2013 (Trines, 2018).

> *Consider This* Developed countries are often the recipients of migrant nurses and developing countries are often the donors. In essence then, developing countries are supporting the health care infrastructure of more developed countries, often at the expense of their own country.

In addition, a recruiting onslaught affects the ability of developing countries to develop sustainable health care systems and provide appropriate care to their citizens. Indeed, few donor nations are prepared to manage the loss of their nurse workforce to such widespread migration. In addition, developing countries often recruit from each other, including within the same geographical region. Table 7.1 summarizes the current dynamic nature of nurse migration in select countries around the world.

GLOBAL MIGRATION OF NURSES: "PUSH" AND "PULL" FACTORS

To understand what is driving the global migration of nurses, it is first necessary to examine what are known as the "push" and "pull" factors of nursing migration. *Push factors* are those factors that push or drive nurses to want to leave their countries to go to another. Low pay, inadequate opportunities for career advancement or continuing education, sociopolitical instability, and unsafe workplaces

TABLE 7.1	**Effect of Push-Pull Migration on Select Countries**
Africa	Trines (2018) notes that sub-Saharan African countries bear 24% of the world's disease burden today but have only 3% of health workers and less than 1% of the world's financial resources to respond to this burden. Thus, the nursing shortage is more severe and felt more strongly in these source countries. The migration drains these countries of desperately needed skilled personnel.
Australia	Australia has long hired foreign nurses to supplement its health care workforce, and the numbers are only increasing. In fact, 18.2% of nurses in Australia were foreign-trained in 2016, up from 14% in 2009 (Trines, 2018). A new assessment model was introduced in January 2020 requiring foreign nurses entering the country after January 2020, to complete an outcomes-based assessment for employment in Australia (Manish, 2019). The former option of completing a bridging course was removed. The priority of the assessment model is public safety and ensuring that all individuals registered as a nurse or midwife in Australia are meeting the same standards, regardless of where they gained their qualifications (Manish, 2019).
Canada	Canada is both a source and a destination country for international nurse migration, with an estimated net loss of nurses. The United States is a major beneficiary of Canadian nurse emigration, resulting from the reduction of full-time jobs for nurses in Canada because of health system reforms. Each province has different procedures and specifications for nurses applying to work in Canada, but nurses are so highly in demand that there are three major immigration programs that lay an easy-to-navigate pathway for nurses to immigrate to Canada (MDC Canada, 2020).
Caribbean	The migration of Caribbean nurses, particularly to developed countries such as Canada, the United States, and the United Kingdom, is a concern for most countries of this region. With nursing vacancy rates averaging 40%, individual countries and the region overall are challenged to address this issue through the development and implementation of sustainable, feasible strategies (Sands et al., 2020). Unfortunately, many of the nurses who move abroad report they have no intention of returning to their home countries, at least not to work in the nursing profession (Sands et al., 2020).
China	Many Chinese nurses intend to migrate because of limited job opportunities, low salary, and low job satisfaction. Commercial recruiters have expressed a strong interest in recruiting Chinese nurses, but there are limited examples of successful ventures as a result of language and cultural challenges as well as differing role expectations. Still, it is likely that China will become an important source of nurses for developed nations in the coming years.
India	India has the world's highest number of medical schools and is the world's largest source of migrant physicians (Smiley, 2020). An estimated 69,000 Indian-trained physicians worked in the United States, United Kingdom, Canada, and Australia in 2017, according to the Organisation for Economic Co-operation and Development (OECD) (Smiley, 2020). In addition, despite an extremely low nurse-to-population ratio in India, large-scale nurse migration to other countries is increasing. Low wages, heavy workloads, poor working conditions, and a lack of respect are push factors for many Indian nurses to migrate.
Indonesia	Indonesia is recognized as a donor country, with policies that encourage nursing professionals to emigrate abroad. Taiwan is the most common destination for migrant nurses from Indonesia, though the United Arab Emirates, the Netherlands, Kuwait, the United Kingdom, and Saudi Arabia have been other major recipients since the first migration in 1996 (Efendi, 2020; Nursalam et al., 2020). Indonesia itself, however, is suffering from a crisis in nursing capacity and struggles with ensuring adequate health care access for its own populations. The Indonesia–Japan Economic Partnership Agreement attempts to balance domestic health workforce needs, employment, and training opportunities for Indonesian nurses while acknowledging the rights of nurses to freely migrate abroad.
Ireland	As late as 25 years ago, Ireland had an abundant pool of nurses. However, Ireland now actively recruits foreign nurses. Thus, Ireland has moved from being a traditional source of nurses to a recipient.
Lebanon	Lebanon is a source country to the Persian Gulf, North America, and Europe. The primary push factors are unsatisfactory salary or benefits, better work opportunities in other countries, and lack of professional development or career advancement (Alameddine et al., 2020). As a result, there are nursing workforce shortages in Lebanon itself.

TABLE 7.1	**Effect of Push-Pull Migration on Select Countries (*continued*)**
New Zealand	New Zealand has been both a source and destination country since the beginning of the 21st century. However, it currently has 27% of internationally qualified nurses in its workforce, one of the highest rates among countries in the OECD (Smiley, 2020). The movement of New Zealand registered nurses (RNs) to Australia is expedited by the Trans-Tasman Agreement, whereas the entry of foreign RNs to New Zealand is facilitated by nursing being an identified priority occupation.
Pakistan	The burden of chronic and infectious diseases is high in Pakistan. In addition, hospitals are run by nurses, not by doctors, and unfortunately there is an acute shortage of nurses and midwives in Pakistan, where density of nurses and midwives is 0.49 per 1,000 population compared to the recommended threshold of 3.28 per 1,000 population (The News, 2020). Nurse migration from Pakistan to developed countries has contributed to adverse capacity development of nursing in Pakistan.
Philippines	The Philippines is a source country for nurse migration. National opinion has generally focused on the improved quality of life for individual migrants and their families and on the benefits of remittances to the nation; however, a shortage of highly skilled nurses and the massive retraining of physicians to become nurses elsewhere has created severe problems for the Filipino health system, including the closure of some hospitals.
Saudi Arabia	Saudi Arabia has a unique nursing profile, as most of the nursing workforce providing direct patient health care are expatriates (Alshareef et al., 2020). Many of these foreign nurses are from the Philippines. Many identify discrimination as an important contributing factor for their intention to return to the Philippines. Furthermore, migrant nurses report discrimination, a lack of social support from their immediate supervisor, a lack of organizational commitment, and a lack of autonomy as factors encouraging turnover (Alsahareef et al., 2020).
United Kingdom	Both a donor and recipient country, nurse migration is common in the United Kingdom. Indeed, the United Kingdom is now the third most popular destination for overseas nurses in the world (Gillin & Smith, 2020). There has, however, been a notable shift away from active EU recruitment toward overseas recruitment, particularly from the Philippines and India. This has occurred in response to diminishing returns from EU sources, high attrition among EU nurses, and the introduction of English-language tests for EU nurses in July 2016 (Gillin & Smith, 2020).
United States	Nurse immigration to the United States has tripled since 1994. The U.S. health system relies heavily on migrant workers, who make up 17% of all health care workers and represent more than one in four doctors in the country (Narea, 2020).

are examples of push factors. Other factors that act as push factors in some countries include the risk of HIV/AIDS to health system workers, concerns about personal security in areas of conflict, and economic instability.

> *Consider This* Nurses migrate for many reasons and the push/pull factors to migrate are in constant imbalance.

Pull factors are those factors that draw the nurse toward a different country. Pull factors typically include higher pay, further developed career structures, opportunities for further education and professional development, and, in some cases, safety from the threat of violence (more prevalent in less-developed countries). Other pull factors, such as the opportunity to travel or to participate in foreign aid work, also influence some

nurses. A summary of push and pull factors for nurse migration is outlined in Table 7.2.

Destination countries can recruit nurses because of many pull factors. Many internationally recruited nurses suggest, however, that they would have preferred to remain in their home country with family and friends and in a familiar culture and environment, but push and pull factors overwhelmingly influenced their decision to migrate.

Indeed, Ferreira et al. (2020) suggest it is not entirely clear how health care professionals actually balance these push and pull factors in their decisions to work abroad and the interplay between these multilevel factors needs to be further studied. In their research of the factors influencing Portuguese health care professionals to emigrate, the major factor influencing migration was remuneration. In addition, improvements in work quality aimed at promoting work satisfaction and burnout would also have contributed to the retention of these professionals (Research Fuels the Controversy 7.1).

TABLE 7.2   Push and Pull Factors for Nurse Migration

Push Factors	Pull Factors
Low pay	High pay
Inadequate opportunities for career advancement or continuing education	More developed career structures or opportunities for further education and professional development
Sociopolitical instability	Increased quality of life
Unsafe workplaces	Safety from the threat of violence
Practice restrictions	Family members in destination country
High workloads	Adventure/love of travel
Poor living conditions (housing, food, water)	Humanitarian motives
Remittance income	Recognition and status
Economic instability	Political stability

Research Fuels the Controversy 7.1

Drivers for Health Care Migration From Portugal

This research tested an analytic model of the individual drivers for health care professional migration from Portugal, a country known for relatively stable labor conditions. Data were collected through an online questionnaire administered to all 19,563 health care professionals in all 1,212 primary health care functional units in mainland Portugal during the 4 months between January and April of 2018. The number of valid questionnaires obtained amounted to 9.097 (46.4 % response rate).

Source: Ferreira, P. L., Raposo, V., Tavares, A. I., & Correia, T. (2020). Drivers for emigration among healthcare professionals: Testing an analytical model in a primary healthcare setting. *Health Policy, 124*(7), 751–757. https://doi.org/10.1016/j.healthpol.2020.04.009

Study Findings

The number of nurses who reported emigrating from Portugal but not returning was 3.7%. An additional 6.6% were preparing to emigrate. Nurses with higher levels of education or with specialty degrees were more likely to report intention to emigrate than others with standard qualifications.

Most of the professionals who were considering migration reported that their household incomes and salaries were insufficient. Work-related burnout also increased the intention to emigrate. Having children, contract type, self-assessed health status, and dissatisfaction with moral issues at work did not influence the intention to emigrate.

In addition, the decision to emigrate for nurses was gender sensitive, with migration more common among male nurses than their female counterparts. Marriage, living with a partner, and level of education limited the intention of nurses to emigrate.

The researchers concluded that push factors can either include more narrowly work-related experiences or social-demographic variables, but financial issues can mediate these influences. Improving monetary compensation would have a visible impact on reducing the intention to emigrate by health care professionals. Improvements of the work quality aimed at promoting work satisfaction and burnout control would also contribute to the retention of these health care professionals.

EFFECTS OF GLOBAL MIGRATION ON DEVELOPING COUNTRIES

A review of the literature suggests that different countries have experienced different effects because of the push-pull of international nurse migration. In some cases, aggressive recruitment of large numbers of nurses may seriously deplete a single health facility or contract an important number of newly graduated nurses from a single educational institute. This has significant local and regional implications because not only is critical intellectual capital taken away from the developing country but that country's health outcomes are at risk to worsen.

For example, the Philippines (Fig. 7.1) has long been the top country of emigrating nurses worldwide, accounting for roughly 25% of all foreign nurses (Smiley, 2020). About

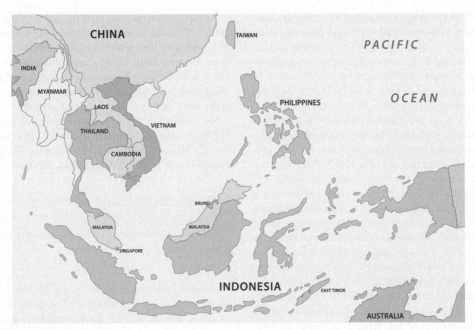

Figure 7.1 Map of Southeast Asia.

85% of employed Filipino nurses work in 1 of more than 50 countries around the world. In the United States, an estimated 20% of all the registered nurses (RNs) in California are Filipino (Smiley, 2020).

The Philippines intentionally encourages more people to become nurses than necessary with the intent of sending them abroad. Starting in the 1960s, the Philippine government created a systematic, state-sponsored system of labor exportation designed to foster economic development through remittances from overseas workers (Trines, 2018). Nurses played a central role in that strategy and were encouraged to emigrate. In addition, in the early 2000s, poorly paid Filipino medical doctors, particularly from rural regions, began to retrain as nurses in order to emigrate (Trines, 2018).

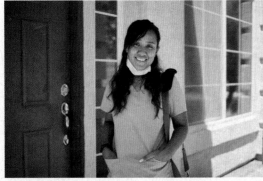

(Joshua Resnick/Shutterstock)

Though intentional, the Philippines is suffering from these widespread migration practices. Castro-Palaganas and colleagues (2017) suggest that the massive expansion in education and training designed specifically for outmigration creates a domestic supply of health workers who cannot be absorbed by a system that is underfunded. This results in a paradox of underservice, especially in rural and remote areas, occurring at the same time as underemployment and outmigration. Policy responses to this paradox have not yet been appropriately aligned to capture the multilayered and complex nature of these intersecting phenomena (Castro-Palaganas et al., 2017).

In addition, the COVID-19 pandemic has furthered the Philippines's inability to meet its own health care needs. Lopez and Jiao (2020, para. 3) noted there was an estimated shortage of 23,000 nurses nationwide as of spring 2020, with the situation so severe that "most Filipinos die without even seeing a medical professional." As a result, in March 2020, the Philippine Overseas Employment Administration (POEA) temporarily suspended the deployment of all health care workers "until the national state of emergency is lifted," freezing the fulfillment of existing contracts with hospitals around the globe (Smiley, 2020). In January 2021, the POEA revalidated overseas employment certificates that had expired during community quarantines (POEA, 2021).

China, with the second largest nursing workforce in the world (2.2 million nurses), is another country actively seeking to send nurses abroad. Yet, a shortage of nurses has haunted China for years. Only a small number of graduates are hired as permanent staff, with most graduates placed on temporary contracts. This leads to instability and uncertainty among the nursing workforce, encouraging many graduates to migrate to other countries.

India is also a donor country, second only to the Philippines in training nurses (Smiley, 2020), despite having an extremely low nurse-to-population ratio. Surveys have shown that Indian migrant nurses, like their counterparts in other countries, are motivated to emigrate by better income prospects abroad, where they can easily earn 10 times more than at home, as well as by the poor working conditions in India (Trines, 2018). Nearly 56,000 Indian-trained nurses work in the United States, the United Kingdom, Canada, and Australia.

Some countries struggle more overtly, however, with their nurse migration. Recent reports from South Africa, Ghana, China, and the Caribbean highlight that a significant outflow of nurses from these countries has reduced the level and quality of health care services available and resulted in a loss of specialist skills. Similarly, African countries, particularly those in sub-Saharan Africa, have lost a substantial proportion of their skilled workforce through migration. Poor working conditions within the health care sector, such as long work hours, high patient loads, inadequate resources, and occupational hazards, influence these nurses to consider migration.

The economic cost of donor countries exporting their mostly highly educated workforce is staggering. Straehle (2017) notes that it costs approximately $65,997 to educate a doctor in Kenya and about $43,180 to educate a nurse. If a doctor leaves, the losses in returns for the training country's investment are estimated to be nearly eight times the cost for training the individual health care practitioner. Public finances deteriorate with the loss in investment return, and the result is that health professionals within the country may then not be hired because of a lack of funds.

> *Consider This* The positive global economic/social/professional development associated with international migration must be weighed against the substantial brain and skills drain experienced by donor countries.

Remittance Income

Some national governments and government agencies encourage the outflow of nurses from their countries; examples include Fiji, Jamaica, India, Mauritius, South Africa, and the Philippines. For many years, the Philippine government actively endorsed and facilitated initiatives aimed at educating, recruiting, training, and placing nurses around the world. This was likely the result of a financial imperative, to encourage the generation of *remittance income.*

In fact, labor is the most profitable export of the Philippines, with about 10 million citizens working around the globe and generating remittance income annually (Philippines Economy 2020, 2020). Castro-Palaganas and team (2017) note that at the household level, migration from the Philippines has engendered increased consumerism and materialism and fostered dependency on overseas remittances. Indeed, Filipino nurses working abroad remit about $1 billion to the Philippines every year, a substantial portion of total remittances that drives 13% of the Philippines's gross domestic product (GDP) (Smiley, 2020).

> *Consider This* Migrating nurses often send remittances back home to support their families and bolster the economy; in addition, some workers later return home with enhanced skills and experience.

Similarly, remittances from migrants are recognized as an important source of resilience for households in African countries. Indeed, in 2019, annual remittance income to low- and middle-income countries was approximately $554 billion, but this fell about 7% in 2020 ($508 billion) due to the economic crisis induced by the COVID-19 pandemic and shutdown (The World Bank, 2020). An additional 7.5% decline to $470 billion is anticipated in 2021.

Brain Drain

It is brain drain, however, that is one of the most critical negative consequences of widespread nursing migration from developing countries. *Brain drain* refers to the loss of skilled personnel and the loss of investment in education that is experienced when those human resources migrate elsewhere. Thus, brain drain typically occurs when the skilled professionals from less-developed countries migrate to more developed countries, resulting in these developing countries losing their most highly skilled and educated workforce. In addition, resource-limited nations have overwhelmingly become donor countries. The consequences of this large-scale and nonstrategic migration are far-reaching, including a breakdown of national health care infrastructures and the inability of many donor countries to meet the health care needs of their own citizens.

For example, Jamaica's Minister of Health noted in 2017 that the brain drain of nurses has "virtually crippled the delivery of certain health care services and has had a dramatic effect on the overall quality of health care" (Trines, 2018, para. 39). He added that the English-speaking Caribbean at large will be facing a shortage of 10,000 nurses over the next 10 years.

Complaints of brain drain are also heard from donor countries such as India, the Philippines, South Africa, and

Zimbabwe. People from these nations argue that their human health care resources are being extracted at a time when they are needed most. This is the case even in many of the countries that have historically encouraged the exportation of their nurses. This suggests that the individual's right to choose where they work cannot be easily negated simply because the donor country does not want to lose its highly educated human resources. Clearly, many nursing organizations and nursing leaders have begun to recognize the negative effects of international migration on the nurses' home countries, but efforts to address the problem have been inadequate.

Finally, one must consider whether recruiting foreign nurses to solve acute staffing shortages is simply a poorly thought-out quick fix to a much greater problem and whether donor nations are being harmed while the issues that led to shortages in the first place are never addressed. Certainly, one must at least question whether wholesale foreign nurse recruitment would even be necessary if recruiting nations made a more concerted effort to improve the working conditions, salaries, empowerment, and recognition of the domestic nurses they already employ.

> *Consider This* Importing foreign nurses to solve the nursing shortage only puts a Band-Aid on the problem. The factors that led to the nursing shortage in the first place still need to be resolved.

> ### Discussion Point
> If the money that is being spent on recruitment and immigration of foreign nurses was instead spent on resolving the domestic nursing issues that led to a shortage in the first place, would international nurse recruitment even be necessary?

GLOBAL NURSE RECRUITMENT AND MIGRATION AS AN ETHICAL ISSUE

Controversy regarding the ethics of international recruitment of nurses is not new. Whenever resources are limited, ethical issues regarding their allocation are likely to arise. In the case of global nurse recruitment and migration, the ethical principles of autonomy, utility, and justice seem most relevant. Certainly, there must be some sort of a balance between the right of individual nurses to choose to migrate (autonomy), particularly when push factors are overwhelming, and the more utilitarian concern for the donor nations' health as a result of losing scarce nursing resources.

International law clearly guarantees an individual the right to freedom of movement and residence as established in the Universal Declaration of Human Rights (United Nations General Assembly, 1948) and the International Covenant on Civil and Political Rights (Office of the United Nations High Commissioner for Human Rights, 1976). The individual's right to migrate is central to self-determination. But how do countries experiencing health care provider anemia balance the need for self-preservation with the right to freedom of movement?

> ### Discussion Point
> Should the right for the individual nurse to migrate (autonomy and self-determination) override what might be best for the donor nation (utilitarianism)?

Justice, or fairness, is another ethical principle appropriate to this discussion because it examines how social and material goods are distributed to or withheld from members of a group or society, particularly in relation to fairness. Both recipient and donor countries have strong moral obligations to work toward fairer distributions of health care services as the fate of other communities cannot be ignored. Straehle (2017) concurs, suggesting that the right to migrate should be tied to the duties of justice that need to be satisfied before benefiting from migration. Societies would then be justified in restricting individual freedom of movement if it limits minimum access to health care for all.

> *Consider This* The majority of countries hiring foreign nurses are primarily White, and donor nations typically export nurses of color. The issue of race and ethnicity and the global economics of nursing should be examined in terms of effect on both recipient and donor countries.

In addition, migration numbers have increasingly become feminized. This impacts negatively on key education and health indicators including infant and child mortality and school enrollment rate by gender.

The following question then must be asked: Does global recruitment violate the principle of justice, particularly if such migration does not solve the underlying shortage and when such retention is done at the expense of the donor country? Clearly, donor countries have an ethical obligation to do what they can to provide their nurses with a safe, satisfying, and economically rewarding work environment. Recruiting countries have an ethical obligation to do what is necessary to be more self-reliant in meeting their professional workforce needs and to avoid recruiting nurses from those countries that can least afford to lose their most experienced health care workers. Finally, professional health care associations must lead the way in addressing how best to respond to these ethical concerns.

PROFESSIONAL ORGANIZATIONS RESPOND

Given the current extent of nurse migration and the many ethical dilemmas associated with it, many professional organizations representing nurses from around the world have weighed in on the issue. Some have provided formal position statements to guide both donor and recipient countries. Others have attempted to provide guidance to the individual nurse considering global migration.

The International Council of Nurses

One international agency, the International Council of Nurses (ICN, 2021), has issued several position statements arguing for ethics and good employment practices in

---

BOX 7.1   **ICN Position Statement on Nurse Retention, Transfer, and Migration (1999)**

ICN and its member associations firmly believe that quality health care is directly dependent on an adequate supply of qualified nursing personnel.

ICN recognizes the right of individual nurses to migrate, while acknowledging the possible adverse effect that international migration may have on health care quality.

ICN condemns the practice of recruiting nurses to countries where authorities have failed to address human resource planning and problems that cause nurses to leave the profession and discourage them from returning to nursing.

In support of the above, ICN does the following:
* Disseminates information on nursing personnel needs and resources and on the development of fulfilling nursing career structures
* Provides training opportunities in negotiation and socioeconomic welfare–related issues
* Disseminates data on nursing employment worldwide
* Takes action to help reduce the serious effects of any shortage, maldistribution, and misutilization of nursing personnel
* Advocates adherence nationally to international labor standards
* Condemns the recruitment of nurses as a strike-breaking mechanism
* Advocates for open and transparent migration systems (recognizing that some appropriate screening is necessary to ensure public safety)
* Supports a transcultural approach to nursing practice
* Promotes the introduction of transferable benefits, for example, pension
   National nurses associations are urged to do the following:
* Encourage relevant authorities to ensure sound human resources planning for nursing.
* Participate in the development of sound national policies on immigration and emigration of nurses.
* Promote the revision of nursing curricula for basic and post-basic education in nursing and administration to emphasize effective nursing leadership.
* Disseminate information on the working conditions of nurses.
* Discourage nurses from working in other countries where salaries and conditions are not acceptable to nurses and professional associations in those countries.
* Ensure that foreign nurses have conditions of employment equal to those of local nurses in posts requiring the same level of competency and involving the same duties and responsibilities.
* Ensure that there are no distinctions made among foreign nurses from different countries.
* Monitor the activities of recruiting agencies.
* Provide an advisory service to help nurses interpret contracts and assist foreign nurses with personal and work-related problems, such as institutional racism, violence, and sexual harassment.
* Provide orientation for foreign nurses on the local cultural, social, and political values and on the health system and national language.
* Alert nurses to the fact that some diplomas, qualifications, or degrees earned in one country may not be recognized in another.
* Assist nurses with their problems related to international migration and repatriation.

Source: International Council of Nurses. (2007). *Position statement: Nurse retention and migration.* Retrieved August 29, 2020, from http://docplayer.net/25478011-Nurse-retention-and-migration-position-statement.html

international recruitment (Box 7.1). The ICN, a federation of more than 130 national nurses associations, represents more than 20 million nurses worldwide. The *ICN Position Statement: Nurse Retention and Migration* authored in 1999 and revised in 2007 confirms the right of nurses to migrate as well as the potential beneficial outcomes of multicultural practice and learning opportunities supported by migration. Still, it acknowledges potential adverse effects on the quality of health care in donor countries (ICN, 2007).

The ICN (2007) position statement also condemns the practice of recruiting nurses to countries where authorities have failed to implement sound human resource planning and to seriously address problems that cause nurses to leave the profession and discourage them from returning to nursing. The position statement also denounces unethical recruitment practices that exploit nurses or mislead them into accepting job responsibilities and working conditions that are incompatible with their qualifications, skills, and experience. The ICN and its member associations call for a regulated recruitment process based on ethical principles that guide informed decision making and reinforce sound employment policies on the part of governments, employers, and nurses, thereby supporting fair and cost-effective recruitment and retention practices.

In addition, the ICN adopted a second position paper on ethical nurse recruitment in 2001 that was revised and reaffirmed in 2007. This document identifies principles necessary to create a foundation for ethical recruitment, whether international or intranational contexts are considered. Most recently, the ICN (2019) published a position statement on international career mobility and ethical nurse recruitment. Its 12 foundational principles are outlined in Box 7.2.

The International Centre on Nurse Migration

Another organization, the International Centre on Nurse Migration (ICNM), established in 2005, represents a collaborative project launched by the ICN and the Commission on Graduates of Foreign Nursing Schools (CGFNS). The ICNM (n.d.) emphasizes the development, promotion, and dissemination of research, policy, and information on global nurse migration and human resources in nursing. The ICNM website features news, resources, and publications widely available to policymakers, planners, and practitioners.

Voluntary Code of Ethical Conduct for International Nurse Recruitment

Funded through a grant from the John D. and Catherine T. MacArthur Foundation in collaboration with the O'Neill Institute for National and Global Health Law at Georgetown University, a task force of recruiters, hospitals, and foreign-educated nurses met in 2008 to develop draft standards of practice about global nurse recruitment, as well as

---

BOX 7.2   **International Council of Nurses Principles for International Career Mobility and Ethical Nurse Recruitment**

As a global voice of nursing, the ICN called for governments and organizations, including employers, recruiters, and nongovernmental organizations, to systematically adopt the following foundational principles, which consider the needs of multiple stakeholders, to guide informed workforce planning and decision making resulting in regulated, ethical, and cost-effective recruitment processes, both domestically and internationally:

1. Comprehensive and effective nursing regulation
2. Access to full and flexible employment opportunities
3. Freedom of movement
4. Freedom from discrimination
5. Good faith contracting
6. Equal pay for work of equal value
7. Access to grievance procedures
8. Safe work environment
9. Effective orientation/mentoring/supervision
10. Freedom of association
11. Regulation of recruitment
12. National self-sustainability

Source: Data from International Council of Nurses. (2019). *Position statement: International career mobility and ethical nurse recruitment.* Retrieved August 29, 2020, from https://www.icn.ch/system/files/documents/2019-11/PS_C_International%20career%20mobility%20and%20ethical%20nurse%20recruitment_En.pdf

recommendations on how to institutionalize these standards. This collaboration led to the release of a *Voluntary Code of Ethical Conduct for the Recruitment of Foreign-Educated Nurses to the United States* (n.d.). The code was designed to increase transparency and accountability throughout the process of international recruitment and ensure adequate orientation for foreign-educated nurses. It also provided guidance on ways to ensure recruitment is not harmful to source countries. This document was endorsed by the National Council of State Boards of Nursing (NCSBN).

The World Health Organization

Another international organization involved in establishing guidelines for nurse migration is the WHO (2021). To balance the right of workers to migrate with a need to ensure that global health care needs are met, the WHO launched the *Health Worker Migration Policy Initiative* in 2007. The initiative brought together professional organizations and other groups to create a code, to emphasize the positive benefits of health worker migration, minimize its negative impacts, and spread the benefits of health worker migration more equitably among developed and developing nations.

In addition, in 2011, the Sixty-Third World Health Assembly unanimously passed a resolution to adopt the *Global Code of Practice on the International Recruitment of Health Personnel*, acknowledging the global dimensions and complexities of the health workforce crisis and the interconnected nature of both the problems and the solutions (WHO, 2021). The code was the first of its kind on a global scale for migration. In addition, the 2004 WHO Resolution 57.19 urged member states to mitigate the adverse effects of health care worker migration by forming country and regional agreements such as the South Africa/United Kingdom Memorandum of Understanding, the Pacific Code, and the Caribbean Community agreement.

THE MISTREATMENT OF FOREIGN NURSES

Despite the costs and investment of time and energy that goes into recruiting foreign nurses, some health care organizations treat foreign nurses poorly once they arrive. Some migrant nurses receive substandard jobs or wages or are subjected to illegal practices by their employers.

In addition, some recruiting firms charge foreign nurses an upfront fee, a practice that has been found illegal in connection with the recruitment of temporary farm workers in the United States and that is prohibited in the U.K. Code of Practice for the International Recruitment of Health Care Professionals. In addition, many recruiters charge migrant nurses a "buyout" or breach fee for resigning before the end

| BOX 7.3 | **Questionable Practices Reported by International Nurses** |

- Changing contracts from the time a nurse departs home country and on arrival in sponsor country without consent
- Paying lower wages than the prevailing rate or less than the hours worked
- Charging high breach fees
- Inadequate orientation to clinical agencies
- Imposing excessive work demands or mandatory overtime
- Retaining green cards, delays in processing social security numbers and RN permits
- Threats that nurses will be reported to immigration authorities
- Providing substandard housing

of their employment contract. This is because placement agencies often charge health care organizations a significant fee, depending on the state and the nurse's experience, to bring in a foreign nurse.

There are also reports that overzealous recruiters have made false promises to foreign nurses regarding job opportunities and wages and virtually forced the newly migrated nurses to work long hours in substandard working conditions. Part of the reason for this is that private for-profit agencies have increasingly become involved in the search for nursing personnel, and there is generally no designated body that regulates or monitors the content of contracts offered. Internationally recruited nurses may be particularly at risk for exploitation or abuse because of the difficulty of verifying the terms of employment because of distance, language barriers, cost, and naiveté. These questionable hiring or employment practices are summarized in Box 7.3.

Consider This   Because of the lack of regulatory oversight of global nurse migration contracting, foreign nurses are at increased risk for employment under false pretenses and may be misled as to the conditions of work, remuneration, and benefits.

Discussion Point

Should there be greater regulatory oversight of foreign nurse recruitment? If so, who should be charged with this responsibility?

ASSIMILATING THE FOREIGN NURSE THROUGH SOCIALIZATION

The ethical obligation to the foreign nurse does not end with their arrival in a new country. The move from one cultural context to another can be stressful. Many migrant nurses are afraid to express dissatisfaction or to ask for help for fear they will no longer have a job or of being sent home. In addition, many of the families left behind in donor countries count on the migrant nurse sending money home to improve their living standards. All of these factors place migrant nurses at increased risk for abuse and failure to assimilate. As a result, recruiting countries must do whatever they can to see that migrant nurses are appropriately assimilated into new work environments.

Pung and Goh (2017) suggest there are seven broad categories of transitional challenges faced by international nurses who migrate: difficulty orientating (cultural disorientation); a longing for what is missing; professional development and devaluing; communication barriers; discrimination and marginalization; personal and professional differences; and a meaningful support system (Box 7.4).

Difficulty orientating and executing routine daily activities (shopping, banking, transportation, paying bills, etc.) in their new countries may be difficult for foreign nurses. In addition, orientation programs offered by their new workplaces may be insufficient in helping them adjust to their new work environments. A longing for what is missing can result from cultural uprooting. The sudden change in the social environment often brings some yearning as well as sadness for what has been left behind.

In addition, professional development and devaluing is a reality for many migrant nurses in their new countries.

Some migrant nurses report a feeling of being undermined, belittled, and disrespected. In addition, they report a drop in occupational status after arriving in their host countries.

Communication barriers, however, may be the most challenging issue facing foreign nurses. Not only do most foreign nurses have an inadequacy of language preparation but they are also unfamiliar with accents, slang, and other language nuances. As a result, they find it difficult to relate to some patients, families, and other health care team members, to speak up for themselves, and to advocate for their patients.

Discrimination and marginalization are also challenging for the migrant nurse. Some migrant nurses experience unfair treatment (such as higher patient loads than others or being passed over for promotions) and racism, which results in stereotyping and rejection by patients and peers. In addition, the risk of being bullied is higher among this population.

Personal and professional differences among international nurses and native nurses may result in disagreements and conflicts. Professional differences may include differences in nursing expectations, communication expectations, and values and beliefs toward patient care. In Asia, family members are expected to provide basic care to patients, and nurses usually follow doctors' orders with little questioning, while critical thinking and independent decision making are emphasized in Western countries.

Finally, the migrant nurse often experiences a lack of a meaningful support system. With family and friends left behind, adjustment may be slow and lonely, and feelings of isolation, depression, and loss are common. When migrant nurses can establish a good relationship with their colleagues, the nurses are more motivated to stay in their work and the safety and quality of patient care is increased.

BOX 7.4 **Broad Categories of Transitional Challenges Facing International Nurse Migrants**

1. Difficulty orientating (cultural disorientation)
2. Communication barriers
3. A longing for what is missing
4. Professional development and devaluing
5. Discrimination and marginalization
6. Personal and professional differences
7. Lack of a meaningful support system

Source: Pung, L. X., & Goh, Y. S. (2017, March). Challenges faced by international nurses when migrating: An integrative literature review. *International Nursing Review, 64*(1), 146–165. https://doi.org/10.1111/inr.12306

THE INTERNATIONAL COMMUNITY ADDRESSES THE PROBLEM

The nursing shortage and resulting global migration issues have led several nations' governments to intervene, and, as a result, some countries have made progress in tackling the ethical issues associated with global recruitment and migration of nurses.

Some Governments Respond

Within the last few years, many countries, including the United States, have published national nursing strategies for dealing with staff shortages. Norway has issued a policy statement on the ethics of international recruitment. The Netherlands, Ireland, and the Scandinavian countries also have practice guidelines on international recruitment or are looking at developing guidelines. The United Kingdom, until the COVID pandemic began, had been implementing tighter immigration and professional registration policies while allowing all nurses free movement rights. Indeed, in 2005, the United Kingdom began limiting nurse recruitment to the EU countries and only granting work permits to nurses from non-EU countries if National Health Services institutions showed that jobs could not be filled by U.K. or EU applications. This U.K. Code of Practice is one of the oldest Codes of Practice in existence. In addition, the United Kingdom's vote to leave the European Union (Brexit) halted the free movement of labor between the United Kingdom and European Economic Area (EEA) countries. All workers arriving from EEA and non-EEA countries were subject to the same immigration rules after January 1, 2021 (Holmes, 2021). However, the U.K. government has committed to recruiting an additional 12,000 nurses from overseas by 2024 to 2025 (Holmes, 2021). This commitment will require an immigration policy that is supportive of ethical international recruitment if it is to be realized.

Other countries have initiated or examined various policy responses to reduce outflow, such as requiring nurses to work in their home countries for a certain amount of time after education completion or by charging the nurse a fee to migrate to another country. Another response has been to recognize that outflow cannot be halted if principles of individual freedom are to be upheld but that the outflow that does occur must be managed and moderated. The "managed migration" initiative being undertaken in the Caribbean, which has provided regional support for addressing the nursing shortage crisis and developed initiatives such as training for export and temporary migration, is one example of a coordinated intervention to minimize the negative effects of outflow while realizing at least some benefit from the process.

Indonesia has adopted international principles to protect Indonesian nurses who migrate as well as the country's own participation with Japan in a bilateral trade and investment agreement, known as the *Indonesia–Japan Economic Partnership Agreement*.

> **Consider This** Recruiting internationally may be a quick-fix solution, but it is far from clear that it is always a cost-effective solution.

U.S. Immigration Policy

On April 22, 2020, U.S. President Donald Trump signed an Executive Order to pause immigration due to COVID-19, but it exempted physicians and nurses (Smiley, 2020).

Currently, foreign nurses who want to work in the United States must have a valid job offer from an employer, and the employer must obtain Department of Labor (DOL) approval for that hire. In addition, the employer must file a special petition with the U.S. Citizenship and Immigration Services (USCIS).

In addition, like most national governments, the U.S. government continues to play a pivotal role in the nurse migration issue with its ability to issue travel visas. The reality is that a finite number of visas are available, and caps exist on how many permanent visas are issued. Clearly, commercial recruiters and employers would like to see fewer restrictions on nurse migration, but labor certification laws and rules regarding the issuance of visas are complex and ever changing.

A permanent labor certification issued by the U.S. DOL allows an employer to hire a foreign worker to work permanently in the United States. In most instances, before the U.S. employer can submit an immigration petition to the USCIS, the employer must obtain a certified labor certification application from the DOL's Employment and Training Administration (ETA). The DOL must certify to the USCIS that there are not enough U.S. workers "able, willing, qualified, and available to accept the job opportunity in the area of intended employment and that employment of the foreign worker will not adversely affect the wages and working conditions of similarly employed U.S. workers" (U.S. DOL, n.d., para. 2).

The main purpose of this legal provision has been to protect the domestic labor market; however, the immigration laws have provided preferential provisions for members of certain professions in the national interest of the United States, and as a result, the government has created a list of occupations and professions, including nursing, that do not require labor certification. Because nursing has been classified as one of the shortage areas in the U.S. economy, a so-called *blanket waiver* of the labor certification is in place.

In addition, from 1962 to 1989, foreign nurses were regarded as professionals under U.S. immigration laws and could therefore seek an H-1 temporary work visa in the United States. In 1989, the Immigration Nursing Relief Act (INRA) created a 5-year pilot program. The INRA stipulated that only health care facilities with "attestations" approved by the Department of Health could obtain H-1A occupation visas to employ nurses on a temporary basis. Consequently, other occupations that formerly fell into the H-1 category became part of the new H-1B category. In addition, in 1990, Congress passed the Immigration and Nationality Act, which is the legal foundation for current immigration policies. In this act, nursing continued to be listed as a shortage area.

In 1999, the Nursing Relief for Disadvantaged Areas Act created H-1C occupational visas, which were perceived largely as an effort to renew the INRA of 1989 but with more restrictions. These temporary visas were created for foreign nurse graduates seeking employment in designated U.S. facilities (serving primarily poor patients in inner cities and some rural areas). This visa classification expired in 2009.

Currently, there are no specific nurse visas available in the United States; however, some foreign nurses apply to work under the H-1B visa for skilled workers (open to individuals from countries other than Canada or Mexico). The H-1B is a nonimmigrant visa that allows recruiting of professionals in shortage areas into jobs that require theoretical and practical application of a body of highly specialized knowledge requiring completion of a specific course of higher education (at least a bachelor's degree).

At first glance, the H-1B might look like a good match for foreign nurses because they are for temporary workers in specialty occupations, and nurses are both educated and specialized (Knapp, 2020). In addition, the United States has nursing jobs that need to be filled. The reality, however, is that many nurses do not qualify for the H-1B visa; a Fifth Circuit Court ruled in 2000 that RN hospital jobs do not currently require a bachelor's degree in nursing, regardless of recruiter requirements. Nurses can still apply for the H-1B status, however, if they have a specialized skill, particularly in intensive care, management, and specialty nursing areas or if U.S. employers can convince immigration officials that specific jobs do meet the H-1B requirement on a case-by-case basis. Other nurses more likely to earn an H-1B visa are those prepared for nurse manager or advanced practice roles, which require a Bachelor of Science in nursing or a Master of Science degree (Knapp, 2020).

In addition, the H-1B visa has an annual numerical limit "cap" of 65,000 visas each fiscal year. The first 20,000 petitions filed on behalf of beneficiaries with a U.S. master's degree or higher will be exempt from this cap in 2021 (USCIS, 2020).

Discussion Point

Does the increased recruitment of foreign nurses directly or indirectly affect the prevailing wages of domestic RNs?

Still, other foreign nurses have sought employment in the United States in accordance with the North American Free Trade Agreement (NAFTA), enacted in December 1993. NAFTA established a reciprocal trading relationship between the United States, Canada, and Mexico and allowed for a nonimmigrant class of admission exclusively for business and service trade individuals entering the United States.

In January 2020, however, President Trump signed a new United States–Mexico–Canada Agreement (USMCA), a renegotiated version of NAFTA (Foreign Worker Canada, 2020). Despite many changes, the new agreement left NAFTA provisions for work visas untouched. This was significant for workers in over 60 professional categories, including nurses, and for employers across the continent, who will continue to have access to labor from all three countries (Foreign Worker Canada, 2020). Many feared that President Trump would eliminate the visas entirely as a result of his "Buy American, Hire American" initiative.

In addition, the USCIS requires foreign-educated health care professionals, including nurses, who are seeking temporary or permanent occupational visas as well as those who are seeking NAFTA status to successfully complete a screening program before receiving an occupational visa or a permanent (green card) visa. This screening, completed by the CGFNS, includes an assessment of an applicant's education to ensure that it is comparable to that of a nursing graduate in the United States, verification that licenses are valid and unencumbered, successful completion of an English-language proficiency examination, and verification that the nurse has either earned certification by the CGFNS or passed the NCLEX-RN.

Another way nurses get work visas in the United States has been under the immigrant *E3 to I-140 status* ("green card" or Alien Registration Receipt Card). Migrant RNs enter into the United States and become permanent residents through petition to the Immigration and Naturalization Service. A problem with this visa status is that it does not require labor certification, so the DOL does not have to certify that the wage offered to the nurse is the prevailing wage. However, the law does state that foreign nurses entering under I-140 cannot have a negative effect on domestic wages.

ENSURING COMPETENCY OF FOREIGN NURSES: COMMISSION ON GRADUATES OF FOREIGN NURSING SCHOOLS AND THE NCLEX-RN EXAMINATION

Nursing is one of the most highly regulated health professions in the United States, and a license is required to practice in all 50 states and U.S. territories. Before 1977, endorsement and taking the State Board Test Pool Examination (SBTPE) were the two ways for foreign nurses to obtain a license. The SBTPE tested the foreign graduate's English-language proficiency and knowledge of U.S. nursing practice, but, alarmingly, only a small percentage (15%–20%) of foreign RNs typically passed the NCLEX-RN.

As a result of this high failure rate and a concern for patient safety, the American Nurses Association and the National League of Nursing, with collaboration from the DOL and the Immigration and Naturalization Service (INS), established CGFNS in 1977 as an independent, nonprofit organization. CGFNS is an immigration neutral nonprofit organization that helps foreign-educated health care professionals live and work in their country of choice by assessing and validating their academic and professional credentials (CGFNS, 2021a, para. 1–3).

The strategies CGFNS uses to accomplish this mission are to evaluate and test foreign graduates via a certification program before they leave their home countries to ensure that there is a reasonable chance for them to pass the NCLEX-RN needed for licensure in the United States. Through a contract with the National League for Nursing (NLN), which designed the NCLEX-RN, a CGFNS-qualifying examination was developed. The examination consists of two parts to test the applicant's knowledge of nursing and English-language proficiency (both written and oral).

To be eligible to take the examination, RNs must have completed sufficient classroom instruction and clinical practice and hold an initial as well as current license/registration as a first-level general nurse in their country of education (CGFNS, 2021b). In addition, a credentials review of secondary and nursing education, registration, and licensure is required to earn the CGFNS certificate. At the federal level, the CGFNS Qualifying Exam component satisfies the examination requirement of the VisaScreen: Visa Credentials Assessment for immigration. (CGFNS, 2021b).

The CGFNS examination, however, should not be mistaken as a substitute for the state board licensing examination. Indeed, most states in the United States require foreign nurses to pass the CGFNS certification before they can take the NCLEX-RN. Of the 9,303 internationally educated nurses who took the NCLEX-RN as first-time test takers in 2020, the pass rate was only 44.32% (NCSBN, 2020). For the 13,879 internationally educated students repeating the exam, the pass rate was only 25.56%. The examination specifications and passing standards are the same for foreign nurses as they are for students taking the NCLEX in the United States.

The NCSBN has also taken steps to make it easier for foreign RNs to take the NCLEX-RN. Until 2005, the NCLEX-RN was offered only in the United States and its territories. In fact, before 2005, the only option foreign nurses had was to earn the CGFNS certificate, secure a job offer from a U.S. employer, and take the NCLEX-RN only after they arrived in the United States with their green cards. Now the examination is offered in numerous countries and nonmember board territories. These locations were selected based on national security, examination security, and similarity with U.S. intellectual property and copyright laws.

CONCLUSIONS

Nurse migration and its associated ethical dilemmas are among the most serious issues facing the nursing profession, and there is little sign that the issue will abate any time soon. Clearly, developed countries have an advantage in terms of pull factors to recruit migrant nurses from less-developed countries, and less-developed countries are the ones most likely to suffer the devastating effects of brain drain. One must ask, however, whether this quick-fix solution to the nursing shortage has become too commonplace and too easy. Does it keep recruiter countries from dealing with the issues that led to their shortage in the first place? Does it negatively affect prevailing domestic wages and artificially alter what should be normal supply/demand curves in the health care marketplace? Of even greater concern is the lack of regulatory oversight of contracting with foreign nurses, placing them at risk for unethical, if not illegal, employment practices in their host country.

Both destination and home countries are challenged by poorly controlled nurse migration. Destination countries must address the ethical implications of aggressive recruitment and their lack of developing a sustainable self-sufficient domestic workforce. Source countries struggle to fund and educate adequate numbers of nurses for domestic needs and migrant replacement.

Some countries and professional nursing organizations are beginning to address these issues. So too are national governments and regulatory agencies in an effort to protect both the migrant nurses and the public those nurses will serve. Yet, in the meantime, large numbers of nurses are migrating internationally, and the potentially negative effects of this increasing trend on both the migrant nurse and the donor nation are becoming ever more apparent.

For Additional Discussion

1. Are the requirements for foreign nurses to get visas in the United States adequate?

2. Does achieving CGFNS certification and passing the NCLEX-RN examination in the United States ensure competency of the foreign nurse graduate?

3. As long as international nurse recruitment is a viable option, will the problems that lead to a nursing shortage in the first place be addressed?

4. Should donor countries develop nurse migration policy efforts that limit human resource drains?

5. How can government and professional nursing organizations work together to ensure that recruitment practices of foreign nurses are both ethical and appropriate?

6. How does the ethical principle of veracity (truth telling) apply to the zealous recruiting efforts of foreign nurses, particularly in developing countries?

7. Is government regulatory oversight of foreign nurse recruitment efforts in conflict with America's value of capitalistic, free enterprise?

References

Alameddine, M., Kharroubi, S. A., Dumit, N. Y., Kassas, S., Diab-El-Harake, M., & Richa, N. (2020, March). What made Lebanese emigrant nurses leave and what would bring them back? A cross-sectional survey. *International Journal of Nursing Studies, 103*, 103497. https://doi.org/10.1016/j.ijnurstu.2019.103497

Alshareef, A. G., Wraith, D., Dingle, K., & Mays, J. (2020). Identifying the factors influencing Saudi Arabian nurses' turnover. *Journal of Nursing Management, 28*(5), 1030–1040. https://doi.org/10.1111/jonm.13028

Castro-Palaganas, E., Spitzer, D. L., Kabamalan, M. M., Sanchez, M. C., Caricativo, R., Runnels, V., Labonté, R., Murphy, G. T., & Bourgeault, I. L. (2017, March 31). An examination of the causes, consequences, and policy responses to the migration of highly trained health personnel from the Philippines: The high cost of living/leaving-a mixed method study. *Human Resources for Health, 15*, 1–14. https://doi.org/10.1186/s12960-017-0198-z

Commission on Graduates of Foreign Nursing Schools. (2021a). *About us*. Retrieved January 19, 2021, from http://www.cgfns.org/sections/about/

Commission on Graduates of Foreign Nursing Schools. (2021b). *Certification*. Retrieved January 19, 2021, from https://www.cgfns.org/services/certification/

Efendi, F. (2020). Career choice for Indonesian nurses after placement abroad. *UNAIR News*. Retrieved August 30, 2020, from http://news.unair.ac.id/en/2019/09/02/career-choice-for-indonesian-nurses-after-placement-abroad/

Ferreira, P. L., Raposo, V., Tavares, A. I., & Correia, T. (2020). Drivers for emigration among healthcare professionals: Testing an analytical model in a primary healthcare setting. *Health Policy, 124*(7), 751–757. https://doi.org/10.1016/j.healthpol.2020.04.009

Foreign Worker Canada. (2020). *Skilled workers and professionals keep visa rights under new USMCA trade deal*. Retrieved August 30, 2020, from https://www.canadianimmigration.net/news-articles/skilled-workers-and-professionals-keep-visa-rights-under-new-usmca-trade-deal/

Gillin, N., & Smith, D. (2020, January). Overseas recruitment activities of NHS Trusts 2015–2018: Findings from FOI requests to 19 acute NHS trusts in England. *Nursing Inquiry, 27*(1), e12320. https://doi.org/10.1111/nin.12320

Holmes, J. (2021, January 11). *Brexit and the end of the transition period: What does it mean for the health and care system?* Retrieved January 19, 2021, from https://www.kingsfund.org.uk/publications/articles/brexit-end-of-transition-period-impact-health-care-system

International Centre on Nurse Migration. (n.d.). *About*. Retrieved August 29, 2020, from http://www.intlnursemigration.org/about/

International Council of Nurses. (2007). *Position statement: Nurse retention and migration*. Retrieved August 29, 2020, from http://docplayer.net/25478011-Nurse-retention-and-migration-position-statement.html

International Council of Nurses. (2019). *Position statement: International career mobility and ethical nurse recruitment*. Retrieved August 29, 2020, from https://www.icn.ch/system/files/documents/2019-11/PS_C_International%20career%20mobility%20and%20ethical%20nurse%20recruitment_En.pdf

International Council of Nurses. (2021). *Who we are*. Retrieved August 29, 2020, from http://www.icn.ch/who-we-are/who-we-are/

Knapp, K. (2020). *When nurses can qualify for an H-1B visa to the U.S.* Nolo. Retrieved August 29, 2020, from https://www.nolo.com/legal-encyclopedia/when-nurses-can-qualify-h-1b-visa-the-us.html

Lopez, D. B., & Jiao, C. (2020, April 23). *Supplier of world's nurses struggles to fight virus at home.* Retrieved August 30, 2020, from https://www.bloomberg.com/news/articles/2020-04-23/philippines-sends-nurses-around-the-world-but-lacks-them-at-home

Manish, S. (2019, September 9). *Australia moves to new assessment model for international nurses.* Retrieved September 1, 2020, from https://www.sbs.com.au/language/english/australia-moves-to-new-assessment-model-for-international-nurses

MDC Canada. (2020, May 12). *Immigrate to Canada as a nurse in 2020.* Retrieved August 29, 2020, from https://mdccanada.ca/news/live-in-canada/immigrate-to-canada-as-a-nurse-in-2020/

Narea, N. (2020, March 30). *The US needs foreign doctors and nurses to fight coronavirus. Immigration policy isn't helping.* Retrieved September 1, 2020, from https://www.vox.com/2020/3/30/21190971/foreign-immigrant-doctor-nurse-coronavirus

National Council of State Boards of Nursing. (2020, October 16). *2020: Number of candidates taking NCLEX examination and percent passing, by type of candidate.* Retrieved January 19, 2021, from https://www.ncsbn.org/Table_of_Pass_Rates_2020_Q3.pdf

Nursalam, N., Chen, C. M., Efendi, F., Has, E. M., Hidayati, L., & Hadisuyatmana, S. (2020, April). The lived experiences of Indonesian nurses who worked as care workers in Taiwan. *Journal of Nursing Research, 28*(2), e78. https://journals.lww.com/jnr-twna/fulltext/2020/04000/the_lived_experiences_of_indonesian_nurses_who.7.aspx

Office of the United Nations High Commissioner for Human Rights. (1976). *International covenant on civil and political rights.* Retrieved August 29, 2020, from http://www.ohchr.org/EN/ProfessionalInterest/Pages/CCPR.aspx

Philippine Overseas Employment Administration. (2021, January 11). *Advisory No. 06. Series of 2021.* Retrieved January 19, 2021, from http://www.poea.gov.ph/advisories/2021/Advisory-06-2021.pdf

Philippines Economy 2020. (2020, January 27). *Economy: Overview.* Retrieved August 29, 2020, from http://www.theodora.com/wfbcurrent/philippines/philippines_economy.html

Pung, L. X., & Goh, Y. S. (2017, March). Challenges faced by international nurses when migrating: An integrative literature review. *International Nursing Review, 64*(1), 146–165. https://doi.org/10.1111/inr.12306

Sands, S. R., Ingraham, K., & Salami, B. O. (2020, March 16). Caribbean nurse migration—A scoping review. *Human Resources for Health, 18,* Article number 19. Retrieved August 30, 2020, from https://link.springer.com/article/10.1186/s12960-020-00466-y

Smiley, S. (2020, May 4). *Developed countries are the largest importers of healthcare professionals.* Global Trade. Retrieved August 29, 2020, from https://www.globaltrademag.com/developed-countries-are-the-largest-importers-of-healthcare-professionals/

Straehle, C. (2017, April). Debating brain drain—May governments restrict emigration? *Developing World Bioethics, 17*(1), 59–60. https://doi.org/10.1111/dewb.12111

Stringer, H. (2020, June 10). *Report: Global nursing workforce needs significant bump in numbers.* Retrieved August 29, 2020, from https://www.nurse.com/blog/2020/06/10/report-global-nursing-workforce-needs-significant-bump-in-numbers/

The News. (2020). *WHO chief calls for doubling the number of nurses in Pakistan.* Retrieved August 30, 2020, from https://www.thenews.com.pk/print/640948-who-chief-calls-for-doubling-the-number-of-nurses-in-pakistan

The World Bank. (2020, October 29). *COVID-19: Remittance flows to shrink 14% by 2021.* Press release. Retrieved August 10, 2021, from https://www.worldbank.org/en/news/press-release/2020/10/29/covid-19-remittance-flows-to-shrink-14-by-2021

Trines, S. (2018, March 6). Mobile nurses: Trends in international labor migration in the nursing field. *World Education News + Review.* Retrieved August 28, 2020, from https://wenr.wes.org/2018/03/mobile-nurses-trends-in-international-labor-migration-in-the-nursing-field

United Nations General Assembly. (1948). *The universal declaration of human rights.* Retrieved August 29, 2020, from http://www.un.org/en/documents/udhr/

U.S. Citizenship and Immigration Services. (2020, May 29). *H-1B Cap Season: The H-1B program.* Retrieved August 29, 2020, from https://www.uscis.gov/working-in-the-united-states/temporary-workers/h-1b-specialty-occupations-and-fashion-models/h-1b-fiscal-year-fy-2021-cap-season

U.S. Department of Labor. (n.d.). *Permanent labor certification.* Retrieved August 29, 2020, from https://www.dol.gov/agencies/eta/foreign-labor/programs/permanent

Voluntary code of ethical conduct for the recruitment of foreign-educated nurses to the United States. (n.d.). Retrieved August 29, 2020, from https://assets.aspeninstitute.org/content/uploads/files/content/images/CodeofConductforRecruitmentofForeignEducatedNurses.pdf

World Health Organization. (2021). *Task force on migration: Health worker migration policy initiative.* Retrieved August 29, 2020, from http://www.who.int/workforcealliance/about/taskforces/migration/en/

Zolot, J. (2019, June). International nurse migration. *American Journal of Nursing, 119*(6), 16. https://doi.org/10.1097/01.NAJ.0000559791.78619.8b

Unlicensed Assistive Personnel and the Registered Nurse

Carol J. Huston

LEARNING OBJECTIVES

The learner will be able to:

1. Identify driving forces behind the increased use of unlicensed assistive personnel (UAP) beginning in the early 1990s.

2. Name common job titles for UAP.

3. Differentiate between the minimum mandated educational preparation of certified nurse aides (CNAs) and UAP.

4. Discuss how the role of the registered nurse (RN) as delegator has changed with the increased use of UAP.

5. Analyze current research that explores the effect of increased UAP use on costs and patient outcomes.

6. Examine how the role of delegator and supervisor of UAP increases the scope of liability for the RN.

7. Identify the sources of increased legal liability an RN and their employer face when health care institutions allow RNs to work beneath their scope of practice as UAP.

8. Identify safeguards that health care organizations can use to increase the likelihood that UAP are used both effectively and appropriately as members of the health care team.

9. Explore strategies for restructuring work environments and clarifying role expectations so that professional nurses spend less time on non-nursing tasks and UAP have role clarity.

10. Discuss factors contributing to both the current and projected shortages of UAP, particularly in long-term care settings.

11. Reflect on the self-confidence and skill that an RN might need to successfully delegate to a UAP.

INTRODUCTION

In an effort to contain spiraling health care costs, many health care providers in the 1990s restructured their organizations by eliminating registered nurse (RN) positions and/or by replacing licensed professional nurses with *unlicensed assistive personnel* (UAP). UAP are unlicensed individuals who provide low-risk, assistive care not requiring the judgment or training of a licensed professional while working under the direct supervision of an RN. The term includes, but is not limited to, nurse aides, nurse extenders, health care aides, technicians, patient care technicians, orderlies, assistants, and attendants. Although the term "UAP" is generally used throughout this chapter, it is noteworthy that in 2007, the American Nurses Association (ANA) stopped using the term "UAP" and replaced it with "nursing assistive personnel" (NAP), suggesting that many NAP are now licensed or formally recognized in some manner.

Regardless of nomenclature, unlicensed workers are a significant part of the health care landscape and have been for some time. By the late 1990s, hospitals began actively recruiting the RNs who had been let go just a few years before. RNs who had lost their jobs, however, were slow to return to the acute care setting despite a widespread, worsening nursing shortage. As a result, hospitals again increased their use of UAP early in the 21st century in an effort to supplement their licensed nursing staff.

Both as a result of the restructuring of the 1990s and subsequent nursing shortages, the skill mix in some hospitals still includes a significant percentage of UAP. According to the U.S. Department of Labor, Bureau of Labor Statistics (2021a), 1.5 million nursing assistants (NAs) were employed in the United States in 2019. Of the UAP, 27% worked in hospitals, 37% in skilled nursing facilities, 11% in continuing care retirement communities and assisted living facilities for older adults, 5% in home care, and 4% for the government (U.S. Department of Labor, Bureau of Labor Statistics, 2021a).

Several reasons are commonly cited for the increased use of UAP. The primary argument for using UAP instead of licensed personnel is usually cost savings, though professional nursing shortages are a contributing factor (Marquis & Huston, 2021). Another widely recognized benefit is that they can free professional nurses from tasks and assignments (specifically, non-nursing functions) that can be completed by personnel with lower levels of training at a lower cost.

So why has the increased use of UAP created so much controversy? The answer is that in many institutions, UAP are not supplements to but replacements of professional RN staff. This is of concern because empirical research exists regarding what percentage of the staffing mix can safely be represented by UAP without negatively affecting patient outcomes. In addition, minimum national educational and training requirements have not been established for UAP, and their scope of practice varies from institution to institution. These issues raise serious questions as to whether greater use of UAP represents an effective solution to dwindling health care resources or whether it is an economically driven, short-term response that could lead to compromised patient outcomes.

> ***Consider This*** Given the lack of national regulatory standards regarding the scope of practice for UAP, some health care institutions allow UAP to complete tasks traditionally reserved for licensed practitioners.

This chapter, however, does not argue for the elimination of UAP. Instead, it addresses what safeguards must be incorporated in the use of UAP so that safe, accessible, and affordable nursing care is possible.

MOTIVATION TO USE UAP

Maximizing RN Time With Patients

UAP can maximize human resources because they free professional nurses from tasks and assignments that do not require independent thinking and professional judgment. This is significant because much of a typical nurse's time is spent on *non-nursing tasks* and functions. Non-nursing tasks and functions are those routine or standardized activities that can be done by an individual with minimal training and do not require a great deal of individual patient assessment, independent thought, or decision making. Examples of non-nursing activities include making a bed, taking vital signs, feeding patients, measuring intakes and outputs, and obtaining a weight or height.

Just how much time is spent by nurses doing non-nursing activities is, however, unclear. Anecdotal reports of significant time spent away from the bedside filling out redundant paperwork and searching for supplies are common among nurses working in acute care settings. So too are concerns about time spent documenting care, answering the phone, and entering and reviewing orders. Clearly, time spent on non-priority items or on tasks that could be done by someone with lesser training, reduce the amount of time that can be spent in direct patient care that improves patient outcomes.

> ### Discussion Point
> Why are professional RNs still completing so many non-nursing tasks? Are they reluctant to delegate them to ancillary personnel or are there inadequate support personnel to take on these tasks?

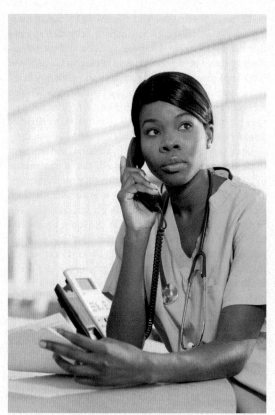

(spwidoff/Shutterstock)

Cost Savings

Cost savings associated with UAP use—the second argument for increased UAP use—are less clear. Studies completed early in the 21st century show conflicting findings, with some suggesting significant cost savings with UAP and others suggesting no cost savings due to the costs of supervision, high UAP turnover rates, and medical errors. Current research is limited. It is this lack of evidence, however, that has led some hospitals to resume reliance on UAP as the primary component of their staffing mix.

EDUCATIONAL REQUIREMENTS FOR UAP

Some monitoring of the regulation, education, and use of UAP has been ongoing since the early 1950s; however, most of this has been for *certified nurse's aides*. The Omnibus Budget Reconciliation Act of 1987 established regulations for the education and certification of nurse's aides- a minimum of 75 hours of state-approved theory and practice and successful completion of a competency examination in both areas.

No federal or community standards have been established, however, for training the more broadly defined UAP. Indeed, the health care industry provides many job opportunities for individuals without specialized training. This does not mean, however, that all UAP are undereducated and unprepared for the roles they have been asked to fill. Indeed, UAP educational levels vary from less than that of a high school graduate to those holding advanced degrees. It does suggest, however, that RNs, in delegating to UAP, must make no assumptions about the educational preparation or training of that UAP. Instead, the RN must carefully assess what skills and knowledge each UAP has, or risk increased personal liability for the failure to do so.

Discussion Point

Is work experience an appropriate substitution for formal education and training for UAP? Can this be determined by an experienced RN?

Far too often, the education and training of UAP in acute care settings is inadequate. In fact, there are no required educational standards or guidelines for the use of UAP in acute care settings. Instead, UAP educational and training requirements for acute care settings are generally facility based. This is important to remember when UAP transfer from one facility to another because no assumption should be made about UAP competency levels to perform certain tasks despite their work experience.

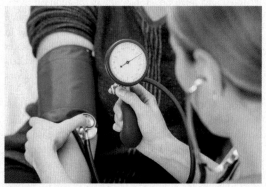

(Bencemor/Shutterstock)

The reality is that UAP training is often completed by the employing facility and occurs without formal certification. Formal training programs that do exist are typically completed at vocational schools and community colleges and focus on long-term care, providing certifications only as necessary to meet state requirements. Often, this training is inadequate and does not prepare UAP with the competencies they need to work in a dynamic health care environment, which is different from that which existed even a decade ago. For efficiency and safety, standardized curricula that address the skill sets needed in many settings where nurse aides are used should be implemented.

Discussion Point

What happens when the condition of a patient changes? Is the training of UAP adequate to recognize changes in patients' conditions that warrant seeking intervention from the licensed nurse?

UAP SCOPE OF PRACTICE

In some health care agencies, UAP assist with dressing changes, parenteral therapy, and urinary catheter insertion and perform numerous other tasks typically reserved for licensed personnel. The skill assumed by UAP, however, that has garnered the greatest concern, is administering medications. UAP who administer medications are also known as *unlicensed medication administration personnel, medication aides,* or *medication assistant technicians.*

For years, medication administration was considered a professional nursing function, requiring assessment and clinical judgment, but during the past decade, many states granted unlicensed personnel the right to administer medications, particularly in schools, assisted living facilities, and correctional institutions. In addition, *certified medicine aides* have worked in licensed nursing home settings, residential care settings, and adult day services in this country for almost four decades. As of 2019, 36 states permitted the administration of medications in select settings by assistive personnel once the requisite training was complete (ANA, n.d.).

However, the ANA (n.d.) suggests that despite the number of states that recognize this practice, there remains sufficient concern that the training is inadequate to ensure safe administration. The delegation of medication administration to UAP may be perceived by many RNs as delegating a professional nursing task that potentially places their license at risk. Indeed, many states lack clear and adequate provisions for nurse oversight of UAP who administer medications.

UAP also administer drugs in school settings when a school nurse is not present. It is the position of the National Association of School Nurses (2019) that when necessary and permitted by law, the registered professional school nurse can implement safe and effective delegation of nursing tasks to UAP at school. Safe nursing delegation requires that the school nurse is knowledgeable about the profession's guidance on delegation, state nurse practice acts, and other applicable federal and state laws and district policies. It also requires communication and collaboration between the school nurse, health care providers, school administrators, parents, teachers, and UAP (National Association of School Nurses, 2019).

Many school nurses and the organizations that represent them, however, are waging a battle to stop the expansion of UAP practice in terms of the drugs they can administer. They argue that the administration of medications is much more than dispensing a pill, handing a student an inhaler, or giving a subcutaneous injection. It requires high-level assessment skills; an understanding of drug actions, interactions, and side effects; and the highly developed critical thinking skills needed to intervene when problems occur. In addition, the practice of nursing clearly requires a license under the Nurse Practice Act.

As a result, numerous lawsuits have been filed in the last decade questioning the use of UAP to administer drugs such as insulin to school children. Indeed, in a landmark May 2013 case, the California Supreme Court was asked to make a ruling on whether allowing UAP to administer insulin to school children was unlawful since it sidestepped the Nurse Practice Act (California Healthline, 1998–2021). The California Nurse Practice Act specifically defines the act of medication administration as a licensed nursing function. The court ruled that California law does permit trained UAP to administer prescription medications, including insulin, in accordance with written statements of individual students' treating physicians and with parental consent (California Healthline, 1998–2021). Other states have followed.

In addition, the American Diabetes Association (ADA, 1995–2021, para. 2) notes that "Federal law gives students the right to receive the diabetes care they need to be safe and participate in school activities just like any other child." Thus, schools cannot require family members to go to school to care for a student's diabetes. Instead, the ADA encourages all schools to arrange for the training of staff members in necessary diabetes procedures like insulin injection and glucagon administration (ADA, 1995–2021).

There are those, however, who suggest that the use of UAP to administer drugs to school children is not only appropriate but also essential in today's economic climate with limited resources and increasing health care needs. The American Academy of Pediatrics (AAP, 2009), the National Association of School Nurses, and the ANA suggest that trained and supervised UAP, who have the required knowledge, skills, and composure to deliver specific school health services under the guidance of a licensed RN, should be allowed to do so. The AAP suggests that UAP can provide standardized, routine health services under the supervision of the nurse and on the basis of physician guidance and school nursing assessment of the unique needs of the individual child and the suitability of delegation of specific nursing tasks. Any delegation of nursing duties must be consistent with the requirements of state nurse practice acts, state regulations, and guidelines provided by professional nursing organizations (AAP, 2009).

> **Consider This** Many patients given direct care by UAP assume that UAP are licensed nurses. This confusion is promulgated when health care professionals do not include their credentials on their nametags or introduce themselves to patients according to their actual job titles.

Similarly, the Association of Women's Health, Obstetric and Neonatal Nurses (AWHONN) recognizes that UAP can function as supportive members of the health care team under the direction of the professional RN, but notes that it is the professional RN who is ultimately responsible for the coordination and delivery of nursing care to women and newborns (AWHONN, 2021).

The reality, then, is that in many settings, some UAP are performing functions that are within the legal practice of nursing. This may be a violation of the state nursing practice act and poses a possible threat to public safety. Clearly, certain professional responsibilities related to nursing care must never be delegated.

Therefore, it is critical that RNs never lose sight of their ultimate responsibility for ensuring that patients receive appropriate, high-quality care. This means that although the UAP may complete non-nursing functions such as bathing the patient, taking vital signs, and measuring and recording intake and output, it is the RN who must analyze that information using highly developed critical thinking skills and then use the nursing process to see that desired patient outcomes are achieved. Only RNs have the formal authority to practice nursing, and activities that rely on the nursing process or require specialized skill, expert knowledge, or professional judgment should never be delegated.

The UAP should be accountable for knowing how to properly perform their segment of assigned care and for knowing when other workers should be called in for tasks beyond the limits of their knowledge and training. As such, UAP do bear some personal accountability for their actions, despite the legal doctrine of *respondeat superior* (the

employer can be held legally liable for the conduct of employees whose actions they have a right to direct or control).

Regulatory Oversight of UAP

The increased use of UAP, called by some the "deskilling of the nursing workforce," has raised concern among professional organizations, consumers, and legislators alike. In the early 1990s, the ANA took the position that the control and monitoring of assistive personnel in clinical settings should be performed using existing mechanisms that regulate nursing practice. Typically, this includes the state board of nursing, institutional policies, and external agency standards.

Legislation has been introduced at the state level to regulate UAP use and scope of practice. Some states have attempted to regulate UAP practice through registration and certification. Others have proposed direct regulation of UAP by passing legislation that requires UAP to be certified by meeting education and competency requirements. Still others require the state boards of nursing or the department of health to register or certify UAP. Thus, regulation by state and jurisdiction varies widely, and getting all states to agree to uniform regulations is unlikely.

> **Discussion Point**
>
> Why has the movement to regulate UAP education and training occurred primarily at the state level? Why has there been no national movement to do the same?

Some state boards of nursing have issued recommendations regarding scope of practice for UAP or attempted to delineate the relationship between RNs and UAP. Few states, however, used the ANA or National Council of State Boards of Nursing definitions for delegation, supervision, or assignment. Most states also report that there are no standardized curricula in place for UAP employed in acute care hospitals. The states have not been able to reach a consensus regarding the education, training, and scope of practice needed for UAP to safely practice either. The result, then, is that there is no universally accepted scope of practice for UAP.

In addition to existing state regulations regarding UAP education and training, as well as required competencies, many professional nursing organizations have studied the use and effect of UAP and are adopting position statements regarding their use. The AWHONN (2021) has suggested eight actions that should be taken when UAP/NAP

<table>
<tr><td>

BOX 8.1

</td><td>

The Association of Women's Health, Obstetric and Neonatal Nurses' (AWHONN) Recommendations for the Use of UAP

</td></tr>
</table>

- Define UAP/NAP as unlicensed personnel who are not professional RNs but who are accountable to and work under the direct supervision of a professional RN to implement specifically delegated patient care activities.
- Evaluate the individual state's current Nurse Practice Act to ensure that UAP/NAP job descriptions and delegated activities are consistent with established rules, regulations, and statutes.
- Provide written job descriptions that clearly delineate duties, responsibilities, qualifications, skills, and supervision of UAP/NAP.
- Ensure that UAP/NAP are readily identifiable by the patient as nonlicensed.
- Establish competence-based performance expectations and systems for ongoing performance appraisals.
- Provide orientation and education for UAP/NAP, including didactic content as needed and appropriate for the clinical setting, evaluation of knowledge, and verification of clinical skills consistent with performance expectations and role responsibilities.
- Clearly define parameters in writing to ensure that all UAP/NAP are supervised directly by and responsible to professional RNs.
- Monitor and evaluate adherence of UAP/NAP to patient care guidelines and their effect on patient outcomes.

Source: Association of Women's Health, Obstetric and Neonatal Nurses. (2020). *The role of unlicensed assistive personnel (nursing assistive personnel) in the care of women and newborns.* Retrieved August 22, 2020, from https://www.jognn.org/article/S0884-2175(15)00018-0/fulltext Copyright © 2016 AWHONN, the Association of Women's Health, Obstetric and Neonatal Nurses. Published by Elsevier Inc. All rights reserved.

participate in direct care (Box 8.1). They also suggest that parameters for the education and supervision of these nursing support personnel must be in place.

In addition, to address the problem, some state boards of nursing have issued task lists for UAP (lists of activities considered to be within the scope of practice for UAP). However, in creating such a list, an unofficial scope of practice is created, and this suggests that such individuals will be performing activities independently. Task lists also suggest there is no need for delegation in that UAP already have a list of nursing activities that they may perform without waiting for the delegation process (Marquis & Huston, 2021).

In addition, at the institutional level, most health care organizations interpret regulations broadly, allowing UAP a broader scope of practice than that advocated by professional nursing associations or state boards of nursing. In addition, although some institutions limit the scope of practice for UAP to non-nursing functions, many organizations allow the UAP to perform skills traditionally reserved for the licensed nurse.

Liability is based on a supervisor's failure to determine which patient needs could safely be assigned to a subordinate or for failing to closely monitor a subordinate who requires such supervision. Experienced nurses have traditionally been expected to work with minimal supervision. The RN who delegates care to another competent RN does not have the same legal obligation to closely supervise that person's work as when the care is delegated to UAP.

Consider This The UAP has no license to lose for "exceeding scope of practice," and nationally established standards to state what the limits should be for UAP in terms of scope of practice do not exist. It is the RN who bears the legal liability for allowing UAP to perform tasks that should be accomplished only by a licensed health care professional.

In assigning tasks to UAP then, the RN must be aware of the job description, knowledge base, and demonstrated skills of each person. Thus, the need for nurses to have highly developed delegation skills has never been greater than it is today. The ability to use delegation skills appropriately will help reduce the personal liability associated with supervising and delegating to UAP. It will also ensure that patients' needs are met, and their safety is not jeopardized.

In addition, communication between the RN and UAP dyad is a critical factor in direct patient care and thus in patient safety. The bottom line is that delegating to UAP is like delegating to other types of health care workers. RNs are always accountable for the care provided and must be responsible for instructing UAP as to the patients who need care and when. The ANA has identified general principles for RNs to use in delegating to NAP; these are shown in Box 8.2.

> **BOX 8.2**   **American Nurses Association's Delegation Principles for RNs Who Work With Nursing Assistive Personnel**
>
> - The RN takes accountability and responsibility for all nursing care performed by the RN or a UAP.
> - The RN directs care and determines the appropriate utilization of any assistant involved in providing direct patient care.
> - The RN may delegate components of care but does not delegate the nursing process itself. The practice-pervasive functions of assessment, planning, evaluation, and nursing judgment cannot be delegated.
> - The decision of whether or not to delegate or assign is based on the RN's judgment concerning the condition of the patient, the competence of all members of the nursing team, and the degree of supervision that will be required of the RN if a task is delegated.
> - The RN delegates only those tasks for which they believe the other health care worker has the knowledge and skill to perform, taking into consideration training, cultural competence, experience, and facility/agency policies and procedures.
> - The RN individualizes communication regarding the delegation to the NAP and patient situation, and the communication should be clear, concise, correct, and complete. The RN verifies comprehension with the NAP and that the assistant accepts the delegation and the responsibility that accompanies it.
> - Communication must be a two-way process. The NAP should have the opportunity to ask questions and/or for clarification of expectations.
> - The RN uses critical thinking and professional judgment when following the "five rights of delegation" to be sure that the delegation or assignment is:
>   1. The right task.
>   2. Under the right circumstances.
>   3. To the right person.
>   4. With the right directions and communication.
>   5. Under the right supervision and evaluation.
> - Chief nursing officers are accountable for establishing systems to assess, monitor, verify, and communicate ongoing competence requirements in areas related to delegation.
>
> *Source:* American Nurses Association & National Council of State Boards of Nursing. (n.d.). *Joint statement on delegation.* Retrieved June 15, 2021, from https://www.ncsbn.org/Delegation_joint_statement_NCSBN-ANA.pdf

UAP AND PATIENT OUTCOMES

Because UAP are often involved in providing direct patient care activities, they directly influence not only the quality of care but also the care recipient's quality of life. A well-trained, caring, and competent UAP can be a vital and contributing member of the health care team.

At some point, though, given the increasing complexity of health care and the increasing acuity of patient illnesses, there is a maximum representation of UAP in the staffing mix that should not be breached. Those levels have not yet been determined. Considerable evidence does exist, however, that demonstrates a direct link between decreased RN staffing and declines in patient outcomes. Some of these declines in patient outcomes are nurse sensitive and include an increased incidence of patient falls, nosocomial infections, increased physical restraint use, and medication errors.

RN LIABILITY FOR SUPERVISION OF AND DELEGATION TO UAP

Delegation has long been a function of registered nursing, though the scope of delegation and the tasks being delegated have changed dramatically over the last three decades with the increased use of UAP in acute care settings. As a result, the RN role has changed in many acute care institutions from one of direct care provider to one requiring delegation of patient care to others.

This role of delegator and supervisor has increased the scope of legal liability for the RN. Although there is limited case law involving nursing delegation and supervision, it is generally accepted that the RN is responsible for adequate supervision of the person to whom an assignment has been delegated. Although nurses are not automatically held liable for all acts of negligence on the part of those they supervise, they may be held liable if they were negligent in the supervision of those employees at the time that those employees committed the negligent acts (Marquis & Huston, 2021). In addition, the nurse should never ask UAP to perform any activities on a patient whose status is unstable—activities that require assessment, problem solving, judgment, or evaluation (Wojciechowski, 2019).

The most common potential violations related to delegation to UAP are failure to supervise those under the supervision of the nurse and inappropriate delegation when the nurse may have reason to know the UAP was not qualified to perform the task (Wojciechowski, 2019). In either case, in a malpractice lawsuit, the nurse's actions or failure to act would be judged against professional practice standards in their state.

UAP, however, must recognize the responsibility and accountability that exist within their role as a care provider. The UAP are responsible both for the tasks they take on as well as the tasks they choose not to do. UAP must have a good understanding of what tasks are within their scope of practice.

> ### Discussion Point
>
> Do most UAP believe they can be held legally liable and accountable for their actions if they are delegated to do something by an RN that is beyond their scope of practice or training?

Marquis and Huston (2021) suggest that the bottom line is that RNs are always accountable for the care given and must be responsible for instructing NAP as to which patients need care, what type of care is needed, and when that care should be provided. NAP should be accountable for knowing how to properly perform their segment of assigned care and for knowing when other workers should be called in for tasks beyond the limits of their knowledge and training. Indeed, NAP must refuse to carry out a delegated task if they feel they do not have the skills, knowledge, and experience to carry it out safely; if the task is something they haven't done before or isn't a part of their normal duties; or if the supervision provided is inadequate. As such, the UAP do bear some personal accountability for their actions. This does not, however, negate accountability for the RN who delegated the task(s). The RN continues to be accountable for the care they deliver and for what is delegated.

RNS WORKING AS UAP: A LIABILITY ISSUE

It must also be noted that during economic downturns, some employers have hired new graduate RNs into UAP positions. Many of these transitional employees secured employment in these positions while students in nursing programs. Though this practice provides employment opportunities for new graduate nurses, it does raise several matters of legality. First, these RNs are not able to provide care to the level of their expertise. Instead, they must perform only direct care duties and remain in the scope of practice of an unlicensed person. This violates numerous statutes that govern scope of practice, because these statutes suggest that licensees are held to the level of practice associated with their licensure, regardless of employment status. Thus, licensed nurses are held liable to provide care to the level of their existing scope of practice and face risk of charges of negligence or malpractice if they provide care only to the level of the UAP. Working then in a capacity beneath the level of licensure appears to greatly increase the potential for legal liability for both the nurse and their employer and revocation of license for the nurse.

CREATING A SAFE WORK ENVIRONMENT

There are strategies health care organizations can use to increase the likelihood that UAP are used both effectively and appropriately as members of the health care team. First, the organization must have a clearly defined organization structure in which RNs are recognized as leaders of the health care team. This organization structure must facilitate RN evaluation of UAP job performance and encourage UAP accountability to the RN.

Health care agencies must also develop job descriptions that clearly define the roles and responsibilities of all categories of caregivers. These descriptions should be consistent with that state's nurse practice legislation as well as with community standards of care, and they should reflect differences between the roles of licensed and unlicensed personnel. Policies should facilitate adequate supervision of UAP by RNs and restrict UAP to simple tasks that can be performed safely. In addition, worker credentials should be readily apparent on the nametags worn by nursing health care personnel.

Unfortunately, in many health care settings, the UAP's job remains misunderstood and underexplored. Indeed, research by Band-Winterstein et al. (2019) found that the boundaries between what the UAP and the RN may do are often blurred or breached (Research Fuels the Controversy 8.1). Therefore, each care setting finds itself establishing internal guidelines and policies to address these issues within the limited scope of their unique setting. Researchers concluded that the dynamic and changing roles of health care assistants vis-à-vis professional nursing staff make it difficult to better frame formal policies in the field.

Research Fuels the Controversy 8.1

Job Analysis of UAP Employed in Nursing Homes

The aim of this qualitative, phenomenologic study was to describe and analyze how professionals, residents, and UAP themselves perceive the components of the actual work carried out by UAP in nursing homes. Data were collected from 50 semistructured in-depth interviews with 18 UAP, 15 certified nurses, and 17 older nursing home residents.

Source: Band-Winterstein, W. T., Doron, I., Zisberg, L., Shulyaev, K., & Zisberg, A. (2019). The meanings of the unlicensed assistive personnel role in nursing homes: A triadic job analysis perspective. *Journal of Nursing Management, 27*(3), 575–583. https://doi.org/10.1111/jonm.12713

Study Findings

Six content dimensions were identified in the participants' descriptions regarding the meanings of the roles and duties of the UAP: (a) care for the physical environment, (b) bodily physical care, (c) psychosocial interpersonal care, (d) professional hierarchy and boundaries, (e) UAP personal traits, and (f) UAP skills, or the need for training and professional education.

Findings revealed that on the day-to-day level, UAP provide important care services to older residents. These services range from cleaning and organizing rooms, bathing and dressing patients, and spending social time with the residents. UAP reported that while these tasks may seem nonprofessional in their essence, they all included some older adult-specific elements that need professional knowledge to be performed properly.

In terms of professional hierarchy and boundaries, UAP reported their position was complex and that they were located under a managerial level that sought to extend or broaden their roles and responsibilities to reduce the costs associated with other workers. They reported, however, that they were also located under the supervision of professional nurses, who viewed themselves as solely responsible for the health and physical conditions of the residents but who also needed the UAP to be able to fulfill their professional responsibilities.

There was an internal tension between the UAP and the nurses about how professional boundaries were drawn and acted upon. While it was clear to all participants that some jobs need to be done only by nurses and others only by UAP, the borders in real life, as described by the participants, were often blurred or breached. Residents were aware of this tension but accepted or understood the constraints that demanded compromises to daily practices. The researchers concluded that while their study takes a step forward in better defining the professional boundaries delineating the meaning of the UAP position, the dynamic and changing roles of health care assistants vis-à-vis professional nursing staff makes it difficult to better frame formal policies in the field.

Second, uniform training and orientation programs for UAP must be established to ensure that preparation is adequate to provide at least minimum standards of safe patient care. These training and orientation programs should be based on clearly defined job descriptions for UAP. In addition, organizational education programs must be developed for all personnel to learn the roles and responsibilities of distinct categories of caregivers. In addition, to protect their patients and their professional license, RNs must continue to seek current information regarding national efforts to standardize scope of practice for UAP and professional guidelines regarding what can be safely delegated to UAP.

In addition, there must be adequate program development in leadership and delegation skills for RNs before UAP are introduced. Delegation is a learned skill, and much can be done to better prepare RNs for this role. Educational programs that produce graduate nurses must explore the nature of the RN's role, with a focus on professional nurse leadership roles, to better prepare them to meet the challenges of working in restructured health care settings. Practicing RNs should have opportunities for continuing education in the principles of delegation and supervision. This will allow them not only to recognize the limitations of UAP's scope of practice but also to gain confidence in differentiating between skills requiring licensure and those that do not.

UAP SHORTAGES

Finally, if all the issues related to the education, training, scope of practice, and delegation to UAP are resolved, there may be an even greater problem. There may not be enough UAP to meet future demand. The U.S. Department of Labor, Bureau of Labor Statistics (2021b) projects that the need for UAP will grow 8% from 2019 to 2029, about as fast as the average for all occupations, predominantly in response to the long-term care needs of an increasing older adult population.

In addition, hospitals will continue to be pressured to discharge patients as soon as possible because of diminishing reimbursement, and this will boost admissions to nursing and residential care facilities. Modern medical technology will also drive the demand for UAP because as technology saves and extends more lives, the need for long-term care provided by UAP increases.

The reality is that the demand for UAP as direct caregivers is already growing and the population of individuals who have traditionally filled these jobs is declining. Indeed, there is a nationwide shortage of well-trained UAP in all settings, and although many states report recruitment and retention of support personnel as a major area of concern, few are actively addressing the situation.

These shortages grew worse with the COVID-19 pandemic in the United States (Flynn, 2021). Indeed, Flynn (2021, para. 3) notes that in a Congressional hearing held in summer 2020, one CNA was adamant that UAP staffing shortages were a problem well before the pandemic, telling representatives that "the only thing COVID did was rip the doors open." Similarly, a report by National Public Radio noted that record unemployment rates in the United States, the demands of caregiving in communities facing COVID-19 outbreaks, and continued shortages of UAP, were deeply felt in 2020 (Caremerge, 2021).

As a result, some UAP decided to leave their high-risk jobs and collect the enhanced unemployment benefits offered during the pandemic instead (Caremerge, 2021). Emanuel (2020) agrees, noting that some long-term care workers found they could make more from unemployment benefits than working, given the $600 extra per week from the federal government on top of typical state unemployment benefits while staying safer from infection. Nursing homes and long-term care facilities were accounting for 60% of COVID-19 deaths as of mid-2020, so many long-term care workers felt the pay they were offered to work did not match the risk (Emanuel, 2020). Indeed, a 2020 survey of nearly 2,400 nursing home workers revealed that almost 80% believed that going to work put their lives at risk (Mason, 2020).

UAP in Long-Term Care Settings

Another problem contributing to the UAP shortage is the high turnover rate, particularly in long-term care. The reasons for this high turnover rate are varied, but long hours, inadequate staffing, the low status of the job, exposure to infectious agents and drug-resistant infections, and the physical and emotional demands of the job contribute to it. In addition, Mason (2020) notes that most long-term care workers identify as women, in particular women of color and those from immigrant communities. This adds vulnerability for being taken advantage of in the workplace.

Working conditions are also often less than ideal. Because of high UAP turnover and absenteeism, UAP must often work shorthanded, leading to greater stress. In addition, many nursing home workers reported shortages of personal protective equipment (PPE) during the COVID-19 pandemic in 2020, and many reported having to reuse what should have been single-use PPE (Mason, 2020).

In addition, patients in nursing homes can require much more complex care than many people may imagine, and UAP should be appreciated for handling a combination of routine care as well as unexpected events. The skill needed to address the complexity of these care requirements may go unnoticed or be taken for granted. Hatcher (2020) notes that because NAs work directly with long-term care residents regularly, they typically are closely attuned to their patients' health statuses. Thus, they are often the first to recognize a condition change, such as loss of appetite, problems sleeping, new or different behaviors, and signs of pain.

It is also important to note that long-term care facilities, the most common employment site for UAP, are required to meet only minimum government standards for staffing and few facilities are cited for violations, even when understaffing occurs. For example, federal standards only require certified nursing homes that provide Medicare and Medicaid services to have a full-time director of nursing (DON), an RN on duty for 8 consecutive hours 7 days a week (this may be the DON), and one RN and licensed nurse (either an RN or licensed vocational nurse [LVN]/LPN) for the two remaining shifts, regardless of its size or the acuity of its patients ("State-Level Minimum," 2021). These federal regulations are out of date and do not reflect new knowledge on safe staffing levels. Many states have higher standards.

> **Consider This**   The brunt of work in long-term care settings typically falls on lowly paid, unlicensed workers who have a tremendous impact on patient satisfaction and the quality of care provided.

Low pay is also an issue. The U.S. Department of Labor, Bureau of Labor Statistics (2021c) noted that the median annual wage for NAs was $30,850 in May 2020. The median wage for UAP was highest in government facilities ($37,240) followed by hospitals ($32,160). Skilled nursing facilities were lower at $30,120 (U.S. Department of Labor, Bureau of Labor Statistics, 2021c).

The Governor of Nebraska announced in early 2018 that 20% pay increases would be granted to NAs at state veterans homes, saying that their wages had fallen behind peer states (Hammel, 2019). This pay increase was the result of a staff turnover of 110% in 2017 that required mandatory overtime and the use of private staffing agencies to fill positions, further increasing costs.

In addition, few employers provide UAP employer-paid benefits such as health insurance coverage, retirement benefits, or childcare. Furthermore, there are limited career paths or advancement opportunities for UAP who do not want to achieve a licensed job category (e.g., LPN, RN), and they often have little direct input into organizational decision making.

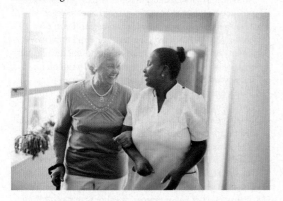

CONCLUSIONS

The increased use of UAP presents both opportunities and challenges for the American health care system. Clearly, UAP play an increasingly integral role in safe and resource-efficient care delivery in this country, particularly in long-term care settings, and they can be successfully used to augment the health care team. With increasing patient loads and an emerging nursing shortage, however, many health care organizations and the RNs who work within them will be tempted to allow UAP to perform tasks that should be limited to professional nursing practice.

The challenge then continues to be to use UAP only to provide personal care needs or nursing tasks that do not require the skill and judgment of the RN. Nurses must remember that the responsibility for ensuring that patients are protected and that UAP do not exceed their scope of practice ultimately falls on the RN. When UAP are allowed to encroach into professional nursing care, patients are placed at risk.

For Additional Discussion

1. Is cost or nursing shortages a greater driving force in increased UAP use in acute care hospitals today?

2. Is institutional training and certification of UAP a precursor to future initiatives for institutional licensure of RNs?

3. Are the cost savings associated with increased UAP use offset by the need for greater supervision by RNs and potential declines in patient outcomes?

4. Should UAP be allowed to administer medications, perform intravenous cannulation, and change sterile dressings?

5. Do you believe that patients are typically aware whether it is the UAP or licensed nurse who is caring for them?

6. How comfortable do you believe most RNs are in the role of delegator to UAP?

7. Do you believe most RNs are clear regarding role differentiation between the RN and the UAP?

8. Should the training and certification of UAP fall under the purview of state boards of registered nursing?

References

American Academy of Pediatrics. (2009). Policy statement— Guidance for the administration of medication in school. *Pediatrics, 124*(4), 1244–1251. Retrieved June 15, 2021, from http://pediatrics.aappublications.org/content/124/4/1244.abstract

American Diabetes Association. (1995–2021). *Know your rights. Safe at school.* Retrieved June 15, 2021, from https://www.diabetes.org/resources/know-your-rights/safe-at-school-state-laws

American Nurses Association. (n.d.). *Medication aides, assistants, technicians.* Retrieved June 15, 2021, from https://www.nursingworld.org/practice-policy/medication-aides—assistants—technicians

Association of Women's Health, Obstetric and Neonatal Nurses. (2021). *The role of unlicensed assistive personnel (nursing assistive personnel) in the care of women and newborns.* Retrieved June 15, 2021, from https://www.jognn.org/article/S0884-2175(15)00018-0/fulltext

Band-Winterstein, W. T., Doron, I., Zisberg, L., Shulyaev, K., & Zisberg, A. (2019). The meanings of the unlicensed assistive personnel role in nursing homes: A triadic job analysis perspective. *Journal of Nursing Management, 27*(3), 575–583. https://doi.org/10.1111/jonm.12713

California Healthline. (1998–2021). *Calif. Supreme Court rules school staffers can administer Rx drugs.* Retrieved June 15, 2021, from http://californiahealthline.org/morning-breakout/calif-supreme-court-rules-school-staffers-can-administer-rx-drugs

Caremerge. (2021). *How COVID-19 has shaped the CNA shortage & why better tech can make a difference.* Retrieved June 15, 2021, from https://caremerge.com/how-covid-19-has-shaped-the-cna-shortage-why-better-tech-can-make-a-difference/

Emanuel, G. (2020, June 15). *Many nursing home employees can make more on unemployment. Experts say this is causing staff shortages.* Retrieved August 23, 2020, from https://www.wgbh.org/news/local-news/2020/06/15/many-nursing-home-employees-can-make-more-on-unemployment-experts-say-this-is-causing-staff-shortages

Flynn, M. (2021, May 3). *To address staff shortages, nursing homes should follow home care's recruiting lead.* Skilled Nursing News. Retrieved June 15, 2021, from https://skillednursingnews.com/2021/05/to-address-staff-shortages-nursing-homes-should-follow-home-cares-recruiting-lead/

Hammel, P. (2019, October 16 [updated]). *Ricketts announces 20 percent pay bump for nursing assistants at state veterans homes.* Live Well Nebraska. Retrieved August 22, 2020, from http://www.omaha.com/livewellnebraska/ricketts-announces-percent-pay-bump-for-nursing-assistants-at-state/article_43d29e7a-f4c5-11e7-b19e-939c5efce6aa.html

Hatcher, T. L. (2020, June 23). *Delegating effectively to nursing assistants in post-acute care.* Retrieved August 23, 2020, from https://www.relias.com/blog/delegating-effectively-nursing-assistants-post-acute

Marquis, B., & Huston, C. (2021). *Leadership roles and management functions in nursing* (10th ed.). Wolters Kluwer.

Mason, A. (2020, June 14). *'They don't respect our job': Critical nursing home workers bear the brunt of the pandemic.* Retrieved June 15, 2021, from https://www.wbur.org/commonhealth/2020/06/14/coronavirus-nursing-home-employees-challenges

National Association of School Nurses. (2019). *Nursing delegation in the school setting.* Retrieved June 15, 2021, from https://www.nasn.org/nasn/advocacy/professional-practice-documents/position-statements/ps-delegation

State-level minimum nurse staffing requirements for nursing homes. (2021). Retrieved June 15, 2021, from http://www.countyhealthrankings.org/take-action-to-improve-health/what-works-for-health/policies/state-level-minimum-nurse-staffing-requirements-for-nursing-homes

U.S. Department of Labor, Bureau of Labor Statistics. (2021a). *Nursing assistants and orderlies: Work environment.* Retrieved August 22, 2020, from https://www.bls.gov/ooh/healthcare/nursing-assistants.htm#tab-3

U.S. Department of Labor, Bureau of Labor Statistics. (2021b). *Nursing assistants and orderlies: Job outlook.* Retrieved August 22, 2020, from https://www.bls.gov/ooh/healthcare/nursing-assistants.htm#tab-6

U.S. Department of Labor, Bureau of Labor Statistics. (2021c). *Nursing assistants and orderlies: Pay.* Retrieved August 22, 2020, from https://www.bls.gov/ooh/healthcare/nursing-assistants.htm#tab-5

Wojciechowski, M. (2019, February 6). *The risks of wrongful delegation.* Retrieved June 15, 2021, from https://dailynurse.com/the-risks-of-wrongful-delegation/

Diversity in the Nursing Workforce

Carol J. Huston

ADDITIONAL RESOURCES

Visit thePoint for additional helpful resources.
- eBook
- Journal Articles
- Web Links

CHAPTER OUTLINE

LEARNING OBJECTIVES

The learner will be able to:

1. Examine the relationship between health disparities and a lack of diversity in health care.

2. Identify common barriers faced in both recruiting and retaining students and faculty from minority backgrounds in higher education.

3. Suggest individual, organizational, and professional strategies to increase ethnic and gender diversity in nursing.

4. Compare opportunities for career advancement at senior levels of health care management between White and non-White individuals.

5. Investigate stereotypes of male nurses that both hinder the recruitment and retention of men into nursing and pose socialization and acceptance challenges for them.

6. Compare economic and advancement opportunities for men and women in nursing.

7. Identify at least three professional nursing associations that are directed at serving the needs of a specific racial or ethnic population.

8. Analyze research exploring generational differences in work values and preferences among registered nurses and explore the challenges inherent in having up to four generations work in the same profession at the same time.

9. Argue for or against the need for affirmative action to bring more men into the nursing profession.

INTRODUCTION

Diversity has been defined as the differences among groups or between individuals, and it comes in many forms, including differences in age, gender, religion, customs, sexual orientation, physical size, physical and mental capabilities, beliefs, culture, ethnicity, and skin color. Yet, despite increasing diversity (particularly ethnic and cultural diversity) in the United States, the nursing workforce continues to be fairly homogeneous, at least in terms of ethnicity and gender; nurses are predominantly White, female, and middle aged.

This lack of ethnic, gender, and gender diversity is a significant concern, not only for the nursing profession but also for its patients because a lack of diversity in the workforce has been linked to health disparities. A diverse nursing workforce that understands cultural influences related to illness and wellness and can adapt nursing interventions accordingly increases the likelihood that patients will receive culturally competent care (Williams et al., 2018). Young et al. (2020) agree, noting that a diverse nursing workforce will improve communication, tolerance, trust, and decision making between patients and providers, leading to expanded health care access and improved quality outcomes.

> *Consider This* For far too long, health care environments were thought of as neutral territories where patients were expected to be "good houseguests" who fit in, rather than recognizing and welcoming their diversity (Rauen et al., 2018, para. 1).

The nursing workforce then must strive to be at least as diverse as the population it serves. Rozelle (2018) agrees, suggesting that diverse health care teams are now considered critical for cultural competence and that organizations that promote diversity and inclusion are more successful than those that do not. That is because inclusive environments accept people for who they are and send a message that no one should feel like they have to change who they are to fit into the group. Indeed, a clamor for greater diversity in the profession continues to occur, and this is apparent in a review of the literature. Historically though, despite this stated need for and appreciation of the benefits of a diverse health care workforce, efforts to increase the number of professionals from nondominant backgrounds have not been as successful as hoped.

> ## Discussion Point
> For nursing care to be culturally and ethnically sensitive, must it be provided by a culturally and ethnically diverse nursing population?

This chapter focuses primarily on three aspects of diversity in the nursing workforce: ethnicity, gender, and age (generational factors), though as Cole (2020) notes, increased attention must also be given to diversity in sexual orientation and identity. Current literature on diversity often fails to address the 4% of the population self-identifying as lesbian, gay, bisexual, transgender, and/or queer (LGBTQ) (Cole, 2020). In addition, LGBTQ and intersex (LGBTQI+) people experience high rates of discrimination in health care settings worldwide, which have been linked to poor health outcomes and delays in seeking care (Sherman et al., 2021).

Factors leading to the lack of diversity in nursing are explored in this chapter, as are individual and organizational strategies to address the problem. In addition, the efforts of health care stakeholders, the federal government, states, and current professional nursing organizations to increase diversity in the profession are examined. Finally, the effect of generational diversity on workers and workplace functioning is presented.

ETHNIC DIVERSITY IN THE UNITED STATES

Demographic data from the U.S. Census Bureau continue to show increased diversification of the U.S. population, a trend that began almost 35 years ago. As of July 2019, 60.1% of the population was identified as White (not Hispanic or Latino origin) (U.S. Census Bureau, 2019). Hispanic individuals continue to be the largest minority group at 18.5% and are the fastest growing population group. Black individuals are the second largest minority group (13.4%), followed by Asian individuals (5.9%), Native Americans and Alaskan Natives (1.3%), and Native Hawaiians and other Pacific Islanders (0.2%) (U.S. Census Bureau, 2019).

ETHNIC DIVERSITY IN NURSING

There are significant differences, however, between the ethnic and gender demographics of the U.S. population and those of the nursing workforce in the United States (Table 9.1). Although the number of nurses from underrepresented backgrounds continues to rise in the United States, it is considerably lower than that of the general population.

According to 2017 data from the National Council of State Boards of Nursing and the Forum of State Nursing Workforce Centers, nurses from minority backgrounds represent just 19.2% of the registered nurse (RN) workforce, with the RN population identifying as 80.8% White, 6.2% African American, 7.5% Asian, 5.3% Hispanic, 0.4% Native American/Alaskan Native, 0.5% Native Hawaiian/Pacific Islander, 1.7% two or more races, and 2.9% other nurses. These figures show only small increases over the

TABLE 9.1   Comparison of U.S. Population and Registered Nurse Workforce in Terms of Ethnicity and Gender

Characteristic	Year 2019 U.S. Census Data (% Representation)	Year 2017 Registered Nurse Workforce (% Representation)
Gender: Male	49.2	9.1
Gender: Female	50.8	90.9
White (non-Hispanic and non-Latino)	60.1	80.8
Black/African American	13.4	6.2
Asian	5.9	7.5
Native Hawaiian/Pacific Islander	0.2	0.5
Native American/Alaskan Native	1.3	0.4
Hispanic/Latino	18.5	5.3
Persons responding to two or more races	2.6	1.7 (other)
Other	Not available	2.9

Source: American Association of Colleges of Nursing. (2019). *Enhancing diversity in the workforce.* Retrieved July 17, 2021, from http://www.aacnnursing.org/News-Information/Fact-Sheets/Enhancing-Diversity; U.S. Census Bureau. (2019). *Quick facts: United States.* Retrieved July 18, 2021, from https://www.census.gov/quickfacts/

past decade (American Association of Colleges of Nursing [AACN], 2019).

Nursing on Point (2021) suggests the numbers are even worse, with recent survey data showing that only about 15% of RNs are of racial or ethnic minority backgrounds as compared to about one-third of the general U.S. population. In addition, the attrition rate for nurses from minority backgrounds is higher, which makes it harder to predict the long-term percentage of nurses from minority backgrounds.

Similarly, Kovner et al. (2018) found only small increases in the number of White Hispanic nurses as well as males in the profession when comparing 2006 and 2016 data. These small gains did not meet the Institute of Medicine's (IOM, 2010) *Future of Nursing* recommendations related to increasing age, gender, and ethnic and racial diversity in the profession.

Recruiting and Retaining Students With Minority Backgrounds in Nursing

Clearly, increasing diversity in the nursing profession must begin with the aggressive recruitment and retention of minority students. The literature reports that individuals from *underrepresented minority* backgrounds in nursing programs encounter multiple recruitment and retention barriers to academic success including financial constraints, inflexible admission practices, a lack of mentoring, discrimination, a lack of guidance about program requirements,

and role stereotypes (i.e., the public's perception of what a nurse is "supposed to look like") (Kilburn et al., 2019; Nelson, 2019; Nursing on Point, 2021; Williams et al., 2018).

One significant barrier faced by underrepresented groups is that they may receive inferior preparatory education, which makes it more difficult for them to compete for nursing program enrollment (Gleeson, 2019a). This occurs because funding for education in the United States is typically heavily dependent on property taxes, with the wealthiest neighborhoods getting the highest funding for education (Gleeson, 2019b). Underrepresented groups are more likely to come from economically disadvantaged backgrounds and poorer neighborhoods. Since the property tax base for educational funding is lower in poorer neighborhoods, these students are often taught by less qualified and/or less experienced teachers in overcrowded classrooms. Indeed, on average, schools in the poorest school districts receive 15% less per pupil than schools in wealthier districts (Gleeson, 2019b). This inferiority of the educational experience then can cause students of color to underperform White students (Gleeson, 2019a).

In addition, because many students of color may be the first in their families to attend college, it may be difficult for family members to understand and be supportive of the challenges of higher education, the rigor of academic coursework, or the discrimination students of color may report experiencing. Indeed, Black students enrolled in higher education report higher levels of isolation, despair, disengagement, and alienation; more often consider dropping out; and have more difficulty relating to faculty than do White students of similar socioeconomic backgrounds and with similar grade point averages (Nelson, 2019). They also face greater challenges in achieving satisfactory grades than do White students of similar economic backgrounds (Nelson, 2019).

Patterson (2020) agrees, noting that Black male nursing students, one of the most underrepresented groups in the profession, often report feeling isolated, lonely, or alienated. Being one of only a few Black men in a classroom may heighten feelings of isolation, loneliness, and alienation, which in turn can decrease their sense of belonging. A sense of belonging has been positively associated with persistence and program success (Patterson, 2020).

In addition, a lack of diversity in faculty role models and mentors can contribute to the social isolation of students of color. When Black and indigenous people of color (BIPOC) have high-quality relationships with diverse faculty members, they benefit in terms of well-being, performance, and persistence (Hoobler & Washington, 2021). In K-12 programs in the United States, 44% of the students are of color, but 83% of the teachers are White (Gleeson, 2019b). Just 9% of the female faculty in higher education identify as American Indian, Asian/Pacific Islander, Black, or Hispanic, and the figures improve little even when they reflect both male and female faculty (Hoobler & Washington, 2021).

The reality is that White students continue to dominate ethnicity in many nursing programs in the United States. Only 34.2% of nursing students in entry-level baccalaureate programs in 2018 to 2019 were from minority backgrounds (AACN, 2019). In addition, about 34.7% of master's students and 33% of students in research-focused doctoral programs were from minority backgrounds (AACN, 2019). These numbers reflect only small percentage increases over the past decade, suggesting that although some strides have been made in recruiting and graduating nurses from minority backgrounds, more must be done before representation in line with the general population is realized.

Discussion Point

Should more resources (e.g., time, energy, money) be devoted to the recruitment and retention of underrepresented students? Is a two-pronged approach (emphasizing both recruitment and retention) necessary? Why or why not?

The key to recruiting more underrepresented students into nursing is likely creating learning environments that integrate diversity and cultural competence across academic programs and demonstrate an appreciation and respect of the students themselves. For example, Young et al. (2020) described efforts by Akron Children's Hospital to restructure an existing nurse technician program into one that would recruit nursing students of diverse backgrounds. The new program, *Assuring Success with a Commitment to Enhance Nurse Diversity* (ASCEND), targets the recruitment of nurses from underrepresented racial, ethnic, gender, and LGBTQ groups to complete an internship at the hospital with the goal of hiring them into the organization's workforce upon graduation.

Similarly, Kilburn et al. (2019) described both individual- and social-level recruitment strategies used over three 12-month periods to target candidates of color nearing eligibility for applying to certified registered nurse anesthetist (CRNA) programs at two entry points: colleges and workplaces. Strategies included developing information sessions and workshops, partnering with diversity organizations, gaining institutional support for diversity initiatives, creating inclusive marketing materials, and using targeted recruiting efforts. Program outcomes reflected that 24.5% of candidates (24 out of 98) for the 2016 to 2018 cohort identified as non-White—an increase of 100% over the previous year. Subsequent years' candidate pools reflected a similar increase in racial and ethnic diversity over baseline data.

Consider This Recruitment and retention of underrepresented nursing students could improve if these students were given solid secondary academic preparation and if the environments in which they are educated were more accepting of and hospitable to students from diverse backgrounds.

Finances are also often a barrier for students from disadvantaged backgrounds, many of whom must work at least part-time to subsidize the cost of their college education. To address the need for financial support for individuals from disadvantaged backgrounds, the U.S. Health Resources and Services Administration (HRSA, 2021) began offering the *Nursing Workforce Diversity* (NWD) program in 1998. This program provides grants or contracts to projects that provide student stipends or scholarships, stipends for diploma or associate degree nurses to enter a bridge or degree completion program, student scholarships or stipends for accelerated nursing degree programs, pre-entry preparation, advanced education preparation, and retention activities. In addition, the NWD program strengthens and expands the comprehensive use of evidence-based strategies shown to increase the recruitment, enrollment, retention, and graduation of students from disadvantaged backgrounds in schools of nursing (HRSA, 2021).

Consider This It is the retention and graduation of non-White students that will begin to change the cultural face of nursing.

Retention efforts, however, are at least as important as recruitment. Given that students who do not perceive any barriers to completing their nursing program are three times more likely to pass the NCLEX (National Council Licensure Examination) on the first attempt, significant attention must be given to retention efforts of underrepresented students (Williams et al., 2018).

In addressing retention of underrepresented minority and disadvantaged students in a baccalaureate nursing program, the University of Delaware School of Nursing (UDSON) developed a grant-funded multipronged program of recruitment and retention, comprising four pillars: economic support; academic support; social, emotional, and cultural support; and leadership and professional development (Diefenbeck & Klemm, 2021). Despite attempts to sustain the essential elements of the program after the grant concluded, student persistence outcomes lagged with the elimination of a dedicated retention coordinator.

Similarly, Opsahl and Townsend (2021) described the targeted inclusion of undergraduate nursing students from ethnic minority and socioeconomically disadvantaged backgrounds to participate in an honors research mentoring program. Study participants who were mentored for 3 years had a retention rate of 98% compared to a rate of 73% in the year before the start of the initiative. NCLEX-RN pass rates were 95% for those in the mentoring program compared to 84% for those not mentored.

Consider This Although most nurse educators and nursing students support the abstract notion of cultural diversity and its inclusion in nursing education in principle, their practices and behaviors may differ in action.

Diefenbeck et al. (2016) suggest that the responsibility for greater diversity in the nursing student population extends to nursing and university faculty, staff, and administration. Strategies they can and must use include implementing diversity training for faculty and students; ensuring cultural competency of the curriculum; fostering formal support structures such as minority student organizations; providing academic supports; facilitating affordability of college; and engaging family support as retention measures for racially and ethnically underrepresented students.

In addition, Pitts et al. (2020) note that all organizations should have a diversity and inclusivity statement that demonstrates their commitment to the value of people from all backgrounds. It should include language that emphasizes the value of diverse cultures, experiences, thoughts, and contributions and be clearly communicated to all the organizations' stakeholders.

Consider This Barriers to increasing the number of health care professionals from minority backgrounds include, but are not limited to, racism, discrimination, and a lack of commitment to changing the situation.

A summary of some of the barriers that students from underrepresented minority backgrounds face in completing their nursing education is shown in Box 9.1.

Nurse Educators From Minority Backgrounds

The underrepresentation of nurse faculty from minority backgrounds is also well documented. Lowery (2020) notes that faculty of color continue to represent less than 13% of nursing faculty. Although the number of diverse nursing faculty has made small but continuous gains over the past decade, the fact is that far too few nurses from racial or ethnic minority groups with advanced nursing degrees pursue faculty careers.

In an effort to increase the number of minority nurse scholars, the American Association of Colleges of Nursing (AACN) and the Johnson & Johnson Campaign for Nursing's Future launched a national scholarship program in 2007 to increase the number of nursing faculty from ethnic minority backgrounds (AACN, 2021). (There was no application cycle in 2019.) This scholarship program supports fulltime nursing students in doctoral or master's degree programs, with a preference given to those completing a doctorate. Scholarship recipients must agree to teach in a U.S. school of nursing after completing their advanced

BOX 9.1	**Common Barriers for Minority Students in Academic Nursing Programs**

1. Inferior academic preparation
2. Financial problems
3. Inadequate social support
4. A lack of mentoring opportunities
5. Inconsistent faculty and institutional support
6. Inadequate numbers of faculty role models from minority backgrounds

degree. Five scholarship recipients are selected annually, with each receiving a $18,000 scholarship.

Another opportunity to support minority faculty is the HRSA *Minority Faculty Fellowship Program* grants. These program grants provide stipends to educational programs to increase the number of faculty representing racial and ethnic minorities. This stipend provides up to 50% of the faculty salary, which is matched or exceeded by the employing institution.

DIVERSITY IN THE C-SUITE

Rosin (2020) notes that a diverse leadership team is important to the realization of strategic goals and objectives for businesses in any industry, yet across all industries, minorities continue to be underrepresented in top leadership positions. A recent study of Fortune 100 companies showed that only 25% of total C-suite (executive level) positions were held by women (Posner, 2020). Only seven companies had a female chief executive officer (CEO) and 9 of the 100 had no women directly reporting to the CEO (i.e., the C+1 level).

The C-suite was even less diverse when it came to race. Racially diverse executives of the Fortune 100 companies held only 16% of total C-suite positions and only 16 had a non-White CEO (Posner, 2020). Of the Fortune 100 companies, 26 had no ethnic diversity at the C+1 level, and 6 had no ethnic or gender diversity at this level. The chief financial officer (CFO) role was the least racially diverse position in the C-suite, with only four non-White CFOs (Posner, 2020).

Sahadi (2020) shares equally dismal numbers in her assertion that Black professionals in 2018 held just 3.3% of all executive or senior leadership roles, defined as within two reporting levels of the CEO, according to the U.S. Equal Employment Opportunity Commission. Among Fortune 500 companies, less than 1% of CEOs are Black. As of July 2020, there were only 4, down from a high of 6 in 2012, and over the past two decades, there have only been 17 Black CEOs in total (Sahadi, 2020).

Diversity in Health Care Administration

Like other industries, health care is struggling to increase diversity in leadership jobs as well. Although improving diversity is a priority to many health care organizations, progress is slow. Although one-third of patients are from minority backgrounds, only 11% of executive leadership positions, 19% of first and middle-level management positions, and 14% of board members are currently filled by individuals from these backgrounds (Butcher, 2017).

The National Association for the Advancement of Colored People (NAACP) suggests there are three primary challenges to increasing diversity in the health care industry, including a lack of diversification in upper management positions and critical pathways to skilled and leadership employment opportunities, as well as a lack of mentoring diversity procurement ("NAACP Grades 6," 2020) (Box 9.2). Indeed, the NAACP graded the six largest health care systems in the country in 2020 to assess the diversity of the workforce and supply chains of each. Dignity Health in San Francisco, California, achieved a letter grade of B, but the other five received letter grades of C or below ("NAACP Grades 6," 2020).

The problem is typically not a lack of highly qualified candidates with minority backgrounds to fill these top jobs. More often, it is that organizations fail to view these talented people as potential leaders. Linda Hill, a professor of business administration at Harvard Business School, suggests this may occur because there are "*demographic invisibles*"— people who, because of their gender, ethnicity, nationality, or even age, don't have access to tools like social networks, fast-track training courses, and stretch assignments—that can prepare them for positions of authority and influence (Hemp, 2008, p. 125). Hill also suggested that other potential leaders are missed because they are viewed as "*stylistic invisibles*"—individuals who don't fit the conventional

---

BOX 9.2 **Three Challenges Identified by the NAACP to Increasing Diversity in the Health Care Industry**

1. Despite a long history of diversity in health care areas related to patient care, diversification in upper management positions continues to lag.
2. As hospitals and health systems face pressure to reduce costs through automation, critical pathways to skilled and leadership employment opportunities may be closed off to diverse candidates.
3. Monitoring diversity procurement is lacking or "rudimentary" at best and a blind spot in the health care industry that is more pronounced than in any other industry the NAACP has surveyed thus far.

Source: NAACP grades 6 large health systems for diversity efforts. (2020). *Becker's Hospital Review*. ASC Communications. Retrieved August 17, 2020, from https://www.beckershospitalreview.com/hospital-physician-relationships/naacp-grades-6-large-health-systems-for-diversity-efforts.html

image of a leader because they don't exhibit take-charge, direction-setting behavior (Hemp, 2008, p. 125). This may also be partly attributed to cultural differences in styles more than leadership ability.

In addition, Sahadi (2020) notes that the culture of promotion sometimes excludes qualified candidates from minority backgrounds, who may not be part of the social networks that board members and CEOs often use to vet candidates. And since boards are typically risk averse, they tend to go for the same types of candidates, such as active or retired CEOs and executives who have already served on boards. Since there are so few executives with minority backgrounds in those categories to begin with, the same professionals with these backgrounds tend to be chosen again and again (Sahadi, 2020).

There are also differences in perceptions between White and non-White individuals and among genders as to how quickly the diversity leadership gap is narrowing. In a 2015 survey, nearly twice as many respondents felt that health care organizations had made headway compared to respondents in 2011 (Rosin, 2020; Research Fuels the Controversy 9.1). However, White respondents were more likely to say diversity had improved than non-White respondents (57% and 26%, respectively); respondents identifying as male were more likely to think diversity has improved (48%) than were respondents identifying as female (32%). Results also suggested an ongoing need to further improve diversity in the C-suite since multiple barriers still exist, slowing efforts to diversify health care management teams.

There is hope, however. The drive to bring more diversity to the leadership ranks and reduce health care disparities spurred the American College of Healthcare Executives, American Hospital Association, Association of American Medical Colleges, Catholic Health Association,

Research Fuels the Controversy 9.1

Diversity in the Health Care C-Suite

Witt/Kieffer distributed an online survey to a broad range of its executive clients in the summer of 2015. (The same survey had been distributed in 2011.) The company also conducted phone interviews with executives who participated in the survey. Of the 311 participants, 75% identified themselves as CEOs or other C-suite executives and vice presidents; 55% identified themselves using the study terminology as Caucasian, whereas 45% identified themselves using the study terminology as racially or ethnically diverse individuals; and 31% identified as female and 69% identified as male.

Source: Rosin, T. (2020). *5 findings on diversity—Or lack thereof—In the healthcare C-suite.* Becker's *Hospital Review.* Retrieved August 17, 2020, from http://www.beckershospitalreview.com/hospital-management-administration/5-findings-on-diversity-or-lack-thereof-in-the-healthcare-c-suite.html

Study Findings

- Two-thirds of respondents (66%) agreed that diversity recruiting enables an organization to reach its strategic goals, whereas 71% of respondents said cultural differences among executives support successful decision making. Another 72% of respondents agreed that a diverse workforce enhances the equity of care.
- Compared with 2011, both White respondents and non-White respondents agreed health care organizations' executive teams today are more racially diverse. However, just 26% of White respondents and 10% of non-White respondents agreed that executives from minority backgrounds are well represented today in health care management teams.
- Although slightly more respondents felt the diversity of management teams today reflect their patient demographics compared with respondents in 2011, the vast majority of respondents still disagreed. Asian respondents were most likely to disagree (90%), followed by Hispanic respondents (88%), Black respondents (77%), and White respondents (69%).
- White respondents were most likely to name lack of access to diverse candidates (indicated by 83% of White respondents), lack of diverse candidates to promote from within (81%), and lack of diverse candidates participating in the executive search process (77%) as the biggest barriers. Non-White respondents were most likely to cite a lack of commitment by top management (indicated by 85% of respondents), lack of commitment by the board (72%), and individual resistance to placing diverse candidates (64%) as the primary barriers.
- Survey respondents agreed that promoting minorities from within (indicated by 83% of all respondents), hiring executives from minority backgrounds for senior management jobs (73%), communicating the value of cultural differences (70%), seeking out candidates from minority backgrounds from professional organizations (67%), and seeking regular input about the organization's diversity initiatives (52%) could support efforts to diversify the senior management team.

and America's Essential Hospitals to form the *Equity of Care Committee* in 2011. This committee put together a set of best practices for building a leadership diversity program that includes the creation of diversity dashboards to determine how an organization is performing.

But even more effort is needed; companies need to offer those from minority backgrounds opportunities to shadow senior executives and should recruit at schools with diverse student populations. Marquis and Huston (2021) agree, suggesting that health care organizations must be more open-minded about who health care's future leaders might be and begin to prepare more diverse candidates to be effective leaders. This will require the formal education and training that are a part of most management development programs, as well as a development of appropriate attitudes through social learning.

Consider This Increasing the number of individuals from minority backgrounds in executive health care positions will require an intentional commitment to do so and a well-planned development program that includes the same type of mentoring activities that White individuals have long enjoyed and benefited from.

GENDER DIVERSITY IN NURSING

Diversity goals in nursing are not just directed at ethnicity; they also frequently include increasing the number of men in nursing. Decades of legal barriers kept men out of the profession, and some nursing schools refused to admit men until a 1981 U.S. Supreme Court ruling (Heitz, 2019). As a result, just 9.1% of U.S. nurses identified as men in 2019, a percentage that has climbed slowly but steadily since 1980 (AACN, 2019). The American Assembly for Men in Nursing hoped to bump that statistic up to 20% by 2020, but that goal was not reached (Heitz, 2019).

There are, however, efforts under way to increase the number of men in nursing. Some suggest that recruitment campaigns are not enough and that affirmative action, similar to the efforts used to increase the number of women in medicine and engineering, will be required before there will be any significant increase in the number of male nurses. Yet, despite a call to increase the number of men in nursing, progress in this regard has been slow.

A lack of male role models and mentors, sexism in nursing education and the media, and negative stereotypes of male nurses have contributed to the problem. Indeed, many Americans would describe nursing as a "female" occupation, and young men often report they never even considered a career as a nurse. The media also perpetuate the image of the nurse as female. Many media sources refer to the comforting caregiver nurse as "she," suggesting that male nurses are unable to demonstrate caring behavior and touch like their female counterparts. In addition, male nurses may be stereotyped as effeminate or predatory. These stigmatizing discourses may deter men's entry into nursing.

Consider This Caregiving is not exclusively a feminine act.

Stuesse and Stuesse (2017) suggest that notions about gender roles in the workplace need to be addressed through education at a young age. Stereotypical gender role choices need to be eliminated, and young minds need to be opened through education to career possibilities once dismissed as "not for men" or "not for women."

Consider This RN Frank Poliafico says one of the first things to know about men in nursing is what to call them—"I'm not a male nurse. I'm a nurse" (English, 2017).

Clearly, stereotypes that suggest male nurses are less capable of therapeutic caring, compassion, and nurturing than female nurses hurt the profession as well as society in general. Sometimes because of these stereotypes, some patients prefer female nurses when male nurses can provide the same level of care.

This seems to be particularly true for nurses employed in labor and delivery settings. As recently as 20 years ago, some states, like California, legally banned men from working as nurses on obstetric units. Today, states and hospitals cannot deny a male entry into a nursing profession simply based on gender. However, court cases have confused the issue further. In some cases, the courts have ruled that female gender identification is a legitimate qualification for labor and delivery nurses while other courts have found these qualifications to be discriminatory.

Is There a Male Advantage in Nursing?

Despite the barriers that male nurses face, their minority status may give them advantages in hiring, promotion, and pay—unlike women in male-dominated professions. Indeed, men in nursing often rise more rapidly into management positions and earn more money than their female counterparts. Paton (2021) notes that 2020 survey data found that male nurse salaries were on average 9% higher than female nurse salaries even when adjusted for factors like hours worked, education, and experience. Male nurses earned an average of $79,688 compared to $73,090 for women, a difference of $6,598 per year.

Similarly, the 2019 Medscape Compensation Report for Advanced Practice Nurses found that male nurse practitioners reported earning about 7% more than their female counterparts and male CRNAs reported earning about 11% more (Stokowski et al., 2019). The report did note that more male advance practice nurses were employed in higher wage acute care settings than their female counterparts, were more likely to be self-employed, and were more likely to seek out overtime.

Indeed, some experts have suggested that the more rapid career trajectory and relatively higher pay for male nurses likely reflects the historical trend that more men are employed fulltime in their career paths, while women tend to experience career gaps related to childbearing or family caregiving and often work fewer hours. There is limited research, however, to support this.

Some differences in work motivation were noted, however, in research by Muench et al. (2016) which found that female RNs moved less often across states and changed employers less frequently than did male RNs. In addition, male RNs were more likely to change jobs for pay, though no gender differences were associated with changing jobs for promotions. Gender pay differences, however, existed early in new graduate nurses' careers, negating the argument that pay differences were a result of men working more hours. This observation is disconcerting because gender differences in salary early in a career typically increase the gap over time. In addition, the gap also existed for female nurses who did not have children. Thus, a "motherhood penalty" is not a primary driver of the earnings gap in nursing (Muench et al., 2016).

> *Consider This* Many experts suggest that the power of the profession would be elevated if more men were to become nurses. However, men in nursing hold a disproportionately larger share of the high-income jobs and have higher salaries than their female counterparts.

In addition, some male nurses report a "male comradery" with male physicians that do not extend to their female counterparts. Research by Smith et al. (2020) suggested that male nurses report that male physicians treat them with more respect and value their opinions more than those of their female coworkers. Respondents reported that the difference in treatment was so profound that at times their female coworkers have asked them to approach physicians to discuss conflicts or debates that had arisen (Research Fuels the Controversy 9.2).

PROFESSIONAL ASSOCIATIONS SERVING MINORITY GROUPS IN NURSING

There is a professional association for almost every minority ethnic group in nursing. Several of these organizations include the National Black Nurses Association (NBNA), the National Association of Hispanic Nurses, the Philippine Nurses Association, the National Alaska Native American Indian Nurses Association, and the Asian American/Pacific Islander Nurses Association Incorporated. Indeed, the National Coalition of Ethnic Minority Nurse Associations (NCEMNA) (2021) was incorporated in 1998 to provide a unified force for all five of these associations to advocate for equity and justice in nursing and health care for ethnic minority populations. See Box 9.3 for more information about these groups.

> **Discussion Point**
> If our goal is to better appreciate and merge cultural and ethnic diversity in nursing, what reasons might there be for culturally and ethnically diverse professional nursing organizations?

GENERATIONAL DIVERSITY IN NURSING

Age has also come to the forefront as a diversity issue during the last decade. The problem is not that the nursing workforce lacks generational diversity but that in the past four generations have not worked at the same time in the profession. This climate offers challenges and opportunities for leaders. Opportunities include having a workforce that more closely resembles the diversity of patients served and the opportunity to benefit from different perspectives. Challenges include the complexities that result when productivity and efficiency are dependent on diverse team members who may have different generational goals, attitudes, beliefs, and values working together effectively.

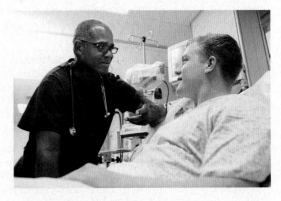

According to the 2018 National Sample Survey of Registered Nurses conducted by the HRSA, the average age for an

Research Fuels the Controversy 9.2

Men in Nursing

The aim of this interpretive descriptive study was to investigate the lived experiences of male nurses in today's health care environment to understand the persistently low numbers of men in nursing. Participants (N=11) were recruited through the American Association for Men in Nursing using purposive sampling. Focused interviews were conducted between May 2018 and June 2018. Interviews were semi-structured, guided by open-ended questions.

Source: Smith, C. M., Lane, S. H., Brackney, D. E., & Horne, C. E. (2020). Role expectations and workplace relations experienced by men in nursing: A qualitative study through an interpretive description lens. *Journal of Advanced Nursing, 76*(5), 1211–1220. https://doi.org/10.1111/jan.14330

Study Findings

Study findings suggested that both shared similar and distinctly individual experiences of the participants in primarily female-dominated clinical and academic work environments. Thematic categories of findings included role expectations and workplace relations. Role expectations were influenced by sociocultural views, professional acceptance, and patient/family perceptions. Workplace relations were associated with being male, social cliques, and peer support.

Participants frequently talked about the public's perception of male nurses. They agreed that the way society defines nurses has had a negative impact on men in nursing and contributed to persistently low numbers of men entering nursing by reinforcing a stereotype that equates nursing with identifying as female. Yet, most participants talked about the acceptance and support received from their female peers. All participants said they felt accepted throughout their careers, and most reported they felt valued by upper management and physicians more so than their female coworkers.

Indeed, some participants discussed that being male was sometimes an advantage. They believed that male physicians typically treated them with more respect and valued their opinions more than their female coworkers. They explained how the difference in treatment had been so profound that at times their female coworkers had asked them to approach physicians to discuss a conflict or debate. Participants attributed this preferential treatment to "male comradery."

In addition, participants' experiences with patients and families were varied and situation dependent. Much of the discussion focused on their interactions with female patients. More than half of the participants expressed having routinely encountered female patients who did not want to be cared for by a male nurse. These instances were usually related to patient concerns about a male nurse performing intimate care such as bathing or urinary catheter insertion. Most of the men expressed hesitancy and caution related to providing intimate care to female patients.

The researchers concluded that there has been progress toward increasing the number of men in nursing. However, increased efforts to recruit more men into nursing education and practice settings are needed to make nursing a more inclusive profession for men.

BOX 9.3   Ethnic Professional Associations in Nursing

Support groups and professional associations abound among nurses in the United States. Some of the groups formed to address specific issues related to ethnic diversity in nursing include the following:

National Black Nurses Association

The National Black Nurses Association (NBNA, 2021), founded in 1971, represents approximately 200,000 African American nurses from the United States, Canada, Eastern Caribbean, and Africa with 115 chartered chapters nationwide. The mission of the NBNA is to "provide a forum for collective action by African American nurses to represent and provide a forum for Black nurses to advocate for and implement strategies to ensure access to the highest quality of health care for persons of color" (NBNA, 2021, para. 4).

National Association of Hispanic Nurses

The National Association of Hispanic Nurses (NAHN, 2021) was founded in 1975 by Ildaura Murillo-Rohde and evolved out of the Ad Hoc Committee of the Spanish-Speaking/Spanish Surname Nurses' Caucus, which was formed during the American Nurses Association (ANA) convention in San Francisco in 1974. In 1976, the organization became the National Association of Spanish-Speaking/Spanish-Surnamed Nurses, which was renamed as the National Association of Hispanic Nurses in 1979. The NAHN is committed to advancing health in Hispanic communities and to lead, promote, and advocate the educational, professional, and leadership opportunities for Hispanic nurses.

| BOX 9.3 | **Ethnic Professional Associations in Nursing (*continued*)** |

Philippine Nurses Association, Inc.

Founded on September 2, 1922, as the Filipino Nurses Association (FNA), the FNA was incorporated in 1924 (Philippine Nurses Association [PNA], 2021). The International Council of Nurses accepted the FNA as one of the member organizations in July 1929. The FNA became the PNA in 1966. The mission of the PNA is to promote professional growth toward the attainment of the highest standards of nursing.

National Alaska Native American Indian Nurses Association

The National Alaska Native American Indian Nurses Association (NANAINA, 2021) was founded on its predecessor organization, the American Indian Nurses Association and later the American Indian Alaska Native Nurses Association. The NANAINA is dedicated to supporting Alaska Native/American Indian (AN/AI) students, nurses, and allied health professionals and exemplifies excellence in nursing through outreach, self-determination, and research by using traditions and innovation to achieve health equity. In addition, the mission is to unite AN/AI nurses and those who care for AN/AI people to improve the health and well-being of AN/AI people.

Asian American/Pacific Islander Nurses Association, Inc.

The Asian American/Pacific Islander Nurses Association, Inc. (AAPINA, 2018–2019) serves as the unified voice for Asian American Pacific Islander (AAPI) nurses around the world. AAPINA strives to positively affect the health and well-being of AAPIs and their communities by supporting AAPI nurses and nursing students around the world through research, practice, and education; facilitating and promoting networking and collaborative partnerships; and influencing health policy through individual and community actions.

RN is 50 years, which may signal a large wave of retirement over the next 15 years (AACN, 2020). Given the need to both retain older nurses and to recruit new, young nurses into the field, generational issues must be examined further.

Defining the Generations

Research increasingly indicates that the different generations represented in nursing today have different attitudes and value systems that may greatly impact the settings in which they work. They may also have significantly different career socialization experiences and expectations regarding their chosen profession and employer. In addition, workplace relationships are often influenced by these generational differences.

Most experts identify four generational groups in today's workforce: the veteran generation (also called the *silent generation*), the baby boomers, Generation X, and Generation Y (also called the *millennials*). The veteran generation is typically recognized as those nurses born between 1925 and 1942. Having lived through several international military conflicts (World War II, the Korean War, and the Vietnam War) and the Great Depression, they are often risk averse (particularly in regard to personal finances), respectful of authority, and supportive of hierarchy. They are also called the silent generation because they tend to support the status quo rather than protest or push for rapid change. As a result, these nurses are less likely to question organizational practices and more likely to seek employment in structured settings (Marquis & Huston, 2021). Their work values are

traditional, and they are often recognized for their loyalty to their employers.

Baby boomers (born between 1943 and 1960) also display traditional work values; however, they tend to be more materialistic and present oriented than the earlier generation and are thus willing to work long hours at their jobs to try to get ahead. They are personally gratified when they perform well at work. This is also a competitive cohort that insists that their work is done to the best of their ability, often beating deadlines. Nurses born in this generation may be best suited for work that requires flexibility, independent thinking, and creativity.

In contrast, Generation Xers (born between 1961 and 1981), a much smaller cohort than the baby boomers who preceded them or the Generation Yers who follow them, may lack the interest in lifetime employment at one place that prior generations have valued, instead valuing greater work-hour flexibility and opportunities for time off. They often put a high emphasis on family and leisure time and tend to be less economically driven than prior generations.

Generation Y (born between 1982 and 1999) are known for their optimism, self-confidence, relationship orientation, volunteer mindedness, and social consciousness. In addition, they are highly sophisticated in their use of technology; therefore, those who were born into homes with personal computers are considered "digital natives."

Although this type of generational diversity poses management challenges, it also provides a variety of perspectives and outlooks that can enhance productivity and result in the generation of new ideas. Although the literature often focuses on differences between and negative attributes of the generations, particularly for Generations X and Y, a more balanced view is needed. Generational diversity allows patients to receive care from both the most experienced nurses and those with the most recent education and likely greater technology expertise.

The key to integrating all these generations in the workforce at the same time is to foster a culture of inclusivity and encourage staff to learn, understand, and appreciate the generational differences. Thus, an appreciation of differences is fostered while focusing on shared goals.

THE CLAMOR FOR DIVERSITY: PROFESSIONAL ORGANIZATIONS SPEAK OUT

Although the need for diversity in nursing is not new, the need to successfully address this issue has never been greater. In response, the government, professional organizations, coalitions, and other health care stakeholders have introduced initiatives and funding to address the issue and bring attention to the lack of diversity.

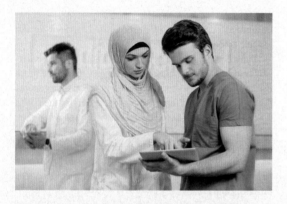

For example, in 2013, the AACN and the Robert Wood Johnson Foundation initiated the Doctoral Advancement in Nursing (DAN) Project to enhance the number of nurses with minority backgrounds completing PhD and Doctor of Nursing Practice (DNP) degrees. DAN's expert committee developed a white paper featuring successful student recruitment and retention strategies to be used by schools of nursing; comprehensive approaches to leadership and scholarship development for students; and suggestions for model doctoral curriculum. The DAN project has also created faculty and student toolkits to guide the process of gaining entry into doctoral programs.

In 2018, AACN (2019) launched the *Diversity, Equity, and Inclusion Group* (DEIG) to provide expert guidance to AACN and member schools on meeting strategic diversity goals. DEIG members work together to explore innovative approaches to enhancing diversity, equity, and inclusion

in academic nursing and the nursing workforce. Group members share evidence-based practices, engage with the membership, convene networking forums, and mentor new diversity officers in nursing schools.

Even more recently, The Joint Commission (2021) released a Quick Safety advisory entitled "Understanding the Needs of Diverse Populations in Your Community" that provided four strategies and actions to help hospitals and medical centers better support their diverse communities. One of these strategies noted that leadership should make equity a strategic priority within its institution. The IOM (2010) report, *The Future of Nursing*, suggested that to improve the quality of patient care, more emphasis was needed to make the nursing workforce diverse, particularly in the areas of gender and race.

In addition, in 2021, leading nursing organizations, including the American Nurses Association (ANA), NBNA, NCEMNA, and NAHN convened for the inaugural meeting to launch the *National Commission to Address Racism in Nursing* (the *Commission*). The Commission will examine the issue of racism within nursing nationwide and describe the impact on nurses, patients, communities, and health care systems to motivate all nurses to confront systemic racism (ANA, 2021).

In addition, many professional nursing organizations have issued position statements or recommendations on diversity. In 2017, AACN, the national voice for baccalaureate and higher degree education programs, drafted a position statement that recognizes diversity, inclusion, and equity as critical to nursing education and fundamental to developing a nursing workforce able to provide high-quality, culturally appropriate, and congruent health care in partnership with individuals, families, communities, and populations ("AACN Position Statement," 2017). The position statement suggests that to improve the quality of nursing education, ameliorate health inequities, and advance leadership in the profession and society at large, the values and principles of diversity, inclusion, and equity must remain mission central.

Similarly, the National League for Nursing (NLN) issued a vision statement in 2016 that suggested that diversity and quality health care are inseparable, and that together, they can create a path to increased access and improved health and the elimination of health disparities ("NLN Releases a Vision," 2016). The NLN affirmed its commitment to the education of exemplary nurses who value and embody the richness of difference and inclusion to advance the health of the nation and the global community.

The *ANA Code of Ethics for Nurses* also advocates for diversity in its assertion that the nurse, in all professional relationships, practices with compassion and respect for the inherent dignity, worth, and uniqueness of every individual, unrestricted by considerations of social or economic status, personal attributes, or the nature of health problems.

The American Organization of Nurse Executives (now American Organization for Nursing Leadership) also developed a diversity statement in 2005. This statement suggests that the success of nursing leadership as a profession depends on reflecting the diversity of the communities it serves and that diversity is one of the essential building blocks of a healthful practice and work environment. In contrast, the International Council of Nurses does not have a diversity statement but rather has embedded diversity in its policy and practice. For example, the organization promotes the principles of equal opportunity employment, pay equity, and occupational desegregation.

CONCLUSIONS

Although nursing has made strides in recruiting and graduating students from minority and disadvantaged backgrounds, the United States remains far from achieving the goal of a nursing workforce that mirrors the nation's diverse population (Spencer, 2020). Even though projections suggest that current ethnic minorities are likely to become a majority in the U.S. population in the coming decades, this diversity is not reflected in the nursing workforce or in schools of nursing.

Similarly, men are underrepresented in nursing, and efforts to increase the number of men in the nursing profession are even fewer than those directed at increasing ethnic diversity. Finally, generational diversity is present in all

health care organizations; however, few organizations have directly confronted the implications of how to deal with its challenges and opportunities or examined the impact it has on the quality of care provided.

Using incremental change strategies to address the lack of ethnic and gender diversity in nursing has been ineffective. Clearly, proactive, well-thought-out strategies are needed at multiple levels and by multiple parties before diversity in the nursing profession mirrors that of the public it serves. Barrier (2020, p. 14) agrees, noting that "committing to diversity, inclusion, and equity poses continuous challenges, but must start with crucial conversations and observable strategies that produce new knowledge to best meet the needs of the academic institutions, practice organizations, and the health care population." Barrier notes the nursing profession must be called to action to make diversity, equity, and inclusion a strategic initiative.

In addition, diversity, equity, and parity must be moral imperatives. Malone (2020) points out that the goal must not be just achieving diversity. It must be about inclusivity. "Diversity with inclusion affirms the uniquenesses of people and differences among them—their ideas and values as well as their ethnicities. The leader achieves a culture of diversity when inclusiveness, willingness, and yearning to understand ourselves and one another move beyond simple tolerance to embracing and celebrating the richness of each individual, with the understanding that we are all more similar than different" (Malone, 2020, p. 226).

For Additional Discussion

1. What are the strongest driving and restraining forces for increasing ethnic diversity in nursing, increasing gender diversity in nursing, and having a multigenerational nursing workforce?

2. What are the advantages and disadvantages of intergenerational nurses working together?

3. Should funding for diversity initiatives come from federal or state governments or from corporate partnerships?

4. Should the institutions that reap the benefits of a diverse workforce share the costs to make that happen?

5. Should there be different nursing school entry requirements for students from nondominant backgrounds than for their White counterparts?

6. Is an affirmative action approach needed to increase the number of both men and minorities in the nursing profession?

7. Will having more men in nursing raise the status of the profession?

8. What are the potential barriers to having more men in the nursing profession?

9. Why have women been better able to further their numbers in medicine than men have in nursing?

10. How does the use of mentors assist in both the recruitment and the retention of nurses from ethnic and gender minority backgrounds?

11. Does a multigenerational nursing workforce improve patient care? If so, how?

12. Which health disparities do you think would be more positively impacted if the nursing workforce was more diverse?

References

AACN position statement on diversity, inclusion, & equity in academic nursing. (2017). *Journal of Professional Nursing, 33*(3), 173–174. https://nursing.utexas.edu/sites/default/files/AACN_Position_Statement.pdf

American Association of Colleges of Nursing. (2019). *Enhancing diversity in the workforce.* Retrieved July 17, 2021, from http://www.aacnnursing.org/News-Information/Fact-Sheets/Enhancing-Diversity

American Association of Colleges of Nursing. (2020). *Nursing shortage.* Retrieved July 17, 2021, from https://www.aacnnursing.org/News-Information/Fact-Sheets/Nursing-Shortage

American Association of Colleges of Nursing. (2021). *Johnson Johnson/AACN minority nurse faculty scholars.* Retrieved July 17, 2021, from http://www.aacnnursing.org/Students/Financial-Aid-Scholarships/Minority-Nurse-Faculty-Scholarship

American Nurses Association. (2021, January 25). *Leading nursing organizations launch the National Commission to address racism in nursing.* Retrieved July 19, 2021, from https://www.nursingworld.org/news/news-releases/2021/leading-nursing-organizations-launch-the-national-commission-to-address-racism-in-nursing/

Asian American/Pacific Islander Nurses Association, Inc. (2018–2019). *About us.* Retrieved July 17, 2021, from https://aapina.org/our-history/

Barrier, K. (2020, July/August/September). The future of nursing: What does diversity, inclusion, and equity mean? *Pelican News, 76*(3), 14.

Butcher, L. (2017, September). Enhancing diversity. *H&HN: Hospitals & Health Networks, 91*(9), 18–23.

Cole, K. A. (2020). Health disparities and diversity in the nursing workforce: A call to action. *Kansas Nurse, 95*(1), 18–20.

Diefenbeck, C., Michalec, B., & Alexander, R. (2016, January). Lived experiences of racially and ethnically underrepresented minority BSN students: A case study specifically exploring issues related to recruitment and retention. *Nursing Education Perspectives (National League for Nursing), 37*(1), 41–44. https://doi.org/10.5480/13-1183

Diefenbeck, C. A., & Klemm, P. R. (2021). Outcomes of a workforce diversity retention program for underrepresented minority and disadvantaged students in a baccalaureate nursing program. *Journal of Professional Nursing, 37*(1), 169–176. https://doi.org/10.1016/j.profnurs.2020.06.001

English, T. (2017, February 1). I am not a male nurse. I am a nurse. *The Journal of Nursing.* Retrieved August 17, 2020, from https://www.asrn.org/journal-nursing/february1-2017.html

Gleeson, P. (2019a, June 11). *Why minority students get bad grades: The Pygmalion effect.* Retrieved July 17, 2021, from https://exclusive.multibriefs.com/content/why-minority-students-get-bad-grades-the-pygmalion-effect/education

Gleeson, P. (2019b, June 5). *Why minority students get inferior educations: School funds and teacher expectations.* Retrieved July 17, 2021, from https://exclusive.multibriefs.com/content/why-minority-students-get-inferior-educations-school-funds-and-teacher-expe/education

Heitz, D. (2019, August 1). Male nurses are on the rise—Filling a need and making a living. *Healthline.* Retrieved July 18, 2021, from http://www.healthline.com/health-news/male-nurses-are-on-the-rise-filling-a-need-and-making-a-living-042215#1

Hemp, P. (2008). Where will we find tomorrow's leaders? A conversation with Linda A. Hill by Paul Hemp. *Harvard Business Review.* Retrieved July 18, 2021, from https://hbr.org/2008/01/where-will-we-find-tomorrows-leaders

Hoobler, J. M., & Washington, A. S. (2021, June 14). *Myths of the diversity dilemma.* Retrieved July 17, 2021, from https://aacsb.edu/insights/2021/june/myths-of-the-diversity-dilemma

Institute of Medicine. (2010, October). *The future of nursing: Leading change, advancing health.* Retrieved August 18, 2020, from http://thefutureofnursing.org/IOM-Report

Kilburn, F., Hill, L., Porter, M. D., & Pell, C. (2019). Inclusive recruitment and admissions strategies increase diversity in CRNA educational programs. *AANA Journal, 87*(5), 379–389.

Kovner, C. T., Djukic, M., Jun, J., Fletcher, J., Fatehi, F. K., & Brewer, C. S. (2018, March). Diversity and education of the nursing workforce 2006–2016. *Nursing Outlook, 66*(2), 160–167. https://doi.org/10.1016/j.outlook.2017.09.002

Lowery, Y. (2020, Jan. 29). The minority nurse faculty shortage. *Minority Nurse.* Retrieved July 18, 2021, from https://minoritynurse.com/the-minority-nurse-faculty-shortage/

Malone, B. (2020). Without diversity, there is no excellence. *Nursing Science Quarterly, 33*(3), 226–228. https://doi.org/10.1177/0894318420920611

Marquis, B., & Huston, C. (2021). *Leadership roles and management functions in nursing* (10th ed.). Wolters Kluwer.

Muench, U., Busch, S. H., Sindelar, J., & Buerhaus, P. I. (2016, September/October). Exploring explanations for the female-male earnings difference among registered nurses in the United States. *Nursing Economics, 34*(5), 214–223.

NAACP grades 6 large health systems for diversity efforts. (2020). *Becker's Hospital Review.* ASC Communications. Retrieved August 17, 2020, from https://www.beckershospitalreview.com/hospital-physician-relationships/naacp-grades-6-large-health-systems-for-diversity-efforts.html

National Association of Hispanic Nurses. (2021). *History.* Retrieved July 18, 2021, from https://www.nahnnet.org/about/history

National Black Nurses Association. (2021). *About NBNA.* Retrieved July 17, 2021, from http://www.nbna.org/about

National Coalition of Ethnic Minority Nurse Associations. (2021). *About.* Retrieved July 17, 2021, from https://ncemna.org/about/

Nelson, E. (2019, April 3). *The case for race-conscious affirmative action.* Retrieved July 17, 2021, from https://daily.jstor.org/the-case-for-race-conscious-affirmative-action/

NLN releases *a vision for achieving diversity and meaningful inclusion in nursing education.* (2016, May/June). *Nursing Education Perspectives (National League for Nursing), 37*(3), 186. https://doi.org/10.1097/01.NEP.0000000000000018

Nursing On Point. (2021). *Diversity in nursing: An overview.* Retrieved July 18, 2021, from https://nursingonpoint.com/about-nursing/nursing-diversity/minorities-in-nursing/

Opsahl, A. G., & Townsend, C. (2021). Mentoring to engage diverse undergraduate nursing students in honors research. *Nursing Forum, 56*(1), 19–23.

Paton, F. (2021, July 12). *Nurse salary 2020: How much do registered nurses make?* Retrieved July 18, 2021, from https://nurseslabs.com/nurse-salary/

Patterson, L. D. (2020). African American males as registered nursing students: A scoping review. *ABNF Journal, 31*(1), 19–30.

Philippine Nurses Association Inc. (2021). *About PNA: History.* Retrieved July 17, 2021, from https://pna-ph.org/the-company/about-pna/history

Pitts, C., Hudson, T., Reeves, G., Christenbery, T., & Johnson, R. (2020, July/August). Writing a diversity and inclusivity statement: Guidelines for nursing programs and faculty. *Nurse Educator, 45*(4), 198–201. https://doi.org/10.1097/NNE.0000000000000754

Posner, C. (2020, May 1). *The sorry state of C-suite diversity.* Retrieved July 17, 2021, from https://cooleypubco.com/2020/05/01/sorry-state-c-suite-diversity/

Rauen, C. A., Knippa, S., Blystone, L., & Roff, H. (2018, April). Response to diversity. *Critical Care Nurse, 38*(2), 76–80. https://doi.org/10.4037/ccn2018435

Rosin, T. (2020). 5 findings on diversity—Or lack thereof—In the healthcare C-suite. *Becker's Hospital Review.* ASC Communications. Retrieved August 17, 2020, from http://www.beckershospitalreview.com/hospital-management-administration/5-findings-on-diversity-or-lack-thereof-in-the-healthcare-c-suite.html

Rozelle, C. (2018, Winter). Exposing students to diverse health care teams. *ABNF Journal, 29*(1), 5–7.

Sahadi, J. (2020, June 2). *After years of talking about diversity, the number of black leaders at US companies is still dismal.* Retrieved July 17, 2021, from https://www.cnn.com/2020/06/02/success/diversity-and-black-leadership-in-corporate-america/index.html

Sherman, A. D. F., Cimino, A. N., Clark, K. D., Smith, K., Klepper, M., & Bower, K. M. (2021, February). LGBTQ+ health education for nurses: An innovative approach to improving nursing curricula. *Nursing Education Today.* Retrieved July 18, 2021, from https://pubmed.ncbi.nlm.nih.gov/33341526/

Smith, C. M., Lane, S. H., Brackney, D. E., & Horne, C. E. (2020). Role expectations and workplace relations experienced by men in nursing: A qualitative study through an interpretive description lens. *Journal of Advanced Nursing, 76*(5), 1211–1220. https://doi.org/10.1111/jan.14330

Spencer, T. D. (2020, July). Improving diversity of the nursing workforce through evidence-based strategies. *Journal of Nursing Education, 59*(7), 363–364. https://doi.org/10.3928/01484834-20200617-01

Stokowski, L. A., McBridge, M., & Berry, E. (2019, November 6). APRN compensation report 2019. *Medscape.* Retrieved August 22, 2020, from https://www.medscape.com/slideshow/2019-aprn-comp-report-6012127#1

Stuesse, E. R., & Stuesse, M. J. (2017). A woman's job? A man's job? *Reflections on Nursing Leadership, 43*(2), 20–23.

The Joint Commission. (2021, July 14). *New Quick Safety advisory on understanding needs of diverse populations to address health and well-being.* Retrieved July 18, 2021, from https://www.jointcommission.org/resources/news-and-multimedia/news/2021/07/new-quick-safety-advisory-on-understanding-needs-of-diverse-populations/

The National Alaska Native American Indian Nurses Association. (2021). *NCEMNA.* Retrieved July 18, 2021, from https://ncemna.org/ourcauses/the-national-alaska-native-american-indian-nurses-association-nanaina

U.S. Census Bureau. (2019). *Quick facts: United States.* Retrieved July 17, 2021, from https://www.census.gov/quickfacts/

U.S. Health Resources and Services Administration. (2021). *Nursing workforce diversity (NWD) program.* Retrieved July 17, 2021, from https://www.hrsa.gov/grants/find-funding/hrsa-21-020

Williams, L., Bourgault, A., Valenti, M., Howie, M., & Mathur, S. (2018, March). Predictors of-underrepresented nursing students' school satisfaction, success, and future education intent. *Journal of Nursing Education, 57*(3), 142–149. https://doi.org/10.3928/01484834-20180221-03

Young, C., Mosca, N., & Aurilio, L. (2020, January 30). *Enhancing diversity in the nursing workforce.* Retrieved August 21, 2020, from https://www.childrenshospitals.org/Newsroom/Childrens-Hospitals-Today/Winter-2020/Articles/Enhancing-Diversity-in-the-Nursing-Workforce

Disaster Planning: Are We Prepared?

Elizabeth O. Dietz

ADDITIONAL RESOURCES

Visit thePoint for additional helpful resources.
- eBook
- Journal Articles
- Web Links

CHAPTER OUTLINE

LEARNING OBJECTIVES

The learner will be able to:

1. Identify the three types of disasters.
2. Define disaster nursing.
3. Differentiate between disaster nursing and emergency nursing.
4. Discuss various roles nurses assume during disasters.
5. Identify nursing functions when caring for clients in shelters.
6. Review standards and guidelines for disaster nursing and planning.
7. Reflect on the importance of both personal and institutional disaster preparedness.
8. Provide examples of self-care when providing disaster nursing.

INTRODUCTION

The last decade has been marked by a broad spectrum of disasters worldwide and this has resulted in changes in how we define and plan for disasters. Indeed, disasters are not "one size fits all." A disaster can be any catastrophic event that causes death to humans and animals as well as damage to a community's infrastructure. Disasters can also cause extensive property damage and, in some cases, the complete destruction of communities.

Disasters also affect acute care hospitals as well as community health and public health agencies. Since many acute care agencies are certified by The Joint Commission (TJC), these entities must have disaster plans as part of their standards and polices. Many community health and public health agencies, however, are not accredited by TJC, and their functions and care during a disaster differ from those of acute care hospitals. In addition, multiple other groups are part of the Voluntary Organizations Active in Disasters (VOAD), a coalition of organizations in community and public health. Their response is also an important part of disaster management.

This chapter begins by detailing classifications of disasters and the need for proactive disaster planning. The primary focus of the chapter, however, is on the roles nurses play in preparing for and responding to disasters, both as employees and as volunteers. Particular attention is given to the multitude of responsibilities disaster nurses hold in preparing and supervising shelters so that vulnerable refugees receive appropriate care. In addition, the need for self-care and personal disaster readiness is emphasized for nurses responding to disasters. Finally, the chapter concludes with a brief overview of the impact of COVID-19 on long-held principles of disaster planning and care.

TYPES OF DISASTERS

The Centers for Disease Control and Prevention (CDC, n.d.) offers many resources that define the types of disasters as well as preparation for, response to, and evaluation of disasters. Before September 2011, however, there were only two classifications of major disasters: *man-made* and *natural*. Since then, however, a *hybrid* classification was added by the CDC. Regardless of the type, all disasters cause severe disruptions in the immediate area of the disaster as well as in adjacent communities.

Man-made disasters include civil unrest, acts of terrorism, active shooter incidents, acts of war, highway and other transportation incidents, chemical emergencies, civil war, government collapse, and other acts of violence. Although wars are considered man-made disasters, they are not covered in this chapter. Examples of the aftermath of man-made acts of violence are listed in Box 10.1. Actions to take following an act of man-made violence are outlined in Box 10.2.

Natural disasters are acts of nature and may include earthquakes, severe storms, tornadoes, hurricanes, landslides and mudslides, and wildfires. From 2005 to 2020, there were over 50 recorded colossal natural disasters, mostly wildfires, tornadoes, hurricanes, and winter storms (Statista Research Department, 2021). Natural disasters may also be associated with seasons. In the United States, hurricane season is late July to November. Wildfire season

---

BOX 10.1   Common Consequences of Man-Made Disasters

- Law enforcement becomes heavily involved at local, state, and federal levels.
- Health and mental health resources in the affected communities are often strained to their limits and may become overwhelmed.
- Extensive media coverage, increased public fear, and international complications and consequences may continue for a prolonged period.
- Workplaces and schools may be closed, and there may be restrictions on domestic and international travel.
- Residents may have to evacuate the area, avoiding roads blocked for safety.
- Clean-up removal of debris and handling of human remains may take many months.
- Locations may become crime scenes and multiple agencies must determine how to best clean up and investigate.

Sources: American National Red Cross. (2021). *Terrorism safety tips*. Retrieved September 13, 2021, from https://www.redcross.org/get-help/how-to-prepare-for-emergencies/types-of-emergencies/terrorism.html; Federal Emergency Management Agency. (2021). *Home page*. Retrieved September 13, 2021, from https://www.fema.gov; Federal Bureau of Investigation. (n.d.). *Resources*. Retrieved September 13, 2021, from https://www.fbi.gov/resources; Federal Emergency Management Agency. (2021, April 28). *Make a plan*. Author. Retrieved from http://www.ready.gov/america/makeaplan/; Federal Emergency Management Agency. (2020, October 1). *FEMA publishes annual preparedness survey: Trends show Americans becoming better prepared*. Retrieved September 13, 2021, from https://www.domesticpreparedness.com/updates/fema-publishes-annual-preparedness-survey-trends-show-americans-becoming-better-prepared/

BOX 10.2 **Actions to Take Following a Man-Made Disaster**

- Remain calm and be patient. Use your senses to determine what is going on around you and what you can do.
- Protect yourself and your fellow staff members if present; survey the scene, and check yourself and then your colleagues for physical injuries.
- Follow the instructions of local emergency officials when they arrive.
- Listen to your radio or television for news and instructions; turn on the radio, cell service, and other communication methods around you.
- If an event occurs near you, check yourself for injuries. Provide first aid and get help for seriously injured people once you know you are not injured.
- If the event occurs near your home while you are there, check for damage using a flashlight. Do not light matches or candles or turn on electrical switches. Check for fires, fire hazards, and other household hazards. Sniff for gas leaks, starting at the water heater. If you smell gas or suspect a leak, turn off the main gas valve, open the windows, and get everyone outside quickly.
- Shut off any damaged utilities.
- Confine or secure your pets and animals. Large farm animals and ranch stock animals are not easy to place; arrangements should be determined in the planning stage. In an emergency, animals that should be separated may need to be placed together.
- Call your family contacts, and then do not use the phone again unless it is a life-threatening emergency.
- Check on your neighbors, especially those who are older or disabled.

can start as early as April and last through October. Tornado season can occur during any time of the year but tends to follow the same pattern as hurricane season. Earthquakes are not seasonal but instead occur when underground tectonic plates shift. Understanding patterns of natural disasters whenever they are known can help in preparation.

Hybrid disasters are made up of multiple specific types of disasters. A hybrid disaster may be a man-made disaster such as the Oklahoma City bombing in April 1995 followed by school shootings, the two bombings of the World Trade Center in New York, and the devastations of September 11, 2001. All disasters involving violence or terrorism are caused by human intervention. These disasters are designed to cause death, injuries, damage, and fear and their effects can be widespread and devastating. In addition, there can be significant numbers of casualties and/or damage to buildings and the infrastructure.

An example of a hybrid disaster is the Fukushima accident or the Fukushima nuclear accident, which occurred in the northern part of Japan in March 2011. A series of earthquakes and tsunami generated waves so strong that the nuclear plant fell apart setting off nuclear material in the plant and surrounding areas. There were multiple explosions with damage from the earthquake and the melting of the nuclear material in the plant.

DISASTER NURSING

Nurses are resources for health care in acute care settings and in the community when responding to disasters. Nurses often fill several key roles in disasters, with many volunteering to serve. In addition, while some nurses do not choose to be involved in disaster nursing, all nurses can play an important part during disaster events. The roles nurses play depend on the nurse's level of education, experience, and desire to participate in the care of the clients involved in the disaster.

Consider This It is important that nurses who want to serve in disasters are adequately prepared to do so.

Wherever nurses' practice, they must have the ability to:

- Provide education to clients and agencies concerning the issues and health needs related to a disaster.
- Assist with a variety of tasks, including first aid, health care delivery, medication administration, triage, and providing mental health care.
- Provide volunteer services to community agencies such as the American Red Cross, U.S. Public Health Service (USPHS), Federal Emergency Management Agency (FEMA), and other Voluntary Agencies Active in Disaster (VOAD) agencies.
- Render service for disasters within their own employment settings.
- Assist with personal, community, and family emergency planning and preparation (Nevada State College, 2018).

Part of a nurse's response to disasters is having knowledge of disaster planning and preparation. There might be rules and regulations within the state, territory, or agency where the nurse works. Nurses must be prepared to determine if they can act effectively during a disaster.

Nurses also need to understand the role of disaster services within their own agencies as well as within organizations that specialize in disaster care and assistance. It is important that the nurse who wants to assist in disaster care understands the appropriate policies, procedures, and rules of any VOAD agencies as well as state and community laws and ordinances. Disaster nurses are often assigned different roles from their normal day-to-day functions. Some nursing roles in a disaster might include establishing triage centers, utilizing the assessment phase of the nursing process to determine client needs, providing first aid, and/or providing or replacing of client medications.

Although there might be organizations that provide payment to nurses in disaster situations, most nurses volunteer through a variety of community agencies. It is up to each nurse to make sure they are appropriately serving within their agency. Developing an understanding of the disaster preparedness and response plans, operational protocols, and security measures can help nurses understand what these agencies expect of them.

In addition, before nurses can provide disaster care they must assess their own personal desire to participate in disaster relief. Many times, the disaster has occurred in a nurse's home area, and they must determine if they are needed for nursing care by their own families, communities, and employment locations. Personal safety is also a critical consideration before any nurse chooses to participate in disaster care. The Society for the Advancement of Disaster Nursing (n.d.) concurs, noting there are many barriers that impact nursing's ability and willingness to respond to disasters. Among them are a lack of personal preparedness, concern or fear for family and pets, effect of the disaster on oneself and one's personal property, transportation obstacles, fear for oneself within the work environment, and the absence of crisis standards of care.

Discussion Point

Have you ever personally been involved in a disaster? If so, did you choose to actively participate in disaster relief? What personal considerations were taken into consideration? Were there factors you should have considered but did not? If you have not personally been involved in a major disaster, what factors would influence your decision to participate in relief efforts?

In addition, nurses should not spontaneously respond to disaster situations. Instead, they should register to volunteer through a disaster relief agency or nongovernmental agency. Otherwise, there may be no record of their knowledge and training by the group they are working with at the disaster site.

Consider This
No one should ever self-deploy to a disaster, but rather join organizations and groups that are officially sanctioned by local, state, and/or federal governments. Nurses and other staff that self-deploy have not verified their presence with the designated disaster groups.

In addition, *workers' compensation* and other types of insurance are not available to most disaster nurse volunteers. Nurses need to work with the organizations from their employers or faith-based and community-based organizations to be a part of disaster relief. It is also important that nurses wait until it is safe to travel to disaster sites to help.

Indeed, nurses can and do encounter many unanticipated challenges while providing disaster relief services (Box 10.3). Working within a disaster scenario then is not for nurses who lack courage, flexibility, adaptability, and even a sense of humor to get through a disaster's unique challenges. Additional information about personal disaster preparedness is presented later in the chapter.

BOX 10.3   Challenges Experienced by Nurses While Providing Disaster Relief Services

- Balancing professional and personal obligations
- Restrictions to volunteering based upon training and immunizations
- Limited resources and supplies
- Potential security and safety threats such as violence or infectious disease
- Legal implications regarding practicing outside of one's specialty area if the nurse is not properly trained
- Uncontrolled physical environments
- Life-and-death situations and difficult ethical decisions

Source: Nevada State College. (2018, July 23). *Nurses play a critical role in disaster response.* Retrieved September 13, 2021, from https://online.nsc.edu/articles/rn-bsn/nurses-critical-role-disaster.aspx

Consider This Nurses involved in disaster planning need to have internal values of common sense, flexibility, and a sense of humor. These attributes may be just as important as clinical and organizational skills.

If a nurse is not prepared for a disaster, has no disaster training, and has not planned for potential disasters at home, responding to a widespread disaster can create a personal disaster. According to the American Nurses Association (ANA, 2008), disaster nurses are often faced with multiple agency and community issues. These are detailed in Box 10.4.

DIFFERENCES BETWEEN DISASTER NURSES AND EMERGENCY NURSES

One key difference between disaster nurses and emergency nurses is how they refer to the audience they are serving. In the acute setting of the emergency room, the nurse cares for patients. In the community setting, disaster nurses care for clients. This differentiation can cause misunderstanding by families and staff in these situations.

BOX 10.4 **Agency and Community Challenges Associated With Disasters**

- Community and personal loss of essential services, including electricity, water, sanitation services, and/ or food supply
- Agency loss of infrastructure, including agency and home facilities or electronic information
- Worker shortages due to lack of transportation, worker or worker family illness/injury, or unwillingness to report to work
- Triage required at a community level
- A sudden increase in the number of patients in agencies employing nurses that occur in marked excess of capacity or surge capacity or with elevated injury severity score or other extreme patient conditions
- Loss of primary health care facilities and forced relocation of care to alternative facilities not fully equipped for patient care
- Need for up-to-date information about the medical needs of employees and how to contact designated next of kin

---

The specific terms used can be very confusing—however, disaster nursing and agencies refer to their people they treat as clients.

Consider This Dr. Leah Curtin (Bonsall, 2016) posed the following differentiation between "patients" and "clients":
Patient: Comes from the Latin word *patior*, which means "to suffer"; "one who suffers"
Client: Comes from the Latin word *clinare*, which means "to lean," "one who is the recipient of a professional service"

Disaster nursing is not emergency room nursing even though nursing care is rendered in emergencies. Emergency room nurses treat patients who are suffering from trauma, injury, or severe medical conditions and require urgent treatment. Since these specialists work in crisis situations, they must be able to quickly identify the best way to stabilize patients and minimize further injury or death.

Emergency room nurses learn to quickly triage patients based on immediate observation and acute assessment skills, then to treat symptoms in order of life-threatening priority. They may immediately start cardiopulmonary resuscitation (CPR) to reverse cardiopulmonary arrest, start the rapid infusion of blood products for a hemorrhaging patient, or work to quickly help identify underlying medical conditions that are less apparent. Emergency room nurses may also be called trauma nurses and critical care nurses. The job is fast-paced, adrenaline-provoking, and completely unpredictable shift to shift; emergency nurses need to be able to think fast and react well under pressure (Hamstra, 2018).

Emergency room nursing usually begins with a process of triage in an indoor or outdoor assessment of the patients coming in for acute care. The focus of care is curative. Resources nurses may use include advanced life support (ALS), telemetry, and laboratory and radiologic equipment. Once assessments are completed, immediate access to surgical rooms exists for patients who need them. There is generally also adequate personal protective equipment (PPE), staff, and other equipment. The emergency room is therefore an environment that is clean and well stocked with consumable supplies. Blood products, medications, and hospital equipment are all generally available upon request. In addition, the roles of the staff are clearly documented.

Disaster nursing is not as organized as emergency nursing, and nursing roles may be less standardized or organized than those in the emergency room. Indeed, nurses in disaster relief organizations typically perform their roles outside of acute care agencies and must provide care in various nonmedical locations such as fairgrounds, gymnasiums, convention halls, recreational vehicle (RV) parks, and hotels or motels.

The primary functions of the disaster nursing team are not always focused on acute care; instead, they include triaging clients that come to a disaster shelter, feeding and clothing survivors, reuniting families, and facilitating temporary living arrangements. In this type of triage, if the client needs acute medical or surgical intervention, they will be sent via the emergency medical system to an acute care hospital emergency room.

In disaster nursing, clients are typically brought to a *temporary evacuation place* (TEP) while decisions are made about setting up disaster shelters. The TEP is meant to protect clients from unsafe conditions while decisions are made about the need for potential sheltering or short-term client placement. Community centers, family centers in the location of the disaster, or other similar places can serve as TEPs. Clients in the TEP are provided with snacks, water, and a place to rest, but it is not set up for 24-hour care. Depending on the location and the disaster, services provided may be extensive or minimal. Immediate care is provided for registration of clients, assessment of the clients' needs, and provision of basic functional needs.

In contrast, the evacuation or emergency shelter itself will provide care for a longer period of time, and clients will be able to sleep in the shelter. The full 24-hour services provided in shelters include dormitory sleeping, food, hygiene, and other appropriate services. Most emergency shelters are open only for 2 to 4 weeks. After that time, the community emergency operations center, government agencies, and nonprofit social service agencies must come together to determine where clients might be best placed. Ideally, community agencies will have worked with sheltering agencies, and short-term or long-term housing arrangements will have been made.

Many times, in large disasters such as wildfires or hurricanes, these housing arrangements can take months and even years to permanently resolve. Hurricanes Katrina, Sandy, and Harvey are examples in which emergency sheltering, short-term sheltering, and, finally, long-term sheltering solutions took years. Specific assessments that need to be completed for clients in these types of shelters are discussed later in this chapter.

THE ROLE OF THE NURSE IN DISASTER MANAGEMENT

There are multiple roles for nurses in disaster planning and response. Some of the roles that nurses take on in responding to disasters are shown in Box 10.5. Nursing functions required in shelters after disasters occur, are shown in Box 10.6.

Care of Clients in Emergency Shelters

One key role assumed by nurses in disaster management is caring for clients in emergency shelters. As clients are evacuated from the specific disaster area, there needs to be a safe and secure location for the clients to stay during the interim. Most of the time, clients will be placed in TEPs or emergency shelters.

Part of the basis for the use of contracts in establishing temporary shelters for clients is the understanding that when the disaster is over, the facility will be returned to the owner in equal or better condition than before the disaster. All personnel who are working with the health care team need to assist in this part of the operation. Shelter facilities that incur damages while being used as a shelter must be repaired, often at great financial burden to the requesting agency. Gymnasium floors can cost over $10,000 to be resurfaced if there is damage. Bathrooms and kitchen faculties need to be repaired if damage has occurred. Water or chemical spills must be cleaned. Trash and other items need to be disposed of appropriately. This is one reason why

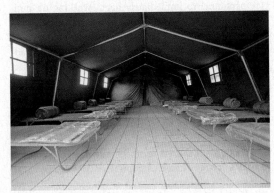

(Baloncini/Shutterstock)

BOX 10.5	Common Roles Assumed by Nurses in Disasters

- Emergency response planning
- Triage
- Leading and directing patients and staff when necessary
- Patient care delivery
- Patient discharge and transfer as well as coordination of transportation and resources for transfer
- Rescuing patients in immediate danger

BOX 10.6

Nursing Functions Required in Shelters After Disasters Occur

- Registration and initial client/family assessments
- Facilitation of living arrangements
- Feeding area setup and cleanup
- Health care, mental health care, and spiritual care services coordination
- Facilities or services for the appropriate care and feeding of service animals
- Provisions for nonservice animals, comfort and therapy animals, and pets
- An information and communication program for clients and staff
- A transportation program for clients, supplies, and staff
- Space for personal possessions
- Coordination with the local public health department and public health nursing departments for inspection

shelter staff need to be present while clients are using the shelter.

Appropriate emergency shelter sites also allow clients to safely park their vehicles, enter the shelter safely, and be able to utilize all the resources within the shelter. Accommodations may need to be made for clients with disabilities who need additional assistance in navigating the shelter.

Assessments and Recordkeeping

In addition, before clients are placed in any disaster living accommodation, an assessment of disability integration and the shelter's accessibility must be done using FEMA's "access and functional needs" form. *Cot-to-cot counts* are a part of this assessment, as well as the need for durable medical equipment. This form also helps the nursing health staff identify and provide appropriate referrals to health services onsite or offsite for emergency medical services and acute care agencies.

The disaster relief team must also identify consumable supplies and health care attendant services for clients. It is recommended that the first assessment be completed within the first 6 hours of the shelter opening as well as every 24 hours while clients are in an acute stage of the disaster. The client record forms and the client referral forms held by nursing staff in the client unit are used to communicate with agencies assisting the shelter.

Legal contracts or memoranda of understanding (MOU) also need to be written and agreed upon before the shelter

site can accommodate disaster clients. This initial assessment can be done using the U.S. Department of Health and Human Services public health emergency CMIST framework: communication, maintaining health, independence, support, and transportation. This framework is used to provide care in shelters and as a basis for referrals to other community health agencies.

In addition, disaster nurses may be involved in completing a daily *disaster health service quality indicator* form. This form is generally due to disaster relief operations leadership by 5 p.m. each day. Information includes client needs for oral medications, emergency department visits by shelter residents, and clients struggling with activities of daily living (ADLs) (American National Red Cross, 2021).

Other required documentation may include a *client assistance memorandum* (Form 1475). This memo form assists with determining what resources need to be spent for a client in any Red Cross setting but usually in congregate or noncongregate shelter sites. These confidential forms are held by nursing staff in the client unit.

In addition, assessments must be made constantly when a shelter is in use for infection prevention and control (IPC). During disasters with limited resources, damaged infrastructure, and involvement of multiple organizations, establishing shelter disease surveillance and IPC is difficult. However, prioritizing this is necessary to prevent, identify, and contain outbreaks.

For example, following California's deadly *Camp Fire* in 2018, shelter IPC assessments revealed gaps in illness surveillance, isolation practices, cleaning, disinfection, and handwashing. Two county health departments collaborated with partner agencies to implement acute gastroenteritis (AGE) screening, institute isolation protocols and 24-hour cleaning services, and promote proper hand hygiene (Chen et al., 2020; Karmarkar et al., 2020). See Research Fuels the Controversy 10.1.

Despite these efforts, outbreaks of norovirus occurred in the Camp Fire shelters, prompting disaster health service personnel to immediately begin working on policies and procedures to combat the outbreak. The health services team also worked with shelter dormitory and food managers to investigate the process to prevent additional outbreaks. As a result, local disaster health services members were able to create materials for changes in standards and procedures during disasters. These new job tools will be put into the protocols for future disasters the agency will respond to (Chen et al., 2020; Karmarkar et al., 2020).

Finally, many shelters maintain individual client health records to document a client's primary complaints and to document. Additional assistance is often required to address lost medications, damaged or lost durable medical

Research Fuels the Controversy 10.1

Norovirus Outbreak Following the Camp Fire in California: The Need for Infection Prevention and Control Assessment and Practices

The Camp Fire, California's deadliest wildfire, began on November 8, 2018, and was extinguished on November 25. The wildfire burned 153,336 acres; destroyed 18,793 structures (including one acute care hospital and three skilled nursing facilities); displaced approximately 52,000 individuals; and killed 85. Nongovernmental organizations (NGOs) opened nine shelters in Butte and Glenn counties that housed a total of approximately 1,100 evacuees. Evacuees stayed in shelter facilities (i.e., indoor evacuees) and shelter-associated parking lots (i.e., outdoor evacuees). On November 10, acute gastroenteritis (AGE) was reported in two evacuation shelters; norovirus illness was suspected, because it is commonly detected in shelter-associated AGE outbreaks. Norovirus is highly contagious and resistant to several disinfectants. The Butte County Public Health Department (BCPHD), assisted by the California Department of Public Health (CDPH), initiated active surveillance to identify cases, confirm the etiology, and assess shelter infection prevention and control (IPC) practices to guide recommendations.

Sources: Karmarkar, E., Jain, S., Higa, J., Fontenot, J., Bertolucci, R., Huynh, T., Hammer, G., Brodkin, A., Thao, M., Brousseau, B., Hopkins, D., Kelly, E., Sheffield, M., Henley, S., Whittaker, H., Herrick, R. L., Pan, C.-Y. Chen, A., Kim, J., … Lewis, L. (2020, May 22). Outbreak of norovirus illness among wildfire evacuation shelter populations—Butte and Glenn Counties, California, November 2018. *MMWR: Morbidity & Mortality Weekly Report, 69*(20), 613–617; Chen, A., Kim, J., & Schaumleffel, L. (2020, May 22). Outbreak of norovirus illness among wildfire evacuation shelter populations—Butte and Glenn Counties, California, November 2018. *MMWR: Morbidity & Mortality Weekly Report, 69*(20), 613–617.

Study Findings

Beginning November 17, CDPH and BCPHD regularly verified the number of patients with AGE and assessed shelter IPC. IPC assessments at six shelters evaluated the availability of physically separate isolation facilities, including toilets; cleaning frequency; and shelter staff members' norovirus IPC knowledge and practices.

Guided by onsite observations, the more comprehensive CDC Shelter Assessment Tool was adapted to focus on six areas: (1) environmental and kitchen practices; (2) illness screening protocols; (3) hand hygiene (including sink access); (4) facility cleanliness; (5) self-service practices for food and beverages; and (6) child play area cleanliness. Teams observed and documented staff member and evacuee adherence to handwashing before meals and before building entry and exit.

A total of 292 patients with AGE were identified among the nine evacuation shelters; norovirus was detected in 16 of 17 unique patient stool specimens. Shelter IPC assessments revealed gaps in illness surveillance, isolation practices, cleaning, disinfection, and handwashing. CDPH and BCPHD collaborated with partner agencies to implement AGE screening, institute isolation protocols and 24-hour cleaning services, and promote proper hand hygiene.

During disasters with limited resources, damaged infrastructure, and involvement of multiple organizations, establishing shelter disease surveillance and IPC is difficult. However, prioritizing effective surveillance and IPC at shelter activation is necessary to prevent, identify, and contain outbreaks of infectious diseases.

equipment (e.g., blood glucose monitors, canes), and to find misplaced hearing aids, eyeglasses, and dentures.

Client Registration

Regardless of the shelter's organizing agency, all clients need to complete a family registration form. Information collected may include family residence, names, phone numbers, and whether family members have health issues, injuries, or deaths due to the disaster. Clients need to sign in and out when leaving and reentering the shelter so that shelter workers know the numbers of who is present and who is returning. This information is used to determine how many meals and snacks will be needed for a potential 24-hour presence in the shelter. It is also used to determine what other equipment and services might be needed.

Congregate Shelters

Dormitory or congregate shelters house large numbers of clients in shared eating and sleeping spaces. Before clients can be admitted to the sleeping area of the shelter, cots and client equipment should be laid out in the dormitory. Cot-to-cot assessments are implemented on a schedule that will be determined by shelter managers. It is normally expected that the assessment should be done at least once a day as a minimum. When there are extenuating circumstances, the cot-to-cot assessment should be done as frequently as the changing needs of the clients in the shelter are noted.

There are written rules and regulations regarding cots and their proper spacing in a congregate shelter. Proper spacing must be maintained between cots to allow clients to move around them as freely as possible. Cot placement, however, is also influenced by the risk of infection spread. For example, during the COVID-19 pandemic beginning in early 2020, basic sheltering principles were affected by infection control needs. All clients and staff needed to wear face masks, the cots needed to be 6 ft apart, and all clients and staff required adequate soap, water, paper towels, and liquid hand sanitizer.

Regular cots are camp cots that are approximately 14 in. off the ground, with a canvas material for clients to sleep on them. Clients who have access and functional needs may be able to obtain special disability cots. Specialty cots are 19 in. off the ground, have a movable back part of the frame to raise or lower clients, have a padded 1- to 2-in. covered mattress, and have portable side rails that allow clients to move more freely while on the cot.

Bathrooms and shower areas need to be inspected for working order and accessibility for clients with access and functional needs. Hygiene items that are available for all clients are placed on cots or in a central area. Hygiene kits and blankets should be replaced every 2 weeks.

The working belief is that most emergency shelters will be closed within a 2-week period of time. The last few years, however, some congregate shelters in response to some disasters remained open longer than expected with adequate numbers of client cots and supplies becoming a problem.

Noncongregate Shelters

Noncongregate dormitory shelters are relatively new and grew in popularity in response to the COVID-19 pandemic. This type of sheltering arrangement usually involves hotels or motels with specific contracts with a sheltering agency. Other types of agencies include college or school dormitories, campgrounds, RV parks, and tent encampments. In other words, noncongregate shelters provide sleeping and perhaps even eating spaces that are separate for individuals and families.

In noncongregate shelters, clients are typically placed in rooms according to their needs. If rooms are used above the first floor, provisions must be made for clients to safely use elevators or well-lit staircases. In addition, the sheltering organization must ensure the delivery of meals, snacks, and beverages throughout the day. Client feeding is generally not provided by the shelter itself.

Health services are also usually provided on an on-call basis from the sheltering agency. Care of the client rooms is left to the clients and generally not the building's staff. Clients may ask for replacement sheets and towels and hygiene supplies from shelter agency employees. In addition, whenever possible, a staff person from the disaster service agency should be available during the daytime hours, and nighttime staff should be on call using cell phone coverage from a central location.

Feeding

All sheltered clients and staff should have three meals a day as well as snacks and water. In the beginning, depending on the disaster and time of day clients arrive at the sheltering site, prepackaged meals or snacks are distributed. As quickly as possible, however, a more comprehensive feeding plan needs to be created and then implemented. All expenses for the feeding program need to be monitored and recorded to address the necessary expenses.

Many sheltering agencies also have MOUs or contracts with feeding agencies that can be put into place. Due to the devastation caused by some disasters, preplanned feeding provisions may not be available. Depending on the sheltering agency's relationship with the local emergency management agencies, emergency military *meals ready to eat* (MREs) might be procured. There are many commercial companies that prepare civilian commercial MREs. These packaged meals contain a variety of foods in a pouch system that can be chemically heated up with the addition of water in the preparation portion of the pouch.

There is usually no provision for a nutritionist on the staff of a sheltering agency and, typically, provisions made for dietary needs of multiple cultures are limited on a short-term basis. All the provisions for meal planning, procurement, distribution, and cleaning of the materials after feeding should be discussed before a disaster occurs, but many times the feeding plan is created and implemented after the fact.

Health Services, Mental Health Services, and Spiritual Care Services

Along with governmental agencies, sheltering organizations must provide for the health care needs of the clients and staff in the shelters. Physical health care should be provided by licensed personnel who are vetted by the sheltering agencies or the government in the sheltering area. Licenses and certifications must be confirmed and documented in the health services area of the shelters.

Consumable over-the-counter medications, first aid supplies, and other health care supplies have to be provided for the health care staff in the shelter. In an American Red Cross shelter, provisions are put into place for replacement of prescriptive medications, supplies, and equipment to be procured and dispensed to shelter clients. Provisions should also be made for durable medical equipment that clients need while in the shelter. Other provisions will be required for clients who use additional health care equipment such as that needed for oxygen therapy.

County- or state-based agencies also need to be part of the sheltering team. *Centers for independent living* should be consulted to help provide assessments of community clients and obtain disability integration or equipment for access and functional abilities. Clients who need outpatient services, such as dialysis and oncologic drug or radiation therapies, also need to have arrangements made with the health staff in the shelter and the community acute care agencies. Transportation systems must be created for these shelter clients.

Mental health services are necessary for shelter clients and staff. Surviving disasters and living in community shelters can be very stressful. Preexisting client health and mental health conditions, such as depression and dementia, will need to be addressed by the mental health staff. Sheltering health care staff providing both physical and mental health care need to work with local public health departments, behavioral health departments, and other community agencies to make connections between the shelter and clients and appropriate community resources.

Spiritual care needs are equally important for clients involved in a disaster. Spiritual needs will depend on the cultures and religious needs of the clients in the disaster. Disasters often bring up many faith-based issues for some clients. Places of worship should be involved depending on the spiritual needs of the clients. Nontraditional worship practices must also be included for clients who have spiritual needs but do not identify with an established religious community.

Information for Clients

Clients become fearful if they do not have appropriate and timely information. Many families have routines in their daily life, and disasters disrupt their typical patterns of family behaviors. Most shelters will have daily meetings or announcements at various times during the day. Governmental agencies may be present and provide specific disaster information, community information, and connection to the world beyond the disaster zone.

Commercial cell phone companies may provide charging stations within the shelter for clients and staff to recharge their phone batteries. Sheltering agencies also generally try to provide computer stations, agency cell phones, and other technology resources. Communication devices that can be utilized by clients with hearing and visual impairment, televisions, gaming consoles, and other equipment are often donated by local community organizations for disaster survivors.

DISASTER PREPAREDNESS TRAINING

It can be argued that disaster preparedness is a moral requisite for nurses. The ANA has established standards and guidelines for professional practice arenas since 2001 as well as its Code of Ethics for Nurses with interpretive statements. These resources indicate an expectation that nurses provide service to vulnerable populations. In addition, a white paper created from an Agency for Healthcare Research and Quality grant outlined *Standards and Guidelines for Disaster Nursing* (ANA, 2008), pointing out the need for nurses to be in a state of readiness for any emergency response. Numerous national organizations have put forth recommendations to improve the nursing profession's readiness for disasters, including TJC, FEMA, the American National Red Cross, ANA, Medical Reserve Corps (MRC), the National Disaster Medical System, and the Department of Veterans Affairs.

In addition, nurses must actively support the communities where they live and work with emergency planning. Awareness of the diversity of the population, cultures, and differences within the community are necessary for effective care during a disaster response. Nurses should be familiar with the disaster plans of the organizations in which they work and should practice implementation of these plans with disaster drills.

The reality is that when disasters strike, health care professionals are often among the first people to respond. Disaster preparedness training for all health care professionals is essential to maintaining an efficient health care system during a disaster, particularly in view of the potentially widespread nature and complex environment of many disasters.

Consider This Disaster preparedness is a process. This process may take many months or years, but every step is a step in the right direction.

In response to these deficiencies, several organizations and groups based mainly in economically developed countries have begun to develop competency-based education and training for members of the health care workforce and other responders. Disaster preparedness training in most countries is based in specialized hospitals, public health schools, and medical schools instead of within nonprofit volunteer disaster agencies. Organizations such as community emergency response team (CERT) programs, the Red Cross, the Salvation Army, and others, however, are prepared to provide education for disaster services in the United States.

Several surveys of recent global disasters by the CDC (2016) and other research groups (Labrague et al., 2018) have noted persistent gaps in education, training, and abilities of health care professionals in managing emergency situations.

The World Health Organization (WHO) recommends that all countries consider training their health care professionals to respond to disasters as a national and local priority. As nurses make up the majority of health care providers, they represent an indispensable workforce during disasters. The nursing staff in acute care hospitals as well as community and public health agencies can provide care to people who are injured or ill, assist individuals and families in dealing with physical and emotional issues, and work to improve the health and well-being within the community. These nurses and their organizations are prepared to provide shelter and other health care services to victims of a disaster.

These attributes require competent nurses who are ready to respond in all situations, including disasters. Nurses must be able to adapt their skills from focusing on individuals to large numbers of patients, both in their delivery of lifesaving and emergency care and in the maintenance of public health. Therefore, disaster training for nurses is vital. Nurses must be involved in all phases of disaster planning in order to increase their understanding of their role and expected contributions in disaster response (Achora & Kamanyire, 2016).

The National VOAD organization (2020) links together states and territories with voluntary organizations that collaborate on disaster preparedness and response. This organization also provides support for preparedness of individuals, nonprofits, faith-based organizations, and small businesses. National VOAD also facilitates coordination of finances, material logistics, and human resources in the total disaster cycle of preparation, response, and recovery. They work with federal, state, and local officials to provide communications and resources for all individuals living in the affected areas. Local and state VOAD agencies continue to communicate and work together to strengthen a coordinated disaster response.

Opportunities need to be created and organized for nurses to safely participate in the disaster operation. All nurses participating in disaster recovery and response must make sure they have a clear assignment in the disaster action and they are always wearing appropriate safety gear and PPE for the specific disaster.

GOOD SAMARITAN LAWS AND VOLUNTEER PROTECTION ACTS

There are times when volunteers are not sure if they have legal protection when performing disaster nursing outside of their normal paid nursing work. This includes nurses volunteering for disaster service agencies. These concerns are valid since legal protection is not fully guaranteed.

All states in the United States provide some legal protection against civil liability. A federal law also protects disaster volunteers from civil liability. In addition, nurse malpractice liability policies may be available from disaster agencies, but agencies are not required to have these policies. Any nurse who volunteers or provides professional nursing services should think about the individual purchase of a malpractice liability policy for full protection.

Most states and territories in the United States, however, have enacted *Good Samaritan Act*s (Association of State and Territorial Health Officials, 2021). These laws encourage health care personnel to provide emergency treatment when they do not have a duty to do so (i.e., they are not working in the health care agency where they are employed). Generally, there are four requirements to have legal coverage under Good Samaritan laws:

1. There needs to be an emergency or disaster.

2. The care provided is free and not subject to a financial charge.

3. The care provided must be in "good faith," using regular standards of care.

4. The health personnel must remain with the disaster victim until the victim is stable or other qualified health care personnel take over (deGuerre, 2004).

Good Samaritan laws, however, do not protect any person who is negligent or reckless in the provision of care. Health personnel are not required to provide care, but once they do provide care, they must continue until the victim is stable or other trained providers take over care.

In addition, multiple states and working agencies have rules that allow for personal care to be provided by nonprofessional staff in a state of emergency. At the time of the disaster, less urgent actions can be delayed, eliminated for some time, or assigned to family members, nonlicensed assistants, or volunteers, including routine care activities (e.g., blood pressure checks in patients who are nonacute, assisted ambulation); providing oral medication and available over-the-counter medications; and documenting care provided.

The Volunteer Protection Act of 1997

In addition to Good Samaritan laws, the Volunteer Protection Act (VPA) is a federal act that protects volunteers against civil liability under certain conditions (Harrigan S, 2018):

- The volunteer was acting within the guidelines of their job description.
- The volunteer had the proper licenses or certifications or was authorized to act, and those acts were within their job description.
- The volunteer did not cause harm by willful or criminal misconduct, gross negligence, reckless misconduct, or a conscious, flagrant indifference to the rights or safety of the individual harmed.
- The volunteer did not inflict harm while using a motor vehicle, aircraft, or other vehicle.
- The volunteer is not protected if the misconduct is a crime of violence, an act of international terrorism, hate crime or misconduct of sexual offense, intoxication, or drug use.

PERSONAL SAFETY IN DISASTERS

Preparation for disasters is critical. Infrastructure destroyed or damaged in any type of disaster may include physical and mental health resources along with other services normally rendered to the affected community. The community may, in fact, become overwhelmed and will need outside assistance to recover. Workplaces and schools may be closed. There may also be restrictions on domestic and international travel to and from the area.

In addition, heavy law enforcement (possibly from local, state, and federal levels) following man-made disasters is common since violence is often involved. Decision making for clients affected by acts of terrorism is by a lead government agency such as local police and fire departments along with the Federal Bureau of Investigation, military, and other agencies. Confusion can occur when many groups are trying to determine who is in charge and how they will relate to the shelter staff and agencies as well as the victims of the terrorist acts.

Families and individuals in an area facing an evacuation should plan in advance how they will evacuate the area to reach safety. It is vital for others to have up-to-date information about each person's medical needs and contact information for the closest living relatives.

It is also important that all people in a disaster area remain calm and be patient. Everyone will need to follow the advice of local emergency officials, National Guard, and fire and police departments. If a terrorism incident occurs where the nurse is, they should check for injuries and give first aid and help to seriously injured individuals. The nurse should provide social, community, and mental health assessments for oneself, one's family, and one's community. The nurse must ensure their surroundings are safe and follow the established chain of command.

If a nurse's home has been damaged or areas nearby are impacted, the nurse can check for damage using flashlights. Using open flames, matches, or candles to assess post disaster damage can be dangerous. The nurse should ensure that electrical switches are turned off and leave the house quickly in the event of fires. In addition, any damaged utilities should be shut off, and no one should try to reestablish any gas lines or other utilities until they have been checked by the local gas and utility companies.

Once safe, it is important that an emergency contact does not attempt contact with landline telephones because they may generate a spark and ignite a fire. The nurse should use a cell phone outside of the home and check for life-threatening emergencies. It is also important to check on neighbors, especially those who are older or have disabilities. Pets should be confined and secured.

SELF-CARE AND PERSONAL PREPAREDNESS FOR DISASTERS

Disaster nursing can be rewarding, but it can also be stressful and challenging. Nurses responding to a disaster may not fully be able to prepare themselves for the emotional aspects. Often, witnessing human suffering, an unusually intense workload, being away from families, and the unique stressors of the specific disaster causes additional personal stress that may be difficult to comprehend.

In addition, when the nurse is not staying at home, living conditions can impede self-care and time to reset. Disaster nurses often say in staff shelters, like client shelters, sleeping on cots, using sleeping bags and camping equipment, eating foods unlike what they eat at home, and not getting enough sleep. Preplanning before responding to a disaster can assist the nurse when away from home. For example, disaster nurses should consider bringing their own bedding or sleeping bag, pillow, and other personal items from home to help with this adjustment.

Discussion Point

Before a disaster, each nurse should consider all aspects of self-care, including emotional, physical, psychological, and spiritual domains. What items might help the nurse with self-care before, during, and after the disaster?

Advance training may also reduce some of the personal stress for disaster volunteers. This includes CPR recertification. Most nurses in professional settings are required to complete this certification every 2 years. In addition, a first aid course should be completed before a disaster strikes. Schools of nursing and nursing employment agencies do not require a first aid course. First aid teaches simple, easy-to-perform tasks to provide aid to families and individuals in the face of an accident or emergency.

Nurses should also complete disaster preparation classes such as those offered by the National Incident Management System (NIMS), State Incident Management System (SIMS), Red Cross, FEMA, MRC, and CERT, and VOAD and Community Organizations Active in Disaster (COAD).

In addition, all nurses should maintain proper health care and immunizations for tetanus, diphtheria, and pertussis (Tdap); influenza; shingles; pneumonia; hepatitis A and B; measles, mumps, and rubella (MMR); and COVID-19. Nurses should also prepare their homes, vehicles, and work sites with safety and disaster supplies, including PPE. In addition, there should be prepacked personal hygiene supplies, extra seasonally appropriate clothing, emergency snacks, and appropriate supplies for medical conditions that the nurses might have. Pet foods and supplies may also be indicated.

One kit should be at home for the nurse and others. A second kit should be placed in the car to protect the nurse in the event that a disaster occurs when the nurse is not at home and traveling between home and the work setting. If the nurse does not have a car, daily items should be kept with the nurses' personal bag in their daily travels. At a place of work in each locker or storage area, disaster supplies should be made available.

There are many premade disaster kits. There are also many resources for what should be included in a disaster kit. One recommendation is for a family to have a disaster kit on wheels; the nurse can buy a 32-gallon plastic trash can on wheels, line it with a 32-gallon trash bag, place all the disaster items inside, close the lid, and label it with paint as a disaster kit and not a trash can. Items can also be in a wheeled duffel backpack or other places that would not be in use during a normal day. Premade kits are available but may be expensive and not contain the specific supplies that a specific nurse may want to have for the disaster preparation.

Another good practice is to create an after-disaster contact list and log for family members and close friends nearby. During a disaster, landline telephones may be overloaded and shut off. Cell phones should be kept charged and everyone should know where in their county, city, or state, the emergency center for cell phones is located.

In addition, part of preparedness is to make sure all household members know where to shut off utilities in the home, including water, gas, and electricity, and how to shut them off. It is ideal to have a fully charged cell phone and other technology charger in the home and bag packed for work each day. Every person should know where fire extinguishers are, and they should be checked for viability on a yearly basis. The nurse may join agencies and community partners to participate in drills and exercises.

Finally, one of the last steps in personal and family planning is practicing a disaster escape from both the home and car. Children and older adults are resilient if they know what to do before a disaster occurs. Family disaster drills can be executed on easy-to-remember dates.

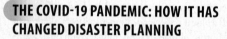

Discussion Point

Disaster preparedness begins with personal preparation. What have you done to be ready for a disaster personally and professionally?

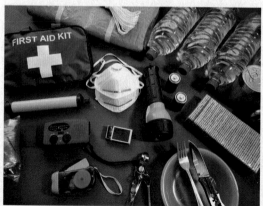

(Roger Brown Photography/Shutterstock)

THE COVID-19 PANDEMIC: HOW IT HAS CHANGED DISASTER PLANNING

As of September 2021, the COVID-19 pandemic, which began in January 2020, continues to be a hybrid disaster with overwhelming consequences. It is not easy to define and discuss this pandemic as it has become politicized beyond the nature of a natural disaster. The disease itself has morphed and mutated with at least five notable variants.

Although public health organizations such as the CDC previously completed extensive planning for influenza outbreaks, there was minimal planning for a pandemic of the scope of COVID-19. The virus caught the public health planning community by surprise, and the world responded by trying to provide direction and planning after the fact.

Airports, cruise ships, and the transportation industry were caught off guard as were acute care hospitals. Supply chain shortages of critical PPE and ventilators threatened the lives of both afflicted patients as well as the staff who were caring for them.

Interventions were put into place in the United States, including stop-gap measures such as travel bans, requesting direct financial help from Congress, and employing expanded use of tele-health for virtual health care. Indeed, many countries experienced social, economic, and educational shutdowns, the likes of which had not been seen in modern times.

In response, the U.S. Congress passed the Coronavirus Aid, Relief, and Economic Security (CARES) Act on March 27, 2020 (Congressional Research Service, 2020). This legislation provided financial assistance to hospitals, small businesses, and state and local governments. In the meantime, the medical community worked feverishly to conduct research about how best to treat and prevent the disease itself.

The usual natural disasters did not stop, though. Hurricanes, floods, earthquakes, single-family and multiple-family fires, and wildfires added to the strain caused by COVID-19. Federal disaster agencies, nonprofit disaster agencies, state emergency management agencies, and the American Red Cross had to suddenly change the way they prepared, responded, and recovered from these additional disasters in the face of COVID-19.

Meetings, conventions, and face-to-face planning and investigation stopped. Communication moved on a widespread scale to virtual platforms like Zoom, Microsoft Teams, Cisco Webex, and Skype to name a few. Companies and disaster agencies had no choice but to quickly implement the use of remote communication technology.

For example, the American Red Cross used *Teams* since the organization was already using the Microsoft Office suite. But smooth transitions were not universal, and many volunteer responders were not prepared to change their entire communications pathways to be fully online. Some volunteers did not have computers and many of those who did had limited knowledge of how to participate using these tools. Schools and other industries suddenly had to stay at home and provide education and instruction online. There were no preventative modalities for COVID-19 during this period of time. Health care was in a reactive mode rather than a clear planning mode.

Methods of caring for staff, volunteers, and clients in disasters literally had to change overnight. This included guidance regarding wearing masks, social distancing, and proper hand and surface cleaning. With evolving research, muddled communications, and politicization, confusion persisted. For instance, people asked if masks were necessary. If so, what type of masks? Where would the masks come from? Who could manufacture the masks when they were in short supply? People questioned social distancing guidelines; should they stay 3 ft apart, 6 ft apart, or 8 ft apart? What products should be used for proper hand and surface hygiene? Early on, it wasn't clear if the virus could be transmitted by contact or if it was airborne? Confusing and conflicting information was often followed by inconsistent and incomplete information. This uncertain environment spilled over into a lack of cohesive and complete protocols and procedures.

The health care community was in a crisis, and critically ill patients kept arriving at acute care agencies. Public health and emergency services continued to provide care but sometimes without the appropriate equipment and services. Capacities were soon strained to the breaking point and beyond. Rationing care became a reality in some areas.

As a result, disaster response to COVID-19 in part shifted from in-person to virtual. Wherever possible, only a few disaster responders were physically present at disaster relief sites. Virtual responses now relied on smartphones and other computer video platforms. This was a significant change for responders as well as clients.

Many communities had to change the way they responded to their citizens. It also meant that there were more clients and staff finding technology challenging. Not everyone had the appropriate hardware, software, or bandwidths. Disaster responders and clients were more emotionally distressed without the ability to communicate as before with in-person responses.

The outcome thus far is that the processes and procedures for providing mass care in a disaster situation have dramatically changed due to COVID-19. National disaster organizations are requiring stakeholders to learn and adhere to new rules and regulations, and there have been major changes in sheltering philosophies from large, in-person congregant shelters. Many communities do not have adequate numbers of appropriate alternatives. In some areas, climate poses additional challenges. For example, campgrounds and tents are not appropriate or safe during the winter or in wet weather.

In addition, sheltering clients from disasters requires more space per person during the pandemic, limiting how cots are placed and how to respond to the health issues of shelter clients. Cleaning and maintaining a safe environment changed due to infectious disease protocols. The specifics of these changes are based upon disaster organizations' new mandates and government standards in specific communities.

This new type of sheltering also mandated increased cleaning and sanitation, more portable bathrooms, and additional shower units. Food services had to change from open, large buffet containers of food to individually wrapped meals, snack items, prepacked liquids, and refreshments. These new meals generally need to be delivered to clients in noncongregant shelter locations, adding to logistic challenges. In addition, other new shelter cleaning protocols have needed to be established such as when to clean, how to clean, and what to do with refuse and trash.

Adapting to the provision of disaster care has always been and will likely always be a challenge. Providing the wide array of necessary services under COVID-19 conditions has made this even more daunting. Fortunately, caregivers and organizations have risen to the challenge to provide the best possible care and services under the circumstances.

CONCLUSIONS

Nurses are reliable, compassionate people who want to respond to health care issues as well as disaster-caused needs. Nurses also have an ethical duty of care to their clients and patients, but before providing care to others, they must make sure they have taken care of the health care issues for themselves and their families. Before any nurse can reach out to help others, they must help themselves first.

Not every nurse will be employed in an emergency room or volunteer in a disaster response agency, but all nurses need to know what to do during a disaster. Disasters can occur whether the nurse is on duty or not, at home or

not, or whether the nurse has planned ahead for a disaster or not.

The most important aspect of disaster nursing is for the nurse, their family, and their colleagues to be prepared for any disasters in the area. A hybrid or man-made disaster can occur at any time, and if the nurse is prepared for predicted natural disasters, they will at least have begun to prepare for any spontaneous ones.

In this chapter, we have discussed some of the most common disasters that can occur, as well as the unprecedented (in modern times) challenges of the COVID-19 global pandemic. Unexpected events can occur at any time. The location of the disaster and the nurse's responsibility in that disaster necessitates the response for everyone to prepare for the disaster, respond appropriately to the disaster, and recover from the disaster as planning and preparation take place for any future disasters.

Regardless of the disaster, nurses play a significant role in disaster response. Nurses are also responsible for the care of their clients in any location. Whether clients or patients are sheltering in mass care shelters or noncongregate living arrangements, nurses must be prepared to respond to their daily health care needs.

Nurses cannot respond to assist in disasters, however, unless they are prepared and maintain their own self-care. Safety of nurses is key to a complete disaster response. There are standards and guidelines to help all nurses in all practice areas of disaster nursing.

For Additional Discussion

1. When educating the community, what disaster preparedness topics need to be included, what resources would be needed, and what take-home pieces would you provide for school-age children, teenagers, young adults, multigenerational families, and older adults?

2. In preparing disaster kits for yourself and family, including personal or family papers, first aid supplies, snack foods, water, medications, money, and technology, which items would be stored in your home, car, workspace, and bag?

3. You are providing health care services in a congregant shelter housed in the gym of a local high school. The school district and the organization managing the shelter both have no-smoking policies. However, one of your clients is in pain and wants to use their prescribed medical cannabis. Can you make an exception for this medical need? Would your response be different if the shelter had a small smoking area for tobacco smokers outside the shelter boundaries?

4. An older adult couple comes to a shelter that has a service animal-only policy. They have a cat in a small carrier. They tell you that they rescued the cat as a kitten many years ago and that they cannot be separated from their pet. Can you accommodate them? Would it matter if they have a note from a mental health therapist validating that they had severe issues when separated from the cat when one of them was hospitalized?

5. In preparation for disaster drills, what skills, tasks, resources, and responsibilities do nursing students, novice nurses, experienced acute care nurses, and nursing educators need to participate in the drill?

For Additional Discussion (*continued*)

6. Describe the disaster agencies and resources in your living area. Contact them and find out how they provide services to the residents of your area.

7. Nancy is a nurse practitioner who has always worked in a community clinic and has a severe allergy to dust of all types, both inside and outside. A wildfire caused significant damage to a community about 10 miles away. The people who have been affected by the fire have been evacuated to a tent complex constructed on a previously empty field where sand is blowing and some smoke from the fire is in the air. What should be Nancy's first concern in her decision-making process? Should she drive over and offer her services? If Nancy cannot work with health issues onsite, what else can she do to help out?

8. Pamela is a nurse in an acute care facility as well as the primary caregiver for her 85-year-old mother who has many medical conditions. Pamela's church group asked her to help out a clinic in a nearby town that has recently experienced a flood. What steps should Pamela take before deciding to help?

9. Fred is a nurse working for a health maintenance organization. One of the conditions of his employment is that he cannot work for another health care agency. If Fred deploys with the Red Cross and works as a volunteer in a shelter at a disaster site, does this violate his employment agreement if the Red Cross pays his expenses such as food and lodging?

10. William is a nurse manager working as the manager of health services in a shelter set up for hurricane evacuees. When the last of the evacuees are sent home, the shelter manager asks William to coordinate the nurses in moving the tables and chairs from their work area to the front of the building so that they can be loaded and taken back to the rental company. Is this a proper assignment of work?

11. If you are deploying to a disaster to provide nursing care, what sort of personal items and professional equipment would you take with you?

References

Achora, S., & Kamanyire, J. K. (2016, February). Disaster preparedness: Need for inclusion in undergraduate nursing education. *Sultan Qaboos University Medical Journal, 16*(1), e15–e19. https://doi.org/10.18295/squmj.2016.16.01.004

American National Red Cross. (2021). *Disaster relief & recovery services.* Retrieved September 13, 2021, from https://www.redcross.org/get-help/disaster-relief-and-recovery-services.html

American Nurses Association (ANA). (2008). *Adapting standards of care under extreme conditions: Guidance for professionals during disasters, pandemics, and other extreme emergencies.* Retrieved September 13, 2021, from https://www.nursingworld.org/~4ade15/globalassets/docs/ana/ascec_whitepaper031008final.pdf

Association of State and Territorial Health Officials. (2021). *Emergency volunteer toolkit.* Retrieved September 13, 2021, from https://www.astho.org/Programs/Preparedness/Public-Health-Emergency-Law/Emergency-Volunteer-Toolkit/Volunteer-Protection-Acts-and-Good-Samaritan-Laws-Fact-Sheet/

Bonsall, L. (2016, April 13). *For whom do you care—Patients or clients?* Retrieved September 13, 2021, from https://www.nursingcenter.com/ncblog/april-2016/for-whom-do-you-care---patients-or-clients

Centers for Disease Control and Prevention. (n.d.) *Homepage.* Retrieved September 13, 2021, from https://www.cdc.gov/

Centers for Disease Control and Prevention (2016, March 16). *Organization of the CDC Center for Global Health.* Retrieved September 27, 2021, from https://www.cdc.gov/globalhealth/organization.htm

Chen, A., Kim, J., & Schaumleffel, L. (2020, May 22). Outbreak of norovirus illness among wildfire evacuation shelter populations—Butte and Glenn Counties, California, November 2018. *MMWR: Morbidity & Mortality Weekly Report, 69*(20), 613–617.

Congressional Research Service. (2020, April 28). *The Coronavirus Aid, Relief, and Economic Security (CARES) Act—Tax relief for individuals and businesses.* Retrieved September 13, 2021, from https://crsreports.congress.gov/product/pdf/R/R46279

deGuerre, C. (2004, April). Good Samaritan statutes: Are medical volunteers protected? *AMA Journal of Ethics.* Retrieved September 13, 2021, from https://journalofethics.ama-assn.org/article/good-samaritan-statutes-are-medical-volunteers-protected/2004-04

Hamstra, B. (2018, April 24). *4 Major differences between ICU and emergency nurses.* Retrieved September 13, 2021, from https://nurse.org/articles/differences-between-icu-er-nurses/

Karmarkar, E., Jain, S., Higa, J., Fontenot, J., Bertolucci, R., et al. (2020, May 22). Outbreak of norovirus illness among wildfire evacuation shelter populations—Butte and Glenn Counties, California, November 2018. *MMWR: Morbidity & Mortality Weekly Report, 69*(20), 613–617. Published online May 2, 2020. doi: 10.15585/mmwr .mm6920a1

Labrague, L. J., Hammad, K., Gloe, D. S., McEnroe-Petitte, D. M., Fronda, D. C., Obeidat, A. A., Leocadio, M. C., Cayaban, A. R., & Mirafuentes, E. C. (2018). Disaster preparedness among nurses: A systematic review of literature. *International Nursing Review, 65*(1), 41–53. https://doi .org/10.1111/inr.12369

National Voluntary Organizations Active in Disaster. (2020). *Home page.* Retrieved September 13, 2021, from https:// www.nvoad.org

Nevada State College. (2018, July 23). *Nurses play a critical role in disaster response.* Retrieved September 13, 2021, from https://online.nsc.edu/articles/rn-bsn/nurses-critical-role-disaster.aspx

Harrigan, S. (2018, June 21). Rue Insurance. *Understanding the Volunteer Protection Act.* Retrieved Oct. 5, 2021, from https://www.rueinsurance.com/understanding-the-volunteer-protection-act/#:~:text=The%20VPA%20protects%20 volunteers%20against%20civil%20liability%20under%20 the%20following%20conditions%3A&text=The%20 volunteer%20did%20not%20cause,safety%20of%20the%20 individual%20harmed

Society for the Advancement of Disaster Nursing. (n.d.). *Personal emergency preparedness: Nurses serving nurses as trusted messengers.* Retrieved September 13, 2021, from https://disasternursing.org

Statista Research Department. (2021, January 21). *Natural disasters in the U.S.—Statistics & facts.* Retrieved September 13, 2021, from https://www.statista.com/ topics/1714/natural-disasters/

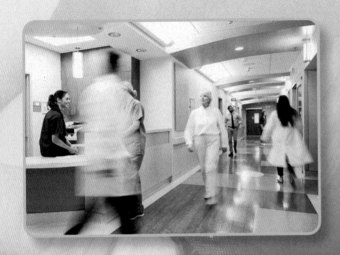

3

WORKPLACE ISSUES

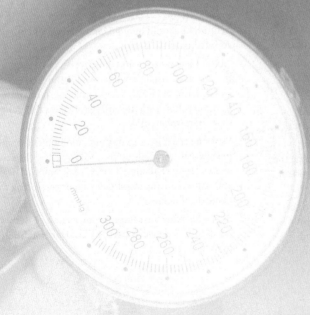

Mandatory Minimum Staffing Ratios

Carol J. Huston

LEARNING OBJECTIVES

The learner will be able to:

1. Explore factors driving legislative mandates for minimum registered nurse (RN) representation in the staffing mix.

2. Investigate the movement and/or progress of states other than California to adopt minimum RN staffing ratios.

3. Debate driving and restraining forces for legislating minimum licensed staffing ratios.

4. Summarize current research findings regarding the effect of staffing ratios and staffing mix on patient outcomes.

5. Describe challenges encountered in conducting empirical research that explores the relationship between staffing and patient outcomes including how outcomes are defined, what operational definitions should be used, and who should be counted in nurse staffing.

6. Assess the efficiency and effectiveness of the processes used by the state of California Department of Health Services to determine initial minimum RN–patient staffing ratios for different types of hospital units.

7. Describe challenges to staffing ratio implementation in California, including the need to define "licensed nurses," legal challenges to the "at all times" clause, and strategies directed at delaying or rescinding the mandate altogether.

8. Argue for or against the appropriateness of the "at all times" clause as part of California's staffing ratio mandate.

9. Assess whether California's 2004 implementation of mandatory minimum RN staffing ratios has met its goals.

10. Identify alternatives to staffing ratio mandates that seek to ensure that staffing resources are adequate to provide safe patient care.

11. Reflect on the staffing ratios used in their work setting and assess, using clearly defined criteria, whether they are adequate to provide quality patient care.

INTRODUCTION

For some time now, economics has been a primary driver in dictating registered nurse (RN) staffing mix in hospitals. As a result, the trend early in the first decade of the 21st century was to reduce RNs in the staffing mix and replace them with less expensive personnel. Empirical research increasingly concludes, however, that the number of RNs in the staffing mix has a direct effect on quality care and specifically on patient outcomes.

Indeed, Griffiths and colleagues (2020) note that multiple reviews of research have established that higher RN staffing levels in hospitals are associated with better patient outcomes and improved care quality, including lower risks of in-hospital mortality, shorter lengths of stay, and fewer omissions of necessary care. Similarly, a recent study by Needleman et al. (2020) found that low RN and nursing support staffing were associated with increased patient mortality (see Research Fuels the Controversy 11.1). In response to this growing evidence, legislators, health care providers, and the public have increasingly demanded adequate staffing ratios of RNs in health care settings.

> *Consider This* There is compelling evidence to suggest that increasing the number of RNs in the staffing mix leads to safer workplaces for nurses and a higher quality of care for patients. As a result, a national (and even international) movement to examine the need for minimum staffing ratios is ongoing.

Research Fuels the Controversy 11.1

Linking Registered Nurse and Support Staffing With Inpatient Hospital Mortality

This study examined the association of inpatient mortality with patients' cumulative exposure to shifts with low RN staffing, low nursing support staffing, and high patient turnover at three U.S. academic medical centers between 2007 and 2012. Staffing below 75% of annual median unit staffing for each staff category and shift type was characterized as low. High patient turnover per day was defined as admissions, discharges, and transfers one standard deviation above unit annual daily averages.

Source: Needleman, J., Jianfang L., Jinjing S., Larson, E. L., & Stone, P. W. (2020). Association of Registered Nurse and nursing support staffing with inpatient hospital mortality. *BMJ Quality & Safety, 29*(1), 10–18. https://doi.org/10.1136/bmjqs-2018-009219

Study Findings

Low RN staffing was found on 10% of day shifts and 9% of night shifts, and low nursing support staffing from licensed practical nurses (LPNs) and nurse assistants on over 20% of day and night shifts. Units also had higher than usual turnover on 8% of shifts. As a result, approximately 30% of admissions had one or more shifts with only low RN staffing; 64% one or more shifts with only low nurse support staffing; 11% one or more shifts on which both RN and nursing support staffing was low; and over half, one or more high turnover shifts.

Low RN and nursing support staffing were associated with increased mortality. No relationship was observed for high patient turnover and mortality.

The researchers concluded that low RN staffing increases patient risk. This risk is intensified when support staffing for nurses is low and may be intensified further when both RN and nursing support staffing are low. Whatever the staffing model at an institution, shortfalls from typical or targeted staffing in both RN and nursing support staffing appeared to have negative consequences for patients. The researchers encouraged hospital administrators and managers to strive for both adequate RN and nursing support staffing every shift to ensure delivery of safe and reliable care.

It is noteworthy, however, that while the U.S. federal government has established minimum standards for licensed nursing in certified nursing homes, it has not done so for acute care hospitals. Several attempts have been made in Congress in the past decade to enact nationwide hospital nurse staffing laws; however, none have been enacted. The most recent effort occurred in May 2021 when a federal bill, the *Nurse Staffing Standards for Hospital Patient Safety and Quality Care Act*, was introduced that would set specific safety limits on the numbers of patients each RN can care for in hospitals throughout the United States (National Nurses United [NNU], 2021). The outcome of that legislation had not been determined as of the writing of this book.

Section 42 of the Code of Federal Regulations (42CFR 482.23[b]) does require Medicare-certified hospitals to have adequate numbers of licensed RNs, licensed practical/vocational nurses (LPNs/LVNs), and other personnel to provide nursing care to all patients as needed ("Title 42," 2021); however, this nebulous language and the lack of national staffing guidelines have left it to states to ensure that staffing is adequate.

Many states in the United States have moved toward imposing mandatory licensed staffing requirements with the backing of some nursing organizations. Many of the states that have adopted legislation regarding staffing guidelines originally sought mandatory staffing ratio legislation. Six states—Florida, Iowa, Minnesota, New Jersey, New York, and Texas—and the District of Columbia were considering enacting mandatory nurse ratio laws at the start of 2021 (NursingLicensure.org, 2021).

As of 2019, however, only 15 states had actually passed some form of *safe staffing laws* (American Nurses Association [ANA], 2019; King University Online, 2019). Some states, however, are active in their pursuit of such legislation. For example, Massachusetts has already passed a law specific to intensive care units requiring a 1:1 or 1:2 nurse-to-patient ratio, depending on stability of the patient, and Minnesota now requires a chief nursing officer or designee to develop a core staffing plan with inputs from others (ANA, 2019).

New York passed "safe staffing" legislation for nursing homes in May 2021, though staffing standards are yet to be established by the Commissioner of Health as well as the civil penalties for nursing homes that fail to adhere to the new minimum standards (Reyes, 2021).

In addition, Pennsylvania nurses went to the state capitol in 2021 to argue for the need for a state policy requiring minimum nurse-to-patient staffing ratios, a need made even more urgent by the COVID-19 pandemic (Sholtis, 2021). As a result, House Bill 106 was introduced, and it was under consideration by the health subcommittee at the time of this writing. This act would amend the act of July 19, 1979 (P.L.130, No. 48), known as the *Health Care Facilities Act*, providing for hospital patient protection (Open States, 2021).

Also in 2021, the Connecticut General Assembly undertook a human resource and cost analysis to consider the adoption of minimum nurse staffing ratios for state nursing homes (Hawk & Sreenivas, 2021). The analysis suggested that Connecticut nursing homes by themselves would be highly unlikely to be able to cover the costs associated with minimum staffing ratios but noted that finding individuals to fill the positions would likely be the most challenging aspect of implementing a minimum staffing threshold. This is because nursing homes must compete with hospitals and others for a workforce that was already low in numbers before the pandemic and has been further dwindling since (Hawk & Sreenivas, 2021).

In addition, eight states (Connecticut, Illinois, Nevada, New York, Ohio, Oregon, Texas, and Washington, DC) now require hospitals to have staffing committees responsible for plans and staffing policy, and five states require some form of disclosure and/or public reporting—Illinois, New Jersey, New York, Rhode Island, and Vermont (ANA, 2019).

> **Consider This** There is wide variation in the skill mix (percentage of licensed to unlicensed workers) and RN-to-patient ratios across the United States.

California, however, is the only state that legally stipulates regulations for required minimum nurse-to-patient ratios in hospitals and long-term care facilities that must be maintained at all times, by unit. The differences between California and other states can be striking. For example, nurses in California take care of two fewer patients on average than nurses in Pennsylvania and New Jersey in general surgery (Daigon, 2020).

Additionally, Massachusetts came close to implementing minimum nurse-to-patient ratios. A November 2018 ballot question would have mandated nurse staffing ratios in the state, but it failed. The Massachusetts Health and Hospital Association argued that mandating nurse staffing ratios would have cost the Massachusetts health care system $1.3 billion in the first year and $900 million each year after that (Schoenberg, 2018). In addition, opponents noted that passing the legislation would have resulted in a shortage of 1,200 nurses statewide and that requiring more nurses per patient would only have made matters worse (Daigon, 2020). Supporters of the ballot question said safe staffing ratios were necessary to ensure that nurses could adequately care for patients. Both sides offered powerful arguments.

This chapter explores both the driving and the restraining forces for legislatively mandated minimum RN representation in the staffing mix. California's experience, as the first and only state to implement minimum staffing ratios, is detailed, as well as its struggle to define appropriate ratios and implement staffing ratios in an era of limited fiscal and human resources. The chapter concludes by looking at the movement of other states toward the adoption of minimum staffing ratios and strategies that have been suggested as alternatives to mandatory staffing ratios.

> **Consider This** Identifying and maintaining the appropriate number and mix of nursing staff is critical to the delivery of quality patient care.

THE RELATIONSHIP BETWEEN STAFFING RATIOS AND PATIENT OUTCOMES

Linda Aiken, a globally influential researcher in nurse staffing, suggests that although most research "has little impact on actual practice, that 20 years of research on the impact of nurse staffing on patient outcomes has made a big difference in the outcomes of patients and nurses, and managerial and clinical practice" (Kerfoot & Douglas, 2013, p. 216). Indeed, hundreds, if not thousands, of studies in the last decade have examined the link between staffing mix and patient outcomes. Many of the studies note a link between the increased representation of RNs in the staffing mix and improved patient outcomes.

Few studies, however, have had as much effect on determining safe staffing ratios as two benchmark research studies published in 2002. The first study was the work of Needleman et al. (2002). This study of 799 hospitals in 11 states found a higher prevalence of infections, such as pneumonia and urinary tract infections, failure to rescue, and shock or cardiac arrest when the nurses' workload was high.

The second study, which is often cited as seminal work in support of establishing minimum staffing ratio legislation at the federal or state level, was completed by Aiken et al. (2002). This study of more than 10,000 nurses and 230,000 patients in 168 hospitals concluded that in hospitals with higher patient-to-nurse ratios, surgical patients had a greater likelihood of dying within 30 days of admission. In addition, they experienced increased odds of failure to rescue (mortality following complications). This occurred because the time nurses have for surveillance, early detection, and timely intervention—particularly with patients who are not at high risk but who are vulnerable to other unfavorable outcomes—has a direct effect on patient outcomes.

In addition, the study found that staffing at six patients per nurse rather than four would result in an additional 2.3 deaths per 1,000 patients and an additional 8.7 deaths per 1,000 patients with complications. Staffing at eight patients per nurse rather than six would incur an additional 2.6 deaths per 1,000 patients and 9.5 deaths per 1,000 patients with complications. Uniformly staffing at eight patients per nurse rather than four was expected to entail five excess deaths per 1,000 patients and 18.2 complications per 1,000 patients. In addition, patients had a 31% higher chance of dying within 30 days of admission (Aiken et al., 2002).

Within days of the study's release, these results were summarized, repeated, and analyzed in detail in almost all relevant public forums and by most professional health care organizations. The message was clear: There was a direct link between nurse-to-patient ratios and mortality rates from preventable complications, and having an inadequate number of RNs places the public at risk. These conclusions were backed up by a 2018 meta-analysis of other research, which found that for every increase of one nurse, patients had a 14% decrease in risk for in-hospital mortality (Driscoll et al., 2018).

> **Discussion Point**
>
> Why did the study by Aiken et al. (2002) garner so much national attention in so many public forums? Were the findings significantly different than those of earlier studies? Was it timing? Was it how "the message" was managed?

Summaries of select recent research studies linking nurse staffing and patient outcomes between 2018 and 2021 are shown in Table 11.1. These mixed and sometimes conflicting research results have made the determination of the optimal nurse-to-patient ratio an ongoing challenge.

Indeed, over the past two decades, research sophistication regarding how best to study the relationship between staffing and patient outcomes has increased dramatically. Still, there are issues related to how outcomes are defined, what operational definitions should be used, and who should be counted in nurse staffing. Perhaps that is why more recent research has raised questions about whether RN staffing levels truly do have an impact on patient outcomes.

Indeed, Wynendaele et al. (2019) raise questions about the empirical nature of current staffing/outcomes-based research. Their systematic review confirmed a relationship between patient–nurse ratios and specific staff-related outcomes but noted that other variables have to be taken into consideration to ensure quality of care (e.g., skill mix, the work environment, patient acuity). The researchers noted that health care organizations should pursue the access and use of reliable data so that the validity and generalizability

TABLE 11.1 Select Research on Nurse Staffing Levels and Patient Clinical Outcomes (2018–2021)

Research	Description
McHugh et al. (2021)	This prospective panel study of 231,902 patients (142,986 in intervention hospitals and 88,916 in comparison hospitals) in Queensland, Australia, assessed the effects of recently established minimum nurse-to-patient ratios on staffing levels and patient outcomes. After implementation, mortality rates were not significantly higher than at baseline in comparison hospitals but were significantly lower than at baseline in intervention hospitals. The majority of change was at intervention hospitals, and staffing improvements by one patient per nurse produced reductions in mortality, readmissions, and length of stay (LOS). In addition to producing better outcomes, the costs avoided due to fewer readmissions and shorter LOS were more than twice the cost of the additional nurse staffing.
Lasater et al. (2021)	Using linked 2017 data sources, the researchers examined the effect of hospital patient-to-nurse staffing ratios and adherence to the early management bundle for patients with severe sepsis/septic shock on patients' odds of in-hospital and 60-day mortality, readmission, and LOS. Each additional patient per nurse was associated with 12% higher odds of in-hospital mortality, 7% higher odds of 60-day mortality, 7% higher odds of 60-day readmission, and longer lengths of stay, even after accounting for patient and hospital covariates including hospital adherence to SEP-1 bundles. Adherence to SEP-1 bundles was associated with lower in-hospital mortality and shorter lengths of stay; however, the effects were markedly smaller than those observed for staffing.
Griffiths et al. (2020)	This systematic scoping review provided an overview of the major approaches to assessing nurse staffing requirements and examined recent evidence to address unanswered questions including the accuracy and effectiveness of staffing tools. The researchers concluded that despite the importance of the question and the large volume of publications, evidence about nurse staffing methods remains highly limited. There was no evidence to support the choice of any particular tool. In addition, researchers noted that little is known about the costs or consequences of widely used tools.
Shang et al. (2019)	Using unit-level cross-sectional data from 2007 to 2012 at a large urban hospital system, the researchers examined the association of nurse staffing (2 days before health care–associated infection [HAI] onset) with HAIs after adjusting for individual risks. Of patient days, 15% had one shift understaffed, defined as staffing below 80% of the unit median for a shift, and 6.2% had both day and night shifts understaffed. Patients on units with both shifts understaffed were significantly more likely to develop HAIs 2 days later. The researchers concluded that understaffing is associated with increased risk of HAIs.
Evans (2019)	This study found that the California mandatory staffing ratios were associated with 55.5 fewer occupational injuries and illnesses per 10,000 RNs per year, a value 31.6% lower than the expected rate without the law. The most probable reduction for LPNs was 33.6%. Analyses of confidence intervals suggest that these reductions were unlikely to be due to chance.
Bridges et al. (2019)	This study using multilevel regression models explored the association between staffing levels, skill mix, and the chance of an interaction being rated as "negative" quality. Of the 3,076 observed interactions, 10% were rated as negative. The odds of a negative interaction increased significantly as the number of patients per RN increased ($p = 0.035$, odds ratio [OR] of 2.82 for ≥8 patients/RN compared with >6 to <8 patients/RN). When RN staffing was low, increases in assistant staff levels were not associated with improved quality of staff–patient interactions.
Kouatly et al. (2018)	This 48-month prospective study assessed the relationship between nurse staffing and six patient outcomes on medical–surgical units and critical care units (CCUs). Nurse staffing was measured by nursing hours per patient day (NHPPD) and skill mix, whereas measured patient outcomes were total falls and injury falls per 1,000 patient days, percent of surveyed patients with hospital-acquired pressure injuries (HAPIs), catheter-associated urinary tract infections, ventilator-associated pneumonia, and central line–associated bloodstream infections (CLABSIs) per 1,000 central line days. The odds for total falls, injury falls, HAPIs, and CLABSIs in the medical–surgical units were higher with lower NHPPD ratios. For the CCUs, lower rates of NHPPD increased the odds for total falls and CLABSIs. Skill mix was associated with total falls in the medical–surgical units but had no effect on patient outcomes in the CCUs.
Driscoll et al. (2018)	This review of 35 cross-sectional research studies, the majority utilizing large administrative databases, found that higher staffing levels were associated with reduced mortality, medication errors, pressure injuries, restraint use, infections, pneumonia, higher aspirin use, and a greater number of patients receiving percutaneous coronary intervention within 90 minutes. The researchers concluded that nurse-to-patient ratios influence many patient outcomes, most markedly in-hospital mortality.
Cho et al. (2018)	This cross-sectional study of 58 hospitals with 100 or more beds in South Korea found that nurse staffing and education were significantly associated with the LOS of surgical patients. A 10% increase in the average number of patients per nurse increased the LOS by 0.284 days ($p = 0.037$).

of evidence-based research can be assessed, which in turn can be converted into policy guidelines.

Williamson (2020) concurs, noting that while many nursing professionals believe adequate staffing numbers are at the heart of care quality and patient safety, mandated ratios might not be the only way to uniformly ensure this. Indeed, there are many questions that still need to be asked and answered before their implementation; several are shown in Box 11.1.

ARE MANDATORY MINIMUM STAFFING RATIOS NEEDED?

One proposed solution to Aiken and team's 2002 research findings was the implementation of minimum mandatory RN–patient staffing ratios in acute care hospitals. Numerous articles have appeared in the media attesting to grossly inadequate staffing in hospitals and nursing homes, and professional nursing organizations, such as the ANA, continue to express concern about the effect poor staffing has both on nurses' health and safety and on patient outcomes.

Proponents of mandated minimum staffing ratios argue that minimum staffing ratios are essential to ensuring that staffing is adequate to promote patient safety and to achieving desired patient outcomes. They also suggest that the use of standardized ratios provides a more consistent approach than acuity-based staffing.

Consider This The bottom line is that minimum staffing ratios would not have been proposed if staffing abuses and the resultant decline in the quality of patient care had not occurred in the past.

Critics, however, suggest that the overall cost of care would increase exponentially if mandatory ratios were imposed nationally and that no guarantee of quality improvement or positive outcomes exists with such ratios. In addition, there is a risk that staffing may actually decline with ratios because they might be used as the ceiling or as ironclad criteria if institutions are unwilling to make adjustments for patient acuity or RN skill level.

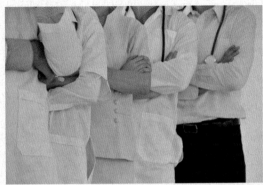

(Supavadee Butradee/Shutterstock)

Another reason cited by opponents of nurse–patient ratios stems from the *law of unintended consequences* (Daigon, 2020). To afford more RNs, some California hospitals reduced the numbers of support staff, creating more work for nurses, not less. Opponents also argue that the need to maintain mandatory ratios at all times interferes with the ability of nurses to schedule their own meals and breaks (Daigon, 2020).

The American Organization for Nursing Leadership (AONL) (formerly the American Organization of Nurse Executives [AONE]) shares these concerns, noting that it does not support mandated nurse staffing ratios because they are a static and ineffective tool that cannot guarantee a safe health care environment or quality level to achieve optimal patient outcomes. AONL suggests such ratios imply a "one-size-fits-all" approach to patient care staffing, ignoring the education, experience, and skill level of the individual nurse.

The Ohio Hospital Association (2017) concurs, arguing that staffing in hospitals is complex due to the constantly

---

BOX 11.1   Questions Surrounding Mandatory Minimum Staffing Ratios

- Are existing patient classification/acuity tools valid and reliable and are their data generalizable across acute care settings?
- Do standardized ratios provide a more consistent approach to safe staffing than acuity-based staffing?
- Does any guarantee of quality improvement or positive outcomes exist with mandatory staffing ratios?
- Can or should staffing be increased when patient acuity suggests more staffing is needed than suggested by the ratios?
- Should RN education, experience, or skill level impact staffing ratios?
- Do minimum mandatory staffing ratios achieve their intended purpose (patient safety and higher quality of care) if there is a concurrent reduction in unlicensed support staff to offset the costs?

Source: Williamson, E. (2020, May 12). *Nurse to patient ratios: Leaders have their work cut out for them.* Retrieved July 23, 2021, from https://www.nurse.com/blog/2020/05/12/nurse-to-patient-ratios-leaders-have-their-work-cut-out-for-them/

changing census and acuity of patients. Mandated staffing ratios restrict hospitals' ability to adjust to the needs of their patients. Furthermore, fixed ratios assume all nurses have the same skill sets and are "interchangeable" in treating patients. The Ohio Hospital Association suggests that hospitals must have greater flexibility than that allowed by mandated ratios, to respond to factors such as patient needs, volume, and acuity, patient satisfaction, resources available, nursing staff competency and skill mix, availability of medical and support staff, and staffing standards set by accrediting bodies, professional societies, and federal and state regulators. This will keep patient safety at the core of staffing decisions.

Aiken also agrees, suggesting that "It's the legislative mandate aspect that is controversial—not so much the actual focus on safe staffing, or the required staffing levels. Americans tend not to like legislative mandates" (Kerfoot & Douglas, 2013, p. 217).

It is cost, though, that is likely most often cited as a deterrent for implementing minimum staffing ratios. An increase in RN staffing is clearly more expensive than using unlicensed staff, but if patient outcomes are better, these increased costs may be offset. Eskes et al. (2020) note that cost must be examined in terms of relative value. *Low-value care* (care that is unlikely to benefit the patient given the harms, costs, available alternatives, or preferences of the patients) may be ineffective, inefficient, or unwanted. Thus, if the care is less expensive but the harms outweigh the benefits of cost savings, the care is neither efficient nor effective.

In addition, empirical evidence regarding the cost of minimum staffing ratios is limited, making it difficult to assess cost-effectiveness. Tung (2019) suggests that imposing ratios would add a cost to the health care system of $2 billion a year, a cost prohibitive to most hospitals that would have to pass on the costs to patients and families in the form of higher health care costs. If this figure is correct, one must question whether what is best for patients can be separated from what is cost-sustainable for the institution.

CALIFORNIA AS THE PROTOTYPE FOR MANDATORY MINIMUM STAFFING RATIOS

Passing the Legislation

California has had a minimum ratio of licensed nurse-to-patient requirement (Title 22 of the California Code of Regulations) for intensive care and coronary care units for almost four decades; however, no minimums were initially established for other types of acute care units. Given

increasing pressure from nursing unions in the state, increasing negative publicity about poor quality care, the increased use of unlicensed assistive personnel as direct care providers, and skyrocketing patient loads for licensed nurses in acute care, California stepped forward as the first state in the nation to implement mandatory minimum staffing ratios.

Under Assembly Bill (A.B.) 394 ("Safe Staffing Law"), passed in 1999 and crafted by the California Nurses Association (CNA), all hospitals in California were to comply with the minimum staffing ratios shown in Table 11.2 by January 1, 2004. These ratios, developed by the California Department of Health Services (CDHS) with assistance from the University of California, Davis, represented the maximum number of patients an RN could be assigned to care for under any circumstance. In addition, this legislation prohibited unlicensed personnel from performing certain procedures such as administering medication, performing venipuncture, providing parenteral or tube feedings, inserting nasogastric tubes, inserting catheters, performing tracheal suctioning, assessing patient conditions, providing patient education, and performing moderately complex laboratory tests.

Determining Appropriate Ratios

Developing draft regulations for minimum staffing ratios was challenging for the CDHS because data were not readily accessible regarding the distribution of nurse staffing in California hospitals, the number of hospitals likely to be affected by the minimum staffing requirements, or the expected costs of this legislation. In addition, the ratios were meant to supplement valid and reliable patient classification systems (PCSs), which had been required in California hospitals since 1996. The problem was that although California hospitals had been required to submit their PCS data to the state, there was no standardization and little guidance about what characterized a valid PCS or what criteria should be used in determining the PCS. Therefore, PCS data yielded little, if any, helpful information to the CDHS for determining appropriate ratios.

Discussion Point

The California Hospital Association (CHA) advocated the use of PCS as the gold standard for staffing decisions rather than staffing ratios. The CNA argued for the reverse. What motives may have driven these positions?

TABLE 11.2   Minimum Registered Nurse (RN) Staffing Ratios for Hospitals in California in 2004 and New National Nurses United (NNU) Recommendations for 2020

Unit	Minimum RN–Patient Ratio Required in California in 2004 as a Result of A.B. 394	Minimum RN–Patient Ratio Recommended by NNU in 2020
Critical care/intensive care unit (ICU)	1:2	1:2
Neonatal ICU	1:2	1:2
Operating room	1:1	1:1 (plus at least one additional scrub assistant)
Postanesthesia		1:2
Labor and delivery	1:2	1:2
Antepartum	1:4	1:3
Postpartum couplets	1:4	1:3
Combined labor and delivery and postpartum		1:3
Well-baby nursery		1:6
Postpartum women only	1:6	
Intermediate-care nursery		1:4
Pediatrics	1:4	1:3
Emergency room (ER)	1:4	1:3
Trauma patient in ER		1:1
ICU patient in ER		1:2
Step-down	1:4 initially; 1:3 as of 2008	1:3
Telemetry		1:3
Medical–surgical	1:6 initially; 1:5 as of 2005	1:4
Oncology	1:5 initially; 1:4 as of 2008	
Coronary care		1:2
Acute respiratory care		1:2
Burn unit		1:2
Other specialty care units		1:4
Psychiatric	1:6	1:4
Rehabilitation		1:5
Skilled nursing facility		1:5

Source: Data from National Nurses United. (2010–2020). *National campaign for safe RN-to-patient staffing ratios.* Retrieved July 23, 2021, from https://www.nationalnursesunited.org/ratios

Cost was also not known. Initial projections by the Public Policy Institute of California suggested that many hospitals in California would experience sharp increases in costs associated with the increase in numbers of licensed staff. At least in part, because of limited empirical data, proposals received by CDHS suggested a wide range of minimum staffing ratios and even more widely differing estimates of cost. CHA, a hospital trade group representing the interests of nearly 500 hospital and health system members in California at that time, called for a minimum staffing ratio of 1 nurse to 10 patients on medical–surgical units, whereas the unions representing the largest numbers of nurses in the state argued for minimum ratios in medical–surgical units of 1:4. The CNA recommended a 1:3 ratio in medical–surgical units.

Following months of waiting and almost 2 years of wrangling, the final minimum staffing ratios were announced in January 2002. In a press conference at St. Vincent's Medical Center in Los Angeles, Governor Gray Davis announced that his administration supported a ratio of one nurse to every six patients in medical–surgical units—twice the number of patients supported by the CNA and four fewer than that favored by the CHA. Regulations were released later that spring with 45 days allocated for public comment. Hospitals in California were also required to continue to keep a PCS in place and to staff according to the PCS if it called for a larger number of nurses than the minimum ratios set by the CDHS.

Delays in Implementation

Implementing the ratio legislation proved to be just as difficult as determining what the ratios should be. The first challenge that arose was interpreting the meaning and intent of the legislation's language in regard to what constituted "licensed nurses." Almost immediately, questions were raised about whether the minimum mandatory ratios had to reflect RN representation in the staffing mix or whether LPNs/LVNs would meet the requirement.

The CNA argued that the intent of the law was to regulate minimum RN staffing, which inflamed the labor unions representing LPNs/LVNs. Amid much controversy, the issues were aired at a public hearing before the Department of Health Services in San Francisco, and a determination was provided that the ratios referred to RNs only and that LPNs/LVNs would be authorized to practice only under the direction of a licensed RN or physician.

Questions were then raised as to whether hospitals could eliminate or reduce their nonlicensed staff to save costs, given that the number of RNs would be increased. The CNA argued that the ratios were based on CDHS surveys of existing hospital staffing patterns and that nonlicensed staff should not be cut if safe patient care was to be ensured. The state, however, chose not to weigh in, arguing that its position was to regulate minimum RN–patient ratios; as a result, many hospitals immediately began reducing the number of support personnel to offset the increased cost of RN staff, and many RNs were forced to assume non-nursing care tasks.

Finally, the CHA, with the help of State Senator Sam Aanestad, introduced new legislation (A.B. 847) to the California State Senate Health and Human Services committee in April 2003 in an attempt to delay implementation of the 1:5 minimum nurse–patient staffing ratio on medical–surgical units until it could be ascertained that adequate RNs were available to meet the ratios. Opponents of the delay argued that this was simply an effort to preclude implementation of the mandate altogether. The bill failed.

The hospitals then persuaded Governor Arnold Schwarzenegger to issue an emergency regulation in November 2004 to overturn emergency room ratios and the improved medical–surgical ratios, citing financial crises (Cortez, 2008). In response, the CNA and the National Nurses Organizing Committee (NNOC) launched more than 100 protests against Schwarzenegger, resulting in a massive grassroots movement and the stinging defeat of four Schwarzenegger ballot initiatives in a 2005 special election (Cortez, 2008). The emergency regulation was ruled illegal in March 2005 by a state superior court judge and overturned. The judge argued that the financial state of hospitals did not give the state the right to delay implementing the law because the law's intent was to improve patient safety. Hospitals were told to comply immediately.

Still, resistance to staffing ratio implementation continued. Hospitals were accused of encouraging management staff to undermine and avoid compliance with the new RN staffing ratios. Nursing unions responded with threats to close down units with inadequate staffing, to delay elective surgeries, and to wage a public relations campaign to garner public support for the nurses.

The Struggle to Implement the Ratios

Despite these efforts and a pervasive, ongoing resistance to staffing ratio implementation, the staffing ratio mandate did go into effect on January 1, 2004. But were hospitals ready and willing to implement these changes? By and large, bigger hospitals in the state were ready to meet the mandate by the time of its implementation. Many smaller hospitals, however, had existing budget deficits and had to seek waivers from the CDHS because of their difficulty in meeting the ratios. Waivers were allowed, but hospitals had to be rural and meet strict conditions.

Discussion Point

Should small rural hospitals be given waivers for the mandatory staffing ratios? Is this justified by the patient population characteristics, or is it simply an economic incentive to keep these hospitals viable?

The dire predictions about reductions in hospital services, increased emergency room diversions, and hospitals in California having to close doors if mandatory staffing ratio legislation passed, never materialized. In fact, most hospitals in California did not have to hire more contracted RNs to comply with the ratios. Nor was there a decrease in skill mix as a result. In fact, nurses from all over the country moved to California for jobs when the staffing ratios legislation passed. Indeed, AHC Media (2019) suggests there was an influx of 110,000 nurses in the first 4 years after the law was passed.

The adverse, unintended consequences of mandatory nurse staffing levels, feared before the implementation of mandated staffing ratios, never materialized. Instead, a large proportion of hospitals continued to have more nurses than required, most nurses reported that their workloads decreased, and when more agency nurses were used, there did not appear to be any negative impacts on quality of care (Kerfoot & Douglas, 2013).

The "At All Times" Clause

Almost immediately after implementation of A.B. 394, legal clarification did become necessary, however, regarding interpretation of the law about ratio coverage "at all times." A ruling by the CDHS blindsided many hospitals in its strict interpretation that ratios had to be maintained at all times, including during breaks and lunches. For many hospitals, this meant hiring additional rotating staff to fill in for nurses when they had to leave the bedside for short periods (breaks, lunch, transporting patients, etc.) or face being noncompliant.

As a result, the CHA filed a lawsuit on December 30, 2003, challenging the ruling and arguing that the "at all times" ruling was impossible to implement. The motion was heard in a Sacramento court on May 14, 2004. In a 10-page ruling issued on May 26, 2004, the judge dismissed the hospital association lawsuit, saying that not adhering to the "at all times" clause would make the nurse-to-patient ratios meaningless. Again, the ruling was an effort to maintain the original intent of the law—to protect patients.

Discussion Point

Is an "at all times" clause necessary?

Have RN Staffing and Patient Outcomes Improved in California Because of Mandatory Minimum Staffing Ratios?

As of January 1, 2008, California's historic staffing law for RN staffing ratios completed its phase-in period, and almost 15 years of data now exist regarding compliance with the staffing ratios as well as any changes in patient outcomes. A synthesis by Donaldson and Shapiro (2010) of 12 studies examining the impact of California's ratios on patient care costs, quality, and outcomes in acute care hospitals revealed that the implementation of minimum nurse-to-patient ratios did reduce the number of patients per licensed nurse and increase the number of worked nursing hours per

patient day in hospitals. There were, however, no significant impacts of these improved staffing measures on measures of nursing quality and patient safety indicators across hospitals. Donaldson and Shapiro emphasized, however, that adverse outcomes did not increase despite the increasing patient severity reflected in case mix index and cautiously posited that this finding might suggest the influence of minimum ratios in preventing adverse events in the presence of increased patient risk.

In addition, Aiken (2010) and the Center for Health Outcomes and Policy Research at the University of Pennsylvania conducted an independent evaluation of California's mandated nurse staffing requirements. This survey of more than 22,000 RNs working in 604 hospitals in California and two comparison states without legislation—Pennsylvania and New Jersey—found that overall, nurses in California cared for an average of one patient fewer than nurses in the two comparison states. On medical and surgical units, California hospital nurses each took care of two fewer patients. In terms of patient outcomes, Aiken studied more than one million patients who had common surgical procedures in these hospitals in 2006, more than 2 years after mandatory nurse staffing was implemented. She found that California hospitals had significantly lower risk-adjusted mortality and were better at rescuing patients who experienced complications than the comparison states, even after accounting for factors other than differences in nurse staffing.

Similarly, a literature review conducted by Serratt (2013b) suggested mixed results, with three studies finding both positive and negative outcomes and five studies reporting no significant changes in patient outcomes. Serratt concluded that some improvements resulted from the implementation of staffing ratios, but the positives were not as significant and widespread as predicted. Another study reported by Serratt (2013a) found an increase in labor costs and some reduction in services with ratio implementation, suggesting a negative financial impact on selected outcomes of California hospitals.

In addition, Munnich (2014) reported that little evidence exists to support the idea that this law was effective in attracting more nurses to the hospital workforce or improving patient outcomes, though nurse-to-patient ratios in medical–surgical units increased substantially following the staffing mandate. Survey data from two nationally representative data sets indicate that the law had no effect on the aggregate number of RNs or the hours they worked in California hospitals, and at most had a modest effect on wages. Munnich cautioned that California's experience with minimum nurse staffing legislation may not be generalizable to states considering similar policies in different hospital markets.

Another literature review by Mark et al. (2013) also noted mixed results in terms of whether mandatory ratios in California improved patient care quality. Although the Agency for Healthcare Research and Quality (AHRQ) reported that its patient safety indicators showed a significant reduction in patient falls, pressure injuries, and restraint use, conflicting data by California hospitals found no significant differences to support AHRQ's findings (Mark et al., 2013).

Yet, Tellez and Seago (2013) note that nurse satisfaction and nurse retention rates did rise after passage of the California staffing law. The significance is that as the nursing workforce ages and retires, there will be a shortage of experienced nurses to care for the increasing demand for health care put forward by the Affordable Care Act. These facts place pressure on the health care system to care for more patients with fewer nurses. California's staffing legislation is serving to counter mounting pressure.

In addition, a study by Leigh (2015) noted that occupational injury and illness rates for California RNs dropped over 30% after implementation of the mandatory ratios. Although the study did not address costs, it is likely that the law resulted in lower workers' compensation costs because employment grew by 15% whereas injuries per employed nurse dropped by 30%.

The answer as to whether mandated ratios have improved care or created new cost burdens for California is still unclear. The CNA says the ratios have improved nurse retention, raised the numbers of qualified nurses willing to work, reduced burnout, and improved morale. Aiken agrees, suggesting that there is good scientific evidence that staffing improved even in safety net hospitals that long had poor staffing (Kerfoot & Douglas, 2013). Aiken also notes that prior to the California staffing legislation, all of the blue-ribbon committees that looked at safe nurse staffing shied away from establishing specific patient-to-nurse ratios. Thus, communicating with stakeholders and the media was difficult without "a recommended number." "The evidence-based benchmark implemented in California of no more than five patients per nurse on medical and surgical units has become the number against which to evaluate hospital staffing" (Kerfoot & Douglas, 2013, p. 217).

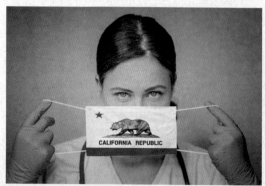

(kovop58/Shutterstock)

> **Consider This**   The answer as to whether mandated ratios have improved care or created new cost burdens for California is still unclear.

Recent Changes to Mandatory Staffing Ratio Enforcement in California

It is noteworthy that for years after the mandated ratios were put into effect, California had limited penalties and enforcement of the ratio legislation. This changed, however, when Senate Bill 227 became effective January 1, 2020, requiring the California Department of Public Health (CDPH) to impose penalties of $15,000 for the first violation and $30,000 for each subsequent violation of nurse staffing ratios (Bartleson & Blanchard-Saiger, 2020). Under the law, multiple staffing violations found on the same inspection constitute a single violation, and any violation that happens more than 3 years after the last violation will be considered a first violation. In addition, hospitals were not subject to penalties only if they could demonstrate that the fluctuation in required staffing levels was unpredictable and uncontrollable; that prompt efforts were made to maintain required staffing levels; and that the hospital immediately used and subsequently exhausted the hospital's on-call list of nurses and the charge nurse (Bartleson & Blanchard-Saiger, 2020).

Unfortunately, just a few months later, as a result of Governor Gavin Newsom's declaration of a state of emergency related to the COVID-19 pandemic, the director of the CDPH authorized a temporary waiver of licensing requirements and suspended regulatory enforcement of all licensing requirements (including Title 22 and nurse-to-patient staffing ratios) for hospitals with a few exceptions (Hughes, 2020). This waiver was extended in July 2020 through March 21, 2021, and then extended again until September 30, 2021. The waiver may be further extended based on updated executive orders or guidance from the Centers for Medicare & Medicaid Services (CMS) or the Centers for Disease Control and Prevention (CDC) (CDPH, 2021). The notification procedures and time frames may only be waived, however, if the hospital is modifying services to address patient surges related to COVID-19.

OTHER ALTERNATIVES

Efforts are also underway, in both California and the rest of the country, to explore alternatives to improving nurse staffing that do not require legislated minimum staffing ratios. The reality is that many leading health care and professional nursing organizations do not support the need for legislated minimum staffing ratios. For example, The Joint Commission, one of the most powerful accrediting bodies for hospitals in the United States, has been reluctant to endorse nationally mandated minimum staffing ratios, suggesting that this would not be flexible enough to encompass the diversity represented in hospitals across the United States.

In addition, the ANA does not support fixed nurse–patient ratios, arguing that a more flexible approach to nurse staffing is needed to allow for nurse-specific factors, which can include factors like a nurse's level of experience, knowledge, education, and skillset, as well as patient-specific factors such as acuity and intensity (Brusie, 2019). To this end, the ANA updated their *Principles for Nurse Staffing* in 2019, which support both nurse- and patient-specific factors in making staffing decisions (ANA, n.d.; Brusie, 2019) (Box 11.2). The ANA argues that this type of approach better accommodates changes in patients' needs, available technology, and the preparation and experience of staff. In addition, the ANA argues that what may be established through legislation today as an appropriate minimum nurse-to-patient ratio may be obsolete by the next shift or 2 years from now and that disclosure of staffing plans without evaluation and recourse for inadequate levels is futile.

In addition, the ANA has been working with federal officials to push for the CMS to provide Congress with information about how the agency assesses "adequate" staffing levels as part of its ongoing budget requests and has been working to maintain National Quality Forum endorsements for two nurse staffing measures: skill mix and nursing hours per patient day (Brusie, 2019).

Aiken also suggests she is not necessarily an advocate of legislative mandates (Kerfoot & Douglas, 2013). Instead, she argues that there are multiple ways to achieve the objectives that have been achieved in California. She continues to support publicly reported nurse staffing and urges nurses to do the same so that greater transparency regarding hospital staffing can occur. She concludes that "even folks who are not in favor of legislative mandates should open their minds to the evidence that the California legislation did work as intended" and that "it is a mistake for nurses to reject evidence if not to their liking for some reason" (Kerfoot & Douglas, 2013, p. 217).

In addition, the Veterans Health Administration (VHA) enacted a staffing methodology model in 2011 that uses expert panels at the unit level to determine inpatient staffing levels based on acuity. These levels are then reported to the facility level. However, implementation of the staffing methodology was delayed in part due to leadership turnover. Preliminary evaluation of the model suggests some empowerment of nurses at the unit level; however, the impact on patient outcomes is not yet available (Fowler & Comeaux, 2017; Taylor et al., 2015).

CONCLUSIONS

Evidence regarding the benefits of staffing ratios is mixed and sometimes contradictory, yet a substantial literature exists, suggesting that increasing RN representation in the staffing mix improves at least some patient outcomes. What is less clear is what the optimal staffing levels are for various patient populations and when costs associated with staffing mix become unreasonable in terms of attempting to improve patient outcomes. In addition, given the lessons that have already been learned with the "RN/LVN debate" and the "at all times" requirement, more thought must be given to how

---

BOX 11.2   **Five Basic Principles Recommended by the American Nurses Association for Nurse Staffing**

1. **Health Care Consumer:** Nurse staffing decisions are based on the number and needs of the patients, families, groups, communities, and populations served.
2. **Interprofessional Teams:** Optimal care is achieved through individual actions and collaboration with other health care team members. Nurses are full partners in the delivery of safe, quality health care.
3. **Workplace Culture:** Organizational leaders must create a workplace environment that values nurses as critical members of the health care team.
4. **Practice Environment:** All nursing care delivery systems must provide the necessary resources to meet each health care consumer's individual needs and the demands of the unit.
5. **Evaluation:** Organizations must have appropriate nurse staffing plans. All settings need well-developed staffing guidelines with measurable nurse-sensitive outcomes.

Source: American Nurses Association. (n.d.). *Principles for nurse staffing.* Retrieved July 23, 2021, from https://www.nursingworld.org/practice-policy/nurse-staffing/staffing-principles/

strictly staffing ratio regulations are to be interpreted and how enforcement can be effective if there are no monetary consequences for breaking rules. In addition, the intermingling roles of state government as a legislator of minimum staffing ratios, compliance officer, disciplinary enforcer, and potential funding source to assist with mandated ratio implementation need further examination and clarification.

Finally, it must be recognized that patient acuity is continuing to rise, and the mandatory minimum staffing ratios adopted in California in 2003 were arguably inadequate just 5 years later, especially when hospitals refused to staff above the ratios when census and acuity call for it (Cortez, 2008). In fact, the NNU (2010–2020) is advocating for even lower ratios (see Table 11.2). These ratios would pose even greater fiscal and human resource challenges to California hospitals in terms of their implementation.

The implementation and subsequent evaluation of mandatory staffing ratios in California should, however, provide some insight into these ongoing issues that will be helpful to other states that choose to follow in California's footsteps. Clearly, the enactment of California's nurse-to-patient ratio law was far from smooth, and concerns continue about the costs of hiring additional licensed staff and the need to meet the "at all times" clause.

It is not clear yet whether California has the resources (both human and fiscal) it would need to lower the staffing ratios further. Some of the initial implementation struggles may have been related to the normal issues that arise whenever a new law takes effect; however, the reality is that California has struggled to maintain the mandate. The fact that it took 5 years from passage of the legislation to mandated implementation is telling. What is even more telling are the number of hospitals in California that continue to report difficulty in meeting staffing ratio requirements and the resistance that continues to be a part of its implementation.

For Additional Discussion

1. Given rising patient acuity levels and increased scope of responsibility for RNs, at what point should California reexamine the adequacy of current staffing ratios?

2. In an effort to cut the costs associated with implementing minimum RN staffing ratios, some hospitals eliminated their support staff. Have RNs gained anything when this is the case?

3. Should LPNs/LVNs be counted to meet minimum mandatory staffing ratio requirements?

4. Does the implementation of mandatory staffing ratios in the midst of an international/national pandemic or nursing shortage make sense? Why or why not?

5. At what point does cost related to staffing mix become so prohibitive that society will be willing to accept some increase in patient morbidity and mortality?

6. What critical lessons should other states learn from California's experience thus far in implementing mandatory staffing ratios?

References

AHC Media. (2019). Mandated nurse-patient ratios protect healthcare workers: Do benefits outweigh the costs? *Hospital Employee Health, 38*(3), 1–4.

Aiken, L. (2010). Safety in numbers. *Nursing Standard, 24*(44), 62–63. https://doi.org/10.7748/ns.24.44.62.s55

Aiken, L. H., Clarke, S. P., Sloane, D., Sochalski, J., & Silber, J. (2002). Effects of nurse-staffing on nurse burnout and job-dissatisfaction and patient deaths. *The Journal of the American Medical Association, 288*, 1987–1993.

American Nurses Association. (2019, July). *Nurse staffing advocacy.* Retrieved July 23, 2021, from https://www.nursingworld.org/practice-policy/nurse-staffing/nurse-staffing-advocacy/

American Nurses Association. (n.d.). *Principles for nurse staffing.* Retrieved July 23, 2021, from https://www.nursingworld.org/practice-policy/nurse-staffing/staffing-principles/

American Organization of Nurse Executives. (2018, October 30). *Policy statement on nurse staffing.* Retrieved July 23, 2021, from https://www.aonl.org/system/files/media/file/2019/04/mandated-staffing-ratios.pdf

Bartleson, B. J., & Blanchard-Saiger, G. (2020, January 21). *CDPH issues notice on mandated fines for hospitals not in compliance with nurse staffing ratios.* Retrieved July 23, 2021, from https://www.calhospital.org/cha-news-article/cdph-issues-notice-mandated-fines-hospitals-not-compliance-nurse-staffing-ratios

Bridges, J., Griffiths, P., Oliver, E., & Pickering, R. M. (2019). Hospital nurse staffing and staff–patient interactions:

An observational study. *BMJ Quality & Safety, 28*(9), 706–713. https://doi.org/10.1136/bmjqs-2018-008948

Brusie, C. (2019, December 4). *ANA updates nurse staffing guidelines to support flexibility.* Retrieved July 23, 2021, from https://nurse.org/articles/nurse-staffing-ana-guidelines/

California Department of Public Health. (2021, July 16). *Suspension of regulatory enforcement of hospital require-ments (This AFL supersedes AFL 20-26.8).* Retrieved July 23, 2021, from https://www.cdph.ca.gov/Programs/CHCQ/LCP/Pages/AFL-20-26.aspx

Cho, E., Park, J., Choi, M., Lee, H. S., & Kim, E. (2018, March). Associations of nurse staffing and education with the length of stay of surgical patients. *Journal of Nursing Scholarship, 50*(2), 210–218. https://doi.org/10.1111/jnu.12366

Cortez, Z. (2008, January 4). *California's nurse-patient ratio law: Saving lives, reducing the nursing shortage.* Retrieved July 20, 2017, from http://www.californiaprogressreport.com/site/california%E2%80%99s-nurse-patient-ratio-law-saving-lives-reducing-nursing-shortage

Daigon, G. (2020, July 15). *Stressed-out nurses say nation's hospitals need more of them to care for patients.* Retrieved July 23, 2021, from https://whowhatwhy.org/2020/07/15/stressed-out-nurses-say-nations-hospitals-need-more-of-them-to-care-for-patients/

Donaldson, N., & Shapiro, S. (2010). Impact of California mandated acute care hospital nurse staffing ratios: A literature synthesis. *Policy, Politics & Nursing Practice, 11*(3), 184–201. https://doi.org/10.1177/1527154410392240

Driscoll, A., Grant, M. J., Carroll, D., Dalton, S., Deaton, C., Jones, I., Lehwaldt, D., McKee, G., Munyombwe, T., & Astin, F. (2018, January). The effect of nurse-to-patient ratios on nurse-sensitive patient outcomes in acute specialist units: A systematic review and meta-analysis. *European Journal of Cardiovascular Nursing, 17*(1), 6–22. https://doi.org/10.1177/1474515117721561

Eskes, E. M., Chabower, W., Nieuwenhoven, P., & Vermeulen, H. (2020). What not to do: Choosing wisely in nursing care. *International Journal of Nursing Studies, 101*, 103420. Retrieved July 23, 2021, from https://reader.elsevier.com/reader/sd/pii/S0020748919302275?token=AB121F8826753 23ABF53A82626A924D15627AD77374BF571A56CBE522 D56D2734254C3D081D2EA02B6406D9B91414B5C

Fowler, D., & Comeaux, Y. (2017). The legislative role in nurse staffing ratios. *Med-Surg Matters, 26*(2), 12–13.

Griffiths, P., Saville, C., Ball, J., Jones, J., Pattison, N., & Monks, T.; On behalf of the Safer Nursing Care Study Group. (2020, March). Nursing workload, nurse staffing methodologies and tools: A systematic scoping review and discussion. *International Journal of Nursing Studies, 103*, 103487. Retrieved July 23, 2021, from https://reader.elsevier.com/reader/sd/pii/S0020748919302949?token=93BCE658922B3 02C1B650392E8C4D17828CB159B75203466A77DBBE08B 655419D9B2BAB5E3A1109200258B025AA677D0

Hawk, T., & Sreenivas, K. (2021, February 12). *Estimating the cost of minimum staffing ratios in Connecticut nursing homes.* Retrieved July 23, 2021, from https://www.cga.ct.gov/2021/appdata/tmy/2021HB-06439-R000303-Barrett,

%20Matthew-CT%20Assoc.%20of%20Health%20Care%20 Facilities-Attachment%20-%20DSS-TMY.PDF

Hughes, K. (2020, April 7). *Nurse-to-patient ratios during the COVID-19 crisis.* Retrieved July 23, 2021, from http://www.nurseallianceca.org/2020/04/07/nurse-to-patient-ratios-during-the-covid-19-crisis/

Kerfoot, K. M., & Douglas, K. S. (2013). The impact of research on staffing: An interview with Linda Aiken, Part 1. *Nursing Economics, 31*(5), 216–253.

King University Online. (2019, March 12). *Nurse-to-patient ratio: How many is too many?* Retrieved July 23, 2021, from https://online.king.edu/news/nurse-to-patient-ratio/

Kouatly, I. A., Nassar, N., Nizam, M., & Badr, L. K. (2018). Evidence on nurse staffing ratios and patient outcomes in a low-income country: Implications for future research and practice. *Worldviews on Evidence-Based Nursing, 15*(5), 353–360. https://doi.org/10.1111/wvn.12316

Lasater, K. B., Sloane, D. M., McHugh, M. D., Cimiotti, J. P., Riman, K. A., Martin, B., Alexander, M., & Aiken, L. H. (2021). Evaluation of hospital nurse-to-patient staffing ratios and sepsis bundles on patient outcomes. Association for Professionals in Infection Control and Epidemiology, Annual Conference (Virtual), 28–30 June, 2021. *American Journal of Infection Control, 49*(7), 868–873. https://doi.org/10.1016/j.ajic.2020.12.002

Leigh, J. P. (2015, March 3). California's nurse-to-patient ratio law reduced nurse injuries by more than 30 percent. *Economic Policy Institute.* Retrieved July 23, 2021, from https://www.epi.org/blog/californias-nurse-to-patient-ratio-law-reduced-nurse-injuries-by-more-than-30-percent/

Mark, B., Harless, D., Spetz, J., Reiter, K., & Pink, G. (2013). California's minimum nurse staffing legislation: Results from a natural experiment. *Health Services Research, 48*(2), 435–454. https://doi.org/10.1111/j.1475-6773.2012.01465.x

McHugh, M. D., Aiken, L. H., Sloane, D. M., Windsor, C., Douglas, C., & Yates, P. (2021, May). Effects of nurse-to-patient ratio legislation on nurse staffing and patient mortality, readmissions, and length of stay: A pro-spective study in a panel of hospitals. *Lancet, 397*(10288), 1905–1913. https://doi.org/10.1016/S0140-6736(21)00768-6

Munnich, E. L. (2014). The labor market effects of California's minimum nurse staffing law. *Health Economics, 23*(8), 935–950. https://doi.org/10.1002/hec.2966

National Nurses United. (2010–2020). *National campaign for safe RN-to-patient staffing ratios.* Retrieved July 23, 2021, from http://www.nationalnursesunited.org/issues/entry/ratios

National Nurses United. (2021, May 12). *RNs applaud introduc-tion of federal legislation to mandate number of patients as-signed to nurses.* Retrieved July 23, 2021, from https://www.nationalnursesunited.org/press/rns-applaud-introduction-of-federal-legislation-to-mandate-number-patients-assigned-to-nurses

Needleman, J., Buerhaus, P., Mattke, S., Stewart, M., & Zelevinsky, K. (2002). Nurse-staffing levels and the quality of care in hospitals. *The New England Journal of Medicine, 346*, 1715–1722. https://doi.org/10.1056/NEJMsa012247

Needleman, J., Jianfang, L., Jinjing S., Larson, E. L., & Stone, P. W. (2020). Association of registered nurse and nursing support staffing with inpatient hospital mortality. *BMJ Quality & Safety, 29*(1), 10–18.

NursingLicensure.org. (2021). *Health experts debate the merits of nurse-staffing ratio law.* Retrieved July 23, 2021, from https://www.nursinglicensure.org/articles/nurse-staffing-ratios.html

Ohio Nurses Association. (2017, May 4). *Nurses say mandatory overtime puts patients at risk.* Retrieved July 23, 2021, from http://www.ohnurses.org/nurses-say-mandatory-overtime-puts-patients-risk

Open States. (2021). *HB 106—An Act amending the act of July 19, 1979 (P.L.130, No.48), known as the Health Care Facilities Act, providing for hospital patient protection. Pennsylvania House Bill. 2021-2022 regular session.* Retrieved July 23, 2021, from https://openstates.org/pa/bills/2021-2022/HB106/

Reyes, A. (2021, May 4). *NYS Assembly and Senate pass 'safe staffing' legislation for nursing homes, hospitals.* Retrieved July 23, 2021, from https://www.wkbw.com/news/state-news/nys-assembly-and-senate-pass-safe-staffing-legislation-for-nursing-homes-hospitals

Schoenberg, S. (2018, May 1). *Nurse staffing ratios: What is the 2018 Massachusetts ballot question all about?* Retrieved July 23, 2021, from http://www.masslive.com/politics/index.ssf/2018/05/nurse_staffing_ratios_what_is.html

Serratt, T. (2013a). California's nurse-to-patient ratios, Part 2: 8 Years later, what do we know about hospital level outcomes? *Journal of Nursing Administration, 43*(10), 549–553. https://doi.org/10.1097/NNA.0b013e3182a3e906

Serratt, T. (2013b). California's nurse-to-patient ratios, Part 3: Eight years later, what do we know about patient level outcomes? *Journal of Nursing Administration, 43*(11), 581–585. https://doi.org/10.1097/01.NNA.0000434505.69428.eb

Shang, J., Needleman, J., Liu, J., Larson, E., & Stone, P. W. (2019). Nurse staffing and healthcare-associated infection, unit-level analysis. *Journal of Nursing Administration, 49*(5), 260–265. https://doi.org/10.1097/NNA.0000000000000748

Sholtis, B. (2021, May 10). *Facing burnout, worker shortages, nurses say COVID-19 shows need for staffing ratios.* Retrieved July 23, 2021, from https://www.wlvr.org/2021/05/facing-burnout-worker-shortages-nurses-say-covid-19-shows-need-for-staffing-ratios/#.YPs4PUBlCUk

Taylor, B., Yankey, N., Robinson, C., Annis, A., Haddock, K. S., Alt-White, A., & Sales, A. (2015). Evaluating the Veterans Health Administration's staffing methodology model: A reliable approach. *Nursing Economics, 33*(1), 36–40, 66.

Tellez, M., & Seago, J. (2013). California nurse staffing law and RN workforce changes. *Nursing Economics, 31*(1), 18–28.

Title 42. Section 483.35. (2021). *483.35 Nursing services. eCFR.* Retrieved August 16, 2020, from https://ecfr.io/Title-42/Section-483.35

Tung, L. (2019, November 29). *Why mandated nurse-to-patient ratios have become one of the most controversial ideas in health care.* Retrieved July 23, 2021, from https://www.witf.org/2019/11/29/why-mandated-nurse-to-patient-ratios-have-become-one-of-the-most-controversial-ideas-in-health-care/

Williamson, E. (2020, May 12). *Nurse to patient ratios: Leaders have their work cut out for them.* Retrieved July 23, 2021, from https://www.nurse.com/blog/2020/05/12/nurse-to-patient-ratios-leaders-have-their-work-cut-out-for-them/

Wynendaele, H., Willems, R., & Trybou, J. (2019). Systematic review: Association between the patient–nurse ratio and nurse outcomes in acute care hospitals. *Journal of Nursing Management, 27*(5), 896–917. https://doi.org/10.1111/jonm.12764

Mandatory Overtime in Nursing

Carol J. Huston

LEARNING OBJECTIVES

The learner will be able to:

1. Explore the current extent of mandatory overtime in nursing as identified in the literature.

2. Identify the strengths and the limitations of the Fair Labor Standards Act of 1938 in terms of protecting workers against mandatory overtime.

3. Identify how changes to federal overtime rules in the past decade and more recent court rulings have affected traditional "white collar" employees, including salaried nurses in the United States.

4. Investigate current federal and state legislative efforts to regulate overtime limits for nurses.

5. Describe the consequences of mandatory overtime in nursing, including fatigue, increased error rates, increased legal liability, threats to the nurse's personal safety, and increased staff turnover rates.

6. Reflect on the number of hours a nurse can safely work before quality of care is potentially compromised.

7. Discuss the limits of the nurse's professional duty and assess how much risk a nurse should assume in fulfilling a professional duty.

8. Know and understand the provisions of the Nurse Practice Act in their state, as well as the position statements or advisory opinions that have been issued by the state board of nursing regarding mandatory overtime and patient abandonment.

9. Identify the criteria that typically must be in place for a nurse to be found guilty of patient abandonment.

INTRODUCTION

A short-term means of dealing with nursing shortages has been to require nurses to work extra shifts, often under threat of "patient abandonment" or punitive measures. *Mandatory overtime*, also called *compulsory* or *forced overtime*, occurs when employees are required to work more hours than are standard (generally 40 hours per week) or risk employer reprisals if they refuse to do so. Mandatory overtime may result from many unexpected events such as natural or human-caused disasters, sudden job vacancies, staff absences on account of illness, or rapid changes in patient care requirements. Alternately, it may be a standard staffing practice.

A review of the literature suggests that the use of mandatory overtime in nursing varies greatly from institution to institution and from state to state. Some health care employers have suggested that manpower shortages are the cause of mandatory overtime in their facilities. The consensus, however, is that working overtime among nurses is a prevalent practice used to control chronic understaffing and normal variations in the patient census. Increasingly, nurses are reporting that mandatory overtime has become standard operating procedure instead of a last resort to deal with short staffing. In fact, in some hospitals, mandatory overtime is routinely used to keep fewer people on the payroll, as well as to alleviate immediate shortages. Furthermore, American nurses are more likely to work 12-hour shifts, and concerns are being raised about whether there is adequate time for rest and recovery between shifts.

> *Consider This* Nursing overtime, both mandatory and voluntary, is prevalent in the health care industry.

Some nursing specialty units are known, however, to have more mandatory overtime than others, such as the operating room and postanesthesia care units. This occurs because of emergent and dynamic patient needs, unpredictable delays in surgical procedures, and significant differences in the efficiency of members of the operating room staff. To create guidelines for safe practice in the perioperative setting, the Association of periOperative Registered Nurses (AORN) created their "AORN Position Statement on Perioperative Safe Staffing and On-Call Practices" in 2014 (AORN, 2014). Excerpts from this document are shown in Box 12.1.

BOX 12.1   **Summary of the Association of PeriOperative Registered Nurses (AORN) Position Statement on Perioperative Safe Staffing and On-Call Practices**

The AORN, recognizing the potential negative consequences of sleep deprivation and sustained work hours and further recognizing that adequate rest and recuperation periods are essential to patient and perioperative personnel safety, suggests the following strategies:

1. On-call staffing plans should
   * support perioperative teams to recognize fatigue as a risk to patient and employee safety rather than a sign of a worker's dedication to the job
   * minimize extended work hours
   * provide rest periods between scheduled shifts
   * maintain a qualified perioperative RN as circulator
   * be provided in accordance with both standards of perioperative and perianesthesia nursing practice
   * not require perioperative team members to work in direct patient care for more than 12 consecutive hours in a 24-hour period and not more than 60 hours in a 7-day work week
   * include all work hours (i.e., regular hours and call hours worked) in calculating total work hours
2. Strategies for developing a safe on-call schedule should include
   * provisions for off-duty periods of uninterrupted 8-hour sleep cycle, a break from continuous professional responsibilities, and time to perform individual activities of daily living
   * calculating to identify when it is cost-effective to replace on-call staff with a scheduled shift (return on investment [ROI], cost analysis)
   * relieving perioperative team members who have worked hours on-call and are scheduled to work a subsequent shift
   * making exceptions to the 12-hour limit only under extreme conditions (i.e., internal or external disasters) and having an organizational policy that outlines the events that would create exceptions to the 12-hour limitation
   * an orientation to on-call responsibilities that is accomplished using the preceptor system (i.e., having an experienced perioperative RN serve as an immediate resource for the orientee)

Other units known to have more mandatory overtime are critical care units. These units tend to rely more on overtime hours to maintain adequate staffing due to their requirements for specialized nurses and higher staffing ratios. In a study by Lobo et al. (2018), in 10 of the 11 intensive care units where study participants worked, overtime hours were offered to nurses on nearly every scheduled day off. Often, these nurses worked these extra shifts despite their fatigue so as not to let coworkers down. Nurses who refused overtime said the high-stress critical care environments drained their resources and they needed time away from work for rest, recuperation, and the maintenance of an appropriate work–life balance.

It should be noted that the Department of Transportation (DOT) and the Federal Aviation Administration (FAA) regulate how long pilots, air traffic controllers, engineers, flight attendants, airline mechanics, and other employees can work in order to maintain airline safety standards and protect crew and passengers. Similarly, the DOT and the Federal Motor Carrier Safety Administration regulate the number of consecutive hours truck drivers may work. In contrast, there is no federal regulation of the hours a nurse may work.

> *Consider This* Federal regulations have used transportation laws to place limits on the amount of time that can safely be worked in aviation and trucking to avoid accident and injury. It seems appropriate to at least examine the need to create similar safety parameters around mandatory overtime in nursing.

In fact, Miller (2020) calls the United States the most overworked developed nation in the world. That is because 85.8% of men and 66.5% of women in the United States work more than 40 hours per week. In comparison, Americans work 137 more hours per year than Japanese workers, 260 more hours per year than British workers, and 499 more hours per year than French workers (Miller, 2020).

In addition, the United States is the only industrialized country in the world that has no legally mandated annual leave, and in every country except Canada and Japan (and the United States, which averages 13 days per year), workers get at least 20 paid vacation days a year. In France and Finland, they get 30—an entire paid month off every year (Miller, 2020).

For some Americans, hard work may be perceived as a badge of honor, or it may be the means of accommodating lifestyles that increasingly require two wage earners in a household. It may also be that Americans are working this hard because they are afraid not to. In the United States, unlike most other countries, employment is *at will*, meaning that employers can dismiss employees for any reason (aside from those of gender, race, age, or disability) or for no reason at all. Thus, employees who refuse to work overtime can lose their jobs or face other reprisals.

Nurses argue, however, that mandatory overtime in nursing is not comparable with other fields because the consequences of being overly fatigued for the nurse may literally have life-and-death consequences. Proponents of mandatory overtime argue that it is an economic reality given how limited labor health care resources are, particularly considering the international nursing shortage. The problem is that both positions are at times correct.

> *Consider This* Many nurses report a dramatic increase in the use of mandatory overtime to solve staffing problems and fear potential consequences for safety and quality of care for their patients.

MANDATORY OVERTIME AS A WAY OF LIFE IN THE UNITED STATES

Although nurses bemoan mandatory overtime in the profession, the reality is that mandatory overtime is not new, nor is it restricted to nursing. While the work week has been shrinking in many countries, the United States continues to be well above average in the number of hours its people work each year, with more worked hours than other developed countries like Australia, Canada, Germany, and the United Kingdom. Indeed, Americans typically work more hours and take fewer vacations than workers in other peer economies.

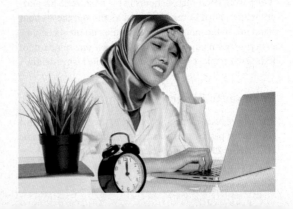

This chapter defines mandatory overtime, examines the extent of its use in nursing, and discusses the consequences of mandatory overtime in nursing as identified in the literature.

LEGISLATING MANDATORY OVERTIME

The Fair Labor Standards Act

The definition of what constitutes overtime in the United States or how it should be calculated has historically varied from state to state and from industry to industry. There are, however, national standards in terms of the *Fair Labor Standards Act* (FLSA) of 1938. This act, which regulates overtime, does not impose limits on overtime hours or prohibit dismissal or any other sanction for declining overtime work. It does, however, require that payroll employees (those who are not "exempt" from the overtime requirements of the FLSA) be paid an overtime premium of at least one-and-a-half times the regular rate of pay for each hour worked more than 40 in a week (U.S. Department of Labor, n.d.).

> *Consider This* Labor laws such as the FLSA need to be amended to protect workers against excessive work hours and mandatory overtime and to protect the public from the dangers of an overburdened, stressed workforce.

The FLSA does, however, contain language that permits the health care industry to use a different overtime standard than the 40-hour work week since scheduling occurs 24 hours a day, 365 days a year. Historically, this overtime standard required that hospitals and residential care facilities pay overtime after either 8 hours in a day or 80 hours in a 14-day pay period. It also permits employees to work more than 40 hours in a week and not be paid overtime provided they do not work more than 8 hours in a shift or if they work fewer than 40 hours in the next week. Employers are permitted to use both the 40-hour and the 80-hour standards in the same facility, depending on the scheduling patterns for employees, but they must use one standard for individual employees, and it must be applied consistently.

Changes to Federal Overtime Rules

There have been changes, however, to the federal overtime rules in the past two decades. Some changes, which became effective in 2004, defined exemptions from the FLSA for what were traditionally called "white collar" employees. The

new rules increased the amount of money employees could earn before they were no longer eligible to receive overtime pay; however, employees who directed and supervised two or more other fulltime employees fell under the executive exemption. Similarly, the new rules excluded employees who had the authority to hire, fire, and promote employees or whose primary duties involved the performance of office or nonmanual work and the exercise of discretion and independent judgment (U.S. Department of Labor, 2019).

Almost immediately, nursing leaders expressed concern that the language in the new rules opened the door for employer attempts to reclassify nurses as exempt from overtime protections historically given to workers under the FLSA. Concerns about the exemption of health care workers from protection under the FLSA were borne out in a June 2007 Supreme Court ruling that the U.S. Department of Labor had acted appropriately in denying FLSA protection to 10 home care workers even when employed by large, third-party home care agencies (Dawson, 2007). In the case of *Long Island Care at Home, LTD. versus Coke*, "the Court ruled that Ms. Evelyn Coke, a home care aide from Queens, New York, deserved neither overtime pay nor minimum wage, although she was frequently asked to work up to 70 hours per week" (Dawson, 2007, para. 1). This ruling occurred because of an exemption to the FLSA that applied to companions and housekeepers who work in the homes of their patients. New rules enacted in 2016, however, extended minimum wage and overtime protections to direct care workers. These are the same protections provided to most U.S. workers including those who perform the same work in nursing homes.

In addition, it is important to note that nurses are eligible for overtime pay and protection under the FLSA if they are classified by employers as hourly—not salaried—employees, because salaried employees are not eligible for overtime. Thus, salaried employees and nurses who are considered exempt under the FLSA have virtually no rights under these new overtime rules. They are entitled only to their base salary less deductions by law and may be held to whatever schedule an employer demands because there are no restrictions on mandatory overtime in the FLSA.

Legislating Limits on Nursing Overtime
Federal and State Efforts

Although a multiplicity of evidence exists suggesting mandatory overtime can lead to negative outcomes, efforts over the past decade to introduce national legislation directed at prohibiting employers from requiring licensed health care employees to work more than 8 hours in a single workday or 80 hours in any 14-day work period—except in the case of a natural disaster or declaration of emergency by federal, state, or local government officials—have not been successful.

States are, however, increasingly taking a role in both defining mandatory overtime and putting limits on its use. Every nurse should know and understand the provisions of the Nurse Practice Act in their state, as well as the position statements or advisory opinions that have been issued by the state board of nursing on mandatory overtime and patient abandonment.

As of 2018, 18 states had restrictions in law or regulations on the use of mandatory overtime for nurses (Alaska, California, Connecticut, Illinois, Maine, Maryland, Massachusetts, Minnesota, Missouri, New Hampshire, New Jersey, New York, Oregon, Pennsylvania, Rhode Island, Texas, West Virginia, and Washington, DC) (Johnson// Becker PLLC et al., 2018).

Alaska passed mandatory overtime restrictions for nurses in health care settings in 2010 (became effective in 2011), preceded by Texas in 2009. In Alaska, the law states that a registered nurse or licensed practical nurse in a health care facility who is not employed in a federal or tribal facility may not be required or coerced, directly or indirectly, to work beyond their agreed-upon regular shift or accept overtime if, in the judgment of the nurse, the overtime would jeopardize patient or employee safety ("Summary of Overtime Limitations," 2018). In addition, the nurse cannot work more than 14 consecutive hours except under specific conditions such as a nurse voluntarily working overtime on an aircraft in use for medical transport or a nurse participating in the performance of a medical procedure that has begun but not been completed. On-call time is not counted in the 14 hours unless the nurse is actually called back into work ("Summary of Overtime Limitations," 2018).

Likewise, Pennsylvania enacted the Prohibition of Excessive Overtime in Health Care Act (Act 102) in 2008. This law stated that a health care facility could not require an employee to work in excess of an agreed to, predetermined, and regularly scheduled daily work shift unless there was an unforeseeable declared national, state, or municipal emergency or a catastrophic event that was unpredictable or unavoidable and that substantially affected or increased the need for health care services (Commonwealth of Pennsylvania, 2021). This law did not preclude employees from voluntarily accepting overtime, and it did not apply to those workers compensated for on-call time.

Discussion Point

What position statement or advisory opinion has your state board of nursing issued regarding mandatory overtime and patient abandonment? Do you feel that it is adequate to protect both nurses and patients from unsafe working conditions?

New York enacted legislation in 2009 prohibiting health care employers (excluding home care facilities) from forcing nurses to work overtime, except during health care disasters that increased the need for health care personnel unexpectedly or when a health care employer determined that there was an emergency and had made a good faith effort to have overtime covered on a voluntary basis (New York, State Department of Labor, n.d.). Although the New York legislation provides a good example of how states can reduce the risk of mandatory overtime for nurses, it should be noted that the New York Nurses Association first proposed legislation to ban mandatory overtime in 2000. Eight years were required to gain enough support from patient advocacy groups and other unions that represent nurses.

Minnesota successfully passed legislation in 2007 that prohibited nurses from being disciplined for refusing overtime if, in the nurse's judgment, it would be unsafe for the patient (Minnesota Nurses Association, 2021).

Similar legislation became effective in New Hampshire in 2008. This legislation prohibited an employer from disciplining or removing any right, benefit, or privilege of a registered nurse, licensed practical nurse, or licensed nursing assistant for refusing to work more than 12 consecutive hours except under specific circumstances such as a nurse participating in surgery until the surgery is completed or a nurse working in a critical care unit until another employee beginning a scheduled work shift relieves them. Other exceptions include a nurse working in a home health care setting until another qualified nurse or customary caregiver relieves them; a public health emergency; or a nurse covered by a collective bargaining agreement containing provisions addressing the issue of mandatory overtime (Lore Law Firm, n.d.). A nurse might face disciplinary action for refusing to work mandatory overtime in these situations.

Professional Association Efforts

In addition, the American Nurses Association (ANA) has added mandatory overtime to its Nationwide State Legislative Agenda, supporting the enactment of mandatory overtime legislation by state legislatures and the attention to such issues by regulatory agencies. The ANA also authored a position statement in 2006 arguing that nursing employers should ensure that sufficient system resources exist to (1) provide the individual registered nurse in all roles and settings with a work schedule that provides for adequate rest and recuperation between scheduled work and (2) provide sufficient compensation and appropriate staffing systems that foster a safe and healthful environment in which the registered nurse does not feel compelled to seek supplemental income through overtime, extra shifts, and other practices that contribute to worker fatigue (ANA, 2006).

In addition, the Academy of Medical-Surgical Nurses (AMSN, 2020) issued a position statement in 2020 suggesting that overtime should be offered only on a voluntary basis and only after all other attempts to provide adequate staffing have failed. In addition, the AMSN notes that nurses should never be required to work beyond their individual physical and mental capacity.

Discussion Point

Is increasing the use of mandatory overtime perpetuating nursing shortages? Do you think nurses who no longer work in nursing roles would be more apt to return to work if they felt they had more control over the hours they worked (i.e., if mandatory overtime were banned)?

THE CONSEQUENCES OF MANDATORY OVERTIME

How long can nurses work safely? Given the variability in each situation, there is no one answer to this question. There is little doubt, however, that after a certain point of protracted work time, fatigue becomes a factor and the likelihood of errors, near errors, mistakes, and lapses in judgment increases. Compounding the difficulty in answering the question, research on the effects of overtime has focused largely on studies of individuals working scheduled 12-hour shifts. However, when staff plan to work 12-hour shifts or additional shifts on a voluntary basis, they are more likely to get plenty of rest immediately before working the extended shift. Overtime mandated by an employer, however, occurs with little or no prior notice, so higher levels of fatigue may occur. In addition, many nurses report working far more than 12 hours when mandatory overtime is involved.

There are, however, numerous studies in leading journals that suggest that when nurses work more than 8 hours a day, patients are at risk. This is because more medication errors and sentinel events occur when nurses are fatigued, and the numbers rise exponentially when nurses work past 12 hours (Bucceri Androus, 2021). These findings were confirmed in a recent study by Bae (2021), who found a conclusive relationship between excessive nurse work hours (more than 40 hours per week or 12 hours per day) and adverse patient outcomes, such as medication errors, nosocomial infections, falls with injuries, and errors or near misses. Bae concluded that nursing shifts longer than 12 hours should be prohibited.

In addition, most nurses who work 12-hour shifts do not get enough sleep, tallying around 5.5 hours per night and even less for night-shift workers. Lack of sleep and fatigue are known to cause poor judgment and significantly high rates of errors (Bucceri Androus, 2021).

Working abnormally extended periods in a health care environment may also cause nurses to exceed the safe limits for exposure to a variety of things, including ergonomic stressors and chemical agents and result in increased risks for both mental and physical health conditions (Stasik, n.d.). In addition, drowsy driving following 12-hour night shifts is persistent among nurses, resulting in elevated rates of vehicle crashes and crash-related injuries and deaths (Smith et al., 2020). Indeed, Olson (2021) notes that nursing is among occupations with the highest workplace fatalities (105 incidents per 10,000 fulltime workers), which may be a consequence of long, cumulative work schedules. Fatigue may accumulate across multiple shifts and lead to performance impairments, which in turn may be linked to injury risks.

In another recent large European study involving more than 31,000 nurses in 488 hospitals across 12 countries, hospital nurses who worked 12-hour shifts experienced more adverse outcomes like burnout and job dissatisfaction ("How 12-Hour Nursing Shifts Impact Burnout and Job Satisfaction", 2020). Most notably, nursing shifts of at least 12 hours increased the odds of high emotional exhaustion by 26% compared with nurses working shifts of 8 hours or less. Nurses who worked longer shifts were also more likely to experience high depersonalization (a dreamlike or detached state of mind) and low personal accomplishment.

Similarly, Meinke (2019) notes that 12-hour (or longer) shifts can be detrimental to an individual's health, causing fatigue, sleep disruptions (if working night shift), an increased potential for errors, and issues with social life. In addition, 12-hour shifts can result in long-term health risks due to the limited time before, during, and after shifts to eat healthy meals and exercise properly. Combined with fatigue and other adverse factors, this can result in depression, anxiety, and insomnia (Meinke, 2019).

Discussion Point

How many hours can the typical nurse work before they might be considered unsafe? How much individual leeway is feasible in making this determination?

Likewise, a recent study by Horton Dias and Dawson (2020) suggested that nurses working 10- to 12-hour shifts ate differently than they did at home: sometimes earlier, later, or in the middle of the night, and sometimes not at all. Most nurses working these long shifts did not eat until they returned home, and then due to time constraints, would go to bed with a full stomach. This caused sleep quality compromise, gastric reflux, and weight gain. See Research Fuels the Controversy 12.1.

Research Fuels the Controversy 12.1

Long Shifts and Eating Patterns in Hospital-Employed Nurses

This qualitative, descriptive study examined workplace influences on hospital nurses' dietary behaviors in the southeast region of the United States. Twenty-one participants participated in 16 one-on-one interviews and two focus groups.

Source: Horton Dias, C., & Dawson, R. M. (2020). Hospital and shift work influences on nurses' dietary behaviors: A qualitative study. *Workplace Health & Safety, 6*(8), 374–383. https://doi.org/10.1177/2165079919890351

Study Findings

Study findings revealed that hospital food was unhealthy, that free food influenced consumption, and that long shift work was a major barrier to healthy eating. The eating patterns of nurses while at work were significantly different from home, largely because of lengthy shifts. Working 10- to 12-hour shifts caused nurses to eat earlier, later, or in the middle of the night. Often, they did not eat at all. Most nurses ate when they returned home, and due to time constraints imposed by long shifts, would then go to bed with a full stomach. Subsequently, nurses suffered from sleep quality compromise, gastric reflux, and weight gain.

Overeating was reported as a common occurrence due to exhaustion and extreme hunger after lengthy shifts and long periods without food. In addition, nurses often used "comfort" foods to cope with job-related stress and exhaustion. Nurses also perceived the need for quick energy to perform their best during long shifts. Fast, high-caloric foods and caffeine were commonly used during busy times and during slow times to ward off boredom or sleepiness.

The hospital food environment also posed particularly challenging barriers to healthy eating. The abundance of unhealthy foods that were accessible nearby at all hours and often for free combined with the lack of healthy food options, required nurses to bring food from home if they wanted to eat healthfully. Shift work and family responsibilities restricted personal time to the degree that having to plan and prepare healthy meals becomes exceedingly burdensome. For nurses exhausted from hospital shift work, the healthy choice quickly became the difficult choice.

All these findings reinforce those of a report of the Board on Health Care Services and the Institute of Medicine (2004), *Keeping Patients Safe: Transforming the Work Environment of Nurses*, which said that nurses' long working hours pose a serious threat to patient safety. In fact, the report argued that limiting the number of hours worked per day and consecutive days of work by nursing staff, as is done in other safety-sensitive industries, is a fundamental safety precaution. Similarly, Marquis and Huston (2021) argue that certain minimum criteria should always be met for safe staffing. These criteria are shown in Box 12.2.

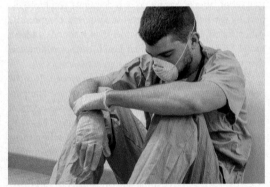

(Deliris/Shutterstock)

BOX 12.2   Minimum Criteria for Staffing Decisions

1. Decisions made must meet state and federal labor laws and organizational policies.
2. Staff must not be demoralized or excessively fatigued by frequent or extended overtime requests.
3. Long-term as well as short-term solutions to staffing shortages must be sought.
4. Patient care must not be jeopardized.

Source: Marquis, B., & Huston, C. (2021). *Leadership roles and management functions in nursing* (10th ed.). Wolters Kluwer.

PROFESSIONAL DUTY AND CONSCIENCE

Mandatory overtime and patient abandonment must also be examined in terms of professional duty. A *professional duty* is the direct result of others having welfare rights, such as the right to safe care. Because people have a right to such care, nurses have an associated duty to ensure that they accept patient care assignments only if they are mentally and physically able to provide, at minimum, safe care.

The problem is that there is great variability in terms of how many hours a nurse can work and still provide competent safe care. For example, the practice of mandatory overtime is grounded in the commitment to prevent harm to patients by guaranteeing adequate nurse–patient ratios, yet the overfatigued nurse may pose even greater risk of harm to patients by agreeing to work. Each nurse must carefully consider their level of fatigue when deciding to accept any assignment extending beyond the regularly scheduled workday or work week.

> ### Discussion Point
>
> Who bears the risk or the consequences of risk when an overworked nurse makes errors that contribute to patient harm?

What happens when nurses determine they must refuse to work additional hours because of safety concerns related to level of fatigue? Saying no to a desperate employer, especially when the fear that short staffing may compromise patient safety, is likely much harder than it sounds. Indeed, moral dilemmas abound when health care providers feel they must refuse a patient care assignment.

When this occurs, some nurses feel compelled to file their refusal to work as a *conscientious objection*. The purpose of conscientious objection is to protect the rights of employees who refuse to participate in procedures based on conscience. The issue of whether a nurse can refuse mandatory overtime based on conscience, however, has limited case law precedent.

The ANA's (2015) *Code of Ethics* might be helpful to some nurses in resolving potential ethical conflicts between their professional duty to provide care and their conscience, or the realization that providing such care may actually place patients at risk for harm. The *Code of Ethics*, however, could potentiate the dilemma because it states that nurses should care for all people in need without discrimination. The problem is that it also says that the nurse is to maintain conditions of employment that are conducive to high-quality nursing care.

The ANA also recommends the *Nurses Bill of Rights* as a tool for dialogue to resolve concerns that nurses may have about work environments that might not support professional practice. The Nurses Bill of Rights was conceived to support nurses in an array of workplace situations, including mandatory overtime and suggests that nurses must bring these workplace issues to the attention of employers to meet their responsibilities to their patients and to themselves (ANA, n.d.).

Patient Abandonment

One of the most common reasons nurses cite for working mandatory overtime is the threat that refusal to do so could be construed as *patient abandonment*, a charge that can result in loss of licensure. Therefore, many nurses believe that they have no choice when confronted by a request for overtime, even though they might be working a shift more than 12 hours.

> *Consider This* In some facilities, nurses are being threatened with dismissal or with the charge of patient abandonment if they refuse to accept overtime.

Despite this perception, the ANA does not support the forced overtime of nurses, and their position is that a nurse should not be held accountable for patient abandonment if the nurse turned down an assignment that could be unsafe to patients or themselves. In fact, most state boards of nursing maintain that refusal to work mandatory overtime is not patient abandonment; in a situation in which a nurse has accepted a patient or assignment, the nurse must simply notify the supervisor that they are leaving and report off to another nurse.

Clearly, this was the case in a recent complaint filed with the Oregon Board of Nursing, in which an employer accused a nurse of patient abandonment (Gamble et al., 2019). The Oregon Board of Nursing's investigation revealed that the nurse submitted the resignation to be effective after the shift ended, had followed correct procedures regarding the follow-up of delegated activities, and had met the standards for documentation. The board determined that the nurse's actions did not violate the Oregon Nurse Practice Act and dismissed the case. The decision was consistent with the board's interpretive statement on patient abandonment that specifies a "nurse who has completed their assigned shift and notifies the employer that she/he is ending the employment relationship with the employer without prior notice, including when the nurse doesn't provide sufficient time for the employer to obtain a replacement, does not commit patient abandonment" (Gamble et al., 2019, p. 15).

It should be noted, however, that nurses have less likelihood of losing their license or being reprimanded if an assignment (mandatory overtime) was never accepted in the first place than if the assignment was accepted and then the nurse changed their mind. This is because accepting the assignment suggests that a nurse–patient relationship has been established. Thus, patient abandonment is more likely when the nurse accepts a patient assignment and then ceases to provide nursing care without appropriately transferring the responsibility for the patient to another professional nurse. This then becomes a form of negligence in nursing since the termination of the provider–patient relationship was unilateral, despite the patient's continued need for care. Once a nurse begins treating a patient, they are legally bound to care for that patient until another nurse is available to assume responsibility for the patient.

In addition, boards of nursing in several states have developed clear statements differentiating patient abandonment from *employment abandonment*. Typically, these statements define employment abandonment as nurses leaving their places of work to avoid injury to patients or to themselves. This definition is similar to language used by the Maryland Board of Registered Nursing (BRN) in defining patient abandonment; however, the Maryland BRN (n.d.) suggested that there are many variables to be examined in determining whether patient abandonment has occurred. The definition of patient abandonment and these variables are shown in Box 12.3.

> *Consider This* Although boards of nursing often rule that refusing mandatory overtime is not patient abandonment and thus is not cause of loss of licensure, they have no jurisdiction over employment and contract issues. Refusing to work mandatory overtime may still result in termination of a nurse's employment.

Similarly, the Vermont Board of Nursing (2015) defined abandonment as disengagement from the nurse–patient or caregiver–patient relationship without properly notifying appropriate personnel (e.g., supervisor or employer) and/or making reasonable arrangements for continuation of care, or failing to provide adequate patient care until the responsibility for care of the patient is assumed by another nurse, nursing assistant, or other approved provider. Examples of situations that may constitute abandonment are provided in Box 12.4.

BOX 12.3 The Link Between Nurse–Patient Relationships and Patient Abandonment as Outlined by the Maryland Board of Registered Nursing

Abandonment occurs when a licensed nurse terminates the nurse–patient relationship without reasonable notification to the nursing supervisor for the continuation of the patient's care.

The nurse–patient relationship begins when responsibility for nursing care of a patient is accepted by the nurse. Nursing management is accountable for assessing the capabilities of personnel and delegating responsibility or assigning nursing care functions to personnel qualified to assume such responsibility or to perform such functions.

The Variables That Need to Be Examined in Each Alleged Incident of Abandonment Include but Are Not Limited to:

1. What were the licensee's assigned responsibilities for what time frame? What was the clinical setting and what were the resources available to the licensee?
2. Was there an exchange of responsibility from one licensee to another? When did the exchange occur, that is, shift report and so on?
3. What was the time frame of the incident, that is, time licensee arrived, time of exchange of responsibility, and the like?
4. What was the communication process, that is, whom did the licensee inform of their intent to leave, and was it lateral, upward, downward, and so forth?
5. What are the facility's policies, terms of employment, and/or job description regarding the licensee and call-in, refusal to accept an assignment, reassignment to another unit, mandatory overtime, and the like?
6. What is the pattern of practice/events for the licensee and the pattern of management for the unit/facility, that is, is the event of a single isolated occurrence, or is it one event in a series of events?
7. What were the issues/reasons why the licensee could not accept an assignment, continue an assignment, or extend an original assignment, and so forth?

Source: Maryland Board of Registered Nursing. (n.d.). *Abandonment*. Retrieved August 12, 2020, from http://mbon.maryland.gov/Pages/practice-abandonment.aspx

Sample Situations That Might Constitute Patient Abandonment

- Leaving the patient care area without transferring responsibility for patient care to an authorized person
- Remaining unavailable for patient care for a period of time such that patient care may be compromised because of lack of available qualified staff
- Inattention or insufficient observation or contact with a patient
- Sleeping while on duty without the approval of a supervisor in accordance with written facility policy
- Failing to notify a supervisor or employer in a timely fashion if the licensee will not initiate or complete an assignment where the licensee is the sole provider of care
- For the advanced practice nurse, terminating the nurse–patient relationship without providing reasonable notification to the patient and resources for continuity of care

Source: Vermont Board of Nursing. (2015, October). *Vermont Board of Nursing position statement on abandonment.* Retrieved August 12, 2020, from https://sos.vermont.gov/media/ri4a5yt2/ps-abandonment-2015-1012.pdf

UNIONS AND MANDATORY OVERTIME

Because collective bargaining agreements can require greater protections beyond those outlined in the FLSA, the position of most collective bargaining agents is that the practice of mandatory overtime should be eliminated entirely. However, there are differences among union contracts, and the strategies used by unions to reduce mandatory overtime vary greatly.

The American Federation of Teachers (AFT, n.d.) has been on record since 1990 calling for a ban on mandatory overtime through a twofold approach—legislation and contract language. At the federal level, AFT is working with legislators to require facilities receiving Medicare funding to stop mandating overtime and notes that on-call time should be treated as work time. In addition, many local unions have negotiated contract language limiting the practice of mandatory overtime.

The Service Employees International Union (SEIU) has also consistently spoken out against mandatory overtime, and in partnership with the Nurse Alliance, created an Overtime Report Form for nurses, union or nonunion, to document mandatory or pressured overtime. Similarly, the American Federation of State, County, and Municipal Employees (AFSCME, 2021) contends that one of the most significant and risky consequences of insufficient staffing is the routine and widespread use of overtime to fill gaps in scheduling. To address the problem, AFSCME Resolution 25 suggests that AFSCME (2021) will continue to advance legislation at the state and federal levels to limit the ability

of employers to impose mandatory overtime for nurses and to give nurses the right to refuse overtime without fear of discrimination or retaliation.

CONCLUSIONS

In the end, the mandatory overtime dilemma, like so many dilemmas in nursing, comes down to a conflict regarding how best to use limited resources (fiscal and human) to provide safe, quality health care. Most nurses and administrators can agree on two goals: (1) staffing should be at least minimally adequate to ensure that all patients receive safe care and (2) nursing staff should not be placed at personal or legal risk to provide that care.

The problem is that the onus is on management to ensure that there is appropriate staffing, and most health care institutions state that there are simply not enough resources to meet the first goal without jeopardizing the second. Clearly, more alternatives such as shift bidding and pay enhancement programs need to be explored. Neither health care administrators nor nurses should have to choose between meeting the needs of patients and meeting the needs of nurses.

The bottom line is that workers should have the right to refuse overtime without fear of repercussion, especially when staffing shortages and mandated overtime are the norm and not the exception. Unfortunately, as long as nursing shortages exist, mandatory overtime will continue to be used as a means of meeting minimum staffing needs.

For Additional Discussion

1. How does the presence of a collective bargaining agreement affect a hospital's ability to require mandatory overtime? How much power do unions have in negotiating this aspect of working conditions?

2. Would passage of a national ban on mandatory overtime tie the hands of hospitals in ensuring that staffing is at least minimally adequate during periods of acute nursing shortages?

3. Does the use of mandatory overtime really save hospitals money in terms of recruitment and benefits?

4. How do the rates of mandatory overtime in nursing compare with those in other professions?

5. Are other non-nursing health care professionals at risk for loss of licensure if they are found guilty of patient abandonment?

6. Are charges of patient abandonment morally appropriate if a nurse works their required shift but refuses to stay and work longer?

7. Given the severity and scope of the nursing shortage, what is the likelihood that mandatory staffing will continue to be used for both emergency and routine staffing needs?

References

Academy of Medical-Surgical Nurses. (2020, April). *Practice environment advocacy: Position statement.* Retrieved July 26, 2021, from http://dev.amsn.org/sites/default/files/documents/amsn-statement-practice-environment-advocacy.pdf

American Federation of State, County and Municipal Employees, American Federation of Labor and Congress of Industrial Organizations. (2021). *The nurse staffing crisis* (Resolution No. 25). Retrieved July 26, 2021, from https://www.afscme.org/about/governance/conventions/resolutions-amendments/2004/resolutions/the-nurse-staffing-crisis

American Federation of Teachers. (n.d.). *Mandatory overtime.* Retrieved July 26, 2021, from http://www.aft.org/healthcare/mandatory-overtime

American Nurses Association. (2006). *Position statements: Assuring patient safety: Registered nurses' responsibility in all roles and settings to guard against working when fatigued.* Retrieved July 26, 2021, from https://ojin.nursingworld.org/MainMenuCategories/Policy-Advocacy/Positions-and-Resolutions/ANAPositionStatements/Archives/Copy-of-AssuringPatientSafety-1.pdf#:~:text=It%20is%20intended%20that%20this%20position%20statement%20be,to%20refuse%20an%20assignment%20if%20impaired%20by%20fatigue

American Nurses Association. (2015). *Code of ethics for nurses with interpretive statements.* Nurse Books.Org.

American Nurses Association. (n.d.). *Bill of rights FAQs.* Retrieved July 26, 2021, from http://nursingworld.org/NursesBillofRights

Association of periOperative Registered Nurses. (2014). *AORN position statement on perioperative safe staffing and on-call practices.* Retrieved July 26, 2021, from https://www.scribd.com/document/317254444/AORN-Position-Statement-on-Perioperative-Safe-Staffing-and-on-Call-Practices

Bae, S. (2021, August). Relationships between comprehensive characteristics of nurse work schedules and adverse patient outcomes: A systematic literature review. *Journal of Clinical Nursing, 30*(15/16), 2202–2221. https://doi.org/10.1111/jocn.15728

Bucceri Androus, A. (2021, June 28). *Are breaks and the 12-hour shift being dealt a bad hand?* Retrieved July 23, 2021, from https://www.registerednursing.org/are-breaks-12-hour-shift-being-dealt-bad-hand/

Commonwealth of Pennsylvania. (2021). *Act No. 102.* Retrieved July 26, 2021, from https://www.dli.pa.gov/laws-regs/laws/Pages/Prohibition-of-Exceesive-Overtime-in-Health-Care.aspx

Dawson, S. L. (2007). Taking a cue from the Supreme Court. *Nursing Homes: Long Term Care Management, 56*(10), 8–10.

Gamble, J., West, N., & Parish, M. (2019). Disciplinary case studies: Patient abandonment. *Oregon State Board of Nursing Sentinel, 39*(2), 15.

Horton Dias, C., & Dawson, R. M. (2020, August). Hospital and shift work influences on nurses' dietary behaviors: A qualitative study. *Workplace Health & Safety, 6*(8), 374–383. https://doi.org/10.1177/2165079919890351

How 12-hour nursing shifts impact burnout and job satisfaction. (2020, March 26). Retrieved July 26, 2021, from https://dailynurse.com/how-12-hour-nursing-shifts-impact-burnout-and-job-satisfaction/

Institute of Medicine. (2004). *Keeping patients safe: Transforming the work environment of nurses.* The National Academies Press.

Johnson//Becker PLLC, Monheit Law P.C., & Banville Law. (2018). *Mandatory overtime in nursing.* Retrieved July 26, 2021, from http://wageadvocates.com/faq/is-mandatory-overtime-legal/

Lobo, V. M., Ploeg, J., Fisher, A., Peachey, G., & Akhtar-Danesh, N. (2018). Critical care nurses' reasons for working or not working overtime. *Critical Care Nurse, 38*(6), 47–57. https://doi.org/10.4037/ccn2018616

Lore Law Firm. (n.d.). *New Hampshire labor laws.* Retrieved July 26, 2021, from https://www.overtime-flsa.com/new-hampshire-labor-laws/

Marquis, B., & Huston, C. (2021). *Leadership roles and management functions in nursing: Theory and application* (10th ed.). Wolters Kluwer.

Maryland Board of Registered Nursing. (n.d.). *Abandonment.* Retrieved July 26, 2021, from http://mbon.maryland.gov/Pages/practice-abandonment.aspx

Meinke, H. (2019, November 18). *Nurses share the pros and cons of working 12-hour shifts.* Retrieved July 26, 2021, from https://www.rasmussen.edu/degrees/nursing/blog/working-12-hour-shifts/

Miller, G. E. (2020, January 13). *The U.S. is the most overworked developed nation in the world.* Retrieved July 26, 2021, from http://20somethingfinance.com/american-hours-worked-productivity-vacation/

Minnesota Nurses Association. (2021). *Mandatory overtime: Just say no.* Opinion by Mathew Keller RN JD, Regulatory and Policy Nursing Specialist on August 17, 2015. Retrieved July 26, 2021, from https://mnnurses.org/mandatory-overtime-just-say-no/#:~:text=If%20you%E2%80%99ve%20been%20told%20by%20your%20nurse%20manager,judgment%2C%20it%20would%20be%20unsafe%20for%20the%20patient

New York, State Department of Labor. (n.d.). *Mandatory overtime for nurses.* Retrieved July 26, 2021, from https://dol.ny.gov/mandatory-overtime-nurses

Olson, N. (2021, May 19). *Your guide to workplace injury statistics for 2021.* Safesite. Retrieved July 26, 2021, from https://safesitehq.com/2021-workplace-injury-statistics/

Smith, A., McDonald, A. D., & Sasangohar, F. (2020, December). Night-shift nurses and drowsy driving: A qualitative study. *International Journal of Nursing Studies, 112.* https://doi.org/10.1016/j.ijnurstu.2020.103600

Stasik, S. (n.d.). *The dangers of mandated overtime for nurses.* Onward Healthcare. Retrieved July 26, 2019, from https://www.onwardhealthcare.com/nursing-resources/the-dangers-of-mandated-overtime-for-nurses/

Summary of overtime limitations for nurses. Alaska Statute 18.20.400–18.20.499. (2018). Retrieved July 26, 2021, from http://www.labor.alaska.gov/lss/forms/nurse_ot_summ.pdf

U.S. Department of Labor. (2019, September). *Fact Sheet #17A: Exemption for executive, administrative, professional, computer & outside sales employee s under the Fair Labor Standards Act (FLSA).* Retrieved July 26, 2021, from https://www.dol.gov/sites/dolgov/files/WHD/legacy/files/fs17a_overview.pdf

U.S. Department of Labor. (n.d.). *Overtime pay.* Retrieved July 26, 2021, from http://www.dol.gov/dol/topic/wages/overtimepay.htm

Vermont Board of Nursing. (2015, October). *Vermont Board of Nursing position statement on abandonment.* Retrieved July 26, 2021, from https://sos.vermont.gov/media/ri4a5yt2/ps-abandonment-2015-1012.pdf

Promoting Civility and Healthy Work Environments in Nursing and Health Care

Cynthia M. Clark

LEARNING OBJECTIVES

The learner will be able to:

1. Summarize the rationale for fostering civility and healthy work environments in nursing and health care.

2. Recognize incivility, bullying, mobbing, and other workplace aggressions.

3. Identify the impact of incivility and other workplace aggressions on individuals, teams, organizations, and patient care.

4. Discuss the relationship between stress and incivility (pre- and post-COVID).

5. Identify common elements of a healthy work environment.

6. Detail an evidence-based Pathway for Fostering Organizational Civility (PFOC).

INTRODUCTION

Over the past decade, there has been a concerted and organized movement toward fostering civility and healthy work environments (HWEs) in nursing and health care. In 2015, the American Nurses Association (ANA, 2015a) issued a position statement on incivility, bullying, and workplace violence advocating for the adoption and implementation of a zero-tolerance policy for all forms of workplace aggression. The position statement outlined individual and shared roles and responsibilities of nurses and employers to create and sustain a culture of respect across the health care continuum, emphasizing the ethical, moral, and legal responsibility of health care employers to create healthy and safe work environments for nurses, health care team members, patients, families, and communities.

That same year, the ANA published the revised Code of Ethics for Nurses (2015b) stating that all nurses have a moral obligation and ethical imperative to create and sustain HWEs and to foster an atmosphere of dignity and respect. Specifically, Provision 1.5 requires nurses

> to create an ethical environment and culture of civility and kindness, treating colleagues, coworkers, employees, students, and others with dignity and respect ... and that any form of bullying, harassment, intimidation, manipulation, threats or violence will not be tolerated. (p. 4)

The ANA Code of Ethics is consistent with the International Council of Nurses (ICN) Code of Ethics (2012), which emphasizes the nurse's obligation to respect human rights, treat people with dignity and respect, and provide respectful and unrestricted care. Additionally, in their workplace violence position statement, the ICN (2017) supported zero-tolerance policies for violence in any form, including those associated with workplace bullying and lateral violence among nurses.

In 2016, the American Association of Critical-Care Nurses (AACN) reaffirmed six standards for establishing and sustaining HWEs and concluded that unhealthy work environments and relationship issues "can become the root cause of medical errors, hospital-acquired infections, clinical complications, patient readmissions, and nurse turnover" (AACN, 2016, p. 8). Shortly thereafter, the Tri-Council for Nursing (2017) proclaimed civility as essential to building healthy, inclusive work environments to protect patient safety. In 2018, the National League for Nursing (NLN, 2018a) released a vision statement on ways to build and sustain civil, healthy academic environments in nursing education, underscoring the role of faculty in modeling civility for colleagues and learners.

Although there may be differences in the various international and national definitions of HWEs, there is a mutual emphasis on the physical, mental, and social well-being of all nurses wherever they work or whatever positions they hold. It is also clear it is essential that a HWE has within it a culture of civility.

More than a decade ago, Clark and Carnosso (2008) conducted a concept analysis to construct a common understanding of the concept of civility to clarify its meaning. The operational definition of civility stemming from this analysis noted that "civility is characterized by an authentic respect for others when expressing disagreement, disparity, or controversy. It involves time presence, a willingness to engage in genuine discourse, and a sincere intention to seek common ground" (p. 13).

Since then, Clark, Gorton, and Bentley (in review) set about to update the original concept analysis and formulate a revised operational definition of civility. The revised operational definition of civility stemming from the updated analysis is "choosing to authentically engage in respectful and inclusive ways to foster equity, belonging, community, and connection, including instances when opposing views are expressed." In both concept analyses, civility was found to be synonymous with respect and emphasized an intention to meaningfully engage to resolve disagreements and seek common ground.

Many studies have reported that health care workers, and in particular nurses, have experienced a higher rate of inappropriate behavior in the workplace than other workers have experienced. A health risk appraisal conducted by the ANA (2017) provides an illuminating perspective of the realities of professional life in the health workplace. Over a 3-year period, the survey responses from more than 14,000 registered nurses and nursing students provided a national cross-section of the health risks experienced in a variety of settings and locations. The summary results showed:

- Workplace stress was identified as the top work environment health and safety risk, with 82% of participants saying they are at a "significant level of risk for workplace stress."
- Up to half of respondents had been bullied in some manner in the workplace.
- Of participants, 25% had been physically assaulted at work by a patient or patient's family member.
- Of participants, 9% were concerned for their physical safety at work (ANA, 2017, p. 4).

The ANA (2017) executive summary further reports:

- Of respondents, 90% were familiar with safety guidelines and policies.
- Of respondents, 80% expressed the belief that their employer values their health and safety.

- Of respondents, 78% felt treated with dignity and respect (ANA, 2017, p. 4).

Sokol-Hessner and colleagues (2018) concluded that harm from disrespect (e.g., incivility) in health care is associated with patients reporting a poorer experience, lower likelihood of perceiving care as high quality, and lower likelihood of seeking care again in the same facility. There was also a higher risk of physical harm to both patients and workers and higher levels of staff disengagement, absenteeism, and turnover. Ulrich and team (2019) conducted a study with 8,080 critical care nurses in the United States to evaluate the current state of critical care nurses' work environments. While the study provided evidence of positive outcomes when implementing HWE standards (AACN, 2016), other findings included:

- Reports of 198,340 incidents of physical and mental well-being issues from 6,017 participants.
- Reports that a third of respondents expressed an intent to leave their current position within the next 12 months.
- Physical and mental safety issues that included verbal abuse, physical abuse, and sexual harassment and discrimination.
- Patients and families were the most frequently reported source of abuse; however, 41% of respondents reported at least one incident from physicians, 34% from at least one other nurse, and 15% from other health care personnel.

While measuring respect and meaningful recognition was only one part of the study, the authors concluded that respect was positively associated with job satisfaction, communication, and intent to stay in one's current position. The authors further concluded that respect is required for effective communication and collaboration and a critical element for patient safety. Results from the AACN study are a critical call to action to improve the physical and mental safety of nurses. Therefore, creating HWEs where nurses are empowered to speak up, have the confidence to be heard, and actions are taken to resolve unsafe conditions is essential.

Discussion Point

What role do you think nurses play in fostering civility and creating HWEs?

Many factors that may contribute to an unhealthy work environment, which are discussed later in this chapter, often go unreported, in part because they may not be physical in nature. In addition, these contributing factors may not be acted upon when they are reported and can have a damaging effect on individuals, colleagues, teams, organizations, and patient care outcomes.

This chapter describes incivility, bullying, mobbing, and other workplace aggressions and their impact on individuals, teams, organizations, and patient care; the relationship between stress and incivility; elements of a HWE; and the evidence-based Pathway for Fostering Organizational Civility (PFOC; Clark, 2017, 2019).

BEHAVIORS AND FACTORS THAT CONTRIBUTE TO UNHEALTHY WORK ENVIRONMENTS

There are several terms in the nursing literature used to describe undesirable and intimidating behaviors and interactions that occur between and among nurses and other health care workers. This section provides working definitions for three of the more common examples—incivility, bullying, and workplace mobbing.

Incivility

Clark (2017) defines incivility as a range of rude or disruptive behaviors that can result in psychological or physiologic distress for the people involved. If uncivil behaviors are left unchecked or unaddressed, they may progress into unsafe or threatening situations. Uncivil acts may range from nonverbal gestures and behaviors such as eye rolling, refusing to listen, and walking away to more overt behaviors such as making demeaning and belittling remarks or refusing to assist a colleague. Incivility also includes silently standing by while others are treated with disrespect and failing to intervene, especially when patient safety is at risk (ANA, 2015a).

In a recent study, Rehder and colleagues (2020) found that over half of health care workers reported exposure to an array of disruptive behaviors, ranging from hanging up the phone before a conversation was over to physical aggression toward others. The authors found a significant unfavorable association between the reported prevalence of uncivil behaviors and various workplace issues, including safety, teamwork climate, job satisfaction, work–life balance, and staff burnout and depression. In addition to high numbers of health care workers exposed to uncivil and disruptive behaviors on a routine basis, there was a lack of recognition of incivility as a safety risk, avoidance of conflict, and fears of retribution leading to potential underreporting of disruptive behaviors. The authors concluded that unprofessional and disruptive behaviors have wide-reaching negative effects on both staff and patients.

Incivility in nursing education is also a serious concern, and several studies have explored their detrimental effects. Clark and Fey (2020) described how incivility experienced by students can trigger fear and humiliation; impair clinical judgment; reduce psychological safety; and increase cognitive load, making students less likely to speak up when a practice error or patient safety issue occurs. The authors concluded that whether uncivil acts are instigated by faculty, peers, or nurses in practice, the detrimental impact of incivility can start a cascade of deleterious events leading to impaired learning and delivery of unsafe patient care. In a national study designed to examine nursing faculty's and academic nurse leaders' perceptions of incivility in nursing education programs, half (50.5%) of 1,074 respondents representing a broad range of nursing education programs in the United States reported incivility as a moderate to serious problem (Clark et al., 2021). Most (85%) stated they avoided dealing with incivility for a number of reasons including fear of retaliation, lack of supervisor or administrator support, or the belief that addressing incivility "makes matters worse." Top contributors to academic incivility included stress, unclear roles and expectations, and demanding workloads.

New graduate nurses are particularly vulnerable to incivility and its effects. Kerber et al. (2015) found that new graduate nurses who observed incivility reported negative effects on their emotional, professional, and physical well-being, and described how uncivil acts in the patient care environment negatively affected patient safety. Laschinger and Read (2016) found that new graduate nurses who experienced incivility also reported lower career satisfaction and greater intent to leave.

Bullying

There is no universally accepted definition for workplace bullying. Terms that may be used interchangeably with bullying are "horizontal violence" and "lateral violence" as well as "relational aggression." A key factor used in identifying bullying is the presence of a real or perceived power imbalance. That is, there is an ongoing misuse of power in workplace relationships, mainly experienced by the targeted person through repeated verbal, physical, and/or social behaviors. In most cases, the closer the power relationship, the greater the effect on the targeted person.

The ANA identifies bullying as a serious issue that threatens patient safety, nurse safety, and the nursing profession altogether (ANA, 2015a). According to the Workplace Bullying Institute (WBI, 2020), workplace bullying is repeated, health-harming mistreatment of a target or targets perpetrated by one or more offenders. The WBI describes workplace bullying is abusive, threatening, humiliating, or intimidating conduct that interferes with a productive work environment and behavior analogous to domestic violence at work. While definitions of bullying vary, most current definitions typically combine three components, including a negative *action* that is *repeated* resulting in *harm* (Hartin, 2020; Hartin et al., 2019).

Edmonson and Zelonka (2019) described nurse bullying as a systemic, pervasive problem that often continues throughout a nurse's career, causing a significant percentage of nurses to leave their first jobs due to the negative behaviors by colleagues. A nurse bullying culture contributes to an unhealthy work environment, increased risk to patients, lower patient satisfaction scores, and hospital nurse turnover costs averaging $4 million to $7 million a year.

Sauer and McCoy (2017) found a statistically significant association between workplace bullying against nurses and adverse patient outcomes. A higher incidence of nurse bullying was associated with lower physical and mental health scores among nurses, which negatively impacted their quality of life and ability to provide safe patient care. The authors noted that prolonged exposure to bullying at work may result in chronic stress levels that hinder nurses' capacity to fully focus on providing optimal patient care. Similar conclusions were drawn from an integrative review conducted to examine the relationship between patient safety and workplace bullying (Houck & Colbert, 2017). The authors found that workplace bullying is associated with negative nursing outcomes such as work dissatisfaction, turnover, and intent to leave. In the same review, several findings related to the impact of workplace bullying on patient safety were identified, including errors in treatment, medication administration, delayed care, and patient falls.

Cyberbullying has also become a major issue in nursing education and practice due to the prevalence of social media. De Gagne and team (2016) described various forms of cyber incivility occurring in nursing including disclosing clinical experiences with enough detail to potentially identify patients, posting pictures of patients on social networking sites, posting sexually provocative pictures of students, and photographs portraying intoxication from drugs and alcohol. Cyberbullying is particularly difficult to address since it often occurs anonymously. Targets may not even be aware of the uncivil postings or they may feel powerless to address the situation. Cyberbullying often creates an intensified and persistent level of anxiety due to the public nature of the internet and its ubiquitous and constant accessibility (Clark & Luparell, 2020). Bullying can be both face-to-face bullying and cyberbullying, for example, in spreading rumors about a nurse. Both forms of bullying can be just as damaging to the targeted person. Unfortunately, what makes cyberbullying different than face-to-face bullying is how intrusive and difficult it is to escape because a nurse can be targeted at any time whether at work or not, day or night. The cyberbully remains anonymous and targets the victim through social media, email, or text messages.

The language of cyberbullying has the possibility to minimize the seriousness of this behavior. For instance, "stalking" is a familiar term and generally understood, and may not be considered bullying. However, in cyberbullying, the same stalking behavior is called "trolling," which has the potential to minimize the seriousness of this behavior. Despite language differences, cyberbullying and face-to-face bullying both can have tragic outcomes.

Mobbing

Leymann (1990) is credited with coining the term workplace mobbing, describing the phenomenon as a form of adult bullying characterized by an employee or a group of employees ganging up on a target employee and subjecting them to psychological harassment, often resulting in severe personal and occupational consequences. Mobbing occurs for various reasons but is often used as an attempt to maintain individual or group control and compliance. According to Bulut (2020), workplace mobbing often occurs due to jealousy or a sense of inadequacy whereby groups or cliques of people will form to hide their insecurities and protect their own self-interests, causing entrenched separations between employees working in an organization.

Discussion Point

Do you agree with Bulut (2020) that workplace mobbing occurs out of jealousy and a sense of inadequacy? If not, why? If so, provide an example.

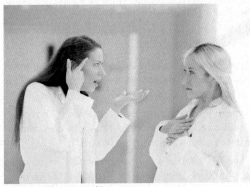

(pathdoc/Shutterstock)

Workplace bullying and other forms of workplace aggression may begin with behaviors that the target may not even know are occurring. Bullies can gossip, spread rumors, or even blame a person without that person's knowledge. This bullying behavior, which starts covertly, may progress to overt bullying but rarely in front of other people. Only in extreme or obvious cases do bullies, who are generally insecure, show their true selves. A bully, for example, may begin by teasing a person, and if the person complains, a bully's response is commonly, "I was only joking." This behavior may escalate over time, however, and eventually the targeted person may withdraw or resign. If they stay, they may develop chronic stress and/or mental health issues.

Incivility and bullying behaviors are reported as a cause for burnout in nursing and job dissatisfaction (Shi et al., 2018). This implies that a specific inappropriate behavior (incivility) may occur in parallel with another inappropriate behavior (bullying). It may also imply that one person's inappropriate behavior (incivility) leads to another person retaliating with inappropriate workplace behavior (bullying).

However, what makes bullying stand out from the other types of inappropriate behaviors in the workplace is the emphasis on the length of time this behavior occurs. Bullying behavior is persistent and repeated over an extended period of time. It is the repetitive nature of bullying that "some sort of vicious circle of events may exist where bullying leads to mental health problems, which may act to worsen the situation for the target or at least worsen the perception the targets make of their work situation" (Einarsen & Nielsen, 2015, p. 133; Nielsen et al., 2016). Studies reveal the connection between bullying and mental distress and medical illness. Social and supervisor support can play a protective role in reducing the negative impact of workplace bullying on health and work ability (Nielsen et al., 2020).

Discussion Point

Is it possible for a person to be bullied once and suffer long-term physical and/or psychological harm? By a group whose deliberate intent is to have the targeted person dismissed? By social media in the workplace? If you answered yes to any of these, consider how this behavior could be prevented.

Stress

According to the American Psychological Association (APA, 2021), stress is a normal reaction to everyday pressures but can become unhealthy when it disrupts an individual's ability to function. All individuals experience stress as a normal part of daily life; however, a stress reaction occurs when perceived demands (stressors) exceed resources or coping mechanisms to meet those demands. Stress can be caused by physical, emotional, environmental, or mental changes that exceed one's ability to effectively cope. Recently, stress related to the COVID-19 pandemic has contributed to disrupting the economy, work and academic settings, relationships, and health care (APA, 2020).

The APA's *Stress in America Report* (2020) revealed that Americans have been profoundly affected by the COVID-19 pandemic, noting that the unusual combination of previously reported stressors such as health care, mass shootings, and climate change along with the persistent pandemic crisis led the APA to assert that Americans are facing a national mental health crisis that could result in serious health and social consequences for years to come. Consequences of the COVID-19 pandemic have caused immense stress and trauma for those who lost loved ones to the disease, those infected and facing long recoveries, and for all Americans who experienced job loss, financial challenges, and uncertain futures. Of survey respondents, 78% say the pandemic is a significant source of stress in their life, nearly half (49%) report their behavior has been negatively affected, and 71% say that the pandemic has caused the lowest point in the nation's history that they can remember.

While nurses have always experienced varying levels of workplace stress, the COVID-19 pandemic has significantly heightened stress levels. The prevalence and novelty of the virus along with its highly infectious nature and associated morbidity and mortality rates place significant demands on nurses and health care professionals worldwide. The nature of the care itself coupled with an increase in the volume and intensity of their work while implementing new protocols create a stressful work environment. Dealing with staff and personal protective equipment (PPE) shortages; navigating an unfamiliar system of care; experiencing psychological conflicts between the responsibility to care for patients and their own right to protect themselves from a potentially lethal virus increase the potential for moral distress and injury, fatigue, and chronic stress levels among nurses (Maben & Bridges, 2020). Given the enormity and widespread effects of COVID-19 and other associated stressors on nurses' mental health, there is a need for a multilayered approach to help nurses prioritize their own health and wellness needs as much as possible, to provide peer support as nurses look after one another, and to develop intentional systematic organizational responses.

Discussion Point

- How has the COVID-19 pandemic affected your stress levels? Provide examples.
- Have you experienced pandemic-related stress in the health care environment?
- How has pandemic-related stress affected your nursing practice?
- How has the pandemic affected your relationship with patients, families, and colleagues?
- What other factors affect your stress level?

VIOLENCE IN NURSING

Over the years, violence in nursing has been a difficult concept to grasp, in part because of people's misunderstanding of what the term "violence" implies as well as the language used to describe this behavior. The confusion derives from a reluctance to expand the meaning of violence to being more than a physical act; it could also be the erroneous perception that such things do not happen to nurses. When people consider violence, they may ignore nonphysical types, such as emotional, financial, and psychological violence against many people who are abused.

Another reason violence in nursing is often misunderstood is the lack of an agreed-upon definition. The terms "horizontal violence," "lateral violence," "bullying," and "mobbing" are used interchangeably when discussing violence in nursing. Although these terms have slightly different connotations depending on context, they all cause harm to another person.

The National Institute for Occupational Safety and Health (NIOSH) (CDC, 2020) defines workplace violence as:

> the act or threat of violence, ranging from verbal abuse to physical assaults directed toward persons at work or on duty. The impact of workplace violence can range from psychological issues to physical injury, or even death. Violence can occur in any workplace and among any type of worker, but the risk for fatal violence is greater for workers in sales, protective services, and transportation, while the risk for nonfatal violence resulting in days away from work is greatest for healthcare and social assistance workers.

According to NIOSH, acts of workplace violence include direct physical assaults (with or without weapons), written or verbal threats, physical or verbal harassment, and homicide. NIOSH has identified four types of workplace violence in health care:

- Type I: Involves "criminal intent": in this type of workplace violence, "individuals with criminal intent have no relationship to the business or its employees."
- Type II: Involves a customer or patient; in this type, an "individual has a relationship with the business and becomes violent while receiving services."
- Type III: Involves a "worker-on-worker" relationship and includes "employees who attack or threaten another employee."
- Type IV: Involves personal relationships; it includes "individuals who have interpersonal relationships with the intended target but no relationship to the business."

Violence from patients or visitors toward nurses (type II) is the most common type; however, many nurses do not report these attacks due to various factors, including a belief that reporting does not effect change; reporting systems that may be too complex or time-consuming for nurses who have many competing demands; nurses excusing violent behavior because their patients are ill; or believing it is part of the job. It is important to understand that violence is not part of a nurse's job and reporting is essential to ending violence against nurses and other health care workers (Benyon, 2019).

The Occupational Safety and Health Act (1970) states that employers have a legal, ethical, and human rights responsibility to provide a safe work environment and HWE, free from discrimination. The organization has a duty of care to all their employees, and "all employers must comply with the safety and health standards issued and enforced pursuant to the OSH Act 1970." In addition, the general duty clause, Section 5(a)(1), "requires employers to provide their workers with a workplace free from recognized hazards that are causing or likely to cause death or serious physical harm." In reference to discrimination, Section 11(c)(1) of the act provides:

No person shall discharge or in any manner discriminate against any employee because such employee has filed any complaint or instituted or caused to be instituted any proceeding under or related to this Act or has testified or is about to testify in any such proceeding or because of the exercise by such employee on behalf of himself or others of any right afforded by this Act.

Reprisal or discrimination against an employee for reporting an incident or injury related to workplace violence is a violation of this legislation. In addition, it prohibits discrimination against an employee for reporting a work-related fatality, injury, or illness. Although it is expected that management would know and be responsible for meeting the requirements of the Occupational Safety and Health Act, all nurses should also be aware of their personal legal responsibility. It is important for all staff to be aware of current workplace risks and hazards. The California Division of Occupational Safety and Health (Cal/OSHA) and NIOSH have identified risk factors that may contribute to violence in the workplace (U.S. Department of Labor, Occupational Safety and Health Administration, 2016, pp. 31–32).

The Canadian Centre for Occupational Health and Safety (CCOHS, 2020) defines workplace violence as any act in which a person is abused, threatened, intimidated, or assaulted in their workplace. These acts may include rumors, swearing, verbal abuse, pranks, arguments, property damage, vandalism, sabotage, pushing, theft, physical assaults, psychological trauma, anger-related incidents, rape, arson, and murder (para. 1).

Discussion Point

Identify your state legislation and regulations aimed at protecting nurses from workplace violence. Does it specifically cover nurses working alone in rural and remote areas? If not, what could you do as an individual or as a member of a professional association to raise awareness to have legislation passed to protect them?

In addition to the lack of a unified definition in describing workplace violence, there is often a lack of agreement on which acts constitute workplace violence. Acts that one person considers a harmful experience may not be every person's experience with or perception of violence. But that does not mean perceiving an act of violence is unique to that person. Additionally, the types of violence that nurses experience are diverse and complex, only adding to the difficulty in addressing this issue. Nevertheless, it is possible to categorize the types of violence nurses and nursing students may experience (Box 13.1).

Although the true extent of violence in nursing is considered greater than the statistics indicate, studies show that violence against nurses who identify as female is greater than that against nurses who identify as male. Compared with the experiences of female nurses, there is a dearth of research into male nurses and their experiences. Studies into violence against men in other contexts tend to focus on rites of initiation of apprentices, college fraternity rites of passage (hazing), and debasing and humiliating initiation practices in the armed services. However, the question of whether violence against male nurses is like violence against female nurses is open to further research. Because the statistics show that men are often the major perpetrators of violence in society and in the workplace (except possibly for internal violence in nursing, that which comes from within the organization), the fear that some male nurses may experience violence could also create more violent incidents in the workplace, generating a recurring cycle of violence.

Boxes 13.2 and 13.3 expand upon the nonphysical and physical aspects of violence in nursing. Box 13.4 lists the potential factors leading to patient–nurse violence, and Box 13.5 suggests variables that may be predictive of patient–nurse violence.

In addition, nurses working in different locations and settings have different issues to address compared to those working in large metropolitan hospital settings. For example, nurses working in home care, rural and remote nursing, or nurses working alone or on night duty must consider the context in which they are working to determine how best to protect themselves (Box 13.6).

BOX 13.1   Types of Violence in Nursing

1. Nurse-to-nurse violence (includes nursing students; horizontal violence, lateral violence)
2. Patient-to-nurse violence (including visitors)
3. Organization-to-nurse violence (vertical downward violence)
4. External perpetrators (strangers, criminal intent)
5. Third-party violence (other health professionals/family members and significant others as well as other health care workers)
6. Impact of mass trauma or natural disasters on nurses (e.g., terrorism, wars, natural disasters)
7. Nurse-to-patient violence
8. Personal violence (e.g., intimate partner violence, family violence, interpersonal violence)

BOX 13.2   Types of Nonviolence Involving Nurses

- Being uncivil, such as exhibiting rudeness, impoliteness, and/or silence
- Condoning inappropriate behavior by being uncooperative or unsupportive
- Social isolation/social exclusion
- Setting someone up for failure, imposing ideas, taking someone's ideas, undermining, embarrassing someone
- Controlling communication—purposefully neglecting to tell someone about a meeting
- Increasing unreasonable workloads and timelines
- Exhibiting threatening behavior—making someone feel intimidated, threatened, or fearful
- Spreading rumors, improperly taking credit, assigning blame or fault
- Stalking
- Defaming
- Cyberbullying

BOX 13.3   Types of Violence Involving Nurses (Predominantly by Patients, Families, and Visitors)

Nonphysical
Verbal
- Swearing
- Yelling
- Shouting
- Making threats
- Calling names

Nonverbal
- Invading personal space
- Threatening gestures
- Constant eye contact
- Facial expressions such as scowling or frowning

Physical
- Hitting, punching, pinching, kicking, scratching, and spitting
- Contact devices such as walking sticks, knives, baseball bats, guns, chemical sprays
- Sexual assaults and rape
- Assault
- Homicide

BOX 13.4   Potential Factors Leading to Patient–Nurse Violence

* Patient in a vulnerable mental state
* Feeling out of control and neglected because of lack of information
* Fear and apprehension
* Lack of assurance from staff
* Lack of privacy
* Negative attitude of staff toward patients
* Limited time to communicate
* Perception that the nurse's approach is aggressive
* Nurses' need to act in controlling ways due to institutional pressures

BOX 13.5   Predicting Patient–Nurse Violence

Does the patient
* indicate a heightened level of anxiety or depression?
* have hostile or aggressive body language?
* continually move around (agitation)?
* have a repetitive speech pattern (I want to go home, I want to go home)?
* complain about the provision of services?
* refuse to cooperate?
* display suicidal tendencies or cries for help?
* have rapid breathing, have clenched fists/teeth, appear restless, or talk loudly?
* swear excessively or use sexually explicit language?
* make verbal threats?
* show noncompliance with requests?

BOX 13.6   Self-Protective Behaviors

* Have an alarm or monitoring system that requires periodic checking in.
* Have a GPS location system turned on at all times on your cell phone or transport.
* Policies, procedures, and training should reflect the nurse's work location.
* Whether working in a group or individually, it is important the nurse is aware of their organization's emergency responses in case of public threats such as terrorist attacks.
* There are some aspects of a policy that would be the same across work settings. For example, it is important to stay calm and not panic; if unable to remove oneself from a potentially dangerous situation, attempt to defuse the situation.
* There may be some aspects that are unique to some work settings. For example, a home or community nurse might need to leave the home as quickly as possible by saying they need to get something for the patient from the car.
* When working alone, have the emergency numbers entered on cell phone speed dial.

Also, a violent person can take their aggression out by using any object near at hand. As well as those outlined in Box 13.3, Box 13.7 includes objects that may be used as potential weapons or cause property damage with violence.

The organizational actions to achieve HWEs include having workplace policies, procedures, and programs that prevent and eliminate workplace violence. For example, achieving a HWE may require constant vigilance against workplace antisocial activities, such as incivility and bullying, as well as awareness of health issues, such as stress and mental health. These measures are above and beyond institutional OSHA requirements.

BOX 13.7   Potential Weapons

- Furniture, such as chairs, tables
- Syringes, sprays, dangerous liquids, gas/oxygen, fire extinguishers
- Equipment in treatment rooms, scissors, scalpels, chemicals
- Equipment that is sharp or blunt
- Telephone, computers, monitors
- Equipment used by patients—walking sticks, walking frames, cutlery, broken glassware, urinals, bedpans
- Guns

Discussion Point

Is there a relationship between nurse-to-nurse violence and patient-to-nurse violence and their environments? Are nursing students more vulnerable to violence in nursing than other nursing staff? What evidence do you have to support your responses?

The high price some nurses have paid for workplace violence over many years is reflected in suicide statistics. Davidson and colleagues (2020) conducted a longitudinal analysis on nurse suicide in the United States and found that nurses of all genders are at a higher risk for suicide than the general U.S. population. The authors also found that nurses who identify as female complete suicide more often with pharmacologic poisoning while those identifying as male do so most commonly with firearms; however, the use of firearms as a method of suicide among female nurses has risen in recent years. Nurse suicide was associated with the presence of known job problems, suggesting that workplace wellness programs focused on reducing stress may improve the problem.

The American Association of Colleges of Nursing (AACN, 2020) released a *Call to Action for Academic Nurse Leaders to Promote Practices to Enhance Optimal Well-being, Resilience, and Suicide Prevention in U.S. Schools of Nursing*. AACN reported that nurses are nearly three times more stressed than the overall American public, and nurse suicide rates are higher than the general population. Workplace stress and burnout (in part, due to the COVID-19 pandemic) are at an high and pose significant health concerns. The need for fostering civility and healthy work and learning environments has never been greater.

CREATING HEALTHY WORK ENVIRONMENTS

The APA Center for Organizational Excellence (n.d.) defines a psychologically healthy workplace as a work environment that fosters employee health and well-being while enhancing organizational performance and productivity. This may be grouped into five categories, including employee involvement; work–life balance; employee growth and development; health and safety; and employee's recognition. Similarly, the AACN (2016) identified six standards for establishing and sustaining HWEs, including skilled communication; true collaboration; effective decision making; appropriate staffing; meaningful recognition; and authentic leadership. AACN's six essential standards provide evidence-based guidelines for success. According to the AACN, HWEs integrate all six standards to help produce effective and sustainable outcomes for both patients and nurses. Harmon and team (2018) recommended that schools of nursing adopt the six AACN HWE standards as well as incorporating a seventh standard of self-care since stress can impede an individual's ability to function well.

The NLN (2018b) updated the Healthful Work Environment Toolkit for academic nursing programs and identified seven key elements of a HWE including establishing safe, civil, and collegial environments; salary; benefits; workload; role development and mentorship; scholarship; and leadership. This framework provides useful resources to improve the health of academic work environments.

Organizations that invest in creating and sustaining HWEs reap the benefits of improved work quality and productivity, lower absenteeism and turnover, improved patient satisfaction and employee engagement, and a better ability to attract and retain top-quality employees. Employees in HWEs enjoy greater job satisfaction, higher morale, better physical and mental health, enhanced motivation, and heightened ability to manage stress (APA, n.d.). Therefore, creating and sustaining a HWE is an imperative for all organizations; however, in nursing and health care, a HWE is also a requisite for safe patient care.

Organizational actions to achieve a HWE include having policies, procedures, and programs in place to foster civility and implementing preventative measures to promote physical and mental health and personal and professional well-being.

Fostering Civility

Fostering civility is an integral part of a positive and productive workplace. An integrative review of nurse-to-nurse incivility, hostility, and workplace violence conducted by Crawford and colleagues (2019) found that a safe and just organizational culture requires a comprehensive, evidence-based, systems-level approach to create civil work environments to ensure optimal patient outcomes and staff relationships.

To maintain or achieve a culture of civility requires strong leadership at all levels of the organization. Executive leaders, nurse managers, academic educators, and students can collaborate to set the tone for civility and an environment that promotes interprofessional teamwork and a consistent, respectful response to uncivil behaviors. All members of the organization must address any form of incivility and lead by example. Organizational change begins with effective leadership and raising awareness about the various ways and degrees incivility and other workplace aggressions are manifested. It requires holding each individual responsible and accountable for ensuring civility throughout the organization. It is important that all members of the organization know the appropriate workplace policies and act accordingly. For example, all staff should be aware that speaking rudely or disrespectfully to a team member or patient is unacceptable behavior. If these behaviors occur, appropriate intervention should be initiated, and if this approach is unsuccessful, then disciplinary action should follow. It is important to remember that it is a nurse's human right to work in a safe and healthy environment.

To build a HWE, leaders and managers may need to address a system-wide cultural change to prevent and address incivility, bullying, and other disruptive behaviors to avoid resultant physical and mental health issues. However, a total work culture change may be too much to achieve at one time. Therefore, another approach may be to plan to use one department or unit that has a successful culture of civility as a model for a HWE. This approach may be less threatening, more manageable, and may achieve more success in implementation and evaluation.

Establishing a Zero-Tolerance Culture

Organizations are called upon to develop zero-tolerance policies for incivility and other forms of workplace aggression. In recent years, there has been a plethora of literature and conference presentations promoting various strategies to address workplace bullying, including implementing zero tolerance for bullying behavior in the workplace (ANA, 2015a; Caristo & Clements, 2019; Crawford et al., 2019). There is also growing awareness about the importance of

speaking out about being bullied. Clark (2020) outlined ways to become an upstander, one who responds and speaks up when bullying behavior or acts of mistreatment or intimidation occur. An upstander takes action to help support someone who is being harmed or harassed. Upstanding does not come easily since some individuals express concern that calling attention to the situation or speaking up may result in retaliation or reprisal or potentially make matters worse. Evidence suggests that when witnesses take safe and effective action to support the target, there is a greater possibility that the behavior will stop. However, without organizational support, nurses may stay silent as a self-protective measure. In organizations where a positive work culture is fostered and reinforced and where upstanding behavior is rewarded, nurses are more empowered to speak up and more likely to intervene when confronted with a bullying situation. Nurse leaders and managers must model the way and set the tone for a HWE and create a safe setting for nurses to speak up. See Research Fuels the Controversy 13.1.

> ### Discussion Point
>
> What are the advantages and disadvantages of a zero-tolerance policy when addressing incivility and bullying in the organization where you work?

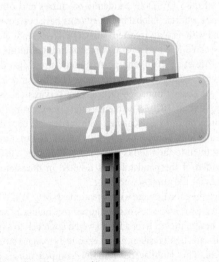

(alexmillos/Shutterstock)

Promoting Stress-Free Work Environments

Organizations should aim to have a healthy, stress-free work environment, or at least to minimize stressors since it may not always be possible to eliminate them completely in health care. Hospitals and other complex health care

Research Fuels the Controversy 13.1

Caring for the Caregiver During COVID-19 Outbreak: Does Inclusive Leadership Improve Psychological Safety and Curb Psychological Distress? A Cross-Sectional Study

This cross-sectional study focused on the relationship between inclusive leadership and nurses' psychological safety and distress.

Source: Zhao, F., Ahmed, F., & Faraz, N. A. (2020). Caring for the caregiver during COVID-19 outbreak: Does inclusive leadership improve psychological safety and curb psychological distress? A cross-sectional study. *International Journal of Nursing Studies, 110.* https://doi. org/10.1016/j.ijnurstu.2020.103725

Study Findings

This cross-sectional study examined the influence of an inclusive leadership style on psychological distress while assessing the mediating role of psychological safety. The researchers recruited 451 on-duty registered nurses from five hospitals providing patient care during a highly infectious phase of COVID-19 in January 2020 in Wuhan, the epicenter at the time of the virus outbreak in China. Results revealed that inclusive leadership had an inverse relationship with psychological distress. Psychological safety mediated the relationship between inclusive leadership and psychological distress. The authors concluded that recurring or prolonged experiences of stress and anxiety at the workplace without a mechanism to counter such effects can culminate into psychological distress. Inclusive leadership style can serve as such a mechanism to curb psychological distress for health care workers by creating a psychologically safe environment.

organizations are by nature perceived as stressful, and the impact of the COVID-19 pandemic has been devastating for individuals, teams, and organizations in health care.

Several studies across the world have examined the impact of the COVID-19 pandemic on nurses and other health care workers. Global health systems have been overwhelmed with patients infected with COVID-19, leading to great psychological pressure on nurses, at times resulting in suicide (Mo et al., 2020) and posttraumatic stress disorder (Wang et al., 2020). The pressures caused by the pandemic have most acutely impacted critical care services (Nayna Schwerdtle et al., 2020). The mental stress of exposure to a highly infectious disease coupled with inadequate supplies of PPE and long hours took a serious toll on nurses, often pushing them to their limits (Rahman & Plummer, 2020). The burden of the pandemic has resulted in devastating outcomes for the nursing workforce.

Given the enormity and widespread effects of COVID-19 and other associated stressors on nurses' psychological and mental health, the need for a multilayered approach to support self-care, build resilience, and effectively manage stress is evident. This multilayered response compels nurses to prioritize their own health and wellness needs as much as possible, provide and accept support from teammates and managers, and establish an intentional systematic organizational response to promote personal and professional wellbeing (Clark, 2020; Maben & Bridges, 2020).

After attempting different stress management strategies, a person may continue to feel stressed. Left untreated, this

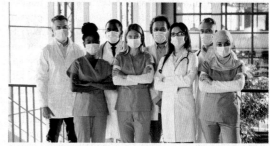

(M_Agency/Shutterstock)

may lead to chronic stress or mental health problems. If the cause of the stress is unresolved, outside professional help may be required. Most organizations have an employee assistance program to offer counseling services and support. The ANA (2021), Sigma Theta Tau International (2021), and the American Holistic Nurses Association (AHNA, 2021) are three of many nursing organizations that provide free and easily accessible resources to build resilience and mental health capacity.

Discussion Point

How would you describe the style of leadership in your department, unit, or nursing program? Do you believe leadership style plays an important role in reducing stress in academic and health care settings?

EVIDENCE-BASED PATHWAY FOR FOSTERING ORGANIZATIONAL CIVILITY

Organizational change requires diligence, commitment, and effective leadership at all levels since incremental changes are generally inadequate to transform a culture. While there is no one-size-fits-all approach for transforming a culture, several essential components can be implemented to increase the potential for doing so. Any model used to foster a HWE must be considered within the context of the organization's unique culture and must be nimble and flexible enough to use in a variety of work environments. The PFOC (Clark, 2017, 2019) is an evidence-based framework to create a HWE. This comprehensive and dynamic approach to workplace improvement provides a systematic step-by-step process to promote a culture of civility and workplace health.

Step 1: Raise Awareness and Enlist Leadership Support

The first step of the PFOC is to raise awareness about the positive impact of civility and educate all members of the organization on the harmful effects of incivility, bullying, and other workplace aggressions as well as to enlist leadership support to implement a system-wide, evidence-based action plan to foster a HWE. Because transformational and sustained change requires broad-based collaboration, individuals need the support from leaders to provide the necessary resources to support the change. Raising awareness about the types and frequency of uncivil behaviors and their harmful effects can be powerful motivators to transform an organization's culture and enlist leadership support. Sharing stories and experiences with incivility and civility is an effective tactic to raise awareness and engage leaders in making a commitment to a culture of respect and dignity (Sokol-Hessner et al., 2018). Enlisting leadership support is essential, not just because they have access to necessary resources but also because they have a vested interest in the organization and frequently possess a broader view of workplace issues. Their knowledge of the workplace and experience with previous and current incivility issues provide insight into possible solutions (Clark, 2019).

Step 2: Assemble and Empower a Civility Team: Seek Broad-Based Support

Note: Steps 2 and 3 can be reversed depending on whether an organizational cultural assessment has already been conducted.

If an assessment has been conducted, installing a civility team can be extremely helpful in moving the civility initiative forward. Results of the assessment(s) provide objective information about the scope of the problem, strengths of the organization, and direction for positive change. The main purpose of the civility team is to lead the transition to a more civil HWE. The team consists of employees who are trusted, committed, and empowered to measure the problem, develop a compelling vision of the organization's future, and carry out the steps of the PFOC. Members of the civility team enlist broad-based support by engaging people at all levels of the organization, communicating the civility mission, and encouraging all members of the organization to participate in the civility initiative. By gaining broad-based support, the civility initiative is more likely to succeed.

Step 3: Assess Organizational Civility at All Levels

A thorough assessment of the organizational culture can yield meaningful information to develop and implement a system-wide, data-driven action plan. Data obtained from the organizational cultural assessment can be used to inform the civility initiative, including development and implementation of strategies, policies, and procedures. Helpful information may also be gathered from formal and informal reports, satisfaction surveys, interviews, focus groups, and open forums. External researchers may be helpful in collecting, analyzing, and reporting the assessment findings, thus establishing a report less likely to be biased.

Step 4: Develop a Data-Driven Action Plan

During this step, the assessment information obtained from Step 3 is synthesized and translated into an evidence-based, data-driven action plan that will be implemented in Step 5. Findings from the assessment are reviewed to identify areas of strength and excellence and to determine specific strategies to improve areas of concern. Each strategy should include clear objectives, expected timelines, and necessary resources (financial, human, time, and organizational) to implement and evaluate the strategies. Establishing policies and procedures to foster workplace civility and a HWE should be included in the action plan.

Step 5: Implement the Data-Driven Action Plan

Step 5 involves implementing evidence-based strategies to foster and sustain a HWE. Key strategies include cocreating and implementing a civility charter with clear norms and ground rules; improving communication skills; developing a conflict-capable workforce; and enhancing teamwork and collaboration. Honing communication and conflict negotiation skills is needed to effectively address incivility in a variety of situations to promote teamwork and protect patient safety. Using staff meeting time, simulation space, and addressing incivility in "real time" will help nurses learn about and practice effective ways of dealing with uncivil encounters, thus increasing the likelihood of success in stopping these behaviors.

Step 6: Evaluation and Reassessment

The PFOC is a cyclical process that includes assessing, planning, educating, strategizing, evaluating, and reassessing. As part of the PFOC cycle, evaluation and reassessment do not complete the pathway, but are necessary steps to review the effectiveness of the change process to foster organizational civility and health. Information gleaned from periodic readministration of the cultural assessment methods can be used to measure progress, goal achievement, and effectiveness of civility interventions. Ongoing assessment data can also be used to make recommendations for continuing the current measures and/or implementing revisions to the PFOC action plan.

Step 8: Expand the Civility Initiative: Sharing Knowledge, Lessons, and Experience

To expand the civility initiative and to sustain organizational transformation, some members of the civility team may remain on the team, while new members may rotate onto the team to continue facilitating the change process and implementing the PFOC initiative. This transition phase may include discussing individual, team, and organizational accomplishments, reviewing progression and assessment of the civility plan, and sharing lessons learned. Policies may be developed and implemented to anchor changes into the organizational culture.

Step 8: Reward Civility and Consolidate Successes

Recognizing and celebrating individual and team accomplishments stimulate enthusiasm and momentum for change. Honoring and rewarding successes, achievements, and accomplishments heightens morale and builds team spirit. Evidence of success includes achieving long- and short-term goals, enjoying increased job satisfaction, improving communication and conflict negotiation skills, giving and receiving meaningful recognition, and increased community visibility and recognition. Celebrations can be formal or informal; the goal is to honor and celebrate successes and acknowledge examples of civility and workplace health.

WHY IS CREATING HEALTHY WORK ENVIRONMENTS SO DIFFICULT IN NURSING?

Not only should we ask the question: "Why is creating a healthy work environment so difficult in nursing?" but also ask: "Why has it taken so long?" According to The Joint Commission (TJC, 2018), only 30% of nurses report incidents of workplace violence. This underreporting is due in part to thinking that violence is "part of the job." Clearly, violence is never part of the job; therefore, this mistaken belief reinforces the need for all health care and academic leaders to foster cultures of safety and respect.

It has been over 30 years since Meissner (1986, p. 52) wrote about the destructive treatment experienced by new nursing students from educators and nursing administrators. However, after a slow acceptance in the 1990s that violence in nursing was occurring, research has evolved rapidly. Until recently, research has focused on the nature and extent of the various forms of workplace violence. This was and remains important work. We now have a good understanding of the nature of violence in nursing and that it is not rare or confined to a single setting but rather experienced by nurses in a wide variety of geographical locations and service areas. Research has shown that nurses can be targeted by other nurses or by other health professionals, patients, visitors, or strangers.

However, as TJC reports (2018), there are difficulties both in gaining accurate statistics on workplace violence and putting streamlined reporting mechanisms in place. Crawford and colleagues (2019) identified various factors contributing to workplace incivility and bullying including ineffective leadership, lack of interpersonal and management skills, avoiding responsibility for staff skill development, tolerating uncivil behavior, and lack of role modeling on ways to effectively prevent and address workplace aggressions. These barriers and others may be removed by hiring and retaining authentic and effective leaders, creating structural empowerment and psychological safety, developing systems to recognize and reward positive behavior, addressing and correcting inappropriate behavior using established guidelines and processes, and reinforcing education regarding expected professional behaviors.

Discussion Point

How could a nurse provide support and understanding to a colleague who has confided that they are being bullied?

The difficulties encountered when attempting to minimize disruptive workplace behaviors are not unique to nursing. Therefore, nurses could learn from other disciplines and organizations that have been successful in their methods of improving their work environment.

Discussion Point

Why is creating HWEs so difficult in nursing? Do nurses want to see change? Are nurses ready for change? Do nurses have the capacity to change? Are nurses ready to unify to protest against workplace violence and bullying? Are nurses prepared to take on a leadership role during the change process?

CONCLUSIONS

There has been a growing interest in organizations working to create HWEs and foster civility. Many changes based on research have already been implemented to improve work environments. However, nurses' work environments do not remain static. Furthermore, current evidence continues to highlight the need for more research and better understanding of the complexity of both positive and negative workplace behaviors. Nevertheless, research is not the only answer. Education that enables nurses to build resilience and feel empowered is another strategy that requires consideration.

Over 30 years ago, Roberts (1983) wrote the seminal work on oppression in nursing. Since the mid-1980s, there has been a major movement by nurses through nursing research, scholarship, and personal experiences, to have a significant role in their ongoing cultural change. These changes have come about by determination and tenacity, which are the same characteristics that persist in nurses today. Nurses and nursing have benefited from these changes. Raising awareness of disruptive behaviors, the causes, and methods for addressing this phenomenon in the workplace has led nurses to be more insightful regarding workplace relationships. More importantly, these changes have come from within the profession, and in the future, nurses will need to continue to drive the change.

For Additional Discussion

1. What does a HWE and organizational culture of civility mean in nursing and health care?

2. What are the characteristics of a HWE?

3. The quality of the organizational culture can create or prevent harmful behavior. Do you agree with this statement, and if not, why not?

4. How does an unhealthy work environment affect patient care?

5. Can a workplace with a toxic culture still provide a high standard of health care?

6. Is it possible to have a HWE in nursing? If not, why not?

7. Can legislation address all disruptive behaviors such as incivility that lead to stressful situations in nurses' work environments?

8. In your opinion, which generally comes first—a stressful situation or incivility?

9. Is it possible for nurses to be immune to influences that affect a HWE?

10. Why might incivility in one department be less disruptive than in another department?

11. How has the COVID-19 pandemic affected the lives of nurses and other health care professionals? What measures might be taken to improve the level of physical and emotional wellness stemming from the pandemic?

References

American Association of Colleges of Nursing. (2020). *A call to action for academic nurse leaders to promote practices to enhance optimal well-being, resilience and suicide prevention in schools of nursing across the U.S.* Retrieved October 15, 2021, from https://www.aacnnursing.org/Portals/42/Downloads/Meetings/2020/ANLC/7-2020-Resolution-For-AACN-Nurse-Wellness-Suicide-Prevention.pdf

American Association of Critical-Care Nurses. (2016). *AACN standards for establishing and sustaining healthy work environments: A journey to excellence* (2nd ed.). Retrieved

October 15, 2021, from http://www.aacn.org/WD/HWE/Docs/HWEStandards.pdf

American Holistic Nurses Association. (2021). *Resources.* Retrieved October 15, 2021, from https://www.ahna.org/Resources

American Nurses Association. (2015a). *Position statement: Incivility, bullying, and workplace violence.* Retrieved October 15, 2021, from nursingworld.org/MainMenuCategories/WorkplaceSafety/Healthy-Nurse/bullyingworkplaceviolence/Incivility-Bullying-and-Workplace-Violence.html

American Nurses Association. (2015b). *Code of ethics for nurses with interpretive statements.* Author.

American Nurses Association. (2017). *Health risk appraisal (HRA) 2013–2016, executive summary.* Retrieved October 15, 2021, from https://www.nursingworld.org/~4aeeeb/globalassets/practiceandpolicy/work-environment/health—safety/ana-healthriskappraisalsummary_2013-2016.pdf

American Nurses Association. (2021). *COVID-19 resource center.* Retrieved October 15, 2021, from https://www.nursingworld.org/practice-policy/work-environment/health-safety/disaster-preparedness/coronavirus/

American Psychological Association. (2020). *Stress in America™ 2020: A National Mental Health Crisis.* Retrieved October 15, 2021, from https://www.apa.org/news/press/releases/stress/2020/report-october

American Psychological Association. (2021). *Stress relief is within reach.* Retrieved October 15, 2021, from https://www.apa.org/topics/stress

American Psychological Association Center for Organizational Excellence. (n.d.). *Creating a psychologically healthy workplace.* Retrieved October 15, 2021, from https://www.apaexcellence.org/resources/creatingahealthyworkplace/

Benyon, B. (2019, August 15). *Violence against nurses: A major issue in healthcare. Oncology Nursing News.* Retrieved October 15, 2021, from https://www.oncnursingnews.com/web-exclusives/violence-against-nurses-a-major-issue-in-healthcare

Bulut, S. (2020). The existing unbearable burden at the workplace: Mobbing. *Journal of Psychology and Clinical Psychiatry, 11*(3), 81–82. https://doi.org/10.15406/jpcpy.2020.11.00676

Canadian Centre for Occupational Health and Safety. (2020, November 20). *Violence and harassment in the workplace.* Retrieved October 15, 2021, from https://www.ccohs.ca/oshanswers/psychosocial/violence.html

Caristo, J., & Clements, P. T. (2019). Let's stop "eating our young." *Nursing Critical Care, 14*(4), 45–48. https://doi.org/10.1097/01.CCN.0000565040.65898.01

Centers for Disease Control and Prevention. (2020, September 22). *National Institute for Occupational Safety and Health (NIOSH). Occupational violence.* Retrieved October 15, 2021, from https://www.cdc.gov/niosh/topics/violence/default.html

Clark, C. M. (2017). *Creating and sustaining civility in nursing education* (2nd ed.). Sigma Theta Tau International Publishing.

Clark, C. M. (2019). Fostering a culture of civility and respect in nursing. *Journal of Nursing Regulation, 10*(1), 44–52. https://doi.org/10.1016/S2155-8256(19)30082-1

Clark, C. M. (2020). An 'upstanding' approach to address bullying in nursing. *American Nurse Journal, 15*(9), 31–34.

https://www.myamericannurse.com/an-upstanding-approach-to-address-bullying-in-nursing/

Clark, C. M., & Carnosso, J. (2008). Civility: A concept analysis. *Journal of Theory Construction and Testing, 12*(1), 11–15.

Clark, C. M., & Fey, M. K. (2020). Fostering civility in learning conversations: Introducing the PAAIL communication strategy. *Nurse Educator. 45*(3), 139–143. https://doi.org/10.1097/NNE.0000000000000731

Clark, C. M., & Luparell, S. (2020). Cyber-incivility, cyber-bullying, and other forms of online aggression: A call to action for nurse educators. *Nurse Education Today, 85.* https://doi.org/10.1016/j.nedt.2019.104310

Clark, C. M., Gorton, K., & Bentley, A. (in review). Civility: A concept analysis revisited. Nursing Outlook.

Clark, C. M., Landis, T., & Barbosa-Leiker, C. (2021). National study on faculty and administrators' perceptions of civility and incivility in nursing education. *Nurse Educator, 46*(5), 276–283. https://doi.org/10.1097/NNE.0000000000000948

Crawford, C. L., Chu, F., Judson, L. H., Cuenca, E., Jadalla, A. A., Tze-Polo, L., Kawar, L. N., Runnels, C., & Garvida, R., Jr. (2019). An integrative review of nurse-to-nurse incivility, hostility, and workplace violence: A GPS for nurse leaders. *Nursing Administration Quarterly, 43*(2), 138–156. https://doi.org/10.1097/NAQ.0000000000000338

Davidson, J. E., Proudfoot, J., Lee, K., Terterian, G., & Zisook, S. (2020). A longitudinal analysis of nurse suicide in the United States (2005–2016) with recommendations for action. *Worldviews on Evidence-Based Nursing, 17*, 6–15. https://doi.org/10.1111/wvn.12419

De Gagne, J. C., Choi, M., Ledbetter, L., Kang, H. S., & Clark, C. M. (2016). An integrative review of cybercivility in health professions education. *Nurse Educator, 41*(5), 239–245. https://doi.org/10.1097/NNE.0000000000000264

Edmonson, C., & Zelonka, C. (2019). Our own worst enemies: The nurse bullying epidemic. *Nursing Administration Quarterly, 43*(3), 274–279. https://doi.org/10.1097/NAQ.0000000000000353

Einarsen, S., & Nielsen, M. B. (2015, February). Workplace bullying as an antecedent of mental health problems: A five-year prospective and representative study. *International Archives of Occupational and Environmental Health, 88*(2), 131–142. https://doi.org/10.1007/s00420-014-0944-7

Harmon, R. B., DeGennaro, G., Norling, M., Kennedy, C., & Fontaine, D. (2018). Implementing healthy work environment standards in an academic workplace: An update. *Journal of Professional Nursing, 34*(1), 20–24. https://doi.org/10.1016/j.profnurs.2017.06.001

Hartin, P. (2020). Bullying in nursing: How has it changed over 4 decades? *Journal of Nursing Management, 28*(7), 1619. https://doi.org/10.1111/jonm.13117

Hartin, P., Birks, M., & Lindsay, D. (2019). Bullying in nursing: Is it in the eye of the beholder? *Policy, Politics, & Nursing Practice, 20*(2), 82–91. https://doi.org/10.1177/1527154419845411

Houck, N. M., & Colbert, A. M. (2017). Patient safety and workplace bullying: An integrative review. *Journal of Nursing Care Quality, 32*(2), 164–171. https://doi.org/10.1097/NCQ.000000000000020

International Council of Nurses. (2012). *ICN code of ethics for nurses.* Retrieved October 15, 2021, from https://www.icn.ch/sites/default/files/inline-files/2012_ICN_Codeofethicsfornurses_%20eng.pdf

International Council of Nurses. (2017). *Position statement: Prevention and management of workplace violence.* Retrieved October 15, 2021, from https://www.icn.ch/sites/default/files/inline-files/ICN_PS_Prevention_and_management_of_workplace_violence.pdf

Kerber, C., Woith, W. M., Jenkins, S. H., & Astroth, K. S. (2015). Perception of new nurses concerning incivility in the workplace. *Journal of Continuing Education, 46*(11), 522–527. https://doi.org/10.3928/00220124-20151020-05

Laschinger, H. K., & Read, E. A. (2016). The effect of authentic leadership, person-job fit, and civility norms on new graduate nurses' experiences of coworker incivility and burnout. *Journal of Nursing Administration, 46*(11), 574–580. https://doi.org/10.1097/NNA.0000000000000407

Leymann, H. (1990). Mobbing and psychological terror at workplaces. *Violence and Victims, 5*(2), 119–126. https://doi.org/10.1891/0886-6708.5.2.119

Maben, J., & Bridges, J. (2020). Covid-19: Supporting nurses' psychological and mental health. *Journal of Clinical Nursing, 29*(15–16), 2742–2750. https://doi.org/10.1111/jocn.15307

Meissner, J. E. (1986, March). Nurses: Are we eating our young? *Nursing, 16*(3), 51–53. https://doi.org/10.1097/00152193-198603000-00014

Mo, Y., Deng, L., & Zhang, L., Lang, Q., Liao, C., Wang, N., Qin, M., & Huang, H. (2020). Work stress among Chinese nurses to support Wuhan in fighting against COVID-19 epidemic. *Journal of Nursing Management, 28*(5), 1002–1009. https://doi.org/10.1111/jonm.13014

National League for Nursing. (2018a). Vision series: Creating community to build a civil and healthy academic work environment. Retrieved October 15, 2021, from http://www.nln.org/newsroom/nln-position-documents/nln-living-documents

National League for Nursing. (2018b). Healthful Work Environment Tool Kit©. Retrieved October 15, 2021, from http://www.nln.org/docs/default-source/professional-development-programs/healthful-work-environment-toolkit.pdf?sfvrsn=20

Nayna Schwerdtle, P., Connell, C. J., Lee, S., Plummer, V., Russo, P. L., Endacott, R., & Kuhn, L. (2020). Nurse expertise: A critical resource in the COVID-19 pandemic response. *Annals of Global Health, 86*(1), 49. https://doi.org/10.5334/aogh.2898

Nielsen, M. B., Christensen, J. O., Finne, L. B., & Stein, K. (2020). Workplace bullying, mental distress, and sickness absence: The protective role of social support. *International Archives of Occupational and Environmental Health, 93*(1), 43–53. https://doi.org/10.1007/s00420-019-01463-y

Nielsen, M. B., Indregard, A. M., & Overland, S. (2016). Workplace bullying and sickness absence—A systematic review and meta-analysis of the research literature. *Scandinavian Journal of Work, Environment, & Health, 42*(5), 359–370. https://doi.org/10.5271/sjweh.3579

Rahman, A., & Plummer, V. (2020). COVID-19 related suicide among hospital nurses; case study evidence from worldwide media reports. *Psychiatry Research, 291,* 113272. https://doi.org/10.1016/j.psychres.2020.113272

Rehder, K. J., Adair, K. C., Hadley, A., McKittrick, K., Frankel, A., Leonard, M., Frankel, T. C., & Sexton, J. B. (2020). Associations between a new disruptive behaviors scale and teamwork, patient safety, work-life balance, burnout, and depression. *Joint Commission Journal on Quality and Patient Safety, 46*(1), 18–26. https://doi.org/10.1016/j.jcjq.2019.09.004

Roberts, S. (1983). Oppressed group behavior: Implications for nursing. *Advances in Nursing Science, 5*(4), 21–30. https://doi.org/10.1097/00012272-198307000-00006

Sauer, P. A., & McCoy, T. P. (2017). Nurse bullying: Impact on nurses' health. *Western Journal of Nursing Research, 39*(12), 1533–1546. https://doi.org/10.1177/0193945916681278

Shi, Y., Guo, H., Zhang, S., Xie, F., Wang, J., Sun, Z., Dong, X., Sun, T., & Fan, L. (2018). Impact of workplace incivility against new nurses on job burn-out: A cross-sectional study in China. *BMJ Open, 8,* e020461. https://doi.org/10.1136/bmjopen-2017-020461

Sigma Theta Tau International. (2021). *Finding your forward: Resources for advocacy and strength resilience.* Retrieved October 15, 2021, from https://nursingcentered.sigmanursing.org/find-your-forward?_ga=2.187355176.1637935552.1606243321-10327058.1606243320

Sokol-Hessner, L., Folcarelli, P. H., Annas, C. L., Brown, S. M., Fernandez, L., Roche, S. D., Lee, B. S., Sands, K. E., & the Practice of Respect Delphi Study Group. (2018). A road map for advancing the practice of respect in health care: The results of an interdisciplinary modified Delphi consensus study. *Joint Commission Journal on Quality and Patient Safety, 44*(8), 463–476. https://doi.org/10.1016/j.jcjq.2018.02.003

The Joint Commission. (2018, May 17). *Sentinel Event Alert 59: Physical and verbal violence against healthcare workers.* Retrieved October 15, 2021, from www.jointcommission.org/sea_issue_59/

Tri-Council for Nursing. (2017, September 26). *Nursing civility proclamation.* Retrieved October 15, 2021, from https://tricouncilfornursing.org/

U.S. Department of Labor, Occupational Safety and Health Administration. (1970). *OSH Act of 1970.* Retrieved October 15, 2021, from https://www.osha.gov/laws-regs/oshact/completeoshact

U.S. Department of Labor, Occupational Safety and Health Administration. (2016). *OSHA 3148-06R. Guidelines for preventing workplace violence for healthcare and social service workers.* Retrieved October 15, 2021, from https://www.osha.gov/Publications/osha3148.pdf

Ulrich, B., Barden, C., Cassidy, L., & Varn-Davis, N. (2019). Critical care nurse work environments 2018: Findings and implications. *Critical Care Nurse, 39*(2), 67–84. https://doi.org/10.4037/ccn2019605

Wang, Y. X., Guo, H. T., Du, X. W., Song, W., Lu, C., & Hao, W. N. (2020). Factors associated with post-traumatic stress disorder of nurses exposed to corona virus disease 2019 in China. *Medicine, 99*(26), e20965. https://doi.org/10.1097/MD.0000000000020965

Workplace Bullying Institute. (2020). Retrieved October 15, 2021, from https://www.workplacebullying.org/

The Use of Social Media in Nursing

Perry M. Gee and Michelle L. Litchman

ADDITIONAL RESOURCES

Visit thePoint for additional helpful resources.
- eBook
- Journal Articles
- Web Links

CHAPTER OUTLINE

LEARNING OBJECTIVES

The learner will be able to:

1. Define social media and social networking.
2. Identify the different types of platforms used for social media.
3. Analyze how social media can be effectively used by the professional nurse.
4. Explore how patients and caregivers are using social media for self-managing illness.
5. Identify the challenges nurses may encounter when using social media.
6. Review the standards and guidelines for safe and effective use of social media by the nurse.

Special thanks to Rachael Katz, MS, for her help with this chapter.

INTRODUCTION

Health care in America is changing—and with a new focus on patient-centered care, value-driven outcomes, health care reform, and the *democratization* of health information and knowledge, the nurse's role is evolving. At the center of this evolution is social media. *Social media* is a method for nurses to share and transmit information as well as knowledge to a far-reaching audience; *social networking* is the process of engaging with that audience using social media. This chapter focuses on the nurse's role with both social media and social networking in practice, administration, education, and research, as well as with consumers who are using these tools for self-management and health promotion.

Among all health care consumers and caregivers (including nurses), the use of social media is rapidly on the rise. Social media is becoming ubiquitous in our society and certainly among patients, caregivers, and their health care provider teams. Nurses interact with patients who are using social media every day; the nurse's understanding of this cultural shift is imperative for promoting health and teaching patients. In fact, social media is starting to play a central role in patient engagement and has the potential to improve health outcomes (Markham et al., 2017; Nguyen et al., 2020). Patients are using social media to learn about health conditions and treatments, connect with other patients, update family members and caregivers, and communicate with members of their health care teams.

Indeed, social media has tremendous power. During the COVID-19 pandemic, social media was used for communication, education, and peer support. For example, the *COVID Resilience for Healthcare Professionals* Facebook group was used by nurses, physicians, and other health care providers to share ideas related to patient care, national trends, and strategies for supporting mental health during the pandemic.

> *Consider This*   Many nurses have shared their real experiences and fears on the front lines of the COVID-19 pandemic through social media. Registered nurse Sydni Lane shared a photo of her face following a 12-hour shift in the emergency department wearing her N95 mask. The image of her red and bruised face and her story of being scared for her own health had a "viral" impact with over 1.2 million likes on Instagram.

Nurses are becoming savvy users of social media in order to (1) enhance their own knowledge; (2) affect health care policy; (3) promote causes and raise money; (4) connect with other nurses; (5) participate in professional organizations; (6) inform patients, caregivers, and the public; (7) communicate with patients and colleagues; (8) conduct research; and (9) just relax and have fun. This chapter explores the important role of social media in nursing, both now and in the future, and provides tools for nurses to successfully navigate this exciting technology. Pitfalls of social media are discussed as well as how nurses can protect themselves from the drawbacks of participating. This chapter begins with an overview of different types of social media.

TYPES OF SOCIAL MEDIA AND HOW IT CAN BE USED FOR NURSING

Social media is currently made up of several different platforms. Each platform has unique strengths, and it is not unusual to combine different platform types into one social media experience. For instance, a single website may contain both social networking and media-sharing capabilities. There are also multiple forms of social media, including social networks, social bookmarking sites, social news, media sharing, microblogging, wikis, messaging tools, and blogs.

Social Networks

Social networks are supported by software that allows individuals to connect and share with others. These networks can take several forms, and the focus can range from personal relationships to professional relationships. Social networks can be called other names, such as virtual networks, virtual communities, or online communities. Note the use of the term *community*; a social media platform gives users access to communities of people outside their geographic boundaries. This access may promote engagement with a nurse in a rural area who wants to have a relationship with other nurses with similar interests, for example. These online communities may also provide a supportive environment for a person with a chronic illness who can learn about self-care activities.

The most widely used social network is *Facebook*. Facebook currently has over 2.8 billion active monthly users worldwide; 1.8 billion people log into Facebook every day (Iqbal, 2021). Even without access to a personal computer, people may access Facebook every day using a smartphone, giving people in remote areas access. Smartphones also facilitate networking on other platforms, access to health care information, and social networking on other platforms. People with similar interests can use Facebook *groups* or *pages* to communicate and engage with peers. Currently, over 1.4 billion people use Facebook groups and many of those groups are devoted to nursing interests or health care (Aslam, 2020).

LinkedIn is an increasingly popular social networking site specifically for the purpose of connecting professionals and hiring and job searching. Nurses can post information about their experience, certifications, and interests, and they can receive public endorsements from others related to their skills and expertise (Brooks, 2019).

Many nursing organizations have groups or pages on Facebook, LinkedIn, and other social media sites to communicate and share information with members and people who are interested. For example, search the American Association of Critical-Care Nurses to access their dedicated page on Facebook.

Patients or health care consumers also use social networking groups on Facebook. For example, the No Nuts Mom Group operates the *NNMG Food Allergic Families* Facebook group, which includes over 33,000 parents and caregivers of children with severe food allergies. Members can use the Facebook page to get health information and tips for day-to-day food allergy management. Social networking is one of the most powerful and widely used components of social media and can, therefore, be important for the professional nurse and the patient.

Discussion Point

It is common for nursing students to set up private Facebook groups for discussion of school-related issues. If negative posts appear in the group about curricula, faculty, or clinical sites, what can be done to keep the discussion from becoming inappropriate?

Social Bookmarking Sites

Bookmarking sites are a way nurses can search, organize, individualize, and comment on lists of internet bookmarks or web pages of interest. There are several popular social bookmarking sites, including *Digg.com*, *Reddit*, and *Pinterest*. Individuals can go to these bookmarking sites and comment on individual links and even critique a site. This may provide a valuable tool for nurses to rapidly find resources important to their areas of interest or the needs of their patients.

Social News

Like social bookmarking, *social news* platforms include user-posted story links that are organized, posted, and voted upon, with the most popular news links appearing at the top of the list. The social news site Reddit (www.reddit.com) helps users find top relevant news articles in nursing by going to the site and performing a search on the word "nursing." Conducting this type of search yields top news stories

voted to be of interest to nursing. Social news sites are another good method for nurses to rapidly stay apprised about what is happening in the world of nursing and health care.

Media Sharing

Media sharing is when users can share photos and/or videos; these sites may also have user profiles and other social components. *YouTube*, *Snapchat*, and *TikTok* are examples of media-sharing platforms. In addition to sharing videos, users can log in, comment, or vote on the videos and see a profile of the person who posted the video. YouTube has over 2 billion users, and every day thousands of videos are uploaded. This includes videos related to nursing and health care topics that are free to view, providing a great opportunity for educating nurses. For example, nurse educator Michael Linares, RN, has a YouTube channel called "Simple Nursing" with hundreds of educational videos geared toward nursing students and seasoned nurses who need refreshers on nearly any clinical topic.

Nurse educators can create videos related to any subject area, upload that video to a media-sharing platform, and send a link to students who can access the video from any computer or smartphone worldwide. Nurses may also want to take advantage of these educational videos when illustrating treatments or procedures to patients and/or their caregivers. Media sharing is a great way to stay current in nursing and to visually share knowledge with others, including patients.

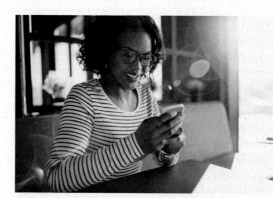

Discussion Point

What is the responsibility of the nurse who encounters a YouTube, TikTok, or other media-sharing site that contains a video of a nursing procedure that would be considered unsafe or even potentially dangerous to patients?

Microblogging

Microblogging is a type of social media platform with which users can post short comments and links to their personal pages and others can view, follow, and comment. *Twitter* is currently the most popular microblogging site. There are over 600 million Twitter users worldwide with over 500 million daily tweets (Smith, 2019). Thousands of nurses have Twitter accounts and so do schools of nursing, nursing organizations, hospitals, governmental health organizations, and patients to write tweets no longer than 280 characters. In addition to text tweets, users can post photos and links to other media. Hashtags are a core part of Twitter to bring conversations about the same topic together; the most popular hashtag is "trend." If one wanted to view a conversation about home care nursing, for example, the hashtag #homecarenursing could be searched to see the conversation about this topic.

Tweet chats are focused conversations on Twitter and typically include four or more questions to generate a dialogue on a specific topic. Engaging in a tweet chat can be exciting and allows for increased perspective based on differences in geographic location, culture, health care stakeholder role, and other factors. #WeNurses is a nursing-specific tweet chat, and #HCLDR is an interdisciplinary health care leader–specific tweet chat. Both occur weekly with a worldwide following.

Wikis

A *wiki* allows multiple users to post internet-based content, modify the content, and create online communities. The largest and most popular wiki is Wikipedia, a crowd-sourced, dynamic, web-based encyclopedia. Wikihealth.com is a wiki site devoted to health care and wellness issues that can be a good source for nurses and patients to access when looking for health resources. However, because of the open-source nature of Wikipedia, the nurse must carefully assess whether clinical content is evidence based to ensure its accuracy and currency.

Messaging

Messaging is an important form of social media. Tools like WhatsApp, Facebook, and Snapchat are communications methods used millions of times each day worldwide. Nurses working in rural Southeast Asia on humanitarian health care teams might use messaging apps to communicate among themselves and with local health officials and providers to coordinate care activities when phone calls are not possible. Simple access to wireless internet can facilitate sending text, voice, and video messages.

Blogs

Blogs ("weblogs") are a social media format on which individuals can write posts of any length about topics of their choice. Typically, bloggers are focused on a specific topic area, for example, public health nursing. Blogs may also promote discussion or engagement and can be set up for free using a software platform like WordPress. Many excellent nursing blogs attract professionals who may read posts, observe others' comments, and post their own.

An example of a well-known, award-winning blog is *Nursology*, which features multiple nursing bloggers with a wide range of experience and expertise discussing issues common to nursing scholarship, practice, and knowledge. During the COVID-19 pandemic, several of Nursology bloggers discussed how nurses could support their own well-being needs.

Discussion Point

Blogging can be an easy, immediate, and free way for nurses to share their important messages. Have you ever thought about writing or hosting a blog? Or being a guest blog contributor?

SOCIAL MEDIA USE BY PATIENTS (HOW NURSES CAN SUPPORT PATIENTS)

Like nurses, health care consumers (both patients and caregivers) more often than not use some form of social media. With all the different types of social media available to patients, nurses have the opportunity to provide guidance. When nurses have a strong understanding of the social media tools available, they can educate patients and caregivers in their selection and use. For instance, eHealth Enhanced Chronic Care Model (CCM) for chronic illness self-managed support has been developed utilizing social media and other eHealth tools. The CCM augments the traditional supportive "community" for a person with chronic illness by providing an "e-community" or online community using social networking (Gee et al., 2015). It also promotes the role of nurses and providers in helping patients choose a useful social network and trains them on effective participation in the group to promote self-management goals.

Discussion Point

Are there appropriate times for the nurse to use social media in the clinical setting? When would it be inappropriate?

Research Fuels the Controversy 14.1

Social Media and Health Care for Adolescents and Young Adults

People affected by diabetes are spending more money to care for the condition than ever. The costs for glucose testing supplies and medications, including insulin, are so high that it has been known to result in a choice between death and debt. People affected by diabetes may need to decide between addressing basic needs that require money (e.g., feeding, clothing, housing) and proper diabetes care.

Source: Litchman, M. L., Oser, T. K., Wawrzynski, S. E., Walker, H. R., & Oser, S. (2019). The underground exchange of diabetes medications and supplies: Donating, trading, and borrowing, oh my! *Journal of Diabetes Science and Technology, 14*(6), 1000–1009. https://doi .org/10.1177/1932296819888215

Study Findings

Out of desperation to manage their diabetes, researchers found that some individuals used social media to engage in an "underground" exchange of diabetes medications and supplies. These exchanges include donating, trading, borrowing, and purchasing insulin, oral medications, glucose strips, insulin pump supplies, and continuous glucose monitoring sensors for survival. The researchers concluded that there is an urgent need to improve access to medications that are essential for life and suggested that the U.S. health care system is failing since such underground exchanges would not be necessary if medications and supplies were accessible.

Social media is used extensively by patients who want to connect with others for help, advice, and social support. Social media can help people with specific conditions and experiences find each other, for example, people with disabilities who are pregnant (Litchman et al., 2019a). In another example, people with diabetes may use online peer support communities to ask questions about the condition, share information, and advocate for their health, resulting in positive health outcomes (Elnaggar et al., 2020; Litchman et al., 2019b, 2020). In addition, people with diabetes may use social media sites to obtain and exchange supplies (see Research Fuels the Controversy 14.1).

The informed "e-patient" may arrive at the health care setting with substantial knowledge about their own condition, possibly even more than the nurse or other members of the provider team. The challenge for the nurse is to find a way to evaluate the patient's knowledge and work together with the patient as a proactive team meets the individual's health care goals.

Virtual Health Communities That Are Consumer Centered

Many patients all over the world are using social media, specifically social networking, in the form of virtual online communities, to find information and support for their health conditions. Historically, many people with rare diseases experienced isolation with limited access to pertinent health information. Now, people with rare conditions can find support using social media. Examples include *PatientsLikeMe* and *Inspire*, which allow patients with various conditions, including rare ones, to engage with and learn from each other (James et al., 2020; Nyman et al., 2020).

Another resource for people with diabetes is the supportive virtual community via the diabetes social media advocacy (#DSMA) tweet chat. #DSMA is a 1-hour weekly tweet chat that was initiated in 2010 by Cherise Shockley, a person living with diabetes. During this tweet chat, a moderator poses diabetes-related questions, and participants (including patients, health care providers, advocacy organizations, etc.) respond to the questions and communicate with each other. An example of #DSMA tweet chats are how individuals with diabetes want to age successfully (Litchman et al., 2018), how online communities support diabetes education, and exploring diabetes stigma (Greenwood et al., 2019). Tweet chats have addressed other areas of health, including cardio-oncology (Conley et al., 2020), advanced planning for brain tumors (Cutshall et al., 2020), and hospice and palliative medicine (Salmi et al., 2020). There is no end to the types of health conditions or demographic makeup of people who can find help from virtual health communities.

Discussion Point

Is there a role for the professional nurse in virtual health communities or would nurses' involvement in the group change the dynamics? What about the nurse who is also a patient and wants to join a virtual health community? What should the nurse disclose?

In addition, the *Society of Participatory Medicine* is a platform where patients, providers, and health researchers can come together using social media to explore treatment options and support health management using the collective wisdom of the group.

The Nurse's Role

Approximately 87% to 88% of nurses are using some form social media (Lefebvre et al., 2020; Surani et al., 2017). Nurses who use social media, either for personal or for professional reasons, must understand the elements of digital citizenship. Digital citizens must encompass the norms of appropriate and responsible technology use. Nurses must not post information about patients or anything that could be linked to patients. Further, nurses should not provide medical advice online. Yet, a recent assessment of nurse "micro-celebrities" on Instagram revealed professional, ethical, and privacy issues (Kerr et al., 2020). Social media has the power to transform how the public views the nursing profession. Nurses should be mindful of how their social media presence reflects not only on themselves but also on the profession.

To help patients traverse the world of these new web-based platforms, nurses should become familiar with the major social media outlets for patients and steer them to evidence-based resources. Nurses must develop the skills to educate patients and caregivers on the use of social media, routinely assessing if their patients are the good candidates for using social media to support their health conditions, then developing an education plan with these assessment findings in mind (Box 14.1).

Another facet nurses should consider is if their patients have access to social media tools. The *digital divide* is the term used for the fact that those of lower socioeconomic status may not have access to the internet or social media tools at all. Compared to White older adults, Hispanic and Black older adults are less likely to use technology for health purposes (Mitchell et al., 2019; Smith, 2014). This is likely tied to socioeconomic status, education levels, and structural racism. Of people who live in rural areas, 58% report access to broadband internet services is a problem (Anderson, 2018). The digital divide has made care during the COVID-19 pandemic more challenging due to disparities in the social determinants of health, including built environments, social and community contexts, education, economic stability, and health care access (Ramsetty & Adams, 2020).

Discussion Point

Should nurses routinely include assessment of social media use and broadband internet access when taking a history and physical examination?

Discussion Point

Nurses are excellent at troubleshooting complicated health care–related technologies, for example, intravenous pumps, cardiac and hemodynamic monitors, defibrillators, and pacemakers. Should nurses be trained to troubleshoot basic internet technology in the patient's home?

BOX 14.1   Potential Patient Education Topics Related to Social Media

- Pros and cons of using social media
- How to choose an appropriate social media for specific health conditions
- Types of hardware, software, and networking needed to participate in social media
- How to join a social network
- How to navigate individual sites
- How to maintain one's privacy on social media
- How to verify if information is credible
- How to protect oneself from scams
- How to formulate a message in a blog or microblog
- How to ask for help from an online community

Cell phones, smartphones, tablets, and other mobile devices are becoming the primary ways many individuals are accessing the internet and the health care system. In fact, 60% of the world's population (4.66 billion people) use the internet, and approximately half of that access is via mobile devices (Johnson, 2021). African Americans, Hispanic Americans, and those with lower incomes rely heavily on smartphones for online access (Perrin & Turner, 2019). These numbers show it is possible to provide mobile access to social media, even though some patients may not have home computers with traditional internet access. Older Americans are also adopting mobile technologies at a rapid pace. Currently, 92% of those over age 65 use a cell phone and 61% own a smartphone, which is a significant increase in the past 5 years; this number is up 24% since the year 2013 (Pew Research, 2021). Nurses should advocate for internet access for their patients and make it part of the assessment process to evaluate web access and individuals' ability to obtain services using the internet.

PITFALLS OF SOCIAL MEDIA AND NURSING

Social media may prove to be a major factor in encouraging patient engagement and in improving health care. However, social media can also be unpredictable, dangerous, and harmful if not used correctly. For example, based on unverified information in social media, some individuals chose to begin taking the drug ivermectin, an antiparasitic deworming agent, as both a prophylactic and curative drug for COVID-19. The drug, however, was not approved by the Food and Drug Administration (FDA) for the treatment of any viral infection in humans, and misinformation has resulted in overdoses and misuse of the drug. As nurses, we must advocate for and protect our patients as they use social media. As professionals, it is imperative for nurses to follow ethical and professional standards as we use this form of media.

Social media can expose nurses and their patients to billions of individuals on the internet. Although this open access may offer endless opportunities, it can also open people up to serious breaches in privacy and exposure to internet predators and criminals who take advantage of users. Because social media allows for a degree of anonymity and no face-to-face interactions, the nurse or patient may believe they are interacting with a highly trained professional or a caring friend and find the person on the other end is not who they say they are. Patients may encounter a social media environment that reports to offer a "cure" for their conditions. Further, nurses may find a group of "experts" who claim to have new standards for nursing care, such as not vaccinating according to the Centers for Disease Control and Prevention (CDC) guidelines. A person's profile on a social media site, such as LinkedIn, may be used for an unsolicited invitation to provide a presentation at a conference or sit on an editorial board that is not legitimate. Social media sites and unsolicited invitations must be carefully analyzed to determine if they are legitimate. This analysis may be an excellent opportunity for the professional nurse to act in an advocacy and education role for their patients.

From students to veteran professionals, nurses have been negatively affected by social media interactions. For example, nurses have unintentionally revealed personally identifiable patient information or revealed patient information in an environment they believed was safe and private but was not.

The privacy laws of the Health Insurance Portability and Accountability Act (HIPAA) equally apply to the world of social media. As an illustration, a young nursing student was being romantically pursued by a patient in the hospital. Later in the shift, the patient was discharged and passed a note expressing affections to the student. Disturbed by the letter, the student wanted to share the note with classmates on a private social media platform. The student scanned a digital image of the note and posted the document to the group; the image of the note also contained the patient's full name. Within hours of the image being posted in the "private" web location, it ended up on a public Facebook page where the patient saw the note and reported the HIPAA infraction to the hospital. The hospital, nursing school, and individual nursing student all suffered serious consequences because of this unintentional breach. This story highlights many pitfalls of social media, starting with the notion that just because a platform says it is private does not mean it will remain private. As a rule, assume anything posted in social media can and will be viewed by all. This is an especially important rule for the nurse to follow. The National Council of State Boards of Nursing's (NCSBN) Implications for Inappropriate Use of Social Media are outlined in Box 14.2.

Discussion Point

What should the nurse do if they witness a post with identifiable patient information on a social media site? What if they live in a different community or even state?

Nurses can face personal liability for inappropriate use of social media. A major concern is that hospitals and health systems typically do not yet have policies on nurses' personal social media use (NCSBN, 2018). Many infractions are due to nurses violating privacy laws and exposing identifiable patient information. The NCSBN has been working with the American Nurses Association and has developed a comprehensive white paper highlighting the appropriate and inappropriate use of social media by the professional nurse (NCSBN, 2018; Box 14.3).

The literature suggests nurses avoid invitations from patients to be "friends" on social media sites. Although some health care providers are known to interact with patients

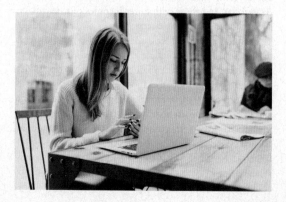

BOX 14.2   National Council of State Boards of Nursing's Implications for Inappropriate Use of Social Media

Instances of inappropriate use of social and electronic media may be reported to the Board of Nursing (BON). The laws outlining the basis for disciplinary action by the BON vary between jurisdictions. Depending on the laws of a jurisdiction, the BON may investigate reports of inappropriate disclosures on social media by a nurse on the grounds of:

- unprofessional conduct
- unethical conduct
- moral turpitude
- mismanagement of patient records
- revealing a privileged communication
- breach of confidentiality

If the allegations are found to be true, the nurse may face disciplinary action by the BON, including a reprimand or sanction, assessment of a monetary fine, or temporary or permanent loss of licensure.

Source: National Council of State Boards of Nursing. (2018). *White paper: A nurse's guide to the use of social media.* Author. https://www .ncsbn.org/NCSBN_SocialMedia.pdf

---

using social media, the standard practice at this time is to keep personal and professional use of these platforms separated with clear boundaries (Grady, 2020). The act of becoming social media "friends" with patients may violate organization policies and violate the boundaries of the nurse–patient relationship (Grady, 2020). Patients may also use social media to give the nurses and other providers bad scores for quality of care, length of the visit, cleanliness of the office, friendliness of the office staff, and even what the provider is wearing. One disgruntled patient can use social media to cause significant damage to the professional's reputation and ability to recruit new patients. This concern holds true for health care businesses and even hospitals. It is prudent for practitioners and health care businesses to routinely examine their web presence for negative comments from consumers.

Discussion Point

Is there ever a time the nurse or other health care provider would want to be social media "friends" with one or more of their patients?

Consider This Monica R. McLemore, PhD, MPH, RN, FAAN (@mclemoremr), and associate professor of family health care nursing at University of California, San Francisco, describes why she engages in Twitter: "In 1998, the Woodhull study named for Nancy Woodhull—the founding editor of *USA Today*—commissioned a study with Sigma Theta Tau International, the Honor Society

in Nursing, that found that nursing voices were cited 4% of the time in print and popular media. TWENTY YEARS LATER, when the study was repeated, they found that number had dropped to 2%. We have been the most trusted of the health professions for decades — and yet, nurses are NOT sought out by the media as the thought leaders, innovators, researchers, or the clinical experts that we are. Social media is one path to correct this and how I choose to use it" (Sieber, Powers, Baggs, Knapp, & Sileo, 1998; Mason, Glickstein, Nixon, Westphaln, Han, & Acquaviva, 2018).

Nurse leaders with large local or national followings need to realize that participation in social media may be great for the promotion of a cause; however, it may also open the individual to personal scrutiny. Recently, the nurse leader of a large health care professional organization was viciously and personally attacked for several days on Twitter for a personal photo that was found on a public social media site. The photo was of the nurse leader holding a cake at a party. This photo was then attached to a tweet to degrade the leader and identify the leader as a hypocrite for promoting unhealthy eating.

In addition, more and more employers are looking at social media as part of the hiring process. In a survey completed in 2018, 70% of employers were using social media sites to screen for potential employees (Driver, 2020). For nursing leadership positions, using the internet is commonplace for human resource specialists, recruiters, or hiring managers to review a candidate's profile, sometimes on LinkedIn. The professional nurse will want to carefully use online platforms and consider steps to evaluate and tidy up their current social media presence. Strategies for keeping a positive social media image and avoiding problems with social media are included in Boxes 14.4 and 14.5, respectively.

SOCIAL MEDIA IN PROFESSIONAL NURSING PRACTICE

Although social media involve risks, they can also enhance practice, education, and research when used properly. Nurses will need to carefully consider their use of social media as a tool and develop knowledge and expertise in its implementation.

Social Media in Nursing Practice

Clinically practicing nurses should be familiar with these social platforms so they can incorporate these tools into their practice. In public and population health, social media has a strong presence in the surveillance of disease. Public health experts used social media and an analysis of its content to identify the rising incidence in COVID-19 during the early days of the outbreak in China; Shen and colleagues (2020) used computer machine learning techniques to identify "sick posts" from social media feeds and accurately predict COVID-19 daily as far as 2 weeks into the future. Other disease surveillance has been developed using algorithms that can identify the differences between "chatter" about the flu and actual incidence of the flu (Science Daily, 2017). Both Google and the CDC evaluate internet searches and social media comments to accurately track to detect outbreaks and incidence of the flu at the state and national levels (visit www.google.org/flutrends/us/#US). In addition, photo surveillance techniques have been used to identify if individuals with diabetes are using their continuous glucose monitors as recommended by the FDA (Litchman & Woodruff, 2017).

Nurses may also use social media to promote self-management for patients with chronic illnesses. For instance, a person with pulmonary fibrosis can be steered toward a social networking site to meet others with the same condition for social support and self-management tips. Online health communities have been shown to increase empowerment, self-management, and social support among those with chronic conditions (Litchman et al., 2019b). Therefore, the opportunity exists for nurses working with patients and caregivers of people with chronic illness to guide them in using social media for engagement and support. Nurses who work with those living with chronic illnesses may want to begin to explore condition-specific social media resources, evaluate the offerings, catalog a list of resources, and make those resources available to patients.

Discussion Point

If the nurse were asked by a patient or caregiver about social media resources for a specific condition, where would the nurse go to find these tools?

To help the nurse who is new to using social media, the American Nurses Association (2011) offers principles for social networking at https://www.nursingworld.org/~4af4f2/globalassets/docs/ana/ethics/social-networking.pdf. Nurses who are part of the policy development process in their organization may want to inform themselves on social media issues and generate unit-based or facility policies to guide nurses new to the organization.

Social Media in Nursing Education

Social media provides an excellent to help in educating nurses, patients, caregivers, and other providers (Lipp et al., 2014). Nurses in large academic medical centers and

BOX 14.4   **Keeping a Positive Social Media Image**

Five tips for nurse job seekers to keep a positive image online:

1. Clean up digital dirt before you begin your job search. Remove any photos, content, and links that can work against you in an employer's eyes.
2. Consider creating your own professional group on sites like Facebook or LinkedIn. It is a great way to establish relationships with leaders, recruiters, and potential referrals.
3. Keep gripes offline. Keep the content you post focused on positive things, whether it is related to professional or personal information. Make sure to highlight specific accomplishments inside and outside work.
4. Be selective about whom you accept as friends. Do not forget others (may be able to) see your friends when they search for you. Monitor comments made by others and consider using the "block comments" feature. Even better, set your profile to "private" so only designated friends can view it.
5. If you are still employed, do not mention your job search in your tweets or status updates. There are multiple examples of people who have gotten fired as a result of doing this. In addition, a potential employer might assume that if you are willing to search for a new job on your current company's time, why would not you do so on theirs?

Source: Haefner, R. (September 10, 2009). *More employers screening candidates via social networking sites.* Career Builder.com. Retrieved October 30, 2020, from http://sites.dreamingcode.com/dccontentnet/Content/Newdata/pdf/75_55Ab.pdf

BOX 14.5   **How to Avoid Problems Using Social Media**

It is important to recognize that instances of inappropriate use of social media can and do occur, but with awareness and caution, nurses can avoid inadvertently disclosing confidential or private information about patients.

The following guidelines are intended to minimize the risks of using social media:

- First and foremost, nurses must recognize that they have an ethical and legal obligation to always maintain patient privacy and confidentiality.
- Nurses are strictly prohibited from transmitting by way of any electronic media any patient-related image. In addition, nurses are restricted from transmitting any information that may be reasonably anticipated to violate patient rights to confidentiality or privacy, or otherwise degrade or embarrass the patient.
- Do not share, post, or otherwise disseminate any information, including images, about a patient or information gained in the nurse–patient relationship with anyone unless there is a patient care–related need to disclose the information or other legal obligation to do so.
- Do not identify patients by name or post or publish information that may lead to the identification of a patient. Limiting access to postings through privacy settings is not sufficient to ensure privacy.
- Do not refer to patients in a disparaging manner, even if the patient is not identified.
- Do not take photos or videos of patients on personal devices, including cell phones. Follow employer policies for taking photographs or video of patients for treatment or other legitimate purposes using employer-provided devices.
- Maintain professional boundaries in the use of electronic media. Like in-person relationships, the nurse has the obligation to establish, communicate, and enforce professional boundaries with patients in the online environment. Use caution when having online social contact with patients or former patients. Online contact with patients or former patients blurs the distinction between a professional and personal relationship. The fact that a patient may initiate contact with the nurse does not permit the nurse to engage in a personal relationship with the patient.
- Consult employer policies or an appropriate leader within the organization for guidance regarding work-related postings.
- Promptly report any identified breach of confidentiality or privacy.
- Be aware of and comply with employer policies regarding use of employer-owned computers, cameras, and other electronic devices and use of personal devices in the workplace.
- Do not make disparaging remarks about employers or coworkers. Do not make threatening, harassing, profane, obscene, sexually explicit, racially derogatory, homophobic, or other offensive comments.
- Do not post content or otherwise speak on behalf of the employer unless authorized to do so, and follow all applicable policies of the employer.

Source: National Council of State Boards of Nursing. (2018). *White paper: A nurse's guide to the use of social media.* Author.

remote areas have access to the exact same clinical reference materials available on social media. For the practicing clinical nurse, there are thousands of videos devoted to nursing skills and the management of illness. Nurse educators may use YouTube to store and distribute videos to nursing students or practicing nurses. Nurse educators can explore available videos for specific skills or management of particular conditions and share that content with students without having to take the time to research and develop the content. Students can learn from a variety of nurses and see care accomplished using a range of different methods. However, faculty and educators need to carefully review the content to be sure the materials are safe, appropriate, and evidence based.

Faculty or nurse researchers can use a wide range of online media tools for education in the classroom, scheduling of meetings, and obtaining survey results. Faculty and nurse educators can use hashtags to keep topics grouped and organized. Social media tools like blogs, microblogs, and wikis offer a wide variety of methods for students to interact with their local cohort or with students in other areas.

> **Consider This** Social media is a way to be "present" and participate in a professional conference or symposium without attending. The COVID-19 pandemic was the impetus for numerous creative ways to participate in nursing conferences that would normally be attended in person. Conferences unattainable in the past now may be cheaper and more accessible for the working registered nurse. Several conferences offer live sessions and the option to watch recorded videos of the presentation's weeks or months after the event. Many conference video systems have live chat features that may give participants a more hands-on experience. The American Association of Critical-Care Nurses offers some guidance for getting the most from a virtual conference at https://www.aacn.org/blog/tips-for-attending-virtual-nursing-conferences/.

Social Media in Nursing Research

To date, there has been paucity of significant research in social media and nursing. However, an analysis of Twitter posts using hashtags examined the public perception of the nursing profession following the wrongful arrest of registered nurse Alex Wubbels was conducted. In this case, a video and multiple news articles of the arrest were circulated on social media, including Twitter. A tweet analysis

indicated that the public perceived Wubbels and the nursing profession at large as trustworthy (Guo et al., 2019; Litchman et al., 2018), consistent with the last 16 Gallup polls (Brenan, 2017). Nurses who are highlighted in the media may support recruitment, retention, and professionalism within the nursing profession; thus, it is important to understand the role nurses play online.

The opportunity exists to further examine how social media can be used to augment health care and professional nursing and how nurses can support patients with their use of social media (Naslund et al., 2020; Pizzuti et al., 2020). Recent research has demonstrated that the use of social media by nurses can help facilitate a faster transition of research evidence into clinical practice and improve the knowledge dissemination process (Barton & Merolli, 2019; Ross & Cross, 2019). Indeed, patients have begun participating in the surveillance research process through social media. For example, using additional software, researchers were able to quantify experiences of hypoglycemia among members of an online community (Weitzman et al., 2013). In addition, social media sites afford the nurse researcher opportunities to connect with colleagues with similar interests using sites like *ResearchGate* where users can share ideas and research literature.

CONCLUSIONS

When properly used, social media is a powerful tool for professional nursing practice and patient support. Nurses must include an understanding of social media in their knowledge base, and nursing education is duty bound to include social media at all levels of curricula. As part of the patient advocate role, nurses must be prepared to use these tools to guide patients who are both new to and experienced in using social media. Nurses can even take the opportunity to learn about these dynamic tools from patients. Finally, the opportunity exists for nurses to conduct research with all forms of social media and use them to rapidly disseminate new nursing evidence.

Social media does come with inherent risks for both nurses and patients. Nurses should review the American Nurses Association *Scope and Standards of Practice* and *Code of Ethics for Nurses* and apply these expectations to the use of social media. The rules remain the same, but the reach and magnitude of the consequences of poor decisions on social media are greatly amplified. Opportunities continue to arise for nursing to embrace new and exciting social media tools to improve the profession and the health of our communities.

FOR ADDITIONAL DISCUSSION

1. What are the three components of social media, and how can they be used by the professional nurse?

2. How might social media be used to promote the nursing profession? Provide examples.

3. How do the HIPAA requirements apply to various types of social media? Are there differences in the legal consequences for a social media breach of confidentiality?

4. What are some examples of using social media for the person with a chronic illness?

5. What is the nurse's role with regard to social media? What is the digital divide, and how can nurses assess its impact related to social media use by patients?

6. Describe two resources available for nurses to explore when considering the implementation of social media projects or interventions.

7. As U.S. population ages, what are some considerations for social media use with the older adult?

References

American Nurses Association. (2011). *ANA's principles for social networking and the nurse.* Author. https://www.nursingworld.org/~4af4f2/globalassets/docs/ana/ethics/social-networking.pdf

Anderson, M. (2018, September 10). *About a quarter of rural Americans say access to high-speed internet is a major problem.* Retrieved August 20, 2021, from https://www.pewresearch.org/fact-tank/2018/09/10/about-a-quarter-of-rural-americans-say-access-to-high-speed-internet-is-a-major-problem/

Aslam, F. (2020). *Facebook by the numbers: State, demographics & fun facts.* https://www.omnicoreagency.com/facebook-statistics/

Barton, C. J., & Merolli, M. A. (2019). It is time to replace publish or perish with get visible or vanish: Opportunities where digital and social media can reshape knowledge translation. *British Journal of Sports Medicine, 53*(10), 594–598. https://doi.org/10.1136/bjsports-2017-098367

Brenan, M. (2017). *Nurses keep healthy lead as most honest, ethical profession. Gallup.* http://news.gallup.com/poll/224639/nurses-keep-healthy-lead-honest-ethical-profession.aspx

Brooks, B. A. (2019). LinkedIn and your professional identity. *Nurse Leader, 17*(3), 173–175. https://doi.org/10.1016/j.mnl.2019.03.001. https://www.nurseleader.com/article/S1541-4612(19)30086-2/abstract

Conley, C. C., Goyal, N. G., & Brown, S. A. (2020). Cardio-Oncology: Twitter chat as a mechanism for increasing awareness of heart health for cancer patients. *Cardio-Oncology, 6*(1), 1–5. https://doi.org/10.1186/s40959-020-00072-w

Cutshall, N. R., Kwan, B. M., Salmi, L., & Lum, H. D. (2020). "It makes people uneasy, but it's necessary.# BTSM": Using Twitter to explore advance care planning among brain tumor stakeholders. *Journal of Palliative Medicine, 23*(1), 121–124. https://doi.org/10.1089/jpm.2019.0077

Driver, S. (2020, March 23). *Keep It Clean: Social media screenings gain in popularity.* Retrieved August 20, 2021, from https://www.businessnewsdaily.com/2377-social-media-hiring.html

Elnaggar, A., Park, V. T., Lee, S. J., Bender, M., Siegmund, L. A., & Park, L. G. (2020). Patients' use of social media for diabetes self-care: Systematic review. *Journal of Medical Internet Research, 22*(4), e14209. https://doi.org/10.2196/14209

Gee, P. M., Greenwood, D. A., Paterniti, D. A., Ward, D., & Miller, L. M. (2015). The e-health enhanced chronic care model: A theory derivation approach. *Journal of Medical Internet Research, 17*(4), e86. https://doi.org/10.2196/jmir.4067

Grady, A. (2020). *Pros and cons of social media for professional healthcare providers.* https://www.melnic.com/pros_and_cons_of_social_media_for_healthcare_providers/

Greenwood, D. A., Litchman, M. L., Ng, A. H., Gee, P. M., Young, H. M., Ferrer, M., Ferrer, J., Memering, C. E., Eichorst, B., Scibilia, R., & Miller, L. M. (2019). Development of the intercultural diabetes online community research council: Codesign and social media processes. *Journal of Diabetes Science and Technology, 13*(2), 176–186.

Guo, J., Tay, D. L., & Litchman, M. L. (2019). Hashtags and heroes: Public perceptions of nursing following a high profile nurse arrest. *Journal of Professional Nursing, 35*(5), 398–404. https://doi.org/10.1016/j.profnurs.2019.02.005

Iqbal, M. (2021, July 06). *Facebook revenue and usage statistics (2021). Business of Apps.* Retrieved August 19, 2021, from https://www.businessofapps.com/data/facebook-statistics/

James, G., Nyman, E., Fitz-Randolph, M., Niklasson, A., Hedman, K., Hedberg, J., Wittbrodt, E. T., Medin, J., Moreno Quinn, C., Allum, A. M., & Emmas, C. (2020). Characteristics, symptom severity, and experiences of patients reporting chronic kidney disease in the PatientsLikeMe online health community: Retrospective and qualitative study. *Journal of Medical Internet Research,* 22(7), e18548. https://doi.org/10.2196/18548

Johnson, J. (2021, September 10). *Internet users in the world 2021.* Retrieved September 30, 2021, from https://www.statista.com/statistics/617136/digital-population-worldwide/

Kerr, H., Booth, R., & Jackson, K. (2020). Exploring the characteristics and behaviors of nurses who have attained microcelebrity status on Instagram: Content analysis. *Journal of Medical Internet Research,* 22(5), e16540. https://doi.org/10.2196/16540

Lefebvre, C., McKinney, K., Glass, C., Cline, D., Franasiak, R., Husain, I., Pariyadath, M., Roberson, A., McLean, A., & Stopyra, J. (2020). Social media usage among nurses: Perceptions and practices. *JONA: The Journal of Nursing Administration,* 50(3), 135–141. https://doi.org/10.1097/nna.0000000000000857

Lipp, A., Davis, R. E., Peter, R., & Davies, J. S. (2014). The use of social media among health care professionals within an online postgraduate diabetes diploma course. *Practical Diabetes,* 31(1), 14a–17a. https://doi.org/10.1002/pdi.1821

Litchman, M. L., & Woodruff, W. (2017, August). *Photosurveillance of non-FDA approved activity in the diabetes online community.* 4th Annual Meeting of the American Association of Diabetes Educators, Indianapolis, IN.

Litchman, M. L., Oser, T. K., Hodgson, L., Heyman, M., Walker, H. R., Deroze, P., Rinker, J., & Warshaw, H. (2020). In-person and technology-mediated peer support in diabetes care: A systematic review of reviews and gap analysis. *The Diabetes Educator,* 46(3), 230–241. https://doi.org/10.1177/0145721720913275

Litchman, M. L., Snyder, C., Edelman, L. S., Wawrzynski, S. E., & Gee, P. M. (2018). Diabetes online community user perceptions of successful aging with diabetes: Analysis of a #DSMA tweet chat. *Journal of Medical Internet Research Aging,* 1(1), e10176. https://doi.org/10.2196/10176. https://aging.jmir.org/2018/1/e10176/

Litchman, M. L., Tran, M. J., Dearden, S., Guo, J., Simonsen, S., & Clark, L. (2019a). What women with disabilities write in personal blogs about pregnancy and early motherhood: A qualitative analysis of blogs. *JMIR Pediatrics and Parenting,* 2(1), e12355. https://doi.org/10.2196/12355

Litchman, M. L., Walker, H. R., Ng, A. H., Wawrzynski, S. E., Oser, S. M., Greenwood, D. A., Gee, P. M., Lackey, M., & Oser, T. K. (2019b). State of the Science: A scoping review and gap analysis of diabetes online communities. *Journal of Diabetes Science and Technology,* 13(3), 466–492. https://doi.org/10.1177/1932296819831042

Markham, M. J., Gentile, D., & Graham, D. L. (2017). Social media for networking, professional development, and patient engagement. *American Society of Clinical Oncology Educational Book,* (37), 782–787. https://doi.org/10.1200/edbk_180077

Mason, D. J., Glickstein, B., Nixon, L., Westphaln, K., Han, S., & Acquaviva, K. (2018). *The Woodhull study revisited: Nurses' representation in health news media.* Center for Health Policy and Media Engagement, The George Washington University.

Mitchell, U. A., Chebli, P. G., Ruggiero, L., & Muramatsu, N. (2019). The digital divide in health-related technology use: The significance of race/ethnicity. *The Gerontologist,* 59(1), 6–14. https://doi.org/10.1093/geront/gny138

Naslund, J. A., Bondre, A., Torous, J., & Aschbrenner, K. A. (2020). Social media and mental health: Benefits, risks, and opportunities for research and practice. *Journal of Technology in Behavioral Science,* 5(3), 245–257. https://doi.org/10.1007/s41347-020-00134-x

National Council of State Boards of Nursing. (2018). *White paper: A nurse's guide to the use of social media.* Author.

Northeastern University. (2017, May 09). *Twitter used to track the flu in real time.* Retrieved September 30, 2021, from https://www.sciencedaily.com/releases/2017/05/170509121952.htm

Nguyen, B. M., Lu, E., Bhuyan, N., Lin, K., & Sevilla, M. (2020). Social media for doctors: Taking professional and patient engagement to the next level. *Family Practice Management,* 27(1), 19–24.

Nyman, E., Vaughan, T., Desta, B., Wang, X., Barut, V., & Emmas, C. (2020). Characteristics and symptom severity of patients reporting systemic lupus erythematosus in the PatientsLikeMe online health community: A retrospective observational study. *Rheumatology and Therapy,* 7(1), 201–213. https://doi.org/10.1007/s40744-020-00195-7

Perrin, A., & Turner, E. (2019). Smartphones help blacks, Hispanics bridge some—But not all—Digital gaps with whites. *Pew Research.* https://www.pewresearch.org/fact-tank/2019/08/20/smartphones-help-blacks-hispanics-bridge-some-but-not-all-digital-gaps-with-whites/

Pew Research. (2021, April 7). *Demographics of mobile device ownership and adoption in the United States.* Retrieved August 20, 2021, from https://www.pewresearch.org/internet/fact-sheet/mobile/

Pizzuti, A. G., Patel, K. H., McCreary, E. K., Heil, E., Bland, C. M., Chinaeke, E., Love, B. L., & Bookstaver, P. B. (2020). Healthcare practitioners' views of social media as an educational resource. *PloS One,* 15(2), e0228372. https://doi.org/10.1371/journal.pone.0228372

Ramsetty, A., & Adams, C. (2020). Impact of the digital divide in the age of COVID-19. *Journal of the American Medical Informatics Association,* 27(7), 1147–1148. https://doi.org/10.1093/jamia/ocaa078

Ross, P., & Cross, R. (2019). Rise of the e-Nurse: The power of social media in nursing. *Contemporary Nurse,* 55(2–3), 211–220. https://doi.org/10.1080/10376178.2019.1641419

Salmi, L., Lum, H. D., Hayden, A., Reblin, M., Otis-Green, S., Venechuk, G., Morris, M. A., Griff, M., & Kwan, B. M. (2020). Stakeholder engagement in research on quality of life and palliative care for brain tumors: A qualitative analysis of# BTSM and# HPM tweet chats. *Neuro-Oncology Practice,* 7(6), 676–684. https://doi.org/10.1093/nop/npaa043

Shen, C., Chen, A., Luo, C., Zhang, J., Feng, B., & Liao, W. (2020). Using reports of symptoms and diagnoses on social media to predict COVID-19 case counts in Mainland China: Observational Infoveillance study. *Journal of Medical Internet Research,* 22(5), e19421. https://doi

.org/10.2196/19421. https://www.sciencedaily.com/releases/2017/05/170509121952.htm

Sieber, J. R., Powers, C. A., Baggs, J. R., Knapp, J. M., & Sileo, C. M. (1998). Missing in action: Nurses in the media. *The American Journal of Nursing*, 98(12), 55–56.

Smith, A. (2014, January 6). *African Americans and technology use*. https://www.pewresearch.org/internet/2014/01/06/african-americans-and-technology-use/

Smith, K. (2019). *126 Amazing social media statistics and facts*. Retrieved November 13, 2020, from https://www.brandwatch.com/blog/amazing-social-media-statistics-and-facts/

Surani, Z., Hirani, R., Elias, A., Quisenberry, L., Varon, J., Surani, S., & Surani, S. (2017). Social media usage among health care providers. *BMC Research Notes, 10*(1), 654. https://doi.org/10.1186/s13104-017-2993-y

Weitzman, E. R., Kelemen, S., Quinn, M., Eggleston, E. M., & Mandl, K. D. (2013). Participatory surveillance of hypoglycemia and harms in an online social network. *JAMA Internal Medicine, 173*(5), 345–351. https://doi.org/10.1001/jamainternmed.2013.2512

Medical Errors

Carol J. Huston

CHAPTER OUTLINE

LEARNING OBJECTIVES

The learner will be able to:

1. Review current research to determine whether organizational, governmental, and national efforts to reduce the incidence of medical errors in the United States have resulted in desired outcomes.

2. Differentiate between the terms "medical error," "medication error," and "adverse event."

3. Describe highly publicized patient cases from the mid- to the late 1990s as well as seminal research studies that brought national attention to the problem of medical errors in the United States.

4. Summarize key findings of the 1999 Institute of Medicine (IOM) report *To Err Is Human*, as well as the multipronged approach identified by the IOM to address the problem of medical errors in the United States.

5. Identify current research studies examining the scope, common causes, and financial/human costs of medical errors in the United States.

6. Identify national committees and groups formed due to governmental or legislative intervention to address the problem of medical errors.

7. Describe the intent and impact of Medicare's Pay for Performance initiatives, as well as Medicare's 2008 decision to no longer reimburse health care

providers for care needed as the result of "never events" or other preventable errors.

8. Identify the meaning of a Six Sigma error failure rate and determine how error rates in health care compare with other industries such as banking and the airlines.

9. Track current federal and state legislative efforts that encourage the voluntary reporting of health care errors by affording confidentiality protections for such reports.

10. Analyze the effect of the medical liability system on systematic efforts to uncover and learn from mistakes that are made in health care.

11. Differentiate among the three evidence-based standards identified by Leapfrog as having the greatest potential to reduce medical errors: computerized physician/provider order entry; evidence-based hospital referral; and intensive care unit physician staffing.

12. Differentiate between workplaces that emphasize a "culture of blame" and those that seek to provide a "just culture" or a "culture of safety management."

13. Reflect on the likelihood that they would self-report their medical errors to their employer, as well as to the involved patients and families.

INTRODUCTION

Quality health care continues to be a critically important yet underachieved goal. Among the most significant threats to achieving quality health care are the scope and prevalence of medical errors. Indeed, preventable medical errors are reported to be the third highest cause of death in the United States, following heart disease and cancer, claiming the lives of 250,000 Americans every year ("Medical Error Statistics," 2020). In addition, every year, roughly 12 million Americans are misdiagnosed, a little more than 4,000 surgical errors occur, and an estimated 7,000 to 9,000 patients die from medication errors ("Medical Error Statistics," 2020).

Similarly, the Canadian Patient Safety Institute notes that medical errors account for 28,000 deaths yearly in Canada (Desjardins, 2019). In fact, someone is injured from unintended harm in Canada every minute and 18 seconds.

Things are no better in England, where more than 237 million medication errors are made every year, costing the National Health Service (NHS) upward of £98 million and more than 1,700 lives every year (BMJ, 2020). The researchers estimated that nearly three out of every four medication errors (72%) were minor, but one in four (just under 26%) had the potential to cause moderate harm, and 2% could have potentially resulted in serious harm.

Discussion Point

Were medical errors historically considered an unavoidable consequence of health care? If so, did this reduce incentives to address the problem?

Surprisingly though, the problem of medical errors did not receive nationwide attention in the United States until several highly publicized cases between the late 1990s and early 2000s. One such case involved Betsy Lehman, a *Boston Globe* reporter, who died following chemotherapy administration errors. The media jumped on the story because it demonstrated repeated widespread communication and dispensing errors despite multiple safeguards in place to keep them from happening.

Libby Zion's case occurred around the same time. Zion, an 18-year-old, died 8 hours after entering a New York emergency department with seemingly minor complaints of fever and earache. Her death from drug interactions brought attention both to the all-too-narrow range between effective and toxic doses of some drugs and the danger of drug–drug interactions, even when all drugs are administered in doses that are considered safe when administered individually. The case also brought attention to the lack of supervision of residents and interns in the United States, as well as the excessive work hours forced on them and the errors that occur as a result.

Another story was of Willie King, a patient with diabetes from Tampa, Florida, who had the wrong leg amputated. This case, which became known as the "wrong leg" case, captured the collective dread of wrong-site surgery, a medical error that occurs too frequently because of the symmetry of the human body.

Finally, there was the story of Lewis Blackman, a healthy, gifted 15-year-old, who slowly bled to death after undergoing a minor surgical procedure at a major university medical center. Despite multiple warning signs, those caring for him repeatedly missed signs and symptoms that he was bleeding internally from a perforated ulcer.

Perhaps it was the clustering of these high-profile cases that made Americans stop and pay attention to the problem of medical errors or maybe it was just time to do so. The result was that an unprecedented number of seminal research studies delving into medical errors took place over the past 30 years to discover how many errors were occurring, what was causing them, and what their financial and human costs were.

The results have been disconcerting to say the least. Most studies have highlighted multiple concerns about quality of care, including high rates of provider-induced injury, unnecessary care, and inappropriate care. Many studies found the number of errors in health care to be unacceptably high. The seminal report of this time, *To Err Is Human*, published in 1999 by the National Academy of Medicine (NAM; formerly the Institute of Medicine [IOM]), a Congressionally chartered independent organization, provided evidence that the public was highly vulnerable to human error in U.S. health care institutions, an arena in which many thought they were safe.

In addition, unlike most health care research, which historically received limited national press, medical error research findings in the late 1990s were published and analyzed in almost every media forum in the country. Consumers were barraged with study findings suggesting that the quality of health care was inadequate and that medical errors were a significant problem leading to increased morbidity and mortality.

As a result, consumers, providers, and legislators stepped forward to voice their concerns and demand, at a minimum, a safer health care system. The government listened and directed providers to reexamine how quality health care was provided, measured, and monitored so that cultures of safety could be developed in all health care organizations.

This chapter examines seminal and current research on medical errors, medication errors, and adverse events, as well as the directives that emerged from their findings. Mechanisms for achieving four goals put forth by the IOM as part of *To Err Is Human* are identified. Finally, strategies for creating a culture of safety management in health care are identified, as are the challenges of changing a system that all too often focuses on individual errors rather than on the need to make system-wide changes.

DEFINING TERMS: MEDICAL ERRORS, MEDICATION ERRORS, AND ADVERSE EVENTS

In reviewing the literature on medical errors, medication errors, and adverse events in health care, it is helpful to first define common terms. *Medical errors* are defined by the *Encyclopedia of Surgery* (2021) as adverse events that could be prevented given the current state of medical knowledge. In addition, the Quality Interagency Coordination (QuIC) Task Force states that medical errors are "the failure of a planned action to be completed as intended or the use of a wrong plan to achieve an aim. Errors can include problems in practice, products, procedures, and systems" (Encyclopedia of Surgery, 2021, para. 3).

Medication errors are the most common type of medical errors and are a significant cause of preventable adverse events. *Medication errors* are defined by the National Coordinating Council for Medication Error Reporting and Prevention (NCC MERP) as:

> Any preventable event that may cause or lead to inappropriate medication use or patient harm while the medication is in the control of the health care professional, patient, or consumer. Such events may be related to professional practice, health care products, procedures, and systems, including prescribing; order communication; product labeling, packaging, and nomenclature; compounding; dispensing; distribution; administration; education; monitoring; and use. (U.S. Food and Drug Administration [FDA], 2020, para. 4)

Tariq et al. (2021) note that 7,000 to 9,000 people die each year in the United States because of a medication error. Additionally, hundreds of thousands of other patients experience an adverse reaction or other complication related to a medication, though many go unreported. In addition, the total cost of treating patients with medication-associated errors exceeds $40 billion each year (Tariq et al., 2021).

Finally, *adverse events* are defined as detrimental changes in health that occur because of treatment. When medications are involved, these are known as adverse drug events.

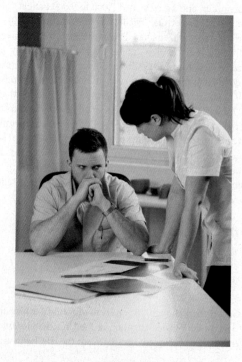

SEMINAL RESEARCH ON MEDICAL ERRORS: 1990 TO 2000

The last decade of the 20th century was marked by a rapid increase in research on medical errors. One of the earliest large-scale studies suggesting that medical errors were a significant problem in health care was published by Brennan and colleagues (1991) in *The New England Journal of Medicine*. This benchmark study involved more than 30,000 hospitalized patients in New York state. Nearly five of every 100 patients suffered an adverse event caused by a medical error of omission or commission. Of these adverse events, approximately one in four involved negligence. The overwhelming majority of iatrogenic occurrences, however, resulted from organization, system, or process failures. This study, extrapolated to the national population, suggested that 1.3 million people were injured each year in hospitals; of that number, 180,000 would die from those injuries. Providing additional cause for alarm, the report suggested that most of those injuries were preventable.

Leape and team (1991) also reported that drug complications represented 19% of these adverse events and that 45% of these adverse events were caused by medical errors. In this study, 30% of the individuals with drug-related injuries died.

In another study, Leape (1994) reported that the average intensive care unit (ICU) patient experienced almost two errors per day. One of five of these errors was potentially serious or fatal. This translates into a level of proficiency of approximately 99%, which seems reasonable. However, if performance levels of 99.9%—substantially better than those found in the ICU by Leape—were applied to the airline and banking industries, it would equate to two dangerous landings per day at Chicago's O'Hare International Airport, or 32,000 checks deducted hourly from the wrong account (Leape, 1994).

Discussion Point

The safety record in health care is a far cry from the enviable record of the similarly complex aviation industry. Should the health care industry be willing to accept higher error rates than the banking or airline industries? Why or why not? Is the public willing to do so?

Another seminal study in the late 1990s involving medical errors was completed by Thomas and colleagues (1999). Their research, based on a chart review of 14,732 medical records from 28 hospitals in Colorado and Utah, found that 265 of 459 (57%) adverse events were preventable. The total cost of adverse events was $661,889,000, with preventable adverse events costing an additional $308,382,000. In addition, the study estimated the national costs of all preventable adverse events to be just under $17 billion (in 1996, not since adjusted for inflation).

To Err Is Human

Many of the studies done in the 1990s laid the foundation for what is perhaps the best known and largest study ever done on the quality of health care: *To Err Is Human* (Kohn et al., 2000). This report, which represented a compilation of more than 30 studies completed by the NAM (formerly IOM), found:

- At least 44,000 Americans die each year as a result of medical errors, and the number may be as high as 98,000.
- Even when using the lower estimate, deaths because of medical errors could be considered the eighth leading cause of death in 1999.
- More people die in a given year as a result of medical errors than from motor vehicle accidents, breast cancer, or AIDS.

The IOM study also examined the types of errors that were occurring. Many of the adverse events were associated with the use of pharmaceutical agents and were potentially preventable. Medication errors alone, both in and out of the hospital, were estimated to account for more than 7,000 deaths in 1993, and one of every 854 inpatient hospital deaths was the result of a medication error. Children experienced harmful medication errors three times more often than adults (5.7% of medication orders for pediatric patients), and the rate was higher yet for neonates in the neonatal ICU. In addition, ICU patients suffered more life-threatening medication errors than any other patient population.

Consider This Pediatric patients are at even greater risk for medication errors than the general population because of weight-based dosing calculations and the misreading of decimal points.

Within a short time of the IOM report's release, some people began to question the numbers, asking whether the problem of medical errors could be as serious as it seemed. The first study to reliably confirm the IOM figures was a 2004 study by the health care ratings company (HealthGrades, 2004). This study looked at 3 years of Medicare data in all 50 states and Washington, DC, and reported that approximately 1.14 million patient safety incidents (PSIs) occurred among the 37 million hospitalizations in the Medicare population for the study period. The most commonly occurring PSIs were failure to rescue, decubitus ulcer, and postoperative sepsis.

Of the total 323,993 deaths among Medicare patients who developed one or more PSIs, 263,864, or 81%, of these deaths were directly attributable to the incidents (Health-Grades, 2004). In addition, one in every four Medicare patients who were hospitalized from 2000 to 2002 and experienced a PSI died. Perhaps most startling, however, was the conclusion that the United States loses more lives to PSIs every 6 months than it did in the entire Vietnam War. This also equates to three fully loaded jumbo jets crashing every other day for the last 5 years. Finally, the study noted that if the Centers for Disease Control and Prevention's (CDC) annual list of leading causes of death included medical errors, it would show up as number six, ahead of diabetes, pneumonia, Alzheimer disease, and renal disease (HealthGrades, 2004).

Additional reports since that time have repeatedly confirmed that the figures suggested in *To Err Is Human* were underreported. Indeed, 2013 study findings released by Patient Safety America suggested that up to 400,000 patients die each year as the result of medical errors (MacDonald, 2013). The lead researcher concluded that

There was much debate after the IOM report about the accuracy of its estimates. In a sense, it does not matter whether the deaths of 100,000, 200,000 or 400,000 Americans each year are associated with preventable adverse events in hospitals. Any of the estimates demand assertive action on the part of providers, legislators and people who will one day become patients. (MacDonald, 2013, para. 6)

Discussion Point

Is the U.S. public aware of the prevalence of medical errors? If not, what could be done to galvanize them to take action?

The Response to the National Academy of Medicine (Institute of Medicine) Report

Within weeks of the release of *To Err Is Human*, the U.S. Senate held its first hearings on the issue, and additional hearings were conducted by committees of both the U.S. House of Representatives and the Senate. Local, state, and national leaders, as well as private and public sector leaders, took immediate action. The significance of the report as a catalyst for change cannot be overstated.

That said, it is important to note that the problems of medical errors and patient safety were not completely unrecognized before *To Err Is Human* was published. Perhaps the most significant aspect of the study was that it summarized the high human cost of medical errors in language that was understandable by the public. In addition, previously an assumption had been made that most patient injuries were the result of negligence, incompetence, or corporate greed. The report indicated, however, that errors are simply a part of the human condition and that the health care system needed to be redesigned so that fewer errors would occur.

Because of these findings, the NAM (IOM) recommended a national goal of reducing the number of medical errors by 50% over 5 years (Kohn et al., 2000). To that end, it outlined a four-pronged approach to reducing medical mistakes nationwide (Box 15.1). The strategies needed to achieve this national goal and attend to each of the four approaches are numerous; however, only a few are detailed in this chapter.

WORKING TO ACHIEVE THE NATIONAL INSTITUTE OF MEDICINE GOALS

The first of the four-pronged approach to reducing medical errors was to "establish a national focus to create leadership, research, tools, and protocols to enhance the knowledge base about safety" (Kohn et al., 2000, p. 6). The second was to "raise standards and expectations for improvements in

BOX 15.1   The Institute of Medicine's Four-Pronged Approach to Reducing Medical Mistakes Nationwide

1. Establish a national focus to create leadership, research, tools, and protocols to enhance the knowledge base about safety.
2. Identify and learn from medical errors through both mandatory and voluntary reporting systems.
3. Raise standards and expectations for improvements in safety through the actions of oversight organizations, group purchasers, and professional groups.
4. Implement safe practices at the delivery level.

Source: Kohn, L. T., Corrigan, J. M., & Donaldson, M. S. (Eds.). (2000). *Executive summary. In To err is human: Building a safer health system* (pp. 1–6). Retrieved August 5, 2020, from https://www.nap.edu/read/9728/chapter/2

safety through the actions of oversight organizations, group purchasers, and professional groups" (Kohn et al., 2000, p. 6). Work to achieve both goals began almost immediately after the IOM report was published. Indeed, several national committees and groups were formed because of governmental or legislative intervention. Some of the committees, groups, and legislative efforts spearheading the task to reduce medical errors are outlined here.

Quality Interagency Coordination Task Force

The QuIC Task Force was established by former President Bill Clinton in 1998 to coordinate federal agencies that provided health care services. In December 1999, the task force began to evaluate the IOM recommendations and develop strategies for identifying threats to patient safety and reducing medical errors.

The final report, *Doing What Counts for Patient Safety: Federal Actions to Reduce Medical Errors and Their Impact*, was delivered in February 2000. The report proposed taking strong action on all the IOM recommendations to reduce errors, implementing a system of public accountability, developing a robust knowledge base about medical errors, and changing the culture in health care organizations to promote the recognition of errors and improvement in patient safety.

The National Forum for Health Care Quality Measurement and Reporting

Consistent with the QuIC's recommendations, the *National Forum for Health Care Quality Measurement and Reporting* was launched by former Vice President Al Gore in 2000. Known as the National Quality Forum (NQF, 2021a, 2021e), it is a broad-based, private, not-for-profit body that establishes standard quality measurement tools to help people better ensure the delivery of quality services. The mission of the NQF is to be the trusted voice driving measurable health improvements (para. 1).

Since its inception, the NQF has endorsed hundreds of performance measures and practices, and many more are either in the early stages of development or moving through the NQF endorsement process. NQF was also the first to create a list of 27 *serious reportable events* (SREs), a list that has grown to 29 as of 2021 (NQF, 2021b; Box 15.2).

In addition, the NQF board of directors approved expansion of their mission in 2008 to include working in partnership with other leadership organizations to establish national priorities and goals for performance measurement and public reporting. The first draft of their core set of national priorities was created in 2008. The National Quality Strategy as of 2021 (last updated in 2017) regarding aims, priorities, and levers is shown in Box 15.3.

Finally, the NQF was identified as the consensus-based entity for implementation of the Affordable Care Act (ACA), which launched in late 2011, including convening a multistakeholder group to provide annual input to the Department of Health and Human Services on the development of a National Quality Strategy (NQF, 2021c). The resulting National Priorities Partnership includes representatives from 51 major national organizations representing public and private sector stakeholder groups in a forum that balances the interests of consumers, purchasers, health plans, clinicians, providers, communities, states, and suppliers (NQF, 2021c).

The National Patient Safety Foundation

The *National Patient Safety Foundation* (NPSF) was also formed in response to the IOM report. The mission of the NPSF, as amended in 2003, is to partner with patients and families, the health care community, and key stakeholders to advance patient safety and health care workforce safety and disseminate strategies to prevent harm (Institute for Healthcare Improvement [IHI], 2021a).

In 2017, the NPSF merged with the IHI, which had been established in the late 1980s by Donald Berwick. The IHI is an independent not-for-profit organization focused on improvement capability; person- and family-centered care; patient safety; quality, cost, and value; and the triple aim for populations—improve care, improve population health, and reduce costs per capita (IHI, 2021a, 2021b). During the annual IHI Forum, the IHI highlights evidence-based best practices to translate research more rapidly into practice. In addition, the group maintains disciplined research and development processes and prototyping projects to pursue health care quality improvements (IHI, 2021c).

The Joint Commission

New organizations were not the only ones that responded to the recommendations of the IOM. *The Joint Commission*, established in 1951, accredits hospitals, long-term care facilities, psychiatric facilities, ambulatory care programs, and home health operations.

The Joint Commission's National Patient Safety Goals, implemented in January 2003, set forth clear, evidence-based recommendations to focus health care organizations on significant documented safety problems. These goals are updated annually for ambulatory care settings, behavioral health settings, hospitals, home care, disease-specific care, laboratories, home-based care, and office-based surgery. The 2021 goals for hospitals are listed in Box 15.4.

BOX 15.2   Serious Reportable Events in Health Care

1. Surgical or invasive procedure events
   - Surgery or other invasive procedure performed on the wrong site
   - Surgery or other invasive procedure performed on the wrong patient
   - Wrong surgical or other invasive procedure performed on a patient
   - Unintended retention of a foreign object in a patient after surgery or other invasive procedure
   - Intraoperative or immediately postoperative/postprocedure death in an American Society of Anesthesiologists Class 1 patient
2. Product or device events
   - Patient death or serious injury associated with the use of contaminated drugs, devices, or biologics provided by the health care setting
   - Patient death or serious injury associated with the use or function of a device in patient care, in which the device is used or functions other than as intended
   - Patient death or serious injury associated with intravascular air embolism that occurs while being cared for in a health care setting
3. Patient protection events
   - Discharge or release of a patient/resident of any age who is unable to make decisions to other than an authorized person
   - Patient death or serious injury associated with patient elopement (disappearance)
   - Patient suicide, attempted suicide, or self-harm that results in serious injury, while being cared for in a health care setting
4. Care management events
   - Patient death or serious injury associated with a medication error (i.e., errors involving the wrong drug, wrong dose, wrong patient, wrong time, wrong rate, wrong preparation, or wrong route of administration)
   - Patient death or serious injury associated with unsafe administration of blood products
   - Maternal death or serious injury associated with labor or delivery in a low-risk pregnancy while being cared for in a health care setting
   - Death or serious injury of a neonate associated with labor or delivery in a low-risk pregnancy
   - Patient death or serious injury associated with a fall while being cared for in a health care setting
   - Any stage 3, stage 4, and unstageable pressure injuries acquired after admission or presentation to a health care setting
   - Artificial insemination with the wrong donor sperm or wrong egg
   - Patient death or serious injury resulting from the irretrievable loss of an irreplaceable biologic specimen
   - Patient death or serious injury resulting from failure to follow up or communicate laboratory, pathology, or radiology test results
5. Environmental events
   - Patient or staff death or serious injury associated with an electric shock in the course of a patient care process in a health care setting
   - Any incident in which systems designated for oxygen or other gas to be delivered to a patient contains no gas, the wrong gas, or is contaminated by toxic substances
   - Patient or staff death or serious injury associated with a burn incurred from any source in the course of a patient care process in a health care setting
   - Patient death or serious injury associated with the use of physical restraints or bed rails while being cared for in a health care setting
6. Radiologic events: Death or serious injury of a patient or staff associated with the introduction of a metallic object into the magnetic resonance imaging area
7. Potential criminal events
   - Any instance of care ordered by or provided by someone impersonating a physician, nurse, pharmacist, or other licensed health care provider
   - Abduction of a patient/resident of any age
   - Sexual abuse/assault on a patient or staff member within or on the grounds of a health care setting
   - Death or serious injury of a patient or staff member resulting from a physical assault (i.e., battery) that occurs within or on the grounds of a health care setting

---

Source: National Quality Forum. (2021a). *NQF's mission, vision, and values.* Retrieved July 27, 2021, from http://www.qualityforum.org/about_nqf/mission_and_vision; National Quality Forum. (2021b). *List of SREs.* Retrieved July 27, 2021, from http://www.qualityforum.org/Topics/SREs/List_of_SREs.aspx

> **BOX 15.3** **The National Quality Strategy (2017): Aims, Priorities, and Levers**
>
> ## Aims
> These aims guide and assess local, state, and national efforts to improve health and the quality of health care.
> * *Better Care*: Improve the overall quality by making health care more patient-centered, reliable, accessible, and safe.
> * *Healthy People/Healthy Communities*: Improve the health of the U.S. population by supporting proven interventions to address behavioral, social, and environmental determinants of health in addition to delivering higher-quality care.
> * *Affordable Care:* Reduce the cost of quality health care for individuals, families, employers, and government.
>
> ## Priorities
> The National Quality Strategy focuses on six priorities:
> 1. Making care safer by reducing harm caused in the delivery of care
> 2. Ensuring that each person and family is engaged as partners in their care
> 3. Promoting effective communication and coordination of care
> 4. Promoting the most effective prevention and treatment practices for the leading causes of mortality, starting with cardiovascular disease
> 5. Working with communities to promote wide use of best practices to enable healthy living
> 6. Making quality care more affordable for individuals, families, employers, and governments by developing and spreading new health care delivery models
>
> ## Levers
> Each of the nine National Quality Strategy levers represents a core business function, resource, and/or action that stakeholders can use to align to the strategy.
> * *Public Reporting*: Compare treatment results, costs, and patient experience for consumers.
> * *Learning and Technical Assistance*: Foster learning environments that offer training, resources, tools, and guidance to help organizations achieve quality improvement goals.
> * *Certification, Accreditation, and Regulation*: Adopt or adhere to approaches to meet safety and quality standards.
> * *Consumer Incentives and Benefit Designs*: Help consumers adopt healthy behaviors and make informed decisions.
> * *Payment*: Reward and incentivize providers to deliver high-quality, patient-centered care.
> * *Health Information Technology*: Improve communication, transparency, and efficiency for better coordinated health and health care.
> * *Innovation and Diffusion*: Foster innovation in health care quality improvement, and facilitate rapid adoption within and across organizations and communities.
> * *Workforce Development*: Invest in people to prepare the next generation of health care professionals and support lifelong learning for providers.
>
> *Source:* National Quality Strategy. (2017). *About the National Quality Strategy (NQS)*. Retrieved July 27, 2021, from https://www.ahrq.gov/workingforquality/about/index.html#aims

> **BOX 15.4** **The Joint Commission 2021 National Patient Safety Goals for Hospitals**
>
> 1. Improve the accuracy of patient identification.
> 2. Improve staff communication.
> 3. Improve the safety of medication administration.
> 4. Reduce patient harm associated with clinical alarm systems.
> 5. Reduce the risk of health care–associated infections.
> 6. Better identify patient safety risks in the hospital.
> 7. Better prevent surgical mistakes.
>
> *Source:* The Joint Commission. (2021). *2021 National patient safety goals*. Retrieved July 27, 2021, from https://www.checklistboards.com/article.cfm?ArticleNumber=177#:~:text=The%20Joint%20Commission%27s%202021%20national%20patient%20safety%20goals,in%20the%20hospital.%207%20Better%20prevent%20surgical%20mistakes

The Joint Commission also maintains one of the nation's most comprehensive databases of sentinel (serious adverse) events by health care professionals and their underlying causes. A *sentinel event* is defined by The Joint Commission (2021) as "a Patient Safety Event (not primarily related to the natural course of the patient's illness or underlying condition), that results in either death, permanent harm, or severe temporary harm and intervention required to sustain life" (para. 2). Such events are called *sentinel* because they signal the need for immediate investigation and response. Information from The Joint Commission sentinel database is regularly shared with accredited organizations to help them take appropriate steps to prevent medical errors.

Another one of The Joint Commission priorities is the development of a *root cause analysis* (RCA) with a plan of correction for the errors that do occur. RCA is a process widely used by health professionals to learn how and why errors occurred. The purpose is to identify system vulnerabilities so that they can be eliminated or mitigated rather than focusing on or addressing individual performance, since individual performance is generally a symptom of larger, systems-based issues (IHI, 2021d).

The Joint Commission's (2021) Sentinel Event Policy requests that organizations that are either voluntarily reporting a sentinel event or responding to The Joint Commission's inquiry about a sentinel event submit their related RCA and action plan electronically to The Joint Commission whenever such events occur. The sentinel event data are then reviewed, and recommendations are made. The Joint Commission defends the confidentiality of the information, if necessary, in court.

Similarly, some organizations use a *failure mode and effects analysis* to examine all possible failures in a design—including sequencing of events, actual and potential risk, points of vulnerability, and areas for improvement (American Society for Quality, 2021).

Consider This National legislation designed to keep such error analyses confidential is a critical but still unrealized step. This discourages error reporting.

Centers for Medicare & Medicaid Services

The Centers for Medicare & Medicaid Services (CMS), formerly the Health Care Financing Administration, also plays an active role in setting standards and measuring quality of health care. With the introduction of the Medicare Quality Initiatives in November 2001, a new era of public reporting on quality began. These diverse initiatives encouraged the public reporting of quality measures for nursing homes, home health agencies, hospitals, and kidney dialysis facilities. These data are then made available to consumers on the Medicare website to assist them in making health care choices or decisions.

Consider This Although few organizations would argue against the benefits of well-developed and well-implemented quality control programs, quality control in health care organizations has evolved primarily from external effects and not as a voluntary monitoring effort.

Medicare also established *pay for performance* (P4P), also known as *quality-based purchasing*, in the middle of the first decade of the 21st century. Because research suggested little relationship between quality of care provided and the cost of that care, P4P initiatives were created to align payment and quality incentives and to reduce costs through improved quality and efficiency.

As part of P4P, the *Physician Quality Reporting Initiative* (PQRI), launched in 2007, allowed for payments to eligible professionals who satisfactorily reported quality information to Medicare. The *Medicare Improvements for Patients and Providers Act* of 2008 made the PQRI program permanent.

With the introduction of the ACA in 2011, the PQRI was changed to the *Physician Quality Reporting System* (PQRS), and incentive payments were established for successfully reporting PQRS measures. An additional incentive payment was possible for providers who qualified for or maintained board certification status, participated in maintenance of certification programs, and successfully completed a qualified maintenance of certification program practice assessment.

The PQRS program, however, ended at the end of 2016, transitioning to the *Merit-Based Incentive Payment System* (MIPS) under the Quality Payment Program (QPP, n.d.). Providers receive incentive pay or payment adjustments depending on the amount and quality of data provided. Thus, PQRS transitioned from incentive payments to penalty charges if quality data are not submitted.

Discussion Point

Should it be necessary to pay health care professionals bonuses to submit quality information? Do you believe incentives or penalty charges are a stronger motivation for provider data submission?

Also as part of the ACA, the CMS has now instituted hospital *value-based purchasing* (VBP). In this program, participating hospitals are paid for inpatient acute care services based on the quality of care, not just quantity of the services they provide. The program uses the hospital quality data reporting infrastructure developed for the *Hospital Inpatient Quality Reporting Program*, which was authorized by Section 501(b) of the Medicare Prescription Drug, Improvement, and Modernization Act of 2003 (CMS, 2021).

The hospital VBP program was funded in 2021 by reducing participating hospitals' base operating Medicare diagnosis-related group payments by 2%. Any leftover funds are redistributed to hospitals based on their *total performance scores*. It is possible for a hospital to earn back a value-based incentive payment percentage that is less than, equal to, or more than the applicable reduction for that fiscal year (CMS, 2021).

In addition, to reduce the number of preventable medical errors, including *never events* (i.e., errors that should never happen, such as removing the wrong limb in surgery, leaving a foreign object inside a patient during surgery, or sending a baby home with the wrong parents), Medicare announced that as of October 1, 2008, it would no longer pay for care that was required as a result of eight specific preventable errors or never events identified by the NQF. Medicaid followed suit in 2011. Private insurance companies are also taking this path. These policies require hospitals to maintain meticulous documentation about what conditions are present on admission to differentiate between preexisting conditions and those that are acquired during the hospital stay (NQF, 2021d; Box 15.5).

Discussion Point

Should public or private insurance plans refuse to pay for care that is extended due to medical errors?

Quality and Safety Education for Nurses Project

The Quality and Safety Education for Nurses (QSEN) project funded by Robert Wood Johnson Foundation began in 2005 with the goal of preparing future nurses who will have the knowledge, skills, and attitudes (KSAs) necessary to continuously improve the quality and safety of the health care systems within which they work (QSEN Institute, 2020a). When nurses have these KSAs, they are better able to identify potential errors and intervene before errors occur.

QSEN is best known, however, for having identified quality and safety competencies for nursing including patient-centered care, teamwork and collaboration, evidence-based practice (EBP), quality improvement, safety, and informatics (QSEN Institute, 2020b). Definitions for these competencies and the KSAs associated with each competency are detailed on the QSEN website (QSEN Institute, 2020b).

HEALTH CARE REPORT CARDS

In response to the demand for objective measures of quality, including the number and type of medical errors, many health plans, health care providers, employer purchasing groups, consumer information organizations, and state governments have begun to formulate health care quality report cards. Most states have laws requiring providers to report some type of data. The Agency for Healthcare Research and Quality (AHRQ) has also been working to create a report card for the nation's health care delivery system. Currently, its website includes an annual National Healthcare Quality and Disparities report (AHRQ, n.d.-a). This report is mandated by Congress to provide a comprehensive

---

BOX 15.5   **The National Quality Forum's Seven Categories of Serious Reportable Events**

1. Surgical or invasive procedure events
2. Product or device events
3. Patient protection events
4. Care management events
5. Environmental events
6. Radiologic events
7. Potential criminal events

Source: National Quality Forum. (2021d). *Serious reportable events.* Retrieved July 27, 2021, from http://www.qualityforum.org/Topics/SREs/Serious_Reportable_Events.aspx

overview of the quality of health care received by the general U.S. population and disparities in care experienced by different racial and socioeconomic groups. The report is produced with the help of an Interagency Work Group led by AHRQ (AHRQ, n.d.-b).

In addition, the National Committee for Quality Assurance's Health Plan Report Card lets an individual create a health plan report card online. In addition, CMS released a proposed rule in June 2011 that would make Medicare information regarding provider cost and quality available to certain organizations.

It is important to remember, however, that many report cards do not contain information about the quality of care rendered by specific clinics, group practices, or physicians in a health plan's network. In addition, most report cards focus on service utilization data and patient satisfaction ratings and have minimal data regarding medical errors.

In addition, Grause (2019) notes that not all report cards are created equal. Each hospital report card, whether it comes from Leapfrog, U.S. News & World Report, or CMS, uses its own approach, deciding which measures to include or exclude and often using different data sources and time frames. Some even use self-reported surveys. This is why health plans may receive conflicting ratings on different report cards.

Grause (2019) also points out that instead of using detailed clinical data from medical records, many report card organizations use administrative information from medical bills to draw conclusions about care quality. The composite measures may not be an accurate representation of hospital quality. To further complicate matters, hospital report cards rely heavily on publicly available data sets based on the mostly age 65 and older Medicare population. These outdated data are often not generalizable to the entire population, particularly for patients looking for maternity care or other services that lend themselves to prior decision making (Grause, 2019).

> **Consider This** "The proliferation of different and sometimes contradictory hospital report cards is confusing patients. People want reliable information to make informed decisions about their care. Instead, they find a cacophony of contradictory reports and ratings."
>
> —Bea Grause, RN, JD, President, Healthcare Association of New York State (Grause, 2019)

Report cards might also not be readily accessible or might be difficult for the average consumer to understand.

Still, there is no doubt that consumers want more access to meaningful quality-of-care information, and it is apparent that such data, which have long been kept secret, are now becoming public.

> **Discussion Point**
>
> Do you consider the care you receive from your primary care provider to be of a high quality? Are your perceptions subjective, or do you have objective data to back up your impression? Have you actively searched for such data on your primary care provider?

CREATING A CULTURE OF SAFETY MANAGEMENT

In response to public forces and professional concerns, patient safety has become one of the nation's most pressing challenges and a mandate for every health care organization. Indeed, the final recommendation of the IOM report was to implement safe practices at the delivery level. The strategies that have been recommended to achieve this goal are overwhelming, both in scope and quantity.

Strategies discussed in this chapter include the *Six Sigma* approach (a customer-based management philosophy) to error management; the mandatory/voluntary reporting of errors; attempts to increase confidentiality of reporting to reduce the fear of legal liability for reporting errors that do occur; the Leapfrog recommendations; the use of bar coding; the development of patient safety solutions by the World Health Organization's (WHO) World Alliance for Patient Safety; and a change in organizational cultures from that of "individual blame" to error identification and system modification.

> **Consider This** Because quality health care is a complex phenomenon, the factors contributing to quality in health care are as varied as the strategies needed to achieve this elusive goal.

A Six Sigma Approach

One approach that has been taken to create a culture of safety management at the institutional level has been the implementation of the Six Sigma approach. *Sigma* is a statistical measurement that reflects how well a product or process is performing. Higher sigma values indicate better performance. Historically, the health care industry has been comfortable striving for three-sigma processes (all data points fall within three standard deviations) in terms of health care quality instead of six. This is one reason why health care has more errors than the banking and airline industries, in which achieving Six Sigma is the expectation. Organizations aim for this lofty target by carefully applying Six Sigma methodology to every aspect of a product or process.

> ### Discussion Point
>
> Is a Six Sigma failure rate a reasonable goal for all health care organizations? Should some health care organizations be expected to have higher failure (defect) rates than others? What variables might affect an organization's ability to achieve this goal?

Mandatory Reporting of Errors

The third prong of the IOM's four-pronged approach to creating a safer health care system was "to identify and learn from medical errors through both mandatory and voluntary reporting systems" (Kohn et al., 2000, p. 6). To accomplish this, the IOM report recommended developing a mandatory reporting system for medical errors and adverse events at both the state and national levels.

> ### Discussion Point
>
> Do you believe the majority of medical errors are reported? Why or why not? Do you believe that error disclosure rates differ between nurses and physicians? If so, which professional group do you believe might be more likely to disclose errors and why?

State mandates for reporting medical errors and adverse events have been slow to materialize, though as of 2020, a total of 25 states required hospitals and/or other medical facilities to report serious medical errors (Lockwood, 2020), and some states also have reporting mandates that apply only to specific types of error, such as hospital-acquired infections. It is important to note that the IOM report did suggest, in addition to mandatory reporting, that more options be created for limited voluntary reporting systems in all 50 states. The IOM also recommended that more research be conducted on how best to develop voluntary reporting systems that complement proposed mandatory reporting systems.

Increased mandatory and voluntary reporting must also occur at the institutional level, as well as by individual providers. As a result, the IOM report suggested that mandatory adverse event reporting should initially be required of hospitals and eventually of other institutional and ambulatory care delivery facilities. This was the impetus for the subsequent The Joint Commission action for sentinel event reporting as part of the accreditation process.

Yet, even when error rates are reported, there is some question as to the accuracy of the reported data. Many hospitals erroneously rely on incident reporting as their key quality and safety measure. It is difficult, however, to enforce greater disclosure and reporting at the individual provider level. Ethical and professional guidelines suggest that providers have a responsibility to disclose medical errors. Yet, the literature continues to suggest that this does not happen because of a fear of legal suits or disciplinary measures by employers. Indeed, recent research by Sattar et al. (2020) noted that full disclosure of adverse events by health care providers often does not occur due to the existence of a blame culture, the fear of litigation, and a lack of skills on how to conduct disclosure (Research Fuels the Controversy 15.1). The ironic part is that full disclosure of errors often reduces the likelihood of legal suit or the extent of patient retribution.

Perhaps this failure to disclose medical errors is a major contributor to the disconnect that exists between consumers' perceptions of the quality of their health care and the actual quality provided. Even consumers who are aware of medical error statistics often report that they believe medical errors to be a problem but believe that such errors will not happen to them because they trust and believe in their own health care providers.

Legal Liability and Medical Error Reporting

If high-quality health care is to be achieved, the medical liability system and our litigious society must be recognized as potential barriers to systematic efforts to uncover and learn from mistakes that are made in health care. One recommendation of the IOM panel was to encourage learning about safety from cross-institutional reporting systems for errors. This reporting is inhibited by fears that such data will be discovered in liability lawsuits.

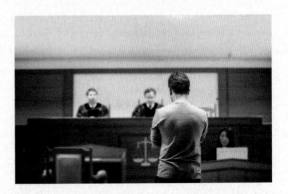

Research Fuels the Controversy 15.1

The Disclosure of Adverse Events

This systematic review of qualitative studies examined the views and experiences of patients, family members, and health care professionals (HCPs) on the disclosure of adverse events. Qualitative data were analyzed using a meta-ethnographic approach, comprising reciprocal syntheses of "patient" and "health care professional" studies, combined to form a lines-of-argument synthesis embodying both perspectives. Fifteen studies were included in the final syntheses.

Source: Sattar, R., Johnson, J., & Lawton, R. (2020). The views and experiences of patients and health-care professionals on the disclosure of adverse events: A systematic review and qualitative meta-ethnographic synthesis. *Health Expectations, 23*(3), 571–583. https://doi .org/10.1111/hex.13029

Findings

The results highlighted differences in attitudes and expectations between patients and HCPs regarding disclosure. Patients/family members expressed a need for information, the importance of sincere regret, and a promise of improvement. A majority of the time, patients did not feel satisfied with the disclosure or felt they were provided with partial disclosure that did not include all the elements they desired.

While HCPs considered disclosure to be a moral and professional duty, they reported barriers to appropriate disclosure, including the difficulty of disclosure in a blame culture, avoidance of litigation, lack of skills on how to conduct disclosure, and inconsistent guidance.

In addition, HCPs assumed that in cases in which the error was not obvious or evident, the patient would rather not be informed. The impact of an error on the patient, whether it resulted in an adverse event, and the severity of the adverse event also influenced whether disclosure occurred. When adverse events were minor or there was no substantial harm resulting from errors, disclosure was not believed to be of importance.

Researchers concluded that a gap exists between the expected communication practices of HCPs regarding disclosure and what is being done. They recommended the development of consistent and transparent policies at the organizational level regarding disclosure as well as the shifting away from a blame culture to facilitate effective disclosure.

Discussion Point

Have you ever encouraged a family member, friend, or colleague to seek compensation for medical errors? If so, do you think this was the most appropriate means of redress?

The provision of stronger confidentiality protections likely would improve the voluntary sharing of data. In 2002, the *Patient Safety Improvement Act* was introduced in the U.S. House of Representatives. This bill provided legal protections for medical error reporting, stating that error information voluntarily submitted to patient safety organizations could not be subpoenaed or used in legal discovery. It also generally required that the information be treated as confidential. After multiple revisions, the final legislation, called the *Patient Safety and Quality Improvement Act of 2005*, was signed into law by former President George W. Bush.

Federal legislation has also been proposed to protect the voluntary reporting of ordinary injuries and "near misses"—errors that did not cause harm this time but easily could the next time. This would be like what is done in aviation, in which near misses are confidentially reported and can be analyzed by anyone.

Dr. Danielle Ofri suggests that the reporting of errors—including the "near misses"—is key to improving the health care system, but she says that shame and guilt prevent medical personnel from admitting their mistakes. "If we don't talk about the emotions that keep doctors and nurses from speaking up, we'll never solve this problem" (Davies, 2020, para. 5).

Consider This "Near misses are the huge iceberg below the surface where all the future errors are occurring," she says. "But we don't know where they are ... so we don't know where to send our resources to fix them or make it less likely to happen" (Davies, 2020, para. 4).

Leapfrog Group

The Leapfrog Group is a conglomeration of non–health care *Fortune 500* leaders dedicated to reducing preventable medical mistakes and improving the quality and affordability of health care. Leapfrog started with a set of simple, focused principles that suggested people should have access to information to make informed decisions about their health care, and purchasers should pay for the best outcomes at the best price (Leapfrog Group, n.d.-a). In addition, the group has advised the health care industry that big leaps in patient safety and customer value can occur if specific evidence-based standards are implemented, including (1) computerized physician (or prescriber) order entry (CPOE); (2) evidence-based hospital referral (EHR); and (3) ICU physician staffing (IPS).

CPOE is a promising technology that allows providers to enter orders into a computer instead of handwriting them. Studies have also shown that CPOE reduces length of stay; reduces repeat tests; reduces turnaround times for laboratory, pharmacy, and radiology requests; and delivers cost savings (Leapfrog Group, n.d.-b). To verify, however, that hospital CPOE systems stay current with changes in available medications and in recordkeeping systems, Leapfrog developed an evaluation tool in collaboration with leading academic researchers. Hospitals enter simulated patient data into their systems and are then given a list of orders—some containing a potentially harmful or even fatal error—to run through their CPOE system.

EHR involves making sure that patients with high-risk conditions are treated at hospitals with characteristics that are associated with better outcomes. Indeed, Leapfrog (2020) notes that three decades of research have consistently demonstrated that patients who have high-risk surgeries at hospitals and by surgeons who have more experience with the procedure have better outcomes, including lower mortality rates, lower complication rates, and shorter lengths of stay than patients who have their surgery done at hospitals or by surgeons with less experience. Leapfrog (2020) notes, however, that lower surgical mortality at high-volume hospitals does not simply reflect more skillful surgeons and fewer technical errors with the procedure itself. More likely, it reflects more proficiency with all aspects of care.

IPS considers the level of training of ICU medical personnel. Evidence suggests that quality of care in hospital ICUs is strongly influenced by whether "intensivists" (those familiar with ICU complications) are providing care and how the staff is organized (Leapfrog Group, n.d.-c). Mortality rates are significantly lower in hospitals with ICUs managed exclusively by board-certified intensivists. "Research has shown that hospitals staffing their ICUs with doctors specializing in critical care medicine can reduce ICU mortality by as much as 40%" (Leapfrog Group, n.d.-c, para. 3).

Barcoding Medications

In addition, Leapfrog has endorsed the use of barcoding to reduce point-of-care medication errors. Per a FDA rule adopted in April 2004, all prescription and over-the-counter medications used in hospitals must contain a national drug code number. The FDA suggested that a barcode system coupled with a CPOE system would greatly enhance the ability of all health care workers to follow the "five rights" of medication administration—that the *right* person receives the *right* drug, in the *right* dose, via the *right* route, at the *right* administration time.

In addition, The Joint Commission originally proposed in its 2005 National Patient Safety Goals and Requirements that accredited organizations would have to implement barcode technology to identify patients and match them to their medications or other treatments by January 2007. Because of implementation concerns, especially in terms of costs, this proposal was abandoned by The Joint Commission in July 2004.

It is noteworthy, however, that although barcode medication administration (BCMA) increases the likelihood of the right patient receiving the right medication at the right dose at the right time, errors still occur. Sometimes, this occurs because the wrong patient is scanned or because staff pursue workarounds that end up causing errors.

Patient Safety Solutions

Recognizing that health care errors affect at least one in every 10 patients around the world, the WHO's World Alliance for Patient Safety and the Collaborating Centre packaged effective solutions called *patient safety solutions* to reduce such errors. A patient safety solution was defined as any system design or intervention that has demonstrated the ability to prevent or mitigate patient harm stemming from the processes of health care and is based on interventions and actions that have reduced problems related to patient safety in some countries (WHO, 2019).

The first package, implemented in 2005, focused on health care–associated infection and hand hygiene in health care. The second package, implemented in 2008, prioritized the use of surgery checklists during the three phases of an operation. The third and most recent package was implemented in 2017 and addressed a number of issues related to medication safety (WHO, 2017). See Box 15.6.

Countries are requested to prioritize action on medication safety, designate leaders to drive action, and devise their own tailored programs centered on local priorities. The WHO will provide support to countries for developing national programs, instigating large-scale international research, providing guidance, and developing practical tools for frontline health workers and patients (WHO, 2019).

Consider This The WHO (2019) notes that globally, the cost associated with medication errors is US$42 billion annually.

Promoting Just Cultures

Perhaps though, the most significant change that must occur before a national culture of safety management can exist is that organizational cultures must be created that remove blame from the individual and instead focus on how the organization can be modified to reduce the likelihood of such errors occurring in the future. Cultures where voluntary reporting is encouraged and constructive feedback is given to those who self-report are often called *just cultures*. Just cultures will be needed to encourage voluntary reporting and reduce the prevalence of errors. Just cultures exhibit "giving constructive feedback and critical analysis in skillful ways, during assessments based on facts, and having respect for the complexity of the situation" (Barry, n.d., para. 5).

This type of intervention encourages people to reveal the errors they have made so that the organization can learn from them.

Consider This Ignoring the problem of medical errors, denying their existence, or blaming the individuals involved in the processes do nothing to eliminate the underlying problems.

CONCLUSIONS

Medical errors are not the only indicator of quality of care. They are, however, a pervasive problem in the current health care system and one of the greatest threats to quality health care. Nurses are uniquely positioned to identify, interrupt, and correct medical errors and to minimize preventable adverse outcomes.

Clearly, a punitive approach to medical errors is not productive, and errors will not be reported if workers fear the consequences. Employees and patients need to feel comfortable and without fear of personal risk in reporting hazards that can affect patient safety.

Efforts to reduce medical errors, however, over the last decade have not resulted in the achievement of desired outcomes. There is a plethora of current studies that suggest that the health care system continues to be riddled with errors and that patient and worker safety is compromised. Yet, movement toward the IOM goals is occurring. It is likely that there has never been another time when the public, providers, and government have worked together so closely to achieve a shared health care goal.

Much, however, remains to be done. Sustained public interest will be needed to create the momentum necessary to systematically change the health care system in a way that

---

BOX 15.6   World Health Organization's Global Patient Safety Challenges Implemented to Date

1. *Clean care is safer care* (implemented 2005): Focuses on health care–associated infection and hand hygiene in health care
2. *Safe surgery saves lives* (implemented 2008): Prioritizes the use of surgery checklists at three phases of an operation: before the induction of anesthesia ("sign in"), before the incision of the skin ("time out"), and before the patient leaves the operating room ("sign out")
3. *Medication without harm* (implemented 2017): Aims to reduce the level of severe, avoidable harm related to medications globally by 50% over 5 years

Source: World Health Organization. (2019). *Patient safety.* Retrieved July 27, 2021, from https://www.who.int/news-room/fact-sheets/detail/patient-safety

reduces patients' vulnerability to medical errors. In addition, although there has been a great deal of talk about using a systems approach to address the problem of medical errors, there has not been much discussion regarding exactly how this integration is to be accomplished. The bottom line is that significant and continuous reform of the health care system will be needed before the problem of medical errors shows any resolution.

For Additional Discussion

1. If cost containment and quality goals conflict, which do you think will take precedence in health care organizations today?

2. Despite stated dissatisfaction levels, why do so many providers feel helpless about reducing medical errors and improving the quality of health care?

3. Why have quality control efforts in health care organizations evolved primarily from external requirements and not as voluntary monitoring efforts?

4. Where does individual provider responsibility and accountability begin and end in a culture in which medical errors are recognized as being a failure of the system?

5. How common is it that medical error documentation is used against employees as part of the performance appraisal process? If so, does this discourage reporting?

6. Does the average consumer have access to and an accurate understanding of health care report cards?

7. Given that most individuals can quickly identify medical errors that have happened to them, a friend, or a family member, why does the U.S. public seem so reluctant to accept that medical errors constitute a threat to the quality of their health care?

8. Has your fear of legal liability ever influenced your decision to report a medical error?

References

Agency for Healthcare Research and Quality. (n.d.-a). *National healthcare quality and disparities reports.* Retrieved July 27, 2021, from https://nhqrnet.ahrq.gov/inhqrdr/state/select

Agency for Healthcare Research and Quality. (n.d.-b). *2019 National healthcare quality and disparities report.* Retrieved July 27, 2021, from https://nhqrnet.ahrq.gov/inhqrdr/reports/qdr

American Society for Quality. (2021). *Failure mode and effects analysis (FMEA).* Retrieved July 27, 2021, from http://asq.org/learn-about-quality/process-analysis-tools/overview/fmea.html

Barry, T. (n.d.). *Patient safety and "just culture."* Retrieved July 28, 2021, from https://www.uclahealth.org/quality/Workfiles/quality/Patient-Safety-and-just-culture.pdf

BMJ. (2020, June 11). *237+ million medication errors made every year in England: Avoidable consequences cost NHS upwards of £98 million and 1700+ lives every year.* Science Daily. Retrieved July 27, 2021, from https://www.sciencedaily.com/releases/2020/06/200611183921.htm

Brennan, T. A., Leape, L. L., Laird, N. M., Hebert, L., Localio, A. R., Lawthers, A. G., Newhouse, J., Weiler, P., & Hiatt, H. H. (1991). Incidence of adverse events and negligence in hospitalized patients: Results from the Harvard Medical Practice Study 1. *The New England Journal of Medicine, 324*(6), 370–376. https://doi.org/10.1056/NEJM199102073240604

Centers for Medicare & Medicaid Services. (2021, February 18). *Hospital value-based purchasing program.* Retrieved July 27, 2021, from https://www.cms.gov/Medicare/Quality-Initiatives-Patient-Assessment-Instruments/HospitalQualityInits/Hospital-Value-Based-Purchasing-.html

Davies, D. (2020, June 30). *A doctor confronts medical errors—And flaws in the system that create mistakes.* NPR Fresh Air. Retrieved July 27, 2021, from https://www.npr.org/sections/health-shots/2020/06/30/885186438/a-doctor-confronts-medical-errors-and-flaws-in-the-system-that-create-mistakes

Desjardins, L. (2019, October 28). *Thousands die from medical errors yearly, notes advocacy group.* Radio Canada International. Retrieved July 27, 2021, from https://www.rcinet.ca/en/2019/10/28/thousands-die-from-medical-errors-yearly-notes-advocacy-group/

Encyclopedia of Surgery. (2021). *Medical errors: Introduction and definitions.* Advameg, Inc. Retrieved July 27, 2021, from http://www.surgeryencyclopedia.com/La-Pa/Medical-Errors.html

Grause, B. (2019, November 20). *Hospitals give report cards a taste of their own medicine.* Becker's Hospital Review. Retrieved July 27, 2021, from https://www.beckershospitalreview.com/rankings-and-ratings/hospitals-give-report-cards-a-taste-of-their-own-medicine.html

HealthGrades. (2004, July). *HealthGrades quality study: Patient safety in American hospitals.* Retrieved July 27, 2021, from http://www.providersedge.com/ehdocs/ehr_articles/Patient_Safety_in_American_Hospitals-2004.pdf

Institute for Healthcare Improvement. (2021a). *About us. Patient safety.* Retrieved July 27, 2021, from http://www.ihi.org/Topics/PatientSafety/Pages/default.aspx

Institute for Healthcare Improvement. (2021b). *About us. History.* Retrieved July 27, 2021, from http://www.ihi.org/about/pages/history.aspx

Institute for Healthcare Improvement. (2021c). *IHI Forum 2021.* Retrieved July 27, 2021 from http://www.ihi.org/education/Conferences/National-Forum/Pages/default.aspx?utm_source=IHI_Homepage&utm_medium=Education_Navigation&utm_campaign=2020_Forum

Institute for Healthcare Improvement. (2021d). *RCA2: Improving root cause analyses and actions to prevent harm.* Retrieved July 27, 2021, from http://www.ihi.org/resources/Pages/Tools/RCA2-Improving-Root-Cause-Analyses-and-Actions-to-Prevent-Harm.aspx

Joint Commission. (2021). *The Sentinel event policy and procedures.* Retrieved July 27, 2021, from https://www.jointcommission.org/sentinel_event_policy_and_procedures

Kohn, L. T., Corrigan, J. M., & Donaldson, M. S. (Eds.). (2000). *Executive summary. To err is human: Building a safer health system* (pp. 1–6). Retrieved July 27, 2021, from https://www.nap.edu/read/9728/chapter/2

Leape, L. L. (1994). Error in medicine. *Journal of the American Medical Association, 272*(23), 1851–1857. https://doi.org/10.1001/jama.1994.03520230061039

Leape, L. L., Brennan, T. A., Laird, N., Lawthers, A. G., Localio, A. R., Barnes, B. A., Hebert, L., Newhouse, J. P., Weiler, P. C., & Hiatt, H. (1991). The nature of adverse events in hospitalized patients: Results of the Harvard Medical Practice Study II. *New England Journal of Medicine, 324*(6), 377–384. https://doi.org/10.1056/NEJM199102073240605

Leapfrog Group. (2020, April 1). *Fact sheet: Inpatient surgery.* Retrieved July 27, 2021, from https://www.leapfroggroup.org/sites/default/files/Files/2020%20Surgical%20Volume-Appropriateness%20Fact%20Sheet.pdf

Leapfrog Group. (n.d.-a). *History.* Retrieved July 27, 2021, from https://www.leapfroggroup.org/about/history

Leapfrog Group. (n.d.-b). *Safe medication ordering.* Retrieved July 27, 2021, from http://www.leapfroggroup.org/ratings-reports/computerized-physician-order-entry

Leapfrog Group. (n.d.-c). *Specially trained doctors care for critical care patients.* Retrieved July 27, 2021, from http://www.leapfroggroup.org/ratings-reports/icu-physician-staffing

Lockwood, W. (2020, April). *Prevention of medical errors and medication errors.* Retrieved July 27, 2021, from http://www.rn.org/courses/coursematerial-135.pdf

MacDonald, I. (2013, September 20). *Hospital medical errors now the third leading cause of death in the U.S.: New study highlights the fact that estimates in "To Err is Human" report were low.* Fierce Healthcare. Retrieved July 27, 2021, from http://www.fiercehealthcare.com/story/hospital-medical-errors-third-leading-cause-death-dispute-to-err-is-human-report/2013-09-20

Medical error statistics. (2020). My Medical Score. Retrieved July 27, 2021, from https://mymedicalscore.com/medical-error-statistics/

National Quality Forum. (2021a). *NQF's mission, vision, and values.* Retrieved July 27, 2021, from http://www.qualityforum.org/about_nqf/mission_and_vision

National Quality Forum. (2021b). *List of SREs.* Retrieved July 27, 2021, from http://www.qualityforum.org/Topics/SREs/List_of_SREs.aspx

National Quality Forum. (2021c). *NQF: National priorities partnership.* Retrieved July 27, 2021, from http://www.qualityforum.org/Show_Content.aspx?id=59894

National Quality Forum. (2021d). *Serious reportable events.* Retrieved August 5, 2020, from http://www.qualityforum.org/Topics/SREs/Serious_Reportable_Events.aspx

National Quality Forum. (2021e). *NQF's history.* Retrieved July 27, 2021, from https://www.qualityforum.org/about_nqf/history/

National Quality Strategy. (2017). *About the National Quality Strategy (NQS).* Retrieved July 27, 2021, from https://www.ahrq.gov/workingforquality/about/index.html#aims

QSEN Institute. (2020a). *Project overview. The evolution of the Quality and Safety Education for Nurses (QSEN) initiative.* Retrieved July 27, 2021, from http://qsen.org/about-qsen/project-overview

QSEN Institute. (2020b). *QSEN Institute competencies.* Retrieved July 27, 2021, from https://qsen.org/competencies/pre-licensure-ksas/

Quality Payment Program. (n.d.). *APMS overview.* Department of Health and Human Services. Retrieved July 27, 2021, from https://qpp.cms.gov/apms/overview

Sattar, R., Johnson, J., & Lawton, R. (2020). The views and experiences of patients and health-care professionals on the disclosure of adverse events: A systematic review and qualitative meta-ethnographic synthesis. *Health Expectations, 23*(3), 571–583. https://doi.org/10.1111/hex.13029

Tariq, R. A., Vashisht, R., & Scherbak, Y. (2021, July 25). *Medication dispensing errors and prevention.* National Center for Biotechnology Information, U.S. National Library of Medicine. Retrieved July 27, 2021, from https://www.ncbi.nlm.nih.gov/books/NBK519065/

Thomas, E. J., Studdert, D. M., Newhouse, J. P., Zbar, B. I. W., Howard, K. M., Williams, E. J., & Brennan, T. A. (1999). Costs of medical injuries in Colorado and Utah in 1992. *Inquiry, 36*(3), 255–264.

U. S. Food & Drug Administration. (2020, November 2). *Medication errors related to CDER-regulated drugs products.* Retrieved July 27, 2021, from https://www.fda.gov/Drugs/DrugSafety/MedicationErrors/default.htm

World Health Organization. (2017). *Global launch of WHO's third global patient safety challenge—Medication without harm.* Retrieved July 27, 2021, from https://www.who.int/news/item/29-03-2017-global-launch-of-who's-third-global-patient-safety-challenge---medication-without-harm

World Health Organization. (2019). *Patient safety.* Retrieved July 27, 2021, from https://www.who.int/news-room/fact-sheets/detail/patient-safety

Resilience and Self-Care in Nursing

Gwen Sherwood

CHAPTER OUTLINE

LEARNING OBJECTIVES

The learner will be able to:

1. Identify defining characteristics and attributes of the concept of resilience in nursing.

2. Examine the evidence base for the impact of resilience in nursing.

3. Describe the impact of stress as related to nursing students.

4. Explore self-care to enable nurses to thrive and build positive work environments.

5. Identify strategies to thrive in academic and clinical environments.

6. Develop an action plan to develop and sustain resilience and self-care practices.

INTRODUCTION

Resilience is one of the most common words used to describe the response of both the public and health care professionals to the impacts of the 2020 COVID-19 pandemic. An unprecedented global pandemic embroiled all aspects of contemporary life in new ways of living each day. Health care professionals experienced a double impact as they attempted to manage their personal lives as well as working on the front lines of managing infections, isolation procedures, visitor restrictions for patient families, and a daily deluge of new information. Concurrently, schools of nursing were forced to pivot from education as usual to remote learning with barely any planning time for instructional delivery new to the majority of nursing faculty and students. Yet, as time went by, schools found new ways to continue with clinical learning, host large classes in virtual formats, and create learning communities. Certainly, some found it difficult to cope and adapt to constantly emerging environments. What helped some thrive while others did not? Many accounts of the experience of nurses and nursing students referred to resilience as a characteristic common to those who continued to thrive in the new normal.

This chapter explores the concept of resilience and self-care to develop and sustain a healthy nursing workforce. First, the chapter examines resilience and why it is so important in nursing. Then, resilience is examined within academic environments, and strategies are suggested for students to develop resilience to thrive in the midst of challenging circumstances. Resilience is also explored as a key strategy for helping create thriving work environments. The chapter concludes by exploring how self-care is the natural counterpart to developing and sustaining resilience with an action plan for a new mindset of thriving.

RESILIENCE

Nursing work is emotionally and physically demanding. Nurses consistently report high levels of work-related stress that can lead to anxiety, dissatisfaction, and burnout

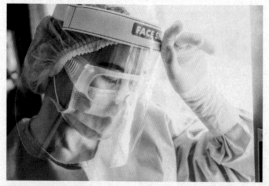

(Boyloso/Shutterstock)

(Gensimore et al., 2020; Wei et al., 2019). Nursing students also report high stress due to demands from their academic programs, time pressures, and the impact of caring for patients as part of clinical learning (Li & Hasson, 2020; McDermott et al., 2020). Resilience is an important part of the educational journey to develop a lifelong mindset of habits for thriving through adversity, coping with emotionally demanding work, and balancing personal and professional priorities. To position resilience as an important part of personal development, nurses need to develop knowledge and practical self-care skills to adapt to complex working environments.

What Is Resilience, and Why Is It Important?

Resilience involves a process of positive adaptation to stress and adversity. Resilience is described variously as an individual ability, a collective capacity, or as an interactive person–environment process (Thusini, 2020). It derives from personal resources, personality traits, cognitive abilities, work views, social support, cultural practices, and spiritual beliefs. Resilience helps health care professionals flourish and thrive even in challenging work circumstances and reduces the possibility of burnout (Gensimore et al., 2020). Jackson and colleagues (2018) defined resilience as (1) adjusting to adversity, (2) maintaining equilibrium, (3) retaining a sense of control over one's environment, and (4) moving constantly in a positive direction.

The view of resilience has evolved over time. Early views of resilience ranged from a continuum of responses to an aggregate of resources such as ego strength, social intimacy, and resourcefulness. One of the earliest applications of resilience in nursing is Polk's Middle Range Theory of Resilience. Polk used the process of concept synthesis to examine the literature on resilience (Polk, 1997) (Box 16.1). Concept synthesis integrates existing knowledge into a new concept to advance theory development that can lead to research. A defining attribute of resilience is being able to rise above adversity. Polk defined *resilience* as the ability to transform adversity into a growth experience and move forward. The model seeks to clarify how some individuals process and overcome adversity and how that contributes to overall well-being and growth.

Polk recognized human beings as more than and different from a sum of their parts that change mutually and simultaneously with the environment, creating a rhythm in which life is an all-at-once multidimensional experience with the meaning in any situation being related to the particular dynamics of that situation, facilitating a feeling of wholeness. Resilience is the basis for the human response to move forward through differing circumstances.

BOX 16.1   **Early Concepts of Resilience Leading to the Middle Range Theory of Resilience**

Resilience was described as four unfolding patterns (Polk, 1997):

1. Dispositional pattern: Physical and ego-related psychosocial attributes
2. Relational pattern: Intrinsic and extrinsic characteristics of roles and the value placed on social relationships and reaching out to confide in others
3. Situational pattern: How one manifests cognitive appraisal skills, problem-solving ability, and a capacity for action in facing tough situations
4. Philosophical pattern: Personal beliefs, self-knowledge, reflection about oneself and surrounding circumstances, meaning in life, and conviction of the contribution of one's purpose

Several recent literature reviews have captured the shifts in defining resilience related to nursing and identified various models and constructs that define and describe resilience (Amsrud et al., 2019; Cleary et al., 2018; Li & Hasson, 2020; McGowan & Murray, 2016; Moloney et al., 2020; Yu et al., 2019). A current view of resilience encompasses these findings into five characteristics (Meyer et al., 2020):

- Equanimity: Maintaining balance in whatever comes
- Perseverance: Persistence and determination to continue in the face of adversity
- Self-reliance: Believing in one's strength and capabilities
- Meaning: Realizing one's purpose, the reason one lives
- Existential aloneness: Recognizing and accepting the path of one's life

Similarly, Etchin et al. (2020) integrated several theories to derive a system theory of stress, resilience, and reintegration. Their work was primarily applied to veterans returning from deployments; however, the theory also helps explain the grounding of resilience in health care as a dynamic buffer mediating stress responses, proving a protective or adaptive resistance to stress.

Resilience encompasses the beliefs, actions, and abilities for coping or adapting to adverse situations; this can build on one's innate resilience for a more deeply ingrained resilience. Positive reactions such as coping skills that build personal growth help to combat chronic stress; resilience builds through social support from friends and family as well as the broader society, the ability to recognize meaning in experiences, and developing one's own self-reliance.

What Is Resilience as Related to Nursing?

Nursing is a helping or service profession, implying an implicit view of nurses as servers or givers. As an art and a science, nursing involves an emotional investment of the self in order to get to know the patient and family, to address needs in an individual and personal way, and an investment in advocating for the patient even in the face of resistance. This energy expenditure can exact a toll on one's capacity to engage in one's work when restorative or renewal strategies are absent from the daily routine. Nursing curricula often focus on empirical content with little attention on fostering self-care and resilience to face the emotional labor of nursing. The COVID-19 pandemic magnified the emotional toll for all health care providers, not only in the sheer numbers of patients in the delivery system but also from the high loss of life that stretched nurses' emotional and physical capacities. Nurses are prepared to put patients first, yet in the pandemic, that came with a calculated risk for infection, lack of personal time, and overwork to ensure an adequate workforce.

Discussion Point

The COVID-19 pandemic beginning in 2020 caused an upheaval in everyday life across the globe. What were disruptions in your life, both personally and professionally? How did you respond to these changes? Pick a one-word metaphor representing how your life was altered during the months of the pandemic. Write a short reflection on how this metaphor was visible in your choices, your responses to the pandemic, and how it is framing lessons learned.

Resilience within nursing is a complex concept whose definition and impact are difficult to pinpoint. Most definitions refer to the capacity for nurses to flourish and thrive in challenging work environments. To understand the application of resilience in nursing, we also need to examine stress in nursing. Nurses accept that their work is whatever the patient presents with that day. Every day nurses are present to help patients grapple with the vulnerability that characterizes illness. Nurses are present when patients need someone to listen to their worries and grief; nurses accept the privileged place of nursing, the vulnerability of getting to know the patient.

Health care is always frontline work for nurses because nurses are the constant presence and they never know what joys and challenges will be part of their work that day. Engaged nurses come to work with a mindset of managing whatever presents in their workload that day. A sense of "just do it" permeates nursing from the moral and ethical commitment to care for anyone and everyone who presents.

Resilience is a part of effective nursing care and was often showcased in stories of the pandemic. Resilience was frequently used to describe nurses, as nurses were the constant bedside presence. COVID-19 stretched that commitment sometimes to a breaking point. The cumulative effects of stress can be damaging (Foster et al., 2019). Undoubtedly, working under such pressure will leave lasting emotional impacts (Thusini, 2020).

The stress many nurses experience contribute to several phenomena. *Compassion fatigue* describes what happens when nurses have no break or effort for self-care to seek work–life balance. Unchecked compassion fatigue can lead to burnout (Abdollahi et al., 2020).

Burnout is a state of emotional exhaustion with feelings of depersonalization that persists over time; it includes sustained feelings of being overwhelmed emotionally and physically and feeling one's personal accomplishments are diminished. In addition, burnout is a predictor of nurses' intent to leave the workforce or a particular place of employment (Gensimore et al., 2020). *Depersonalization* refers to feeling detached and unable to engage in assigned responsibilities (Klein et al., 2020).

Compassion fatigue and burnout are industry concerns as all health care professionals have reported increased stressors from the many changes in health care over the past decade that have stretched capacity. In response, the Institute for Healthcare Improvement (IHI) replaced the "triple aim" of health care quality with the "quadruple aim," emphasizing the well-being of health care workers to help restore joy and meaning in work (Sikka et al., 2015).

Compassion fatigue is different from burnout. Burnout is a state of emotional exhaustion with detachment and depersonalization from responsibilities, while compassion fatigue is an emotional state stemming from prolonged, intense, and continuous care for those with high needs (Abdollahi et al., 2020).

A new mindset can change perspective from compassion fatigue, a negative term, to focus the conversation on what gives meaning and purpose to one's work, thereby building emotional resilience. Rather than focusing on what depletes nurses' spirit, *compassion satisfaction* recognizes confidence in one's competence, satisfaction from work well done, and the practice of reflection to help make sense of events (Sherwood et al., 2017). The spirit of gratitude arising from caregiving is thus an antidote to compassion fatigue (Abdollahi et al., 2020).

Gensimore and team (2020) examined the effect of the work environment on retention and quality of care by surveying nurses' burnout, work characteristics, and resilience. Findings revealed resilience can be a moderator for managing the stress of nurses' work in reducing burnout. Resilience as a personal resource enables one to handle adverse situations in a productive manner (Chambers & Ryder, 2018).

Students enrolled in nursing academic programs also experience challenges from the intense nature of nursing school, which affects psychological well-being and, if unchecked, can contribute to poor performance and academic burnout. Developing skills, such as resilience, within academic nursing programs help prepare learners to deal with the challenges unique to nursing practice.

Resilience often refers to the capacity for individuals to develop strategies to overcome adversity and, therefore, help promote personal responses that emphasize positive ways to support and learn about surviving and thriving. *Resilience* is a term commonly used to describe the ability to turn adversity into opportunities and learn from demanding situations. Kester and Wei (2018) describe resilience as a skill nurses learn to help survive and thrive in adverse circumstances. Resilience allows one to adapt to adversities and maintain hope about the future.

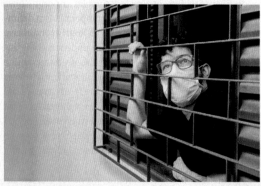

(Julio Ricco/Shutterstock)

Discussion Point

Improving resilience may not always be the answer but reducing stressors can be. Is it fair to offer help to staff or students to improve their resilience and then add additional stressors such as heavier workloads or reduced staffing?

Consider This Multiple instruments are available to
measure resilience:

1. The Resilience Scale: 25 items with a 1- to
   7-point rating scale that measures individual
   resilience, considering a positive personality
   (Wagnild & Young, 1993)
2. The Brief Resilience Scale: Six items measured
   on a 1- to 5-point rating scale; includes items
   like "I have a hard time making it through
   stressful events" (Smith et al., 2008)
3. Connor-Davidson Resilience Scale: Developed
   in 2003 and may be the most frequently used;
   includes 10 items scored on a 1- to 6-point
   rating scale with items like "The quality of
   care on my unit has deteriorated over the
   past year" and "I intend to remain with my
   current employer for at least 1 year" (Connor &
   Davidson, 2003)

Related Terms that Help Understand Resilience

Hardiness is a term frequently aligned with resilience, yet
hardiness notes how individuals bounce back from stressors
and, as a result of the experience, grow in well-being
(McGowan & Murray, 2016). Resilience reflects *elasticity*,
an ability to adapt and return to the state one was in prior
to a particular stressor. Hardiness goes further reflecting
that individuals can bounce back from stressors but grow in
well-being because of the experience.

Meyer and colleagues (2020) explored the relationship
between resilience and *grit*; both help nurses persist in their
goals. Resilience refers to the personal qualities that enable
one to thrive in the face of adversity, while *grit* is the passion and perseverance to pursue long-term goals. Grit is
overcoming challenges and maintaining effort and interest
despite failure; grit means not giving up.

Nursing is a physically and emotionally demanding profession with high role expectations and difficult working conditions. Burnout and resilience represent opposite ends of how
nurses respond to workplace adversity. Burnout is the failure
to manage work-related stressors, while resilience is how one
faces and overcomes work-related adversities (Guo et al., 2018).

Workplace adversity can take many forms and has a
negative impact on nurses. Nurses are constantly at risk
of burnout and stress-related illness, and how they cope
is of immense interest for maintaining the workforce.
COVID-19 magnified the demands of nurses' work and exposed some of the inherent challenges in the current health

care system. Still, nurses continued to deliver high-quality
patient care, retain resilience, progress professionally. This
earned increased public respect for facing adversity.

Creating a Culture to Thrive in Academic Environments: Developing Resilience

As young adults, college students are confronted with
crucial decisions, such as their first independent financial management, career choices, time pressures, new environments, and academic relationships quite different
from high school. Nursing academic programs compound
those stressors with additional unique challenges. Nursing
students must master complex content for immediate application in simulated or real-world clinical learning experiences, confront life and death, and perform interventions
using new skills. Interacting with patients and families at
highly vulnerable times intensifies the stress. Sam and Lee
(2020) assessed perceived stress and resilience in nursing
students as detailed in Research Fuels the Controversy 16.1.

Academic pressures due to a highly prescribed and
academically challenging curriculum are a leading cause
of attrition, especially in the absence of academic success
resources. Emotional exhaustion was the most relevant
dimension of academic burnout when predicting psychological well-being and resilience, both of which have an
important positive effect to mitigate academic distress and
promote well-being (Sam & Lee, 2020).

Several studies support resilience as having an important positive effect on psychological well-being in nursing
students. To promote nursing students' coping strategies
and their general well-being, nurse educators should foster
resilience and courage through various educational interventions. Nurse educators have a responsibility to prepare
students to be more resilient to promote patient safety,
handle professional demands, and function as advocates
for the discipline. Faculty awareness of the importance of
resilience in nursing students can better prepare students
for the role of the professional nurse.

Ebrahimi Ghassemi et al. (2019) recommend educational
interventions that promote resilience during academic studies that will sustain students through the transition to practice and throughout their careers. Jackson and team (2018)
reported that nursing students who more effectively managed
stress also developed a clearer professional identity, challenged poor practice, managed conflict, advocated for others,
and had socially supportive relationships. Further, they were
more able to manage a hostile work environment.

Li and Hasson (2020) conducted an integrative review
of 12 publications to examine resilience, stress, and psychological well-being in nursing students. The high interaction between resilience and stress and well-being led to

Research Fuels the Controversy 16.1

Stress and Resilience Among Undergraduate Nursing Students

Nursing students confront intense human situations through clinical learning experiences producing stress that can have a negative effect or further develop resilience. The study sought to validate and examine the impact of the unique challenges of nursing students by examining the link between stress and resilience. Perceived stress and resilience scales were self-administered by 620 undergraduate nursing students enrolled in a nursing program in southern India.

Source: Sam, P. R., & Lee, P. (2020). Do stress and resilience among undergraduate nursing students exist? *International Journal of Nursing Education, 12*(1), 146–149. https://doi-org.libproxy.lib.unc.edu/10.5958/0974-9357.2020.00032.X

Study Findings

The study reported 46% of students had severe stress but 55% reported low resilience, a weak negative correlation between perceived stress and resilience. The authors concluded there is a need for more robust measures of the two along with a strong recommendation that resilience becomes an intrinsic part of nursing education programs. This would help students develop the strength and endurance needed to helps them enter practice with confidence.

the conclusion that new educational policies and practices would help students develop resilience to promote their well-being and moderate the stressors of nursing school.

Similarly, Amsrud et al. (2019) synthesized qualitative studies to examine how nurse educators can support the development of resilience among nursing students to carry over to strengthen their professional practice. Two overarching analytic themes were identified as making the difference: (1) an educational culture of trustworthiness and (2) readiness to care. Five descriptive themes helped describe how educators applied a variety of strategies:

1. Demonstrating caring relationships
2. Recognizing resources and power
3. Acknowledging uncertainty
4. Reframing burdensome experiences
5. Adjusting frames for learning

Discussion Point

Nursing school is recognized as one of the most challenging among academic programs. Students have heavy course loads scheduled amid demanding clinical learning experiences. What are the major challenges you face as a nursing student? Who have you shared these concerns with? Do you have a self-care plan?

Discussion Point

Resilience may be one factor that influences new graduates' transition to practice. Meyer and Shatto (2018) examined a cohort of direct entry accelerated master's in nursing graduates and compared the relationship over time between their transition to practice experience and their resiliency. New graduates' professional satisfaction fluctuated during the first year of practice. At 12 months postgraduation, resilience accounted for the variance in perspectives. Interventions to improve resilience in new nursing graduates may be one way to positively impact the transition to practice (Meyer & Shatto, 2018). When you think about the transition to practice, what excites and concerns you? How can you prepare for what is often called a stressful time? Since about half of new graduates change jobs in the first year, how could efforts to promote resilience and self-care among new graduates foster retention?

A study by McDermott et al. (2020) also illustrated the complexity of understanding resilience among nursing students. The study revealed three characteristics to promote student success (Research Fuels the Controversy 16.2).

Research Fuels the Controversy 16.2

Nursing Students' Resilience, Depression, Well-Being, and Academic Distress

A sample of 933 nursing students from the national 2017 to 2018 Healthy Minds Study completed measures of resilience, depressive symptoms, intrapersonal well-being for flourishing, interpersonal well-being for belonging, and academic distress to test links between nursing students'

(a) psychological resilience, (b) depressive symptoms, (c) intrapersonal well-being, (d) interpersonal well-being, and (e) academic distress. Their perceptions of campus climate were measured as moderators.

Source: McDermott, R. C., Fruh, S., Williams, S., Hauff, C., Graves, R., Melnyk, B., & Hall, H. (2020). Nursing students' resilience, depression, well-being, and academic distress: Testing a moderated mediation model. *Journal of Advanced Nursing, 76,* 3385–3397. https://doi.org/10.1111/jan.14531

Study Findings

Negative perceptions of campus climate partially erased the mediation of resilience and well-being in managing stress. The study revealed three characteristics to promote student success: (1) build and enhance resilience; (2) create a positive, supportive academic environment; and

(3) identify and reduce depression. Educators should consider contextual factors such as campus climate, initiate resilience training, and improve the identification of mental health issues among students.

Consider This Reflective practice is a systematic self-assessment of one's work. In the context of meaningful recognition, a pillar of the healthy work environment model (American Association of Critical-Care Nurses, 2015), self-recognition does not replace meaningful recognition from other forms of recognition but helps one focus on working according to purpose. It helps acknowledge using one's unique skills and expertise to make a difference. Reflection helps one examine events from a positive perspective to appreciate and value one's work as a positive step in self-recognition of the meaning of one's work, not a boastful pat on the back but honestly thinking about the difference made through work. Meaningful recognition and reflective self-recognition are important parts of a work environment that promote thriving and continuous development for compassion satisfaction (Sherwood, Cherian, Horton-Deutsch, Kitzmiller, & Smith-Miller, 2018).

Sustaining Practice Environments Through Resilience Practice

Regardless of policies regulating nursing work hours, nurses still may feel compelled to work more with less recovery time. Chronic nurse shortages with high work demands deplete nurses' energy and motivation. Most nurses have

had limited opportunities to develop the skills and culture to achieve work–life balance as evident in the high burnout rates. The sustained stress and pressure contribute to emotional fatigue, burnout, and high rates of turnover in the workforce.

Resilience is one of the buffers for the negative impact of workplace stress on nurses. Improving the resiliency of health care workers promotes work satisfaction and career persistence, and its strength has an added impact of contributing to better patient outcomes (Kaplan et al., 2017; Tawfik et al., 2019).

Nurses foster resilience by developing clinical knowledge, skills, and experiences that promote confidence and flexibility that help to confront and adapt in the workplace (Meyer et al., 2020). Resilience has a positive correlation with hardiness, self-esteem, life, and job satisfaction among nurses; it has negative correlations with depression and burnout (Foster, 2020).

The leadership capacity of nurse leaders has a significant impact on nurses' work performance and building nurse resilience and work–life balance (Kester & Wei, 2018). Maintaining work–life balance is an important part of self-care that unit managers and administrators need to monitor to help staff place boundaries.

Work–life conflict is often the source of tensions personally and professionally as staff seek balance. Work–life balance is further associated with better teamwork, a climate of patient safety, and better engagement that is part of staff satisfaction (Kaplan et al., 2017). The cumulative effects of stress from work–life conflict can lead to harmful impacts.

Kester and Wei interviewed nurse leaders as part of a qualitative study and identified seven resilience-building strategies that could likewise be adopted by educators to help students, as described in Box 16.2.

BOX 16.2   Strategies for Building Resilience Among Nurses

Strategy to Create Resilience	Specific Focus	Activity
Facilitating social connections	Create an atmosphere for positive interpersonal relationships. Social connections form the foundation for a resilient nursing workforce.	Break down silos among units (e.g., a multiunit cookie exchange allows nurses to meet other nurses). Random acts of kindness Community service activities
Promoting positivity	Being able to see events from varying perspectives to develop positivity	Role model by starting meetings with naming three positive team wins. End shifts with positivity so that each nurse shares something good that happened. Practice gratitude.
Capitalizing on nurses' strengths	Recognize nurse strengths with opportunities to apply them at work to build self-confidence and work engagement.	Match workflow with strengths of nurses to improve productivity. Delegate to utilize specific talents such as unit social activities or decorating the staff lounge.
Nurturing nurses' growth	Guide and support nurses in developing personally and professionally to create a nonjudgmental environment.	Mentoring Host a breakfast to get to know new nurses and new graduates. Demonstrate caring through an "open door" policy to connect with nurses, get to know nurses, and build trust.
Encouraging nurses' self-care	Affirm the importance of taking time to care for oneself; self-care is not a selfish act. Reinforce positive self-care actions.	Incorporate self-care actions in meetings. Use flexible scheduling. Create homelike break rooms or a caring center in the staff lounge; encourage adequate physical care by using stairs for exercise, for example.
Fostering mindfulness practice	Direct attention away from simply staying busy to focus on the present moment.	Recharge by taking moments of meditation or mindful practice and deep breathing. "Tea for the soul" is a time for nurses to take a moment for tea, drawing, or journaling.
Conveying altruism	Conveys a personal connection between the nurse and the unit leader for a human-to-human bond and promotion of meaningful recognition	Convey caring in word and body language. Listen; be a part of the nurses' world. Recognize and value nurses' work.

Source: Adapted from Kester, K., & Wei, H. (2018). Building nurse resilience. *Nursing Management, 49*(6), 42–45. https://doi.org/10.1097/01.NUMA.0000533768.28005.36

Strategies to Develop and Sustain Resilience

Nurses' work can be rich with purpose and meaning, and nurses enter the profession with a commitment to helping others. However, the demands on one's time and the constant attention to patient needs can be relentless to the point of being unhealthy. Policies may be in place to guide work schedules and responsibilities to manage healthy work–life balance. The complexity of patient needs and high patient census pressure nurses to prioritize work over personal needs. How much nurses can focus on work–life balance is largely dependent on cultural norms in the workplace. Nurses benefit from taking adequate breaks and eating a balanced meal, but they are likely to do so only when cultural norms, supervisors, and surrounding coworkers also demonstrate a commitment to work–life balance.

Feeling supported and receiving feedback on ones' work uplift spirits to create a protective barrier against emotionally exhaustive work (Tawfik et al., 2019). Paying attention to even small changes can reduce stress: reducing interruptions and conflicting demands, developing better teamwork and coordination, and sharing meaningful recognition of everyone's contributions.

Leaders themselves need to attend to their own work–life balance to role model boundaries, efficiency, and smart practices surrounding technology; they may limit the use of mobile devices that do not allow nurses to fully separate themselves from the work environment (Wei et al., 2019).

> **Consider This** *Fika* is a Swedish term that does not have a literal English translation. *Fika* is a daily ritual in Sweden; coworkers or friends gather to have a coffee and a sweet treat and talk about topics other than work. *Fika* provides a mental and physical break from the day-to-day grind and helps create community. It is easy to think one is too busy, but Swedes believe this small 15-minute break shapes the work culture. How might this kind of break with colleagues foster resilience, help restore one's sense of balance, and promote collegiality? What are ways small breaks with colleagues can impact productivity and renewal?

Manomenidis et al. (2019) examined and compared the impact of individual characteristics, external factors, and coping strategies on nurses' resilience in a study of 1,012 Greek nurses working in eight hospitals in northern Greece. Courage and resilience were key aspects of effective patient care delivery. Educational level, anxiety, and the overall use of mental preparation strategies were the main predictors of nurses' resilience. Mental preparation, especially at the start of a shift, paired with reflective practices helped nurses manage vulnerability, engage mindfully in their work, and develop resilience. These findings are similar to the self-care recommendations from Horton-Deutsch et al. (2017) based on mindfulness and reflective practice.

Creating Workplace Cultures for Thriving

Developing resilience and encouraging self-care is a shared responsibility between nurses and the organizations where they work (Moloney et al., 2020). With an international nursing shortage, looming retirements, high stress with absenteeism from adverse health outcomes, and the exhaustion of burnout, organizations have a vested interest in supporting nurses to thrive. The development of knowledge and practical skills in resilience is essential for promoting long and rewarding careers while working in challenging working environments and is of universal significance to nursing. Education about resilience and related terms appears to be an effective approach.

Chambers and Ryder (2018) explain how working on a well-managed team provides a buffer between the team, its individual members, and organizational stressors. Team members are less likely to experience exhaustion and burnout when they feel valued and listened to, work with effective leaders, and take time for reflection. People must believe the team leader has a genuine concern for their well-being, provides honest regular feedback, and recognizes each individual's unique contribution. Offering staff training on the meaning of resilience, mindfulness, and support demonstrates commitment to healthy work environments. Supportive teams also use situational monitoring to ensure no one is overwhelmed, everyone has a lunch break, and all have the chance to participate in social events outside work.

Yu et al. (2019) reviewed 38 articles to conduct a systematic review to identify and describe how personal and work-related factors differed in nurse resilience. Findings revealed that job demands like burnout, stress, and bullying, had a negative impact on resilience. Job resources like coping skills, self-efficacy, social support, job satisfaction, and retention promoted resilience. Proactively promoting nurse resilience positions nurses to anticipate issues to ward off emotional exhaustion. This, in turn, helps increase work engagement, function more effectively, and foster job resources to achieve personal and professional growth.

Consider This Implementing a standardized debriefing following an unanticipated or critical event such as an unsuccessful code or trauma resuscitation is a way to help the care team recognize, acknowledge, and respond to psychological and spiritual needs resulting from an often hectic and fast-paced effort to save a life. Initiated first in emergency departments, some hospitals have expanded the practice throughout the facility. Taking time to debrief encourages a supportive team environment and provides the team a moment to regroup before transitioning back to regular work duties. Adding a moment of silence is a way to express reverence for human life, honor the team's work, and support spiritual care for patients and team members.

Questions often used are:

1. What did the team do well?
2. What is something we should have tried or something we should not have tried?
3. Did we have what we needed?
4. What can we improve?
5. How did we support the patient and family?
6. How are you doing?
7. What do you need to effectively return to work right now? (Copeland & Liska, 2016)

SELF-CARE

Flight attendants on every commercial airline are required to deliver safety information including actions to take should the airplane lose its oxygen source. One statement from this information applies to nurses: put on your own oxygen mask before helping others. This chapter has examined the concept of resilience as a defining characteristic of nurses' survival, but self-care provides the balance to develop resilience. Self-care is a companion concept for balance between work and life (Sherwood et al., 2017).

The high stress of nursing contributes to soaring burnout rates that compromise patient care and contribute to economic burdens for health care organizations. A mindset for self-care can help prioritize strategies for daily renewal and compassion satisfaction even while managing hectic schedules. An action plan for self-care can create a proactive long-term approach with more benefits than short-term crisis responses when nurses are already struggling.

What Is Self-Care, and Why Is It Critical for Nurses?

Self-care is a broad term. One common definition is the process of taking action to engage in activities that establish and maintain one's health and well-being (Andrews et al., 2020). Nurses learn how to educate patients to care for themselves, yet little is included in nursing education and practice on nurses' self-care. Nursing itself is grounded in delivering compassionate care. Nurses face difficult and emotionally laden situations: daily, like births, suffering, and deaths; these situations often pose ethical and moral dilemmas. This can lead to internal conflict, anxiety, and moral distress.

Self-compassion is being able to turn compassion inward to treat oneself with kindness by acknowledging one's own humanity and frailty (Andrews et al., 2020). Developing the capacity for self-compassion can help lower emotional drain, help manage stress, and contribute to well-being (Research Fuels the Controversy 16.3).

The demands of nursing can lead to emotional drain. Emotional resilience is the capacity to experience profound levels of demand without being consumed; emotional resilience is the capacity to intervene and provide for patients' care rather than burying the stress internally. Mindfulness is at the core of self-care, and evidence indicates it is an effective way to develop emotional resilience (Lin et al., 2020). Educational programs and training that emphasize mindfulness, self-care, and emotional intelligence can improve emotional resilience and change life habits that also contribute to better patient care (Foster et al., 2020; Horton-Deutsch et al., 2012).

While self-compassion promotes positive well-being, self-satisfaction, emotional intelligence, and coping, it is ironic that nurses reported feeling the need for permission to treat themselves with compassion and care (Andrews et al., 2020). Impact of the overall work culture, changing leadership, and organizational shifts in priorities affect how nurses feel they can prioritize self-care or be criticized by their peers for taking care of themselves. Many nurses felt called to be a nurse as the central purpose of their lives and therefore struggled with "vocation versus role" in seeking work–life balance while also managing stressful responsibilities.

Self-Care Practices to Thrive, Not Just Survive

Nursing is a demanding profession that offers unique challenges. The reality is that work environments are highly variable and nurse leaders have varying emotional intelligence development and preparation to demonstrate

Research Fuels the Controversy 16.3

Perceived Stress, Self-Compassion, and Job Burnout in Nurses: The Moderating Role of Self-Compassion

Nurses report higher job burnout than other health professions, which has adverse effects on the mental and physical health of both nurses and their patients. This cross-sectional study of 150 Iranian nurses evaluated the associations between job burnout as a dependent variable with perceived stress and self-compassion as an independent variable to test how self-compassion can buffer perceived stress and job burnout.

Source: Abdollahi, A., Taheri, A., & Allen, K. A. (2020). Perceived stress, self-compassion and job burnout in nurses: The moderating role of self-compassion. *Journal of Research in Nursing, 26*(3), 2021. https://doi.org/10.1177/1744987120970612

Study Findings

Participants completed three questionnaires: the Perceived Stress Scale, the Self-Compassion Scale, and the Copenhagen Burnout Inventory. Higher levels of perceived stress were associated with greater levels of job burnout, and greater levels of self-compassion were associated with lower levels of job burnout in nurses. Self-compassion diminished the effect of perceived stress on job burnout in nurses. The results demonstrated a significant association between perceived stress and job burnout in nurses and revealed the buffering role self-compassion can have to mitigate perceived stress and job burnout in nurses.

supportive leadership. The antidote to working in stressful environments is to deploy resilience strategies, such as positive attitudes, healthy lifestyles, and caring for oneself and colleagues.

Emotional intelligence skills foster resilience and help nurses respond to challenges and adversity in their academic programs that can carry over to their future practice (Cleary et al., 2018). Self-awareness is the foundation of emotional intelligence and is likewise a foundation for developing resilience. Being able to recognize one's emotions, strengths, weaknesses, values, and goals is a prelude to self-regulation, the second area of emotional intelligence. Other emotional intelligence skills are developing social skills to help direct others in positive directions and showing empathy to recognize other's emotions and self-motivation.

These skills of emotional intelligence guide nurses' situational awareness in practicing with a consciousness of the self, others, and the overall context (Sherwood et al., 2017). Resilience stems from knowing oneself and having the skills of emotional intelligence to face whatever work brings (Thusini, 2020). With emotional intelligence, resilience becomes a dynamic process that enables one to act in the face of vulnerabilities, adjust, and adapt, that is, to thrive.

From this, nurses can experience satisfaction in one's work through self-recognition (Sherwood et al., 2018). These skills were evident in the COVID-19 pandemic in Thusini's (2020) description of how nurses and other health professionals moved out of their usual tribes and silos to come together in one team with the shared purpose of overcoming COVID-19. This pulling together opened nurses to resilience in the face of severe shortages and threats to their own health.

Thusini related the COVID-19 response to the four attributes cited earlier that define resilience (Jackson et al., 2018):

1. Adjust to adversity.
2. Maintain equilibrium.
3. Retain a feeling of control over the environment.
4. Continue in a positive direction.

Facing unprecedented adversity, many nurses were able to adjust and adapt from a vulnerable state to a new equilibrium. Thusini (2020) shares an example of emotional equilibrium as a shared sense of humor among the team frequently interrupted by a shared sense of loss and sadness as patients separated from loved ones deteriorated.

Inside the COVID-19 intensive care unit (ICU), nurses could not leave or escape from the constant threat, leading Thusini to ponder whether these emotions are similar to the experience of police, firefighters, and other first responders who likewise have to search for resilience to care for the public. The support of the organization's leadership was welcomed as an anchor through the chaos, uncertainty, and constant pressure.

To help maintain a sense of control, staff used standardized procedures as much as possible, constantly updating as emerging evidence came to light. The overarching theme, however, became "mind over matter" to endure the long shifts and safety fears to be able to continue going

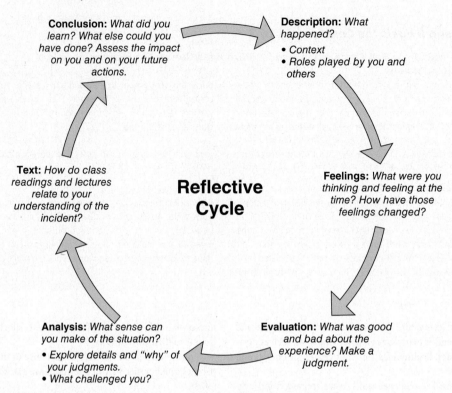

Conclusion: *What did you learn? What else could you have done? Assess the impact on you and on your future actions.*

Description: *What happened?*
• *Context*
• *Roles played by you and others*

Reflective Cycle

Text: *How do class readings and lectures relate to your understanding of the incident?*

Feelings: *What were you thinking and feeling at the time? How have those feelings changed?*

Analysis: *What sense can you make of the situation?*
• *Explore details and "why" of your judgments.*
• *What challenged you?*

Evaluation: *What was good and bad about the experience? Make a judgment.*

Figure 16.1 Developing and sustaining resilience in nursing (based on Jackson et al., 2018).

forward in a positive direction. These dynamics are in a cycle illustrated in Figure 16.1. One does not simply achieve a state of resilience; it involves a mindset of how one approaches one's work to see the meaning and satisfaction of work well done and of realizing that stress and vulnerability are inherent in nursing work and that the human spirit is capable of surviving and thriving even in the midst of adversity.

Reflective Practice: Learning from Experience

Reflective practice is a systematic way of examining oneself and events for sense making, analysis, and reframing (Sherwood et al., 2017). Taking opportunities for reflection helps mitigate exhaustion and burnout. Learning does not come from experience alone, but it happens from reflecting on experiences to understand what happened and reconsider future responses.

Reflective practice is a focused way of thinking about the practice to gain a deeper awareness and understanding. Reflective practice guides purposeful examination of one's role in a critical experience to be able to see things from different perspectives. Reflection examines situations from one's internal compass of values and ethics, applies what one knows, considers previous experience, and helps reformulate future responses (Sherwood et al., 2017, 2018).

The essence of learning through reflection is to surface contradiction between intention and actual practice. A system for developing reflective practices can be framed as reflecting-before-action, reflecting-in-action, and reflecting-on-action.

• Reflection-before-action: Taking the time to mentally prepare, develop a plan, collect needed information, and make sure everyone is on the same page

• Reflection-in-action: Pausing to check on others and clarify procedures

• Reflection-on-action: Considering outcomes to focus on improvement

Reflection can occur in small moments prior to entering a patient's room, before responding to a critical remark, or at the start of a major examination. An easy-to-remember pneumonic is pause, breathe, listen, engage, and reconsider (P-BLER). Taking a moment to consider the patient as a person, to think about what the team really needs, or to think through a difficult negotiation can change the outcome and provide a source of compassion satisfaction.

Both positive and challenging experiences are part of one's growth and development. Taking time to reflect in a systematic way can help to reframe one's perception of the circumstances, make sense of confounding experiences, and celebrate positive experiences. We learn and grow by looking inward to consider how to reframe how we respond to circumstances. All provide lessons to grow personally and professionally. Reflection helps to identify values that guide your choices and align future actions.

Consider This Maintaining a reflective journal of profound experiences can help to shape who you are. Reflective journals help record details that fade with time, document the purpose of an event, clarify your thinking, and explore one's emotions. Secure a notebook or journal, record electronically, or choose one of many apps for your handheld device; the point is your journal must be convenient and easy to use. Set a daily timer to maintain your journal. Use a systematic format such as this one shared by Gibbs (1988) (Fig. 16.2). Some people prefer to write according to a series of prompts such as gratitude, relationships, academic progress, professional lessons, or people who make a difference to you and other imaginative topics to help reconsider important events from your daily life.

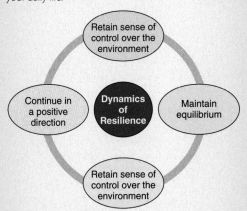

Figure 16.2 Gibbs' (1988) reflective cycle as a guide to reflective practice in journaling.

Discussion Point

Think over the past week. How often did you:

- Fail to eat a meal at regular time?
- Eat a poorly balanced meal?
- Skip breaks during a shift or class day?
- Arrive home late from work?
- Have a restless night?
- Sleep less than 5 hours a night?
- Miss personal and family commitments because of work or school?

If you answered yes to more than three items, look back further to see if this is a recurring problem. Rethink how you can rebalance your priorities. Can you improve time management according to what is most important? Who can you enlist to support you in setting boundaries?

Discussion Point

How could time for reflection impact nurses' resilience and self-care in recovering from a stressful acute event? What are other applications to recognize and honor nurses' work on interprofessional teams?

TAKING ACTION TO DEVELOP AND SUSTAIN RESILIENCE AND SELF-CARE

Nurses must first be aware of the need to take action. Setting an action plan while in academic study helps build a lifelong commitment to self-care, resilience, and well-being to achieve work–life balance. Nurses may manage exposure to stress by denying reality through protecting, processing, decontaminating, and distancing themselves from the experience and potential emotional toll. On the other hand, developing resilience can promote thriving, survival, and balance (Jackson et al., 2018). Faculty and other nurse leaders can intervene to reduce adversity, offer support, and assure policies are in place that guards work–life balance.

An Action Plan: Caring for Oneself to Care for Others

Interventions to foster resilience in nurses include physical exercise, social support systems, engagement with art, and written expressions. Educators can include learning activities for students to develop resilience, such as coping skills, ethics, socialization, stress management, self-care, and reflective journaling. Helping students develop independence, supportive relationships, creativity, optimism, mindfulness, conflict management, stress management, and communication skills are other ways to help establish resilience as a lifelong habit.

As nursing students approach the end of their academic training, it is important to investigate the workplace culture of future employers to choose workplaces that match their own values, priorities, and purpose. Nurses are more likely to experience satisfaction when practicing in places where they feel a cognitive balance between personal and professional goals with a high value for healthy and positive work environments. Wei and Wei (2020) offer a plan for nurses to take charge of their self-care. This ENERGY model of self-care promotes wellness and resilience through six domains to incorporate into a daily routine. Users can create an action plan based on the ENERGY model to instill a mindset to build resilience and self-care (Box 16.3).

Monitoring Progress to Sustain Resilience and Self-Care

To transform behaviors to achieve a goal, a vision board of your overall goals can help you achieve them. Pictures can say more than words. Use pictures or visual art, quotes, or other mediums to illustrate the goals you hope to achieve.

BOX 16.3   The ENERGY Model of Self-Care

Domain	Daily Actions	Reflecting on Actions of Self-Care	What Goals Will You Set for Tomorrow?
Energy source	When today did you experience or offer social support and teamwork? Today did you eat a balanced diet and get adequate sleep?		
Nurturing kindness	How well did you model respect, caring, compassion, and empathy in your interactions with patients and coworkers?		
Emotional hygiene	What are you grateful for today? What did you do for yourself today that illustrates self-valuing? How did you practice mindfulness to help achieve work–life balance?		
Refocusing purpose	How did your work today help you refocus on your meaning and purpose? What actions do you need to take to reconnect with your internal compass of values and attitudes to regain passion for nursing work?		
Germinating positivity	By practicing daily gratitude, were you able to reframe negativity to foster a growth mindset? To whom did you show appreciation today for being a part of your day?		
Your uniqueness	How do you identify the inner power that drives your actions in fulfilling your purpose and addresses your spiritual needs? How can you practice your strengths and acknowledge your limitations as part of practicing resilience?		

Source: Adapted from Wei, H., & Wei, T. (2020). The power of self-care: An ENERGY model to combat clinician burnout. *American Nurse, 15*(10), 28–31.

Maintaining the Course: Creating a Self-Care Vision Board to Stay the Course

1. Design a vision board to document your self-care goals and your resilience in addressing the challenges you face.
2. Reflect on your life and work to clarify what steps you need to take to improve self-care.
3. Define your goals to improve self-care that you hope to accomplish over the next quarter.
4. Focus on each goal to set the actions you need to accomplish that goal.
5. Establish a timetable and post on the vision board to help keep pace.
6. Illustrate your goals and actions with artwork that will serve as motivation to achieve.
7. Be as colorful and creative as you wish such as creating a collage.
8. Integrate words of encouragement and quotes to reinforce your goals.
9. Post in a place for daily inspiration.
10. Add your progress to the vision board and record reflections in your journal.
11. Update each quarter so that you maintain your journey of development.
12. Reflect on the emotions you encounter to examine how they affect achieving your goal of self-care and foster resilience.

Create a unique visual that reminds you of how to meet adversity with resilience and how to manage self-care and workplace stress and well-being. Suggestions for creating a vision board are shown in Box 16.4.

CONCLUSIONS

Resilience is a prominent part of effective nursing practice. Education can help nurses learn resilient practices that foster self-care, satisfaction with practice, and quality care. Nurse faculty need to further integrate resilience training in academic programs to develop the mindset and lifelong habits of reflective practices that contribute to teamwork and self-care. Helping nurses develop a positive mindset contributes to compassion satisfaction and retention to foster healthy workplaces and nurse satisfaction.

Organizations share in the responsibility by preparing leaders to create supportive environments. Emotional intelligence is a core building block for developing resilience. Self-care is a key for keeping nurses in the workforce. Nurse turnover is a concern in most countries, especially in the first year of practice as a new graduate. Nurses are at the heart of every health care setting; therefore, they constitute the largest health care discipline worldwide. The impact of constant recruitment and orientation has a huge economic impact on employers who could better invest the funds in fostering healthy workplaces and recognizing nurses for their constant contributions.

For Additional Discussion

1. How well do you tend to bounce back from distressful events? Think back to the last time you were feeling overwhelmed. How did you manage the situation? After reading this chapter, how would you reframe your response?

2. Do you tend to think more about being well or about not feeling well? How do attitudes influence our perspective, and how we respond?

3. What are you most grateful for in your life? Do you think more about things you are grateful for or worry about the things you do not have? How can you develop an attitude of gratitude?

4. How do you respond to the finding by Andrews et al. (2020) that nurses feel they need permission to practice self-compassion and self-care? What are ways nurses use peer pressure to mentally judge other nurses who seek work–life balance?

5. What are activities you engage in for work–life balance and attend to physical, emotional, social, and spiritual needs?

References

Abdollahi, A., Taheri, A., & Allen, K. A. (2020). Perceived stress, self-compassion and job burnout in nurses: The moderating role of self-compassion. *Journal of Research in Nursing, 26*(3), 2021. https://doi.org/10.1177/1744987120970612

American Association of Critical-Care Nurses. (2015). *AACN Healthy Work Environment assessment*. Retrieved December 20, 2020, from http://www.aacn.org/wd/hwe/content/aboutassessment

Amsrud, K. E., Lyberg, A., & Severinsson, E. (2019). Development of resilience in nursing students: A systematic qualitative review and thematic synthesis. *Nurse Education in Practice, 41*, 102621. https://doi.org/10.1016/j.nepr.2019.102621

Andrews, H., Tierney, S., & Seers, K. (2020). Needing permission: The experience of self-care and self-compassion in nursing: A constructivist grounded theory study. *International Journal of Nursing Studies, 101*, 103436. https://doi .org/10.1016/j.ijnurstu.2019.103436

Chambers, C., & Ryder, E. (2018). *Supporting compassionate healthcare practice: Understanding the role of resilience, positivity and wellbeing.* Routledge. https://doi-org.libproxy.lib .unc.edu/10.4324/9781315107721

Cleary, M., Visentin, D., West, S., Lopez, V., & Kornhaber, R. (2018). Promoting emotional intelligence and resilience in undergraduate nursing students: An integrative review. *Nurse Education Today, 68*, 112–120. https://doi.org/ 10.1016/j.nedt.2018.05.018

Connor, K. M., & Davidson, J. R. (2003). Development of a new resilience scale: The Connor-Davidson Resilience Scale (CD-RISC). *Depression and Anxiety, 18*(2), 76–82. https:// doi.org/10.1002/da.10113

Copeland, D., & Liska, H. (2016). Implementation of a post-code pause: Extending post-event debriefing to include silence. *Journal of Trauma Nursing, 23*(2), 58–64. https://doi.org/10.1097/JTN.0000000000000187

Ebrahimi Ghassemi, A., Zhang, N., & Marigliano, E. (2019). Concepts of courage and resilience in nursing: A proposed conceptual model. *Contemporary Nurse, 55*(4–5), 450–457. https://doi.org/10.1080/10376178.2019.1661786

Etchin, A. G., Fonda, J. R., McGlinchey, R. E., & Howard, E. P. (2020). Toward a system theory of stress, resilience, and reintegration. *Advances in Nursing Science, 43*(1), 75–85. doi: 10.1097/ANS.0000000000000277

Foster, K. (2020). Resilience in the face of adversity: A shared responsibility. *Int J Mental Health Nurs, 29*: 3-4. https://doi .org/10.1111/inm.12688

Foster, K., Roche, M., Delgado, C., Cuzzillo, C., Giandinoto, J., & Furness, T. (2019). Resilience and mental health nursing: An integrative review of international literature. *International Journal of Mental Health Nursing, 28*(1), 71–85. https://doi.org/10.1111/inm.12548

Gensimore, M. M., Maduro, R. S., Morgan, M. K., McGee, G. W., & Zimbro, K. S. (2020). The effect of nurse practice environment on retention and quality of care via burnout, work characteristics, and resilience: A moderated mediation model. *The Journal of Nursing Administration, 50*(10), 546–553. https://doi.org/10.1097/NNA.0000000000000932

Gibbs, G. (1988). *Learning by doing.* Oxford Polytechnic.

Guo, Y. F., Luo, Y. H., Lam, L., Cross, W., Plummer, V., & Zhang, J. P. (2018). Burnout and its association with resilience in nurses: A cross-sectional study. *Journal of Clinical Nursing, 27*(1–2), 441–449. https://doi.org/10.1111/jocn.13952

Horton-Deutsch, S, Drew, B. L., & Beck-Coon, K. (2012). *Engaging educators and learners in reflective practice engaging educators and learners in reflective practice* (pp. 79–99). Sigma Theta Tau International Press.

Horton-Deutsch, S. & Sherwood, G. (Eds.) (2017). Reflective Practice: Transforming Education and Improving Outcomes. 2nd Edition. Indianapolis: Sigma Theta Tau International Press.

Jackson, J., Vandall-Walker, V., Vanderspank-Wright, B., Wishart, P., & Moore, S. L. (2018). Burnout and resilience in critical care nurses: A grounded theory of Managing Exposure. *Intensive & Critical Care Nursing, 48*, 28–35. https:// doi.org/10.1016/j.iccn.2018.07.002

Kaplan, H., Tawfik, D., Adair, K., Sexton, B., & Profit, J. (2017). Context in quality of care: Improving teamwork and resilience. *Clinics in Perinatology, 44*(3), 541–552. doi:10.1016/j .clp.2017.04.004

Kester, K., & Wei, H. (2018). Building nurse resilience. *Nursing Management, 49*(6), 42–45. https://doi.org/10.1097/01 .NUMA.0000533768.28005.36

Klein, C. J., Weinzimmer, L. G., Cooling, M., Lizer, S., Pierce, L., & Dalstrom, M. (2020). Exploring burnout and job stressors among advanced practice providers. *Nursing Outlook, 68*(2), 145–154. https://doi.org/10.1016/j.outlook.2019.09.005

Li, Z. S., & Hasson, F. (2020). Resilience, stress, and psychological well-being in nursing students: A systematic review. *Nurse Education Today, 90*, 104440. Advance online publication. https://doi.org/10.1016/j.nedt.2020.104440

Lin, L., Liu, X., & He, G. (2020). Mindfulness and job satisfaction among hospital nurses: The mediating roles of positive affect and resilience. *Journal of Psychosocial Nursing & Mental Health Services, 58*(6), 46–55. https://doi.org/10.3928/ 02793695-20200406-03

Manomenidis, G., Panagopoulou, E., & Montgomery, A. (2019). Resilience in nursing: The role of internal and external factors. *Journal of Nursing Management, 27*(1), 172–178. https://doi.org/10.1111/jonm.12662

McDermott, R. C., Fruh, S., Williams, S., Hauff, C., Graves, R., Melnyk, B., & Hall, H. (2020). Nursing students' resilience, depression, well-being, and academic distress: Testing a moderated mediation model. *Journal of Advanced Nursing, 76*, 3385–3397. doi:10.1111/jan.14531

McGowan, J. E., & Murray, K. (2016). Exploring resilience in nursing and midwifery students: A literature review. *Journal of Advanced Nursing, 72*(10), 2272–2283. https://doi.org/ 10.1111/jan.12960

Meyer, G., & Shatto, B. (2018). Resilience and transition to practice in Direct Entry nursing graduates. *Nurse Education in Practice, 28*, 276–279. https://doi.org/10.1016/j.nepr.2017 .10.008

Meyer, G., Shatto, B., Kuljeerung, O., Nuccio, L., Bergen, A., & Wilson, C. R. (2020). Exploring the relationship between resilience and grit among nursing students: A correlational research study. *Nurse Education Today, 84*, 104246. https:// doi.org/10.1016/j.nedt.2019.104246

Moloney, W., Fieldes, J., & Jacobs, S. (2020). An integrative review of how healthcare organizations can support hospital nurses to thrive at work. *International Journal of Environmental Research and Public Health, 17*(23), 8757. https://doi .org/10.3390/ijerph17238757

Polk, L. (1997). Toward a middle-range theory of resilience. *Advances in Nursing Science, 19*(3), 1–13. https://doi.org/10 .1097/00012272-199703000-00002

Sam, P. R., & Lee, P. (2020). Do stress and resilience among undergraduate nursing students exist? *International Journal of Nursing Education, 12*(1), 146–149. https://doi.org/10 .5958/0974-9357.2020.00032.X

Sherwood, G., Horton-Deutsch, S., & Giscombe, C. W. (2017). Attention to self as nurse: Caring for patients, caring for self, making sense of practice. In S. Horton-Deutsch, & G. Sherwood (Eds.), *Reflective practice: Transforming education and improving outcomes* (2nd ed.). Sigma Theta Tau International Press.

Sherwood, G., Koshy Cherian, U., Horton-Deutsch, S., Kitzmiller, R., & Smith-Miller, C. (2018). Reflective practices: Meaningful recognition for healthy work environments. *Nursing Management (Harrow, London, England: 1994), 24*(10), 30–34. https://doi.org/10.7748/nm.2018.e1684

Sikka, R., Morath, J. M., & Leape, L. (2015). The quadruple aim: Care, health, cost and meaning in work. *BMJ Quality and Safety, 24,* 608–610. http://dx.doi.org/10.1136/bmjqs-2015-004160

Smith, B. W., Dalen, J., Wiggins, K., Tooley, E., Christopher, P., & Bernard, J. (2008). The brief resilience scale: Assessing the ability to bounce back. *International Journal of Behavioral Medicine, 15*(3), 194–200. https://doi.org/10.1080/10705500802222972

Tawfik, D. S., Scheid, A., Profit, J., Shanafelt, T., Trockel, M., Adair, K. C., Sexton, J. B., & Ioannidis, J. (2019). Evidence relating health care provider burnout and quality of care: A systematic review and meta-analysis. *Annals of Internal Medicine, 171*(8), 555–567. https://doi.org/10.7326/M19-1152

Thusini, S. (2020). Critical care nursing during the COVID-19 pandemic: A story of resilience. *British Journal of Nursing, 29*(21), 1232–1236. https://doi-org.libproxy.lib.unc.edu/10.12968/bjon.2020.29.21.1232

Wagnild, G., & Young, H. (1993). Development and psychometric evaluation of the resilience scale. *Journal of Nursing Measurement, 1*(2), 165–178. PMID: 7850498.

Wei, H., & Wei, T. (2020). The power of self-care: An ENERGY model to combat clinician burnout. *American Nurse, 15*(10), 28–31. https://www.myamericannurse.com/?s=Wei%2C+H.+and+Wei%2C+T.+%282020%29.+The+power+of+self-care%3A+an+ENERGY+model+to+combat+clinician+burnout.+American+Nurse+15%2810%29%3A28-31

Wei, H., Roberts, P., Strickler, J., & Corbett, R. W. (2019). Nurse leaders' strategies to foster nurse resilience. *Journal of Nursing Management, 27*(4), 681–687. https://doi.org/10.1111/jonm.12736

Yu, F., Raphael, D., Mackay, L., Smith, M., & King, A. (2019). Personal and work-related factors associated with nurse resilience: A systematic review. *International Journal of Nursing Studies, 93,* 129–140. https://doi.org/10.1016/j.ijnurstu.2019.02.014

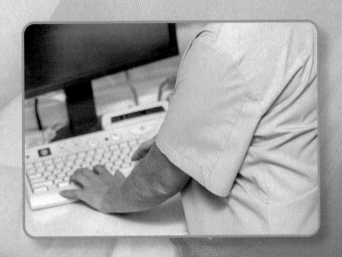

4

LEGAL AND ETHICAL ISSUES

Whistleblowing in Nursing

Carol J. Huston

LEARNING OBJECTIVES

The learner will be able to:

1. Define whistleblowing and differentiate between internal and external whistleblowing.

2. Explore why reactions to whistleblowers are often mixed and why the courage to speak out is something we honor more often in theory than in action.

3. Identify risks and retaliatory consequences frequently experienced by whistleblowers because of their actions.

4. Delineate strategies to create an organizational climate that both discourages the need for whistleblowing and supports the whistleblower when it is necessary for them to come forward.

5. Identify strategies that whistleblowers should use to reduce their likelihood of retaliation as well as legal liability.

6. Examine how cultural background may affect a nurse's willingness to blow the whistle on unsafe practices.

7. Differentiate among the consequentialist, deontologic, and utilitarian viewpoints regarding the purposes of whistleblowing.

8. Analyze how whistleblowing could be considered a failure of organizational ethics.

9. Analyze existing and proposed federal and state legal protections for whistleblowers.

10. Identify the process used by a whistleblower to file a *qui tam* or whistleblower lawsuit under the False Claims Act and the potential benefits of doing so.

11. Identify conditions that should be met before whistleblowing occurs as well as situations in which whistleblowing is clearly indicated.

12. Reflect on their willingness to assume the personal risks associated with whistleblowing should the need arise.

INTRODUCTION

Enron and the artificial manipulation of energy prices; Martha Stewart and insider trading; WorldCom and accounting fraud; Morgan Stanley and overcharging customers; Edward Snowden leaking thousands of pages of documents; long patient wait times and inadequate care at the Department of Veterans Affairs (VA); fraudulent bank loans by Wells Fargo; systemic safety issues with the Boeing 737 MAX. These high-profile cases, alleging some degree of ethical malfeasance, have led the U.S. public to an increased sense of moral awareness about what is right and what is wrong.

Additionally, these cases all came to public attention as the result of *whistleblowing*. The Free Dictionary by Farlex (2003–2021) defines whistleblowing as "the disclosure by a person, usually an employee in a government agency or private enterprise, to the public or to those in authority, of mismanagement, corruption, illegality, or some other wrongdoing" (para. 1). Similarly, Ceva and Bocchiola (2019) describe whistleblowing as the exposure by a member of an organization of episodes of corruption, fraud, or general abuses of power within the organization.

> *Consider This* Most definitions of whistleblowing suggest the importance of advocating for others who may be harmed.

Indeed, the concept of whistleblowing, which began to emerge in the 1970s, has gained significant traction since that time and across all industries and disciplines, including law, management, public administration, sociology, psychology, and health sciences (Gagnon & Perron, 2020). Likewise, according to the 2021 Global Business Ethics survey report, the global median for reporting misconduct via whistleblowing was 81% in 2020; compared with 63% in 2019, employees are whistleblowing more often (DeltaNet International, 2021).

It is generally accepted that there are two types of whistleblowing: internal and external. *Internal whistleblowing* typically involves reporting concerns up the chain of command within an organization in the hope that whatever the problem is, it will be resolved. *External whistleblowing* involves reporting concerns outside the organization and specifically to the media. In many cases, whistleblowing becomes external only if inadequate action is taken at the organizational level to address the concerns of the whistleblower. In some cases, however, whistleblowing becomes external to embarrass an organization publicly or to seek financial redress.

> **Discussion Point**
> Is it ever appropriate to blow the whistle externally before attempting to resolve the problem internally?

In an era of transparency in quality reporting, declining reimbursements, and the ongoing pressure to remain fiscally solvent, the risk of fraud, misrepresentation, and ethical malfeasance in health care organizations has never been higher. As a result, the need for whistleblowing has also likely never been greater.

It is important, however, to remember that whistleblowing should never be considered the first solution to ethically troubling behavior. Indeed, it should be considered only after other prescribed avenues of solving problems have been attempted. This is true, however, only if lives are not at stake. In those cases, immediate action must be taken. In addition, the employee should generally be able to go up the chain of command in reporting their concerns to see them resolved.

There are other general guidelines for blowing the whistle that should also be followed, including carefully documenting all attempts to address the problem and being sure to report facts and not personal interpretations. These guidelines, as well as others, are presented in Box 17.1.

This chapter explores the effect of groupthink on the likelihood that whistleblowers will come forward. In addition, it presents select cases of whistleblowing. Personal risks associated with whistleblowing are described, as are the mixed feelings many individuals hold about whistleblowers. Whistleblowing is also explored as a failure of organizational ethics, and strategies are identified to create an organizational climate that both discourages the need for whistleblowing and supports the whistleblower when it is necessary for them to come forward. Finally, legal protections or the lack thereof for whistleblowing are discussed.

GROUPTHINK AND WHISTLEBLOWING

Being a whistleblower takes great courage and conviction because it requires the whistleblower to avoid *groupthink*—an inappropriate conformity to group norms. Going outside group norms often carries significant personal and professional risks. Unfortunately, these risks are more common than not because whistleblowers may be viewed as disloyal rather than as courageous. That theme is common in the cases detailed in this chapter.

One infamous case of whistleblowing occurred in the early 1970s when Mark Felt, the associate director of the

BOX 17.1   Guidelines for Blowing the Whistle

- Stay calm and think about the risks and outcomes before you act.
- Know your legal rights, because laws protecting whistleblowers vary by state.
- First, make sure that there really is a problem. Check resources such as the medical library, the internet, and institutional policy manuals to be sure.
- Seek validation from colleagues that there is a problem, but do not get swayed by groupthink into not doing anything if you should.
- Follow the chain of command in reporting your concerns whenever possible.
- Confront those accused of the wrongdoing as a group whenever possible.
- Present just the evidence; leave the interpretation of facts to others. Remember that there may be an innocent or good explanation for what is occurring.
- Use internal mechanisms within your organization.
- If internal mechanisms do not work, use external mechanisms.
- Private groups, such as The Joint Commission or the National Committee for Quality Assurance, do not confer protection. You must report to a state or national regulator.
- Although it is not required by every regulatory agency, it is a good rule of thumb to put your complaint in writing.
- Carefully document the problem that you have seen and the steps that you have taken to see that it is addressed.
- Do not lose your temper, even if those who learn of your actions attempt to provoke you.
- Do not expect thanks for your efforts.

Source: American Nurses Association. (n.d.). *Things to know about whistle blowing.* Retrieved July 30, 2021, from https://www.nursingworld.org/practice-policy/workforce/things-to-know-about-whistle-blowing/

Federal Bureau of Investigation (FBI), discovered and reported that five men had broken into the Democratic National Committee headquarters at the Watergate hotel in 1972 for political gain (Coxwell, 2018). After being pressured to not pursue the matter, Felt decided the press was the only way to expose the corruption and the White House's complicity. Using the moniker "Deep Throat," he met regularly with *Washington Post* journalists Bob Woodward and Carl Bernstein, helping them uncover the full story that ultimately led to former President Richard Nixon's resignation (Coxwell, 2018). The impact of this whistleblowing is still being felt in American politics today.

In another infamous case, Colvin (2002) recounted how Sherron Watkins, an accountant, first blew the whistle on Enron's complex "special-purpose entities." She detailed them in a memo to chief executive officer Ken Lay, her boss's boss. She understood that something wrong was going on—something everyone else seemed to accept—and that public revelation would be disastrous.

What Colvin argued was most important in this scandal was that Watkins had access to the same facts as did many other people inside Enron, but she was the one able to escape the groupthink that ensnared her colleagues. Soon after writing the memo, she identified herself as its author and met with Lay. When her memo eventually became public, the wrongness of what happened was apparent even internally (Colvin, 2002).

Colvin (2002) also recounts a similar story at World-Com, where Cynthia Cooper, another internal auditor, saw something that did not look right and took matters into her own hands. In this case, Cooper began investigating some of the company's capital expenditures and discovered bookkeeping entries that would eventually uncover what is likely the largest case of accounting fraud in U.S. history.

Faced with disturbing facts, Cooper discussed her findings with the company's controller and with Scott Sullivan, the chief financial officer. Sullivan tried to explain to her why costs that had previously been expensed were suddenly being capitalized. Then he asked her to stop the audit, which was being conducted early, and to put it off until the third quarter. She did not. Instead, she continued and immediately went over her boss's head to call the chairman of the board's audit committee. He arranged to meet with her and the company's new auditor, KPMG. Two weeks later, WorldCom announced that it would restate earnings by $3.9 billion—the largest restatement ever.

Again, Colvin (2002) suggested that the importance of Cooper's refusal to postpone her audit, as Sullivan had asked, is even greater than it may appear. Facts uncovered about the company, combined with the memo Sullivan wrote to the board in a last-ditch attempt to defend himself, show that if Cooper had been "a good soldier," the whole problem might have been concealed forever.

Consider This "To see what is right, and not do it, is want of courage, or of principles."

—Confucius

Another high-profile case of a whistleblower, Edward Snowden, revealed in 2013 the existence of previously classified mass intelligence-gathering surveillance programs run by the U.S. National Security Agency (NSA) and the United Kingdom's Government Communications Headquarters (GCHQ) (Younger, 1997–2021). To some, Snowden's exposure of NSA surveillance was "un-American," while others viewed him as a hero. Snowden himself felt confident about the positive impact of his disclosures, suggesting that "we live in a better, freer, and safer world because of the revelations of mass surveillance" (Young, 1997–2021, para. 2). Snowden, however, was charged with espionage by the U.S. government and subsequently fled the country in an effort to escape prosecution.

A more recent case of whistleblowing malfeasance involved Wells Fargo Bank. Lewis (2017a) notes that the bank reportedly put heavy pressure on employees to meet sales quotas, and accounts were opened without authorization for customers who were charged fees for accounts they "knew nothing about." Lewis notes that this corruption occurred despite more than 700 whistleblower complaints to the Comptroller of the Currency, the federal banking regulator, before the scandal finally broke. The Comptroller neither "investigated the root cause" nor forced Wells Fargo to probe it. Indeed, Wells Fargo responded to internal ethics complaints from employees by firing them (Lewis, 2017a). Senator Elizabeth Warren suggested the possibility that a system operated by the Financial Industry Regulatory Authority to promote integrity may actually have perversely enabled whistleblower blacklisting (Lewis, 2017a).

Finally, engineer Curtis Ewbank blew the whistle on Boeing Airlines in 2020, alleging in a letter to a U.S. Senate subcommittee that there were serious shortcomings in development of the 737 MAX airplane, asserting that systemic problems with the jet's design had to "be fixed before allowing it to return to service" (Boeing Whistleblower, 2020). His letter went on to say that it was not enough for Boeing to fix the flawed maneuvering characteristics augmentation system (MCAS) known to have brought down aircrafts in two crashes in Indonesia and Ethiopia.

Ewbank alleges that Boeing rejected his recommended safety upgrades because of management's focus on schedule and cost considerations and the insistence that anything that might require more pilot training would not be considered. He also alleged that Boeing pushed regulators at the Federal Aviation Administration (FAA) to relax certification requirements for the airplane, particularly with regard to the cockpit systems for alerting pilots if something was wrong inflight (Gates, 2020). Boeing responded that company officials had not seen the letter, but that it did offer its employees a number of channels for raising concerns and complaints and had rigorous processes in place to ensure complaints receive thorough consideration and protect employee confidentiality (Gates, 2020).

Discussion Point

In the United States, there is some evidence that the events of September 11, 2001, have made people more public-spirited and more inclined to blow the whistle. Do you think this inclination is driven more by fear or by a desire to promote public good?

Perhaps the most frightening aspect of all these cases is that the responses to the whistleblowers are not unique. Many organizations are aware of problem situations but choose to ignore them until a crisis occurs or the problem becomes public.

Some nurses take comfort in thinking that nursing is different and that any moral professional would report substandard care. The reality, however, is often different, and many professionals are torn between what they believe they should do and what they actually do. This is particularly disconcerting, because those who bear witness are required to overcome groupthink despite their moral distress. This is a primary reason why so many whistleblowers delay reporting their concerns outside the organization.

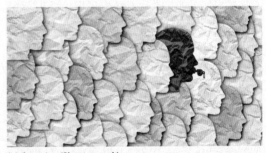

(Lightspring/Shutterstock)

EXAMPLES OF WHISTLEBLOWING IN NURSING

Complaints about unsafe staffing, inadequate equipment, and unlicensed assistive personnel performing nursing tasks outside their scope of practice are fairly common. In addition, some nurses claim that they have been told to participate in illegal or unethical activities such as fraudulently altering medical records, falsifying insurance claims, and covering up the failure to meet mandated staffing ratios. A review of the literature reveals multiple case studies of whistleblowing by nurses.

Mason (2011) shared the story of two nurses, Anne Mitchell and Vicki Galle, who blew the whistle on a physician for a variety of charges, including unprofessional conduct, via what they thought was a confidential report to the state board for medicine. Instead of the physician being investigated, the nurses found themselves the target of unprofessional conduct charges brought by the local sheriff and county attorney, who were friends and business associates of the reported physician. In the end, the nurses, who had a combined 47 years of experience at the hospital, were fired. The charges against Galle and Mitchell were eventually dropped, and the sheriff, county attorney, and hospital administrator were indicted for retaliating against the whistleblowers. Each faced six counts, including misuse of official information and retaliation, which are third-degree felonies (Sack, 2011). The nurses sued the county and settled for a shared $750,000 (Sack, 2011).

Rohner (2015) wrote about a more recent case in Cape Dorset, Nunavut, Canada, following the preventable death of a 3-month-old baby in 2012. The Nunavut government's policies and procedures for nurses state that nurses must examine sick children younger than 1 year old when a parent contacts them after normal working hours. Gwen Slade, the whistleblower nurse, alleged that another nurse told the mother not to bring the baby into the health center, but to bathe the infant instead, and that the accused nurse faced numerous complaints that coworkers and members of the public had filed against her. The territory's health minister ordered an immediate independent review, which in the end was highly critical of the health department, but restrictions were placed on Slade's license by the Registered Nurses Association of the Northwest Territories and Nunavut.

In addition, Slade said she was suspended from her job for speaking out against what she believed to be misdiagnoses and irresponsible behavior by her coworker. An investigation ensued, and Slade was eventually cleared of any wrongdoing; however, she stated that she continued to suffer the consequences of speaking out and was not able to find work in Nunavut as a nurse after the alleged incidents. Slade argued that she was the victim of an extraordinary abuse of power, which brought pain, devastation, and destruction to someone who did nothing wrong.

Similarly, Lewis (2017b) shared the story of Oregon whistleblower Vikki Mata, who reported that officials improperly diverted federal funds intended to provide health care for uninsured children via the Healthy Kids Program to state coffers. An audit Mata requested confirmed her allegation that state officials overstated the number of uninsured children in the state and that those inflated numbers allowed authorities to improperly claim additional federal funds,

thus reducing the money available to aid qualified children. The state later returned $4.5 million to the federal program, where it was again available for its intended purpose thanks to Mata. However, Mata lost her job in the process and was unable to cover the expense of an appeal herself.

Lewis (2017b) notes that Mata's case highlights a flaw in our justice system. "Unlike other witnesses, whistleblowers often must take alleged wrongdoers to court on their own dime. Absurdly, the welfare of millions of people may rely on how much a whistleblower has in his savings account. It's a great incentive for employers to evade accountability by firing whistleblowers and crippling them financially. Americans protect their own interests when they help whistleblowers overcome obstacles imposed by employers and the justice system" (para. 4).

> *Consider This* Advocacy is the foundation and essence of nursing, and nurses have a responsibility to promote human advocacy (Marquis & Huston, 2021).

Most recently, multiple cases of whistleblowing by nurses emerged in response to the COVID-19 pandemic, involving a lack of personal protective equipment (PPE), being asked to work in unsafe conditions, and provision of substandard care. For example, Kenisa Barkai, a nurse employed at Sinai-Grace Hospital in Detroit, Michigan, implored her supervisors to address what she described as a dangerous and severe staffing shortage in March 2020 (Neavling, 2020). When she felt they ignored her, Barkai threatened to alert state authorities and even tried to form a union. She also posted a brief video on social media about the need for more PPE and inpatient beds for an increasing wave of patients infected with COVID-19. The hospital said that the cell phone video violated hospital policy, and Barkai was fired.

Barkai's attorney said the explanation for her termination was a "pretext" to cover up the real reason she was fired—blowing the whistle on the unsafe conditions. A whistleblower lawsuit has since been filed against the hospital on behalf of Barkai (British Virgin Islands, 1995–2021).

In another lawsuit filed on May 20, 2020, Andrea Hinich, a military veteran, alleged she was fired a day after bringing up safety lapses in a meeting at her workplace, Norwood Park senior home (Struett, 2020). Hinich stated she was fired for "insubordination" after refusing to take part in a plan to distribute PPE to staff without required "fit testing." The Norwood administration allegedly told Hinich they "didn't have to do the fit testing" and that the PPE was being given to the staff only to "make them feel better." The suit claims Hinich was fired without warning and given false reasons for her termination that made her the scapegoat for the safety issues she raised (Struett, 2020).

In another case, a Florida nurse-turned-investigative journalist, Erin Marie Olszewski, who worked in New York City at the height of the COVID-19 pandemic, reported she had witnessed negligent practice firsthand at Elmhurst Hospital in Queens. Olszewski alleged the hospital failed to properly isolate patients with COVID-19, intermingling them with COVID-19 rule-out patients (Musto, 2020). In addition, she alleged that Elmhurst did not make use of rapid COVID-19 testing, though resources were not an issue in either situation (Musto, 2020).

In all these cases, the nurse whistleblowers suggested their actions were directed at protecting patients or colleagues. Indeed, patient advocacy has a central role in nursing. So too does professional advocacy, through which nurses are committed to improving the practice of nursing and maintaining the integrity of the health care profession. Both roles suggest that the nurse is accountable for ensuring that at least minimum standards are met. The cases detailed here depict nurses who believe or believed they were acting honorably in the role of advocate. Yet virtually all suffered negative consequences, including job loss. Unfortunately, this is more common than not. Hymas (2020) reports that 7 in 10 whistleblowers are victimized or forced to quit despite laws that exist to protect them.

Consider This The motive of most whistleblowers is advocacy, not troublemaking.

This willingness to speak out requires even greater courage when the whistleblower lacks official power and status. For example, research by Albert et al. (2020) found that nursing students often feel torn between the conflicts of whether to provide ethical care or accept unethical practices, stay silent about patient care neglect, or confront and report it, and provide ethical and quality care or adapt to the culture due to lack of autonomous decision making. Such conflicts can be detrimental to students' professional learning and mental health in clinical settings (see Research Fuels the Controversy 17.1).

Research Fuels the Controversy 17.1

Students Speaking Up

This integrative review of articles published from January 2000 to March 2019 aimed to develop a comprehensive understanding of nursing students' ethical dilemmas regarding patient care in clinical settings.

Source: Albert, J. S., Younas, A., & Sana, S. (2020, May). Nursing students' ethical dilemmas regarding patient care: An integrative review. *Nurse Education Today, 88*, N.PAG.

Study Findings

Three themes emerged: (a) applying learned ethical values versus accepting unethical practices, (b) desiring to provide ethical care but lacking autonomous decision making, and (c) silence versus whistleblowing to address patient care neglect.

The students observed many unethical practices from nurses, physicians, and other nursing students. Common unethical practices included breach of patients' privacy, confidentiality, respect, rights, and dignity; using derogatory and discriminatory statements about patients and their families; unprofessional attitudes toward patients and their families; giving patients insufficient and inappropriate information; and physical and psychological maltreatment of patients. Students considered these unethical practices deviant from the ethical values learned during their education.

Despite noting the discrepancies in learned ethical values and desire to provide ethical care to patients in clinical settings, nursing students struggled to act upon their desire to do the right thing during nursing care. This reluctance to act was attributed to a lack of autonomous decision making, lack of support from management and professional nurses, nursing students' lower position on the hierarchy of health care providers, and perceived oppression in clinical settings.

Students reported staying silent to keep patients' trust and confidence intact in health professionals, fearing hurting professionals and ruining their reputation, and losing personal relationship and rapport with the professionals. The students also reported lacking self-confidence to report these neglects; experiencing fear of unforeseen negative consequences of reporting; feeling that it was not their place to report; feeling that despite reporting, the unethical behaviors would not change; and feeling that they might be wrong.

The researchers concluded that nursing students are mostly observers, analyzers, and reflectors of unethical practices and require support and encouragement from their role models and mentors. It is essential that educators and nursing institutions develop programs to support these students and help them develop ethical competence, decision-making skills, and courage to confront such dilemmas.

THE PERSONAL RISKS OF WHISTLEBLOWING

Being a whistleblower is not without risks. Rather, it is filled with risks. Ceva and Bocchiola (2019) suggest at least part of the reason whistleblowers experience distrust and retaliation is because whistleblowing can be viewed as an instance of civil disobedience. Proponents of this view conceive whistleblowing as an exceptional individual response to some serious organizational wrongdoing that exceeds the standard duties of organizational membership. Thus, it is as an act of individual dissent, even if ordinary organizational reporting mechanisms have proved unviable, unavailable, or inefficient.

Discussion Point

Why is speaking out often honored more in theory than in fact?

Unfortunately, most whistleblowers set out believing their actions will be welcomed only to discover that the problems raised go much deeper than they imagined and the personal consequences can be overwhelming. Such consequences include negative reactions from coworkers, losing one's job, and, in the extreme, legal retaliation. In many cases, whistleblowers are fired from their jobs, especially those who are considered at-will employees.

Lewis (2017a, para. 7) notes that "the experiences of numerous whistleblowers show that reporting wrongdoing internally is a risky endeavor even when federal laws appear to offer whistleblower protection. Court remedies are frequently out of reach for whistleblowers with no source of income. For this reason, many concerned workers choose to report problems anonymously, although staying anonymous is increasingly difficult as surveillance by industry and government continues to grow."

Consider This   Although the U.S. public wants corruption and unethical behavior to be unveiled, the individual reporting such behavior is often looked upon with distrust and considered to be disloyal.

A study out of Tilburg University (2018) in the Netherlands also indicates the personal effects of blowing the whistle can be dramatic. About 80% of whistleblowers reported very negative effects on work and wages, and almost 50% reported very negative effects on family life. About 45% suffered from clinical levels of mental health problems such as anxiety and/or depressive symptoms after blowing the whistle. This prevalence among whistleblowers was about six times higher than among matched controls.

Many nurse whistleblowers are not prepared for this type of impact on their personal, emotional, physical, and professional welfare.

Not all whistleblowing, however, results in repercussions from employers. Employers are increasingly adopting policies encouraging employees to speak up and note practices that do not meet expected standards. In addition, a company's administration must create an organizational culture that supports workers who do speak out. For example, nursing departments within hospitals should provide nurses with an ethics committee chaired by someone with experience in bioethical issues (not one who has a vested interest in promoting administrative or hierarchical constraints). Nurse managers should promote the values inherent in patient advocacy, and the organization should openly support individuals who are willing to take the risk of being a whistleblower. The reality is that if an employee is willing to go to the trouble and risk the repercussions of blowing the whistle, those concerns should be taken seriously and investigated.

The bottom line, though, is that whistleblowers should never assume that doing the right thing will result in a financial incentive or protect them from retaliation. Instead, potential whistleblowers should determine their legal duty for reporting and carefully research the specifics of their protection under the law. They should try to report anonymously when possible. Moreover, they must be prepared to defend their claims, and prospective whistleblowers should always at least try to solve problems internally before going public. When that is impossible and there is a clear indication of serious harm, they must document their actions and go public. They should also seek support and counsel before taking any steps.

Clearly, whistleblowers often face both social- and work-related retaliation, and at times this retaliation can be severe and life-altering. Yet it must be noted that at least some self-satisfaction and pride must come with the recognition that unethical behavior has been exposed and that at least the potential for correction is possible because of the whistleblower's actions. Box 17.2 summarizes some of the pros and cons of whistleblowing.

Consider This   A whistleblower must blow the whistle for the right reason for it to be considered a moral action.

CULTURAL BACKGROUND AND WHISTLEBLOWING

For some nurses from minority backgrounds, cultural issues further complicate the decision to blow the whistle and, if so, how to do it. It is possible that nurses from some

BOX 17.2   **Pros and Cons of Whistleblowing**

Pros
- Protects patients
- Improves quality of care
- Meets professional expectations and standards
- Satisfies ethical duty
- Brings problems out into the open
- Provides validation of concerns and moral rightness

Cons
- Poses personal and professional risks
- Casts doubt on motives
- Can lead to possible job loss or employer retaliation
- Is typically a tiring, anxiety-producing, and often frustrating experience

cultural backgrounds may be more reluctant to blow the whistle because of their respect for authority and hierarchy. Travers (2019) agrees, noting that people from Japan, China, and Taiwan view whistleblowing less favorably than people in the United States. This has to do with "a culture's degree of collectivism, or the degree to which individuals perceive interdependence with their group, with more collectivist groups expressing more negative feelings toward whistleblowing" (Travers, 2019, para. 9).

Consider This   Whistleblowing is viewed less favorably in "collectivist" cultures than in "individualist" cultures (Travers, 2019).

The same is true for nurses whose first language is not English. Whistleblowers need clear and concise communication skills to articulately repeat their concerns to multiple stakeholders. Someone who lacks confidence in their ability to accurately communicate the problems they are observing would likely be more reluctant to undertake whistleblowing.

ETHICAL DIMENSIONS OF WHISTLEBLOWING

Ethical organizations practice in such a way that patients and workers are protected from harm. Sometimes, however, health care organizations fail to provide accountability for the safety and welfare of their patients and workers. Nurses or other employees then feel compelled to take action against the wrongdoing in an effort to fulfill their professional obligations.

Stuart (2020) agrees, noting that whistleblowing is now a full-blown ethical debate since the ideologic camp maintains that whistleblowing is ethical as a form of civil disobedience that aims to protect the public from wrongdoing. The political camp, however, sees whistleblowing as unethical since it requires a breach of confidentiality. "Should people tell the truth or obey orders when these two are in conflict" (Stuart, 2020, para. 9)?

Clearly, whistleblowing can create considerable moral distress for nurses as they weigh the consequences of their actions against the duties of their profession. In other words, they must weigh a consequentialist view based on utilitarianism (greatest good for greatest number of people) with their professional duty and values, which is founded more in a deontologic framework (duty-based reasoning).

Ceva and Bocchiola (2019) note that in a deontologic view, whistleblowing is a dutiful practice (not just an individual conscientious act) that any legitimate organization should implement to monitor its overall performance and the contribution that its members give toward or against it. As such, it directs members of an organization in the ordinary performance of their duties in nonideal conditions.

For example, clearly, nurses are bound to the role of patient advocacy by ethical codes of conduct. The problem is that nurses also have professional commitments to their employers and to other health care professionals, and this loyalty to the employer can be misplaced when it leads to patient harm. All too often, the result is then a conflict between principles and duty. This tension between loyalty to an employer and the need to protect patients is a major reason so many nurses delay blowing the whistle.

A compelling argument can be made, however, for the precedence of the nurse's duty to the patient over their duty to the employer. Indeed, nurses must always remember that their primary professional responsibility is to their patients, not to their employers. As such, the need to uphold the rights of others, to promote fairness, and to provide for the greater good becomes paramount.

Discussion Point

Can you think of a situation in which you have been involved in which utilitarianism (the greater good) would support not blowing the whistle on unethical behavior?

Bashir (2020) states that *fidelity* is another ethical principle that must be examined when considering the implications of whistleblowing. While society could not function if individuals routinely broke their agreements, concealing malpractice or unethical behavior decreases an organization's ability to meet its mission and violates the fidelity owed to the professional code of conduct. *Justice*, the moral obligation to act fairly, must also be considered. At times, however, claims of justice may supersede the claims of fidelity, and one's professional duty sometimes includes a legal and moral duty to report violations, especially if they are being concealed.

The American Nurses Association (ANA) *Code of Ethics for Nurses With Interpretive Statements* may also provide guidance for nurses who are considering becoming whistleblowers. Provision 3 states that the nurse "promotes, advocates for, and strives to protect the health, safety, and rights of the patient" (ANA, 2015, p. 9). In addition, Section 3.5 states:

> When incompetent, unethical, illegal, or impaired practice is not corrected and continues to jeopardize patient well-being and safety, nurses must report the problem to appropriate external authorities such as practice committees or professional organizations, licensing boards, and regulatory or quality assurance agencies. Some situations are sufficiently egregious as to warrant the notification and involvement of all groups and/or law enforcement. (ANA, 2015, p. 12)

Ethical codes of conduct from nursing organizations in Canada, the United Kingdom, Australia, and Japan mandate similar action. Such ethical codes bind nurses to the role of patient advocacy and compel them to act when the rights or safety of patients is jeopardized. The bottom line is that although whistleblowing can result in negative consequences for both the employing institution and the whistleblower, nurses must uphold a professional standard and protect their patients no matter what.

LEGAL PROTECTION FOR WHISTLEBLOWERS

Kohn, Kohn, and Colapinto (2021) note that many countries do not have whistleblower laws, and those that do offer only weak protection. Currently, however, the leader in whistleblower protection laws is the United States.

Yet with more than 50 whistleblower laws in this country (Wolf, 2019), there is no universal legal protection for whistleblowers. Under the 1st and 14th Amendments to the U.S. Constitution, state and local government officials are prohibited from retaliating against whistleblowers. In addition, though they do not fall under the category of "whistleblower" protections, laws protecting individual employees from mistreatment in the workplace, such as Title VII of the Civil Rights Act or the Fair Labor Standards Act, also protect employees from retaliation for asserting their rights under those laws. For example, it is illegal to terminate an employee for reporting sexual harassment or for

challenging an employer's failure to pay overtime (Joseph & Kirschenbaum, LLP, 2020).

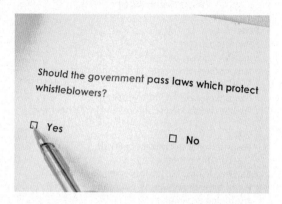

Should the government pass laws which protect whistleblowers?

☐ Yes   ☐ No

The False Claims Act

Some whistleblower legislation has been enacted at the federal level, however, to encourage people to report wrongdoings. One such piece of legislation is the *False Claims Act* (FCA), originally a Civil War statute, that encourages whistleblowers to come forward regarding fraud committed against the federal government and to file a lawsuit seeking lost monies in the government's name.

The individual would file a *qui tam* or whistleblower lawsuit and provide knowledge that a person defrauded the government. A *qui tam* lawsuit is brought by a citizen, known as a "relator" or whistleblower, against a company, person, or entity that they believe is cheating the federal or state government in some way (Whistleblowerlaws, 2020). Since the *qui tam* suit is brought in the name of the whistleblower on behalf of the government, the government may actually join the case and litigate alongside the whistleblower's lawyers. These FCAs or "*qui tam* laws" exist at the federal level. An individual who successfully pursues a *qui tam* action is entitled to a bounty that ranges between 15% and 30% of the government's recovery (Khurana Law Firm, 2020; The Employment Law Group, 2021).

For example, a whistleblower may have knowledge of a colleague inappropriately billing Medicare or Medicaid. The FCA provides protection for government whistleblowers, thereby prohibiting employers from punishing employees who report the fraud or assist in the investigation of the fraud. If the whistleblower is dismissed or discriminated against in any way as a result of the lawsuit, the whistleblower can file a claim against that employer for unlawful retaliation.

To have a case brought to trial under federal law, the whistleblower must first exhaust their internal chain of command and then file a complaint with the Department of Health and Human Services (DHHS). If the DHHS decides that the complaint is valid, the government proceeds with litigation against the employer, and the whistleblower receives a percentage of the damages awarded. The case discussed earlier in this chapter involving the two nurses in Missouri who alleged nursing home abuse and fraud was a FCA *qui tam* lawsuit.

For example, Phoenix-based Banner Health was required to pay more than $18 million as part of an FCA lawsuit to settle whistleblower claims that they admitted patients who could have been treated less expensively at outpatient facilities (Alltucker, 2018). The settlement resolves a complaint brought forth by a former Banner Health employee who claimed a dozen hospitals in Arizona and Colorado overcharged Medicare for brief, inpatient procedures that should have been billed on a less costly outpatient basis. The employee who filed the claim was paid $3.3 million as part of the FCA settlement (Alltucker, 2018).

Are financial incentives the primary driving force for whistleblowers who bring forth FCA claims, or does most whistleblowing occur because of a perceived obligation to address a problem? Dey et al. (2021) suggest that little is known about how financial incentives affect whistleblowers' decisions to report potential misconduct to authorities, but new research suggests that greater incentives increase the number of lawsuits filed with the regulator, the regulator's investigation length, the percentage of intervened lawsuits, and the percentage of settled lawsuits. Dey and team (2021) also note that FCA whistleblowers can expect to receive approximately $140,000 for blowing the whistle.

It is noteworthy, however, that since the FCA was signed into law, it has become the most successful antifraud legislation in the United States. According to the Department of Justice, in fiscal year 2020 alone, the government recovered over $2.2 billion in FCA settlements and judgments. Over $1.6 billion of that can be attributed to whistleblower-initiated cases (Guidance for Whistleblowers, 1997–2021).

Other Legislation Related to Whistleblowing

Another piece of legislation, the *Whistleblower Protection Act of 1989*, protects federal employees who disclose government fraud, abuse, and waste. The *Whistleblower Protection Enhancement Act of 2007* extended the Whistleblower Protection Act of 1989 to federal employees who specialize in national security issues. In addition, the *Paul Revere Freedom to Warn Act* protects federal employee whistleblowers who speak out about abuse, harassment, and unethical behavior in the workplace.

The National Labor Relations Act might protect employees in the private sector from retaliation when employees act as a group to modify working conditions or ask for better wages. The best protection for employees who work for publicly traded companies or companies that are required to file certain reports with the Securities and Exchange Commission (SEC) in the United States at this time, however, is likely the *Sarbanes–Oxley Act of 2002* (further amended by the *Dodd–Frank Wall Street Reform and Consumer Protection Act* in 2010). This act dramatically redesigned federal regulation of public company corporate governance and reporting obligations and provided some protection for whistleblowers who report fraud in publicly traded companies to the proper authorities (Joseph & Kirschenbaum, LLP, 2020).

Employees in these companies who experience retaliation for whistleblowing have 180 days to file a written complaint with the Occupational Safety and Health Administration (OSHA). If the evidence supports an employee's claim of retaliation and a settlement cannot be reached, OSHA will issue an order requiring the employer to reinstate the employee, pay back wages, and restore benefits (OSHA, n.d., para. 7). After OSHA issues its final ruling, either party may request a full hearing before an administrative law judge of the Department of Labor. That decision can then be appealed to the Department's Administrative Review Board for final review.

In 2018, the SEC announced it had awarded more than $262 million to 53 whistleblowers since issuing its first award in 2012 (SEC.gov, 2018). In March 2018, it announced its highest-ever Dodd–Frank whistleblower awards with two whistleblowers sharing a nearly $50 million award and a third whistleblower receiving more than $33 million. In June 2020, SEC announced an award of almost $700,000 to a whistleblower whose significant information helped the agency bring a successful enforcement action that resulted in the return of money to harmed investors (SEC.gov, 2020). And in February 2021, the SEC announced two whistleblower awards totaling almost $3 million, a record start to the 2021 fiscal year (Schweller, 2021). These awards were issued to whistleblowers whose disclosures helped lead to successful enforcement actions.

In 2018, however, the U.S. Supreme Court ruled that whistleblower protections under the Dodd–Frank Act apply only to people who report misconduct directly to the SEC (Nagelle-Piazza, 2018). That is, people who report misconduct internally would not be protected from retaliation. This places increased pressure on company compliance programs to ensure their monitoring, reporting, and investigation policies, procedures, and practices are in a position to sufficiently incentivize and encourage employees to report securities law violations internally (Giampetruzzi et al., 2018).

Because the FCA has been fairly effective in detecting fraud at the federal level, some state versions of the FCA have also passed, though the federal laws contained in the FCA may not be exactly duplicated by state governments (The Employment Law Group, 2021). Under these state laws, whistleblowers can file lawsuits seeking lost monies in the state or local government's name and share in the proceeds. As of 2020, FCAs or "*qui tam* laws" had been adopted by 29 states, the District of Columbia, the city of New York, and the city of Chicago, although a number of other states are considering the introduction of such legislation (Whistleblowerlaws, 2020).

There are some state legal protections for whistleblowers as well. Although some state laws prohibit retaliation, the standards for proving retaliation vary. Employees in most states increase their likelihood of whistleblower protection under general statutes or common law if they meet criteria similar to those established at the federal level:

1. They must be acting in good faith that the employer or its employees are breaking the law in some way.
2. They must complain about that violation either to the employer or to an outside agency.
3. They must refuse to be a party to the violation.
4. They should be willing to assist in any official investigations of the violation.

Discussion Point

What whistleblowing protections, if any, exist in the state where you live? Is any legislation pending?

The Office of Accountability and Whistleblower Protection

In 2017, former President Donald Trump signed an executive order establishing an Office of Accountability and Whistleblower Protection (OAWP) to be led by a special assistant to the secretary (OAWP, 2021). This office was charged with working closely with relevant VA components to ensure swift and effective resolution of veterans' complaints of wrongdoing at the VA and to ensure adequate investigation and correction of wrongdoing throughout the VA. The OAWP also protects employees who lawfully disclose wrongdoing from retaliation.

Still, recent reports suggest that some VA whistleblowers continue to be intimidated, bullied, and threatened with physical violence as they report wrongdoing in their agencies (Diaz, 2018). Reporting wrongdoing through official VA channels like the OAWP can take months, and complaints often go back to the employee's supervisors at work—even when anonymity is supposedly guaranteed (Diaz, 2018).

In addition, Sisk (2020) suggested that a climate of intimidation exists at the OAWP. Citing 20 anonymous current and former staffers at OAWP, a report by the nonprofit Project on Government Oversight (POGO) alleged that an OAWP supervisor was fired and a staff person demoted for refusing orders not to cooperate with investigators from the VA's Office of Inspector General (OIG). The report also alleged a toxic work environment exists.

The VA OIG, which has an oversight role with respect to the OAWP, has acknowledged an oversight report from 2019 that found significant failings at the OAWP, which had a chilling effect on complainants, that to some extent still lingers today. Efforts to address the problem, however, are ongoing, and the OIG has made a commitment to treat all complainants as whistleblowers and to respond respectfully, safeguard confidentiality, and evaluate their concerns (The Department of VA/OIG, 2021).

WHISTLEBLOWING AS AN INTERNATIONAL ISSUE

Whistleblowing cases are not limited to the United States. Whistleblower protection has been recognized as part of international law since 2003, when the United Nations (UN) adopted the Convention Against Corruption (Guidance for Whistleblowers, 1997–2021). This convention was subsequently signed by 140 nations and formally ratified, accepted, approved, or acceded by 137 nations, including the United States. Articles 32 and 33 of the UN Convention also endorse protection for whistleblowers. In addition, the *Foreign Corrupt Practices Act* (FCPA) prohibits thousands of corporations, both American and international, from paying bribes to foreign officials and mandates proper financial recordkeeping (Guidance for Whistleblowers, 1997–2021).

However, the strength of whistleblower laws varies substantially from country to country, and many countries have no laws at all while others offer only weak protections (Guidance for Whistleblowers, 1997–2021). The lack of protection for whistleblowers, then, is a global problem, and mounting pressure exists internationally to adopt whistleblower protection laws to reduce the risk of retaliation to whistleblowers.

Federal law in Canada enacted in 2004 with Section 425.1 of the Criminal Code prohibits employers from retaliating or threatening to take action against employees who provide information to law enforcement officials. The *Public Servants Disclosure Protection Act* has protected whistleblowers in the federal public sector since 2007 (The state of whistleblowing, 2016). Yet legal experts suggest these laws are still too limited to fully protect whistleblowers.

In October 2019, the European Union adopted a directive on the "protection of persons who report breaches of Union law," which provides for the implementation of new comprehensive European Union–wide rules on whistleblower protections (William Cutler Pickering, Hale, and Dorr LLP, 2021). To date, EU countries have offered varying and fragmented standards of protection for those who speak out when they encounter wrongdoing that could harm the public interest. EU member states have until October 2021 to transpose the directive into national law.

Discussion Point

Would international adoption of legislation similar to the FCA increase the likelihood that whistleblowers will both come forward and be protected from recrimination globally?

CONCLUSIONS

As health care professionals, nurses have a responsibility to uncover, openly discuss, and condemn shortcuts that threaten the patients they serve. Clearly, however, there has been a collective silence in many such cases. The reality is that whistleblowing offers no guarantee that the situation will change or the problem will improve, and the literature is replete with horror stories regarding negative consequences endured by whistleblowers. The whistleblower cannot even trust that other health care professionals with similar belief systems about advocacy will value their efforts because the public's feelings about whistleblowers are so mixed. In addition, state laws vary, and protections for the nongovernment employee whistleblower are often limited.

For all these reasons, it takes tremendous courage to come forward as a whistleblower. It also takes a tremendous sense of what is right and what is wrong, as well as a commitment to follow a problem through until an acceptable level of resolution is reached. Whistleblowers are heroes and should be treated as such; their courage is nothing short of exceptional. How unfortunate that we frequently do not treat them that way!

For Additional Discussion

1. Why do Americans have a "love–hate" relationship with whistleblowers? Is this dichotomy prevalent in other countries as well?

2. Which is greater for you personally—your duty to your patients, your duty to your employer, or your duty to yourself? How do you sort out what you should do when these duties are in conflict?

3. Do you believe that most whistleblowing must be external before appropriate action is taken?

4. Should whistleblowers receive compensation under the FCA?

5. Would you be willing to bear the risks of becoming a whistleblower?

6. Do you believe that there is more, less, or the same amount of whistleblowing in health care as in other types of industries?

7. Can you identify a whistleblowing situation in which it might be appropriate to go outside the chain of command in reporting concerns about organizational practice?

References

Albert, J. S., Younas, A., & Sana, S. (2020, May). Nursing students' ethical dilemmas regarding patient care: An integrative review. *Nurse Education Today, 88*, N.PAG.

Alltucker, K. (2018, April 12). *Banner health settles whistleblower case for $18 million.* Retrieved July 29, 2021, from https://www.azcentral.com/story/money/business/health/2018/04/12/banner-health-settles-whistleblower-case-18-million/511848002

American Nurses Association. (2015). *Code of ethics for nurses with interpretive statements.* Author.

Bashir, F. (2020, March 12). Decision making through the lens of fidelity: Ethical dilemma. *Journal of Clinical Research and*

Bioethics. Retrieved July 29, 2021, from https://www
.longdom.org/abstract/decision-making-through-the-lens-
of-fidelity-ethical-dilemma-54578.html

British Virgin Islands. (1995–2021). *A Detroit nurse was fired
after speaking out about her hospital's handling of the coronavirus outbreak. Now she's fighting back*. Retrieved July
29, 2021, from https://bvi.org/a-nurse-was-fired-after-
speaking-out-about-conditions-in-her-hospital-during-the-
coronavirus-outbreak

Ceva, E., & Bocchiola, M. (2019, December 27). Theories of
whistleblowing. *Wiley Online Library*. Retrieved July 29,
2021, from https://onlinelibrary.wiley.com/doi/full/10.1111/
phc3.12642?fbclid=IwAR17UhSIqs3ajRMgCiigEkuKDOq
ZVMUxHSR2KUOZ0b9RuIHtt_QN6ITXMJ4

Colvin, G. (2002). Wonder women of whistleblowing. Is it significant that the prominent heroes to emerge from the two
great business scandals of recent years were women?
Fortune, 146(3). Retrieved July 29, 2021, from http://money
.cnn.com/magazines/fortune/fortune_archive/2002/08/12/
327047/index.htm

Coxwell, M. (2018, February 9). *7 of the most famous whistleblower cases in the U.S.* Retrieved July 29, 2021, from
https://blog.coxwelllaw.com/famous-whistleblower-cases-
in-the-us/

DeltaNet International. (2021, June 23). *Why whistleblowing is
important*. Retrieved July 30, 2021, from https://www.delta-
net.com/blog/2021/06/why-whistleblowing-is-important

Department of Veterans Affairs, Office of Inspector General.
(2021, May 19). Office of Inspector General Department of
Veterans Affairs statement of Christopher A. Wilber Coun-
selor to The Inspector General Office Of Inspector General,
U.S. Department Of Veterans Affairs before The Subcommittee On Oversight And Investigations, U.S. House Of
Representatives Committee On Veterans' Affairs, hearing
on "protecting whistleblowers and promoting accountability: Is VA making progress?" Retrieved July 30, 2021,
from https://www.va.gov/oig/pubs/statements/VAOIG-
statement-20210519-wilber.pdf

Dey, A., Heese, J., & Pérez Cavazos, G. (2021, June 10).
*Cash-for-information whistleblower programs: Effects on
whistleblowing and consequences for whistleblowers. Harvard
Law School Forum on Corporate Governance*. Retrieved July
30, 2021, from https://corpgov.law.harvard.edu/2021/06/10/
cash-for-information-whistleblower-programs-effects-on-
whistleblowing-and-consequences-for-whistleblowers/

Diaz, A. (2018, April 11). *VA whistleblowers, under threat, seek
help from the outside*. Retrieved July 29, 2021, from http://
www.foxnews.com/us/2018/04/10/va-whistleblowers-
under-threat-seek-help-from-outside.html

Gagnon, M., & Perron, A. (2020). Whistleblowing: A concept
analysis. *Nursing & Health Sciences, 22*(2), 381–389. https://
doi.org/10.1111/nhs.12667

Gates, D. (2020, June 18). "*Boeing whistleblower alleges systemic
problems with 737 MAX*." *The Seattle Times*. Retrieved July
29, 2021, from https://www.seattletimes.com/business/
boeing-aerospace/boeing-whistleblower-alleges-systemic-
problems-with-737-max/

Giampetruzzi, G., Montes, J., & Baker, J. (2018, April 19).
*In light of digital realty and the largest ever Dodd-Frank
Whistleblower award, whistleblower risks are up
and-company compliance programs are under pressure. Paul Hastings*. Retrieved July 29, 2021, from
https://www.paulhastings.com/publications-items/
details/?id=e3d88c6a-2334-6428-811c-ff00004cbded

Guidance for whistleblowers outside the U.S. (1997–2021).
National Whistleblower Center. Retrieved August 2, 2020,
from https://www.whistleblowers.org/know-your-rights/
international-whistleblower/

Hymas, C. (2020, June 21). *Seven in ten whistleblowers are
victimised or forced to quit despite laws to protect them*.
Retrieved July 29, 2021, from https://www.telegraph.co.uk/
news/2020/06/21/seven-ten-whistleblowers-victimised-
forced-quit-despite-laws/

Joseph & Kirschenbaum, LLP. (2020). *Whistleblower and
Sarbanes-Oxley claims*. Author. Retrieved July 29, 2021,
from http://www.jhllp.com/lawyer-attorney-1324989.html

Khurana Law Firm. (2020). *Whistleblower and qui tam lawyers battling Medicare fraud*. Retrieved July 28, 2020, from
http://www.medicarewhistleblowercenter.com

Kohn, Kohn, and Colapinto, LLP. (2021). *US Whistleblower
Protection Laws [2021]*. Retrieved July 30, 2021, from
https://kkc.com/frequently-asked-questions/us-whistleblower-
protection-laws/

Lewis, L. (2017a). *Regulator ignored 700 Wells Fargo-
whistleblower complaints. Whistleblowing Today*. Retrieved
July 29, 2021, from http://whistleblowingtoday.org/2017/05/
regulator-ignored-700-wells-fargo-whistleblower-
complaints

Lewis, L. (2017b). *Child health whistleblower Vikki Mata appeals
for donations. Whistleblowing Today*. Retrieved July 29,
2021, from http://whistleblowingtoday.org/2017/01/child-
health-whistleblower-vikki-mata-appeals-for-donations

Marquis, B., & Huston, C. (2021). *Leadership roles and management functions in nursing* (10th ed.). Wolters Kluwer.

Mason, D. J. (2011, January 14). *Public officials indicted in RN
whistleblowing case [Web log post]*. Retrieved July 29, 2021,
from http://www.healthmediapolicy.com/2011/01/14/
public-officials-indicted-in-rn-whistleblowing-case

Musto, J. (2020, June 13). *Undercover nurse: NY hospital didn't
properly isolate coronavirus patients*. Retrieved July 29,
2021, from https://www.foxnews.com/media/undercover-
nurse-ny-hospital-isolate-coronavirus-patients

Nagelle-Piazza, L. (2018, February 22). *Whistleblowers must report to SEC for Dodd-Frank retaliation protection*. Retrieved
August 2, 2020, from https://www.shrm.org/resources
andtools/legal-and-compliance/employment-law/pages/
whistle-blowers-sec-dodd-frank.aspx

Neavling, S. (2020, April 10). *Whistleblowing nurse fired
after complaining of inhumane conditions at Detroit's
Sinai-Grace amid coronavirus outbreak*. Retrieved July
29, 2021, from https://www.metrotimes.com/news-hits/
archives/2020/04/10/whistleblowing-nurse-fired-after-
complaining-of-inhumane-conditions-at-detroits-sinai-
grace-amid-coronavirus-outbreak

Occupational Safety and Health Administration. (n.d.). *OSHA fact sheet: Filing whistleblower complaints under the Sarbanes-Oxley Act.* Retrieved July 29, 2021, from https://www.osha.gov/Publications/osha-factsheet-sox-act.pdf

Office of Accountability and Whistleblower Protection. (2021, July 13). *VA's office of accountability and whistleblower protection.* Retrieved July 29, 2021, from https://www.va.gov/accountability/

Rohner, T. (2015, February 6). *Whistleblowing nurse wants action on Nunavut nursing scandal. Nunatsiaq Online.* Retrieved July 29, 2021, from https://nunatsiaq.com/stories/article/65674whistle-blowing_nurse_wants_action_on_nunavut_nursing_scandal/

Sack, K. (2011, January 14). *Sheriff charged in Texas whistleblowing case. The New York Times.* Retrieved July 29, 2021, from http://www.nytimes.com/2011/01/15/us/15nurses.html?_r=1

Schweller, G. (2021, February 29). *SEC pays whistleblowers $3 million in first awards of new administration.* Retrieved July 30, 2021, from https://whistleblowersblog.org/corporate-whistleblowers/dodd-frank-whistleblowers/sec-pays-whistleblowers-3-million-in-first-awards-of-new-administration/

SEC.gov. (2018, March 19). "*SEC announces its largest-ever whistleblower awards.*" *U.S. Securities and Exchange Commission.* Retrieved July 29, 2021, from https://www.sec.gov/news/press-release/2018-44

SEC.gov. (2020, June 19). "*SEC awards almost $700,000 to whistleblower.*" *U.S. Securities and Exchange Commission.* Retrieved July 29, 2021, from https://www.sec.gov/news/press-release/2020-138

Sisk, R. (2020, March 6). *VA Whistleblower Protection Office retaliated against its own whistleblowers, report claims.* Retrieved July 29, 2021, from https://www.military.com/daily-news/2020/03/06/va-whistleblower-protection-office-retaliated-against-its-own-whistleblowers-report-claims.html

Struett, D. (2020, May 26). *Nurse fired from Norwood Park senior home for pointing out COVID-19 safety issues: Lawsuit.* Retrieved July 29, 2021, from https://chicago.suntimes.com/news/2020/5/26/21270733/andrea-hinch-norwood-park-crossing-nursing-home-lawsuit-ppe-covid-19-coronavirus

Stuart, G. L. (2020, October 23). *The ethics of whistleblowing.* Retrieved July 30, 2021, from https://ethicsofwriting.com/2020/10/ethics-of-whistleblowing/

The Employment Law Group. (2021). *Do you need a whistleblower rewards attorney?* Retrieved July 29, 2021, from https://www.employmentlawgroup.com/what-we-do/whistleblower-protection-rewards/how-our-attorneys-help-whistleblowers/?utm_campaign=Bing%20Whistleblower%20Law&_SR=Bing&_AC=Whistleblower%20Law&_AG=Whistleblower%20Law&_kk=Federal%20%2Bwhistleblower%20Law&_ph=1-888-387-3057&mm_campaign=8f347e770d565c22a9c780b9d17bed34&keyword=Federal%20%2Bwhistleblower%20Law&utm_source=Bing&utm_medium=CPC

The Free Dictionary by Farlex. (2003–2021). *Whistleblowing [Definition].* Retrieved July 29, 2021, from https://legal-dictionary.thefreedictionary.com/Whistleblowing#:~:text=Whistleblowing%20The%20disclosure%20by%20a%20person%2C%20usually%20an,the%20public%20value%20of%20whistle-blowinghas%20been%20increasingly%20recognized

The state of whistleblowing. (2016, Summer). *Canadian Journal of Medical Laboratory Science, 78*(2), 25–27.

Tilburg University. (2018, February 19). *Whistleblowers often suffer from severe psychological problems.* Retrieved July 29, 2021, from https://medicalxpress.com/news/2018-02-whistleblowers-severe-psychological-problems.html

Travers, M. (2019, September 26). *What science tells us about the psychology of whistleblowers.* Retrieved July 29, 2021, from https://www.forbes.com/sites/traversmark/2019/09/26/inside-the-mind-of-a-whistleblower/#47c58d955007

Whistleblowerlaws. (2020). *What is a qui tam? Guttman, Buschner & Brooks PLLC.* Retrieved July 29, 2021, from http://www.whistleblowerlaws.com/what-is-qui-tam

Wilmer Cutler Pickering Hale and Dorr LLP. (2021). *EU adopts new whistleblower protections, but will the UK follow suit and how much comfort do they really provide?* Retrieved July 30, 2021, from https://www.lexology.com/library/detail.aspx?g=1bf5c9d9-7b9e-4a52-be69-9cc44b3819a3

Wolf, Z. B. (2019, November 5). *The law puts Trump in charge of enforcing whistleblower protections.* Retrieved July 29, 2021, from https://www.cnn.com/2019/11/05/politics/whistleblower-identity-trump-legal-obligations/index.html

Younger, N. (1997–2021). *The case of Edward Snowden. National Whistleblower Center.* Retrieved July 29, 2021, from https://www.whistleblowers.org/news/the-case-of-edward-snowden/

Substance Use Disorder in Nursing Practice

Carol J. Huston and Jennifer Lillibridge

CHAPTER OUTLINE

LEARNING OBJECTIVES

The learner will be able to:

1. Examine the prevalence of substance use disorder (SUD) in the nursing profession.

2. Describe early factors that result in an increased risk for SUD in the nursing profession.

3. Explore how nurses and managers can prevent or detect drug diversion in the workplace.

4. Describe challenges and barriers nurses face when confronting and/or helping colleagues with SUD.

5. Identify the state boards of nursing reporting requirements for nurses suspected of SUD or of diverting drugs for personal use.

6. Identify the driving forces that compelled most U.S. state boards of nursing to move from mandatory disciplinary action for nurses with SUD to diversion program treatment.

7. Describe typical components of a state diversion program, as well as a "return-to-work" agreement, for a nurse with SUD.

8. Identify links between national nursing policies about impaired practice and local implementation of strategies to address the problem.

9. Examine the role practice and academic nurse leaders hold in addressing SUD in nursing practice.

10. Examine the role of nursing education in the prevention of SUD in nursing practice.

INTRODUCTION

The American Society of Addiction Medicine (2020) uses the term *impairment* for a functional classification that exists dynamically on a continuum of severity and can change over time rather than being a static phenomenon. In the case of impairment in nursing, this occurs when the nurse is unable to provide safe patient care due to using a mood- or mind-altering substance or having a physical condition or distorted thought process from a psychological condition (Intervention Project for Nurses [IPN], 2001–2016). As a result, the nurse is unable to perform their professional responsibilities and duties consistent with expected nursing standards. This chapter focuses on nurses who are impaired due to substance use disorder (SUD).

The National Council of State Boards of Nursing (NCSBN, 2021) notes that no one is immune to the development of SUD since it can affect anyone regardless of age, ethnicity, gender, economic circumstance, or occupation. This includes nurses. When nurses abuse chemical substances, however, the risk extends from the self to those they care for since SUD in nursing impairs professional judgment and slows reaction time, threatening the ability of the nurse to make safe, appropriate decisions in the provision of quality patient care. In addition, when being cared for by an impaired nurse, patients may not receive their pain medication, or it may be given in a limited dose due to diversion.

The Centers for Disease Control and Prevention (CDC), along with state and local health departments, also note that infection outbreaks have occurred due to drug diversion activities involving health care providers (Morris, 2020). Indeed, Lockwood (2020) reported that in New Hampshire in 2013, David Kwiatkowksi, a hospital worker infected with hepatitis C, injected himself with patients' narcotics and then refilled the syringes with saline and administered the contaminated solution to patients. Forty-six patients were infected in New Hampshire, and nearly 8,000 people across eight states required testing. Lockwood (2020) suggests that similar diversions are taking place in hospitals across the United States every day.

SUD in nursing, however, is not a new problem. Modlin and Montes (1964) first documented drug addiction in the health professions in the late 1940s, though public recognition of the problem did not really begin until the early 1980s. Despite this relatively recent examination of the problem, there is little doubt that SUD has existed as long as alcohol and drugs have. Yet, the problem of impaired practice continues to be poorly understood and underreported with discussion typically raising more questions than answers.

This is because several key issues surround impaired nursing practice. The first is concern for patient safety. Patient safety has been at the forefront of national considerations about professional nursing practice for more than 20 years. Given this agenda, it seems critical that preventing impaired practice and dealing with it proactively when it does occur should be inclusive in all discussions about patient safety.

Another key issue is concern for the health of the impaired nurse. With denial and underreporting common, the problem can go without detection or treatment for years. In addition, the impaired nurse may face the possibility of criminal prosecution, a loss of livelihood and license, overdose, and even death (Morris, 2020). Losing one nurse to SUD is losing one nurse too many. Nursing is a profession known for its caring nature toward others, but we often fail to adequately care for ourselves.

Finally, there are numerous issues for organizations that employ nurses with SUD. There are liability concerns—both civil and regulatory as well as negative publicity that could damage an organization's reputation. In addition, lax institutional controls have led to large fines for some organizations and placed licenses at risk of restriction or revocation (Morris, 2020).

> *Consider This* Most addiction specialists and the American Medical Association view addiction as a chronic medical illness and argue that it should be approached in an analogous way to other disorders like diabetes and asthma.

PREVALENCE OF THE PROBLEM

Some experts suggest the prevalence of SUD in nursing mirrors that of the general population at approximately 10%, but efforts to quantify this prevalence may be skewed since self-disclosure and peer reporting are limited due to fear, stigma, and denial. The Recovery Village (2020) suggests that approximately 10% to 15% of nurses are impaired by or recovering from SUD, including alcohol addiction, a figure commonly found in the literature. Similarly, Taylor (2020) notes that SUD is the principal cause of professional impairment for certified registered nurse anesthetists (CRNAs), with one of every 10 experiencing addiction to drugs or alcohol. Some researchers, however, suggest the numbers are even higher.

> *Consider This* Given current estimates of impaired nursing practice, it is likely that at least 1 of every 10 nurses you work with will struggle with SUD.

Research Fuels the Controversy 18.1

Substance Use Disorders Among Nurses in Medical–Surgical, Long-Term Care, and Outpatient Services

This research was a retrospective, descriptive, secondary analysis of nurses enrolled in the Texas Peer Assistance Program for Nurses (TPAPN) between January 2010 and October 2016.

Source: Mumba, M. N., & Kraemer, K. R. (2019). Substance use disorders among nurses in medical-surgical, long-term care, and outpatient services. *MEDSURG Nursing, 28*(2), 87–118.

Study Findings

Medical–surgical, long-term care, and outpatient services settings were found to have a higher prevalence of nurses with SUD than other work areas in the database. The researchers suggested the reduced accountability and supervision of nurses in long-term care and geriatric specialty areas may be contributing factors in this increased prevalence. In addition, many residents in these facilities may be incapacitated in some way and thus less likely to report they are not receiving their medications when nurses divert from their patients.

In addition, researchers found nurses in the prone area sample showed a greater likelihood than others to have a primary drug of choice of alcohol or stimulants; in addition, a smaller portion of the sample had opioids as the primary drug of choice. Study findings also revealed that alcohol abusers tended to be older than nurses who abused opioids ($p < 0.001$) and nurses who abused cannabis ($p = 0.05$).

In addition, self-reporting was marginally higher among nurses with comorbid psychiatric disorders (18%), compared to nurses without psychiatric comorbidity (11%) (c2 [1, $N = 436$] = 3.77, $p = 0.052$). Self-reporting users were less likely to relapse (4%) compared with non–self-reporting users, and a tendency to relapse was associated with individuals who took longer to enroll in the monitoring program once their abuse was discovered. Indeed, the median time to enroll for individuals who relapsed (67 days) was nearly twice that of the median time to enroll for those who did not relapse (38 days).

Prevalence may also vary among the areas in which nurses work. Mumba and Kraemer (2019) suggest that specialty areas such as medical–surgical, long-term care, and outpatient services demonstrate a higher prevalence of impaired nurses and identify the reduced accountability and supervision of nurses in long-term care and geriatric specialty areas as contributing factors to these higher numbers (Research Fuels the Controversy 18.1).

COMMONLY MISUSED OR ABUSED DRUGS

Although alcohol is the most frequently abused substance, opioid pain relievers, such as Vicodin and OxyContin; stimulants for treating attention-deficit/hyperactivity disorder (ADHD), such as Adderall, Concerta, and Ritalin; and central nervous system (CNS) depressants for relieving anxiety, such as Valium and Xanax, are the three classes of prescription drugs most commonly misused (National Institute on Drug Abuse, 2020). Barbiturates may also replace alcohol in the workplace so that the employee may feel a similar effect without having alcohol detectable on their breath. Indeed, nearly 7% of nurses use prescription drugs for nonmedical purposes, a rate higher than the national average (Gonzales, 2020).

It is the overuse of opioids, however, that has become a leading cause of injury and death due to drug overdose in the United States, and opioids have become a drug of choice for many nurses with SUD. The National Institute on Drug Abuse (2021) notes that in 2019, nearly 50,000 people in the United States died from opioid-involved overdoses. In addition, roughly 21% to 29% of patients prescribed opioids for chronic pain misused them and between 8% and 12% developed an opioid use disorder (National Institute for Drug Abuse, 2021). Similarly, the CDC (2020) reported that more than 81,000 drug overdose deaths occurred in the United States in the 12 months ending in May 2020, the highest number of overdose deaths ever recorded in a 12-month period. The COVID-19 pandemic appears to be a factor in this increase (CDC, 2020).

In addition, over the past few years, the opioid death toll has been exacerbated by the use of heroin and synthetic opioids, most notably fentanyl. Overdose deaths from synthetic opioids increased 38.4% from the 12-month period leading up to June 2019 compared with the 12-month period leading up to May 2020 (CDC, 2020). In addition, 37 of the 38 U.S. jurisdictions with available synthetic opioid data reported increases in synthetic opioid-involved overdose deaths, with 18 of these jurisdictions reporting increases of more than 50%. Ten Western states reported over a 98% increase in synthetic opioid-involved deaths (CDC, 2020). Clearly, the misuse of and addiction to opioids—including prescription pain relievers, heroin, and synthetic opioids—is a serious national crisis that affects public health as well as social and economic welfare (National Institute on Drug Abuse, 2021).

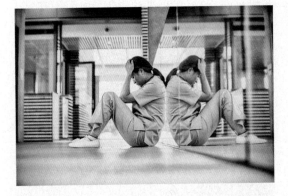

RISK FACTORS FOR SUBSTANCE USE DISORDER IN NURSING

Mirlashari et al. (2020) identify many etiologic factors known to contribute to the initiation and continuation of drug use, including genetic and social factors, family relationships, and poor parenting practices. In addition, although substance use generally begins during the adolescent years, there are known biologic, psychological, social, and environmental factors that contribute to the risk; these may begin accumulating as early as the prenatal period.

Why nurses abuse substances at a rate higher than the general population, however, is not well understood. The NCSBN (2013) suggests several work factors that may increase the risk of substance abuse in nurses, including staffing shortages, increased patient acuity and assignment ratios, demanding administrators and physicians, rotating shifts, and long work hours. Recovery Village (2020) agrees, noting that nursing is a stressful, fast-paced occupation, requiring both physical and mental stamina. In addition, on-the-job injuries are common, and prescription drugs are sometimes the first-line treatment for painful physical injuries. It may be difficult to avoid job strain in the current health care environment.

However, there are many reasons nurses may turn to drugs or alcohol. Co-occurring disorders, such as depression and posttraumatic stress disorder (PTSD), and genetics contribute to substance abuse as does fatigue and stress (Gonzales, 2020). In addition, many nurses are subject to workplace bullying and verbal abuse, contributing to stress and feelings of powerlessness.

In addition, some nurses may believe they are invulnerable to addiction. Because nurses are highly experienced in administering medications to others, they sometimes erroneously believe this allows them to better control their own use of drugs. Certainly, nurses are more apt to self-diagnose and self-medicate. Indeed, one common difference between chemically impaired health professionals with SUD and other individuals with SUD is that nurses and physicians are able to obtain their drugs of choice through channels such as legitimate prescriptions or diversionary measures on the job rather than illegally purchasing them (Marquis & Huston, 2021).

> ***Consider This*** Anne, a 59-year-old Canadian nurse who struggled with addiction for decades, said, "I got this attack of pain and I just helped myself to opioids at work, thinking I could get through my shift." She says, "I knew I was doing something wrong, so ethically, it was really soul-destroying. You rationalize and justify it . . . but once you take the drug, the drug sort of takes you. And I struggled off and on with that all my life" (Contenta, 2019, para. 1).

The very nature of nursing work seems to increase the risk. Nurses have constant access to controlled substances and other drugs of abuse, institutional controls for storing and distributing narcotics may be inadequate. In addition, many nurses have access to medications that nonmedical individuals do not have; for those with SUD, the temptation to divert patient drugs for their own use can be overwhelming (Recovery Village, 2020). All these issues place nurses at higher risk.

> ***Consider This*** "Hospitals are filled with myriad prescription painkillers, which can be problematic for nurses with addictions. These medicines may induce strong cravings and heightened temptations to steal drugs" (Gonzales, 2020, para. 19).

> ### Discussion Point
> Workplace risk factors for nurses include access, stress, lack of education, and attitude. Whose responsibility is it to address these issues?

BOX 18.1   **Common Methods of Diversion**

- Removal of medication when a patient does not need it
- Removal of medication for a discharged patient
- Removal of a duplicate dose
- Removal of fentanyl patches
- Removal of medication without an order
- Removal under a colleague's sign-on
- Substitution of a noncontrolled substance for a controlled substance
- Theft of patient medications brought from home
- Failure to waste when indicated
- Frequent wasting of entire doses

DRUG DIVERSION

When nurses take drugs designated for patient use, it is known as *diversion*. Identifying and investigating drug diversion is critical to consider when examining impaired nursing practice.

Indeed, Morris (2020) suggests there are many ways in which drugs can be diverted by health care providers, including removing medications of discharged patients; taking medications from pumps, drips, or discarded vials in sharps containers; removing larger doses of medication when a smaller dose is available; not documenting administration or waste of medications; utilizing unnecessary overrides to obtain medications; or stealing medications for personal use from a lock box or cabinet, never intending to administer them to patients. The methods continue with theft of home medications, removal under a colleague's sign-in, diluting a dose with water or saline, removal of duplicate doses, and substitution of a dose with other medication, water, or saline (Morris, 2020). Despite narcotic-dispensing machines, introduced to reduce the diversion of these drugs, workplace theft has been identified as the most frequent source of illegally obtained narcotics (Marquis & Huston, 2021). Box 18.1 lists some of the common methods of drug diversion.

Discussion Point

You suspect that a coworker is diverting drugs for personal use. You find yourself covering up for your friend because you know that she is depressed, exhausted, and having family problems. Your supervisor makes a casual comment with similar suspicions. Your first instinct is to make excuses for your friend; what would you do?

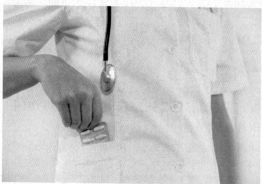
(Tyler Olson/Shutterstock)

IDENTIFYING AN IMPAIRED COLLEAGUE

Although most nurses have finely tuned assessment skills for identifying patient problems, they may be less sensitive to behaviors and actions that may signify chemical impairment in their coworkers (Marquis & Huston, 2021). Before a nurse can be reported or referred to a treatment program, there must be recognition that the nurse needs help. It is not always easy to recognize that a nurse is impaired or diverting drugs, and a lack of knowledge or skill in recognizing substance abuse makes it difficult for some nurses to report.

Indeed, the profile of the impaired nurse may vary greatly, though several behavior patterns and changes are frequently noted. These behavioral changes can be grouped into three primary areas: personality/behavioral changes, job performance changes, and time and attendance changes (Marquis & Huston, 2021). Box 18.2 includes characteristics of these categories.

In the earliest stages of SUD, Marquis and Huston (2021) note that the employee typically uses the addictive substance primarily for pleasure, and although the alcohol or drug use

BOX 18.2   **Characteristic Changes in Chemically Impaired Employees**

Changes in Personality or Behaviors
- Increased irritability with patients and colleagues often followed by extreme calm
- Social isolation; eats alone, avoids unit social functions
- Extreme and rapid mood swings
- Euphoric recall of events or elaborate excuses for behaviors
- Unusually strong interest in narcotics or the narcotic cabinet
- Sudden dramatic change in personal grooming or any other area
- Forgetfulness ranging from simple short-term memory loss to blackouts
- Change in physical appearance, which may include weight loss, flushed face, red or bleary eyes, unsteady gait, slurred speech, tremors, restlessness, diaphoresis, bruises and cigarette burns, jaundice, and ascites
- Extreme defensiveness regarding medication errors

Changes in Job Performance
- Difficulty meeting schedules and deadlines
- Illogical or sloppy charting
- High frequency of medication errors or errors in judgment affecting patient care
- Frequently volunteers to be medication nurse
- Has a high number of assigned patients who complain that their pain medication is ineffective in relieving their pain
- Consistently meeting work performance requirements at minimal levels or doing the minimum amount of work necessary
- Judgment errors
- Sleeping or dozing on duty
- Complaints from other staff members about the quality and quantity of the employee's work
- Disappears from the work area for long periods of time or may spend long periods of time in the bathroom or around the medication cart

Changes in Attendance and Use of Time
- Increasingly absent from work without adequate explanation or notification; most frequent absence on a Monday or Friday
- Long lunch hours
- Excessive use of sick leave or requests for sick leave after days off
- Frequent calling in to request compensatory time
- Arriving at work early or staying late for no apparent reason
- Consistent lateness
- Frequent disappearances from the unit without explanation

Source: Marquis, B., & Huston, C. (2021). *Leadership roles and management functions in nursing* (10th ed.). Wolters Kluwer.

is excessive, it is primarily recreational and social. Thus, substance use usually does not occur during work hours, though some secondary effects of its use may be apparent.

As chemical dependency deepens, the employee develops tolerance to the chemical and must use greater quantities more frequently to achieve the same effect. At this point, the person has made a conscious lifestyle decision to use addictive substances. There is a high use of defense mechanisms, such as justifying, denying, and bargaining about the drug. Often, the employee in this stage begins to use the chemical substance both at and away from work. Work performance generally declines in the areas of attendance,

judgment, quality, and interpersonal relationships. An appreciable decline in unit morale, resulting from an unreliable and unproductive worker, may become apparent.

In the later stages of SUD, the employee must continually use the addictive substance, even though they no longer gain pleasure or gratification. Marquis and Huston (2021) add that as the employee becomes both physically and psychologically addicted, a total disregard for themselves and others often emerges. Because the need for the substance is so great at this point, the employee's personal and professional lives focus on the need for drugs, and the individual typically becomes unpredictable and undependable in the work area. Assignments are incomplete or not done at all, charting may be sloppy or illegible, and frequent judgment errors may occur.

In addition, because the employee in this stage must use drugs frequently, signs of drug use during work hours may be seen. Narcotic vials may be missing. The employee may be absent from the unit for brief periods with no plausible excuse. Mood swings are excessive, and the employee often looks physically ill. Clearly, the behavior and actions of such employees should have been reported long before it has become this extreme.

REPORTING AN IMPAIRED COLLEAGUE

In theory, reporting an impaired nurse seems like a decision that would be easy to make. The position of the American Nurses Association (ANA) Code of Ethics (2015) is clear: it is the ethical and legal duty of a nurse to advocate for public safety, their colleagues, and the profession. This means simply that it is a nurse's job to protect the patient from harm; if that means reporting an impaired colleague, that is what one must do. In practice, however, the situation is anything but clear-cut.

Often, there is a "code of silence" about impaired practice. Gonzales (2020, para. 41) agrees, noting that "some hospitals deny the existence of substance abuse among their workers. Administrators may address the issue behind closed doors and fail to report the situation. Nurses in these situations often move on to new jobs without treating their disorders."

A study of nurses early in their careers (fewer than 5 years of experience) by Stimpfel et al. (2020) using a qualitative, descriptive design also supports the existence of a code of silence. One theme identified by the researchers was "*It's somewhere out there.*" This theme emerged from participants' beliefs that substance use was occurring in great numbers across the profession, including with prescription and over-the-counter medications, as well as other legal and illicit substances. Yet, when asked how widespread substance use was at their workplace or in the nursing profession, participants suggested they did not see or hear about substance use from their peers or have time to discuss it during the workday. In addition, another emerging theme "*See no evil, speak no evil, hear no evil*" suggested that participants were reluctant to discuss substance use beyond legal or socially acceptable types of substances.

Other reasons for silence also exist. Some individuals may assume others are already aware of and addressing a problem. More commonly, however, coworkers may not be aware of the signs and symptoms of SUD in their peers, or they may not understand the process they should use to report their concerns.

In addition to the ethical need to report suspected SUD in colleagues, there may be legal requirements as well, though no uniform agreement exists among the states as to what those reporting requirements are. In many states, if a board of nursing finds that a nurse's impairment was well known to other licensees and no report was made, the board may move to also investigate their compliance with the Nurse Practice Act for not coming forward to protect the public.

It is often a difficult and traumatic experience for a nurse to report an impaired colleague. Most health care organizations have policies in place that include reporting suspicions that do not have to be proven to the appropriate manager. If the manager suspects the employee has SUD, the individual must immediately be removed from the work environment.

Although some employees admit the problem when directly confronted, most use defense mechanisms (including denial) because they may not have admitted the problem to themselves. Indeed, individuals with a history of substance abuse often become effective at deception regarding their drug use (Marquis & Huston, 2021).

Denial and anger should be expected. If the employee denies having a problem, documented evidence demonstrating a decline in work performance should be shared. The manager must be careful to keep the confrontation focused on the employee's performance deficits and not allow the discussion to be directed to the cause of the underlying problem or addiction. These are issues and concerns that should be addressed by others. The manager must also be careful not to preach, moralize, scold, or blame.

Discussion Point

Considering your nursing education, practice experience, and workplace support, how comfortable would you feel about recognizing and reporting an impaired colleague?

Marquis and Huston (2021) also caution that because of the general nature of nursing, many managers find themselves wanting to nurture the impaired employee, much as they would any other person who is sick. However, this nurturing can quickly become enabling. The employee who already has a greatly diminished sense of self-esteem and a perceived loss of self-control may ask the manager to participate actively in their recovery. This is one of the most difficult aspects of working with an employee with SUD. Others who have greater expertise and objectivity should assume this role.

ALTERNATIVE-TO-DISCIPLINE PROGRAMS/ DIVERSION PROGRAMS

Until the 1980s, most nurses were disciplined by their state boards for drug and alcohol abuse, despite researchers identifying SUD as a treatable disease. For most nurses, this meant job loss and revocation of license.

Currently, however, most state boards of nursing recognize addiction as a disease and advocate a nondisciplinary approach that allows nurses with addiction to pursue recovery without worrying about losing their jobs. These voluntary, confidential *diversion programs* (also called intervention or peer assistance programs) protect the public with early identification of impaired nurses and by providing the nurses access to appropriate intervention programs and treatment services (Marquis & Huston, 2021). In addition, public safety is protected with immediate suspension of practice when needed and careful ongoing monitoring of the nurse.

The first treatment program offered in the United States was the IPN (2001–2016) in Florida in 1983. The IPN has a comprehensive website offering information about the history of the program, including frequently asked questions and available services.

California also offers a diversion program through the California Board of Registered Nursing (CBRN, 2021). Established in 1985, its goal is to protect the public by early identification of impaired registered nurses and by providing these nurses access to appropriate intervention programs and treatment services. Impaired nurses can be self-referred or referred by family, coworkers, or the board. All licensed registered nurses residing in California are eligible to enter the program, but they must agree to enter the program voluntarily. Since 1985, more than 2,000 nurses have successfully completed the diversion program in California (CBRN, 2021).

A similar approach is followed in the TPAPN. This program offers services to nurses suffering from chemical dependency, as well as from anxiety and other mental health disorders. It requires abstinence, maintains confidentiality, is strictly voluntary, and is independent of the state licensing board. Information from the TPAPN website includes how and when to make referrals, how the program works, and important links to services and organizations.

Consider This Although most states lean toward treatment rather than discipline for substance use problems, some nurses still attach a stigma and to think that impaired nurses should be punished and not allowed to return to work.

The North Carolina Board of Nursing (2021) also offers an *Alternative Program* for nurses with SUD. Eligible participants submit a signed consent order prepared by the North Carolina Board of Nursing agreeing to a period of abeyance (a state of temporary inactivity), during which they will not work in a licensed nursing position until approved to do so by the board. The impaired nurse is eligible to petition to reenter practice a minimum of 3 months from the date treatment is initiated and is required to follow all recommendations of the treatment facility. Upon receipt of treatment information, the nurse goes to the board for an orientation interview. Within 3 business days of that interview, the nurse is required to submit to random body fluid screens and to continue to do so for the duration of participation. The nurse is also required to attend a minimum of three in-person 12-step meetings each week for the duration of and to participate in aftercare for 1 year, which is a minimum of one treatment meeting per week.

Some state boards of nursing have detailed documents about return-to-work processes, and a small number of board websites offer some information about the reentry process. Most, however, focus primarily on what should be done if someone suspects an impaired colleague, how to report it, the treatment or disciplinary action once impairment is identified, and the specific aspects of each program. A question that is left unanswered is how long the board follows a recovered nurse in terms of random drug testing. Some hospitals or health care agencies already do random drug testing, so the question of invasion of privacy has in some instances already been addressed.

Bettinardi-Angres (2020) cautions, however, that nurses should not think of alternative-to-discipline programs (ADPs) as treatment programs. In fact, they are separate from treatment programs to retain the integrity of the process. ADPs do, however, refer nurses with SUD to programs for treatment and evaluation and continue to be the monitoring entity that randomly tests for substance use through early and sustained remission to ensure the nurse is safe to practice with reasonable skill (Bettinardi-Angres, 2020).

THE RECOVERED NURSE: REENTRY INTO PRACTICE

The eventual goal of most treatment plans is to return the employee to work, though not all practitioners will be able to return to practice. Indeed, Contenta (2019) suggests that the risk of relapse is 20% to 30% and notes that some health care institutions still believe strongly that greater weight needs to be put on the best interests of the patients and residents because that is the purpose of the institutions. "Health care institutions are not there for the purpose of providing job opportunities to people who are addicted to drugs, whether you regard that as a disability or not" (Contenta, 2019, para. 21).

Because impaired nurses recover at varying rates, predicting how long the reentry process should take is difficult. Many experts believe that impaired employees must devote at least 1 year to their recovery without the stresses of drug availability, overtime, and shift rotation (Marquis & Huston, 2021). Success in reentering the workforce depends on factors such as the extent of the recovery process and individual circumstances.

For the employee, return to work usually entails a comprehensive return-to-work agreement or contract with the organization. These *last chance agreements* (LCAs) outline the terms and conditions under which the nurse can return to work. Bettinardi-Angres (2020, p. 8) notes that these "LCAs are gifts to recovering nurses from employers and/or state because it prevents their termination and avoids disciplinary action against their licenses if they adhere to the terms. Most state [boards] will honor the LCA and allow the nurse to continue to practice if there is compliance with all recommendations."

In addition, though standardized guidelines do not exist for reentry guidelines, there are some general guidelines that should be considered by all employers when a recovered nurse returns to work (Box 18.3). In addition, there are important questions that must be asked or things that must be considered before return to work (Box 18.4). These issues include whether the nurse's practice is limited or restricted in some way, how long the nursing board has a right to invade the nurse's privacy to ensure that recovery is ongoing, where organizational responsibility ends, and who bears the cost if the nurse does not return to work at full capacity.

Discussion Point

You just came from a staff meeting at which the nurse manager informed everyone that a recovered nurse would begin working on the unit in a few weeks. Some nurses believed the nurse should not be allowed back to work because they could not be trusted. How would you respond to your colleagues?

To protect patient safety, practice restrictions may be in place for varying lengths of time, depending on the length of the program and whether it was treatment based or disciplinary action occurred. It is important that staff nurses realize the commitment of the recovering nurse to reestablish their career and continue in the profession.

NATIONAL: IMPAIRED PRACTICE POSITION AND POLICIES

Many national nursing organizations have espoused formal position statements and policies about impaired practice. The ANA (2015) position about impaired practice can be found on its website under the updated Code of Ethics with Interpretative Statements, 3.6 Patient Protection and Impaired Practice. The ANA supports treatment rather than discipline and a process that facilitates reentry of the recovered nurse back into practice (ANA, 2015).

The American Association of Colleges of Nursing (AACN, 1998) policy statement focuses on SUD in nursing education. Their policy was written in 1994 and updated in 1998 and has guidelines for the prevention and management of substance abuse for students, faculty, and staff. It also calls attention to confidentiality and legal issues and suggests strategies for identification, intervention, evaluation, treatment, and reentry into practice. The AACN agrees with the ANA regarding the importance of treatment over a reasonable time frame and a process for successful reentry into practice.

The NCSBN (2018) published *Substance Use Disorder in Nursing* to provide practical and evidence-based guidelines for evaluating, treating, and managing nurses with SUD. The NCSBN has also published several brochures (NCSBN, 2018) and videos (NCSBN, 2013) on the topic that serve as "quick guides" for nurses to read and view. As with the AACN and the ANA, the NCSBN supports early detection and treatment of the impaired nurse, with the goal of returning a recovered nurse to work.

LOCAL: IMPAIRED PRACTICE POLICIES IN THE WORKPLACE

In keeping with progress made at the national level, it is imperative that local health care organizations and educational institutions have policies in place that clearly identify the process to be followed if problematic substance use is suspected. A commitment to a drug- and alcohol-free educational setting or workplace environment is a critical part of local practice policies.

Anecdotal evidence, however, suggests that many nurses in clinical practice have no knowledge of such policies and would not know what to do if they suspected a colleague was impaired. Impaired practice policies, including drug diversion prevention, should be introduced during hospital orientation for new employees and during annual renewal of hospital safety procedures. This would highlight the issue for everyone and put the problem clearly in the spotlight, especially if barriers (such as stigma and fear) to reporting

BOX 18.3 Generally Accepted Reentry Guidelines for the Recovering Nurse

- No psychoactive drug use will be tolerated.
- The employee should be assigned to day shift for the first year.
- The employee should be paired with a successfully recovered nurse whenever possible.
- The employee should be willing to consent to random urine screening with toxicology or alcohol screens.
- The employee must give evidence of continuing involvement with support groups such as Alcoholics Anonymous and Narcotics Anonymous. Employees should be encouraged to attend meetings several times each week.
- The employee should be encouraged to participate in a structured aftercare program.
- The employee should be encouraged to seek individual counseling or therapy as needed.

Source: Marquis, B., & Huston, C. (2021). *Leadership roles and management functions in nursing* (10th ed.). Wolters Kluwer.

BOX 18.4 Issues to Consider When the Recovered Nurse Returns to Work

- Should the nurse returning to work following rehabilitation have their practice limited or restricted in some way, such as no exposure to the drug of choice or no access to controlled substances for a period of time?
- How long does the board of nursing have a right to invade the privacy of a recovered nurse?
- Where does the organizational responsibility end?
- Who bears the cost if the recovered nurse is not able to return to work at full capacity?
- Can confidentiality be maintained?
- Should the nurse be allowed to work in stressful practice areas?
- Should the nurse initially be allowed to work fulltime?

an impaired colleague and prevalence of the problem are discussed. Nurses should be allowed to ask questions so that they are clear about the process of reporting and that a nurse with SUD knows where to go for help.

HOW CAN WE STOP LOSING NURSES TO SUBSTANCE USE DISORDER?

Preventative health care is finally receiving much needed attention in the media and in practice. Insurance companies are increasingly paying for prevention and screening procedures, yet many areas of health care still lag behind on ideal preventative practices. The issue of preventing SUD is no exception to this situation. How can nurses individually and as a profession help prevent the cycle of addiction from starting among nurses?

Some of the risk factors for substance abuse that have been identified are difficult to modify. Nurses will always have easy access to narcotics, do shift work, and suffer from fatigue. The ongoing stress that has worked its way into clinical settings seems a long way from dissipating. What, then, can be done to diminish the effects of these factors so that nurses do not turn to substances as an inappropriate coping mechanism?

Perhaps, one avenue is to more fully explore the experiences of nurses who do not turn to substances. Do nurses who use healthy self-care strategies to cope with a stressful work environment and to prevent burnout also use those same strategies to avoid harmful substance use? Perhaps, this information about how nurses navigate difficulties of the workplace when they do not turn to drugs or alcohol will contribute to prevention.

Where does the education about SUD begin? Student nurses need not only to be made aware of the risks of substance abuse but also to be self-aware about their own attitudes and beliefs regarding those who do abuse substances and whether those people are patients or colleagues. Nursing school can be an incredibly stressful time for students. Not only could appropriate education in nursing school help prevent the onset of substance abuse, it might also allow students to explore their feelings and beliefs about impaired practice. This increased self-awareness might help students have empathy toward impaired nurses and encourage them to take the appropriate steps to assist a nurse or fellow student in getting help.

Nursing is going through a tumultuous time. Most nurses struggle daily with low staffing levels and a stressed work setting. How this stress is channeled can lead a nurse to use both positive and negative coping strategies. What are health care institutions doing to acknowledge and diffuse this stress? Are nurses too stressed to seek counsel from each other when they have a particularly bad day? Are nurses debriefing with each other or at home so they can let go of the often traumatic nature of work and move forward? Nurses and nurse managers need to answer these questions for their work settings to know whether they are doing enough for themselves, their colleagues, and their staff.

CONCLUSIONS

The Office of Disease Prevention and Health Promotion (2021) notes that although progress has been made in substantially lowering rates of substance abuse in the United States, the use of mind- and behavior-altering substances continues to take a major toll on the health of individuals, families, and communities nationwide. This is true among health care professionals as well.

Clearly, nurses with active SUD pose a risk to their own health, patient safety, and the integrity of the nursing profession. To achieve the best possible outcomes for safe reentry, prompt identification, appropriate treatment, and professional monitoring are necessary (Bettinardi-Angres, 2020). The American Society of Addiction Medicine (2020) agrees strongly, arguing that the interest and safety of the public are best served when state regulatory agencies and clinicians with expertise in the treatment of addiction in health care professionals work in concert to develop a confidential, nondisciplinary process for SUD, allowing for early intervention, evaluation, treatment, and return to practice with subsequent monitoring of the professional with addiction.

SUD is an enduring and significant problem for nurses, and there is much more we can do to mitigate the risk factors and to promote early detection and treatment. Do we teach our students, new graduates, and seasoned nurses to ask for help when they need it, or do we expect them to "do it all?" Do we create work cultures in which nurses feel informed about the signs and symptoms of SUDs and empowered to act when they suspect a colleague may be chemically impaired? Do most nurses recognize they have an ethical, regulatory, and legal obligation to report suspected SUD in the interest of patient safety? If all nurses are aware of the problem and intervene when they suspect a colleague of impaired practice, we are one step closer to decreasing the incidence of substance abuse in the nursing profession.

Finally, responsibility rests not just with individual nurses. Educators must accept the challenge to teach students about impaired practice and how to recognize it when they see it and to assist them in developing positive coping strategies so they do not turn to substances to deal with stress.

Employers must also accept the challenge to create a safe work environment that supports nurses in dealing with stress successfully, know employees so that confrontation can occur early, increase awareness about substance abuse so that nurses are not afraid to ask for help, support nurses if they do suspect drug diversion or an impaired colleague, ensure that an impaired practice policy is in place, and lastly to provide a process that facilitates reentry into practice following recovery.

For Additional Discussion

1. Explore your attitudes and beliefs about impaired nursing practice. How would you treat a colleague suspected of diverting drugs for personal use? Would you trust a recovered nurse returning to work?

2. What kind of peer support exists in your work setting? How do staff debrief from stressful situations?

3. Should recovered nurses who return to work have a limited practice? If so, for how long, and with what types of limitations?

4. How does this affect the workload of other nurses? What practices are in place in your work setting that could deter a nurse from diverting drugs for personal use?

5. Have you known a colleague who was caught diverting drugs for personal use? If so, how was it handled? Did the nurse seek treatment and return to work? Could it have been managed better?

6. You are a nurse manager for an intensive care unit and have been asked to talk to student nurses about impaired practice. What key points would you make?

7. Does your workplace have an impaired practice policy in place? If so, have you read it and was it discussed during your initial hospital orientation? Is it discussed annually? If not, what might you do to ensure that one is in place?

References

American Association of Colleges of Nursing. (1998). *Policy and guidelines for prevention and management of substance abuse in the nursing education community*. Retrieved August 25, 2021, from https://www.aacnnursing.org/News-Information/Position-Statements-White-Papers/Substance-Abuse

American Nurses Association. (2015). *Code of ethics for nurses with interpretive statements*. https://www.nursingworld.org/practice-policy/nursing-excellence/ethics/code-of-ethics-for-nurses/

American Society of Addiction Medicine. (2020, February 6). *Public policy statement on physicians and other healthcare professionals with addiction*. Retrieved August 25, 2021, from https://www.asam.org/docs/default-source/public-policy-statements/2020-public-policy-statement-on-physicians-and-other-healthcare-professionals-with-addiction_final.pdf?sfvrsn=5ed51c2_0&utm_source=Informz&utm_medium=Email&utm_campaign=Infomz-%20Google%20analytics

Bettinardi-Angres, K. (2020, April). Nurses with substance use disorder: Promoting successful treatment and reentry, 10 years later. *Journal of Nursing Regulation, 11*(1), 5–11. https://doi.org/10.1016/S2155-8256(20)30054-5

California Board of Registered Nursing. (2021). *General information*. Retrieved July 25, 2020, from http://www.rn.ca.gov/intervention/whatisint.shtml

Centers for Disease Control and Prevention (2020, December 17). *Overdose deaths accelerating during COVID-19*. Retrieved August 25, 2021, from https://www.cdc.gov/media/releases/2020/p1218-overdose-deaths-covid-19.html

Contenta, S. (2019, February 15). *"I was an impaired nurse": Three nurses who battled addiction welcome dramatic shift in approach to discipline and treatment*. Retrieved August 25, 2021, from https://www.thestar.com/news/canada/2019/02/15/i-was-an-impaired-nurse-three-nurses-who-battled-addiction-welcome-dramatic-shift-in-approach-to-discipline-and-treatment.html

Gonzales, M. (2020, February 26). *Nurses and addiction*. Retrieved August 25, 2021, from https://www.drugrehab.com/addiction/nurses/

Intervention Project for Nurses. (2001–2016). *IPN history*. Retrieved August 25, 2021, from https://ipnfl.org/about

Lockwood, W. (2020). *Recognizing impairment in the workplace*. Retrieved August 25, 2021, from https://www.rn.org/courses/coursematerial-10023.pdf

Marquis, B., & Huston, C. (2021). *Leadership roles and management functions in nursing* (10th ed.). Wolters Kluwer.

Mirlashari, J., Jahanbani, J., & Begjani, J. (2020). Addiction, childhood experiences and nurse's role in prevention: A qualitative study. *Eastern Mediterranean Health Journal [EMHJ], 26*(2). Retrieved August 25, 2021, from https://applications.emro.who.int/emhj/v26/02/10203397-2020-2602-212-218.pdf

Modlin, H. C., & Montes, A. (1964). Narcotics addiction in physicians. *The American Journal of Psychiatry, 121*, 358–365. https://doi.org/10.1176/ajp.121.4.358

Morris, L. (2020). A real situation: Drug diversion in nursing. *AAACN Viewpoint, 42*(1), 8–9.

Mumba, M. N., & Kraemer, K. R. (2019). Substance use disorders among nurses in medical-surgical, long-term care, and outpatient services. *MEDSURG Nursing, 28*(2), 87–118. https://www.semanticscholar.org/paper/Substance-Use-Disorders-among-Nurses-in-%2C-Long-Term-Mumba-Kraemer/16cff3bb1f8fd856fb1cefa65c78d78bce7acb2d

National Council of State Boards of Nursing. (2013). *Substance use disorder in nursing (video)*. Retrieved August 25, 2021, from https://www.ncsbn.org/333.htm

National Council of State Boards of Nursing. (2018). *A nurse manager's guide to substance use disorder in nursing (-brochure)*. Retrieved July 25, 2020, from https://www.ncsbn.org/3692.htm

National Council of State Boards of Nursing. (2021). *Substance use disorder in nursing*. Retrieved August 25, 2021, from https://www.ncsbn.org/substance-use-in-nursing.htm

National Institute on Drug Abuse. (2020, June). *Misuse of prescription drugs research report*. Retrieved August 25, 2021, from https://www.drugabuse.gov/publications/research-reports/misuse-prescription-drugs/summary

National Institute on Drug Abuse. (2021). *Opioid overdose crisis*. Retrieved August 25, 2021, from https://www.drugabuse.gov/drugs-abuse/opioids/opioid-overdose-crisis

North Carolina Board of Nursing. (2021, August 23). *Drug monitoring programs. Alternative program (AP)*. Retrieved August 25, 2021, from https://www.ncbon.com/discipline-compliance-drug-monitoring-programs

Office of Disease Prevention and Health Promotion. (2021, August 24). *Substance abuse*. Retrieved August 25, 2021, from https://www.healthypeople.gov/2020/leading-health-indicators/2020-lhi-topics/Substance-Abuse

Recovery Village. (2020, February 24). *When nurses abuse drugs: A look at the issues*. Retrieved August 25, 2021, from https://www.therecoveryvillage.com/drug-addiction/related-topics/nurses/

Stimpfel, A. W., Liang, E., & Goldsamt, L. A. (2020, April). Early career nurse reports of work-related substance use. *Journal of Nursing Regulation, 11*(1), 29–35. https://doi.org/10.1016/S2155-8256(20)30058-2

Taylor, L. (2020, June). Substance abuse and misuse identification and prevention: An evidence-based protocol for CRNAs in the workplace. *AANA Journal, 88*(3), 213–221. https://www.researchgate.net/publication/341795661_Substance_Abuse_and_Misuse_Identification_and_Prevention_An_Evidence-Based_Protocol_for_CRNAs_in_the_Workplace

Texas Nurses Association. (n.d.). *Texas peer assistance program for nurses*. Retrieved August 25, 2021, from http://www.texasnurses.org/?page=TPAPN

Academic Integrity in Nursing Education

George C. Pittman

CHAPTER OUTLINE

LEARNING OBJECTIVES

The learner will be able to:

1. Identify types of cheating common in nursing programs.

2. Identify variables that contribute to integrity failures.

3. Discuss possible reasons for academic dishonesty.

4. Discuss the consequences of a lack of academic integrity in nursing programs.

5. Identify methods and strategies to ensure academic integrity and decrease cheating.

6. Analyze conditions that promote academic integrity or that promote cheating.

7. Discuss barriers to self-reporting cheating or reporting others for cheating.

8. Reflect on their individual willingness to report other students for cheating.

INTRODUCTION

Loschiavo (2017) suggests that cheating in college has occurred since the inception of higher education and that much of this cheating appears to take shape in high school, with 64% of 24,000 students at 70 high schools admitting to cheating on a test, 58% admitting to plagiarism, and 95% saying they participated in some form of cheating, whether it was on a test, plagiarism, or copying homework. Data from another large national study indicated that 51% of high school students admit that they have cheated during a test (The Conversation, 2018).

Equally disconcerting, Buchmann (2014) suggests that about 75% of college students admit to cheating and that probably even more than three-quarters of college students have done something against the rules to improve their grades. "With an increasingly competitive atmosphere and a culture that some say is more accepting of cheating than it was in past generations, cheating has sadly become a somewhat expected phenomenon at universities across the country" (Buchmann, 2014, para. 2). For example, the number of students caught cheating at Russell Group universities rose 40% between 2014 to 2015 and 2016 to 2017 (Lodhia, 2018).

Buchmann (2014) notes that in May 2012, a teaching fellow for a government class at Harvard started noticing similarities between students' final exams that shouldn't have been there. The professor brought the case forward, and it was discovered that approximately 125 students—nearly half the entire lecture class—had been cheating. Buchmann (2014) concluded that "if students at Harvard—the most prestigious school in the world—can be caught cheating in large numbers, it's safe to assume that cheating happens on every campus much more often than we would like to think" (para. 1). The trend seems to continue; Farkas, updating a 2017 article in Cleveland.com, discussed a study by Kessler International, a firm that provides investigative and auditing services, that surveyed 300 students from public and private colleges, including online universities. The study found that 86% of the students said they had cheated. Of these, 97% said they had never been caught, and only 12% said they would not cheat because it is an ethical violation (Farkas, 2019).

Similarly, in 2017, students at the prestigious Stuyvesant High School in New York were caught sharing answers to Spanish assignments via a Facebook group. This followed a highly publicized incident that occurred at Stuyvesant several years before, when students were caught cheating on a language examination via text messaging (The Conversation, 2018).

Statistics are similar in online courses. Morgan (2018) suggests that 30% of all online test-takers bring an unpermitted resource (class notes, scratch paper, a calculator, or another unauthorized element) to their exam. This means that without proctor supervision, almost 600,000 items would have gone unnoticed before an exam in 2017 alone.

As the COVID-19 pandemic swept the world beginning in 2020, most in-person learning went online and remote. It seems intuitive that this development would lead to increased cheating, since faculty proctoring of student work became significantly more difficult. The combined effects of the pandemic threats to survival and security would seem to contribute to a "perfect storm" for increased cheating (Gallant, 2020). While to date there is little evidence to support or disprove this development, research into reasons for cheating has found that people tend to make bad decisions when stressed and pressured (Gallant, 2020).

Indeed, in December 2020, the U.S. Military Academy at West Point was rocked by the news of some 73 cadets cheating on a calculus final exam conducted online in May during the institution's closure for the pandemic. Despite the school's honor code, the cheating occurred and was discovered by professors grading the exams who noted irregularities in the work submitted by students. While some reviewers viewed the incident as an example of the school's honor code working, it must be noted that the cheating came to light not because students reported themselves in accordance with the honor code, but due to observant grading by the faculty (Shepherd, 2020).

> **Consider This** "It's no secret that students cheat" (Online Degree Programs, 2012). Indeed, research increasingly suggests that cheating from middle school through college is epidemic.

> **Discussion Point**
> Does a legacy of cheating exist in academia today? Are cheating cultures accepted or even condoned in contemporary secondary and collegiate settings?

CHEATING IN NURSING EDUCATION

Nurses are viewed as among the most trustworthy, ethical, and honest professionals in American society. From 1999 to 2019, *Gallup* polls found between 79% and 85% of respondents viewed the honesty and ethical standards of nurses as high to very high, and from 2016 to 2019, 82% to 85% of respondents rated nurses high or very high for honesty and ethics (Gallup, 2020). It would seem to follow, then, that nursing students would exhibit high or very high ethical standards. The comment of a student who participated in a longitudinal study on academic dishonesty illustrated this view: "I think that … the type of people who choose to go into nursing … results in less cheating than in other disciplines" (McCabe, 2009). Unfortunately, the data don't support this assumption.

Cheating is a concern in any academic discipline. It is of particular concern to nursing educators because nurses hold the well-being and health of their patients in their hands. Lapses of integrity can have grave consequences for patients. It follows, then, that nursing educators and leaders must inculcate the highest standards of honesty and integrity in students to create a culture of trustworthiness in the nurses who graduate from their programs. Although there isn't a great deal of data that defines the link between academic integrity and professional integrity, there is some evidence, beyond the intuitive, that there is a correlation.

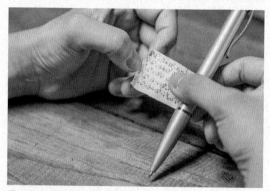

(Toonz Jirana/Shutterstock)

Lapses in academic integrity can take many forms. Cheating in the classroom can include copying answers from another's exam sheet, offering answers to exam questions to another student, soliciting answers to exam questions from students who have already taken the exam, collaborating with other students on assignments when collaboration is not allowed, quoting without appropriate attribution, using disallowed materials to get answers on exams or quizzes, or any of a myriad of practices that pass another's work as one's own. It can also include downloading papers from the internet, taking photos of tests and posting them online, hiring someone to take their online tests, purchasing an instructor's version of a book to get copies of tests and answers, and faking test scores or letters of recommendation for employers or academic pursuits.

In the clinical setting, dishonest practices include recording vital signs that weren't actually taken or recorded accurately, reporting medications as given that were not administered, reporting patient responses to treatment that weren't observed, attempting procedures without adequate

knowledge or asking for guidance from the instructor, breaking sterile technique without reporting it or replacing contaminated items, and discussing protected patient information in public places or with nonmedical personnel (McCrink, 2010).

Discussion Point

Do you believe that students who lack academic integrity are more likely to demonstrate the same behaviors in clinical practice?

OVERVIEW OF THE LITERATURE

Numerous studies of nursing students' academic misconduct have been published in the past 30 years. Two of the earliest studies were by Hilbert in 1985, with a follow-up study in 1987. Other studies that documented academic dishonesty among nursing students were conducted by Bailey (2001), Beasley (2014), Gaberson (1997), Krueger (2014), McCabe (2009), McCrink (2010), Sheer (1989), Stonecypher and Willson (2014), and Woith et al. (2012).

These studies, and others, indicate that nursing students engage in a wide variety of dishonest academic practices in both the classroom and clinical settings. More than just documenting the size of the problem, these studies examined the attitudes among nursing students that caused them to engage in these behaviors as well as the strategies that may be employed to deter such behavior. These studies also suggest that students engage in a variety of rationalizations to explain their misconduct such as time constraints, unfair course assignments, and the unrealistic expectations of nursing faculty, among others (McCrink, 2010).

Prevalence of the Problem in Nursing

The question of whether academic dishonesty is rising among nursing students may not be answerable. However, there is considerable evidence that such behavior is common. McCrink (2010) studied nursing students in two associate degree nursing programs in the northeastern United States (193 respondents) and found a mean score of 21.58 (range 19–95, SD 3.46) for frequency of self-reported misconduct. Krueger (2014) found that of the 335 participants, 216 (64.7%) admitted to engaging in some form of academic dishonesty in the classroom setting and 181 (54%) engaged in academic dishonesty in the clinical setting.

Similarly, disconcerting data were noted in a study by McCabe (2009) that involved nursing students from 12 schools. A request to participate was sent to 6,290 students, and 1,057 responses were received (a return of 16.8%). He found that more than half of the undergraduate students and almost half of the graduate students self-reported engaging in one or more of 16 behaviors identified as classroom cheating. The study by Kessler International reinforces that the problem of nursing students cheating continues (Farkas, 2019).

Clearly, there is cause for concern. Moreover, because all these studies involved self-reporting of academic dishonesty, there is likely considerable underreporting. As one of McCabe's (2009) participants put it, "I think that you may have difficulty generating accurate statistics. I don't think that people who cheat are willing to give out that information." In an article in the *British Journal of Nursing*, Glasper reported that 1,700 (2.6%) nursing students of a population of 64,000 student nurses over a 3-year period had been found guilty of cheating (Glasper, 2016). Although it might seem that British nursing students are more honest than American nursing students, it's important to note that Glasper was writing about nursing students convicted of cheating, while McCrink, Krueger, and McCabe studied nursing students who self-reported cheating by themselves or their peers, without necessarily being caught and found guilty.

There also seems to be a correlation between self-reported cheating in the classroom and self-reported cheating in the clinical setting. Krueger (2014) found a statistically significant correlation between the two behaviors ($r = 0.42$, $p < 0.01$). Krueger's study included more than 300 nursing students and found there was a clear relationship between cheating in the classroom and ethical lapses in the clinical setting. This correlation suggests that students who cheat in the classroom are likely to cheat in the clinical setting as well.

McCrink's (2010) data recorded the most common self-reported behaviors of academic dishonesty as discussing patients in public or with nonmedical personnel (35.3%), paraphrasing material without appropriate attribution (35.2%), working collaboratively when it was not allowed (24.3%), obtaining test questions from other students

(21.8%), and recording vital signs that were not taken or recorded accurately (13%; Box 19.1). Moreover, 8.8% of McCrink's (2010) respondents reported recording patient treatments that were neither performed nor observed, 6.7% reported they'd recorded patient responses to treatment they hadn't observed, and 2.1% reported they'd recorded administration of medications that had not been administered.

Discussion Point

What do you believe is driving these significant numbers of self-reported academic dishonesty? Is it a quest for a higher grade? For recognition of success? Is it driven by more intrinsic or extrinsic factors?

Another finding by Krueger (2014) was also disturbing. In her study of 335 participants in two associate degree nursing programs in the Midwest, 329 (98.2%) participants believed that plagiarism occurs at their college, and 97 (28.9%) participants reported witnessing another student cheating. Furthermore, of these 329 participants, 291 (88.4%) said they'd never reported an incident of cheating and 74 (22.3%) believed that the typical student would never report an incident of cheating they observed. In a recent student survey of graduating students in the author's nursing program, graduating students rated the academic integrity of their classmates at a mean of 3.58, the lowest score of the questions related to how these students viewed their classmates. Students who had reported cheating to the faculty were extremely reluctant to name the students they'd observed cheating. This, of course, makes taking action against the perpetrators even more difficult. Another consequence of this reluctance is that a policy to assure academic integrity by catching and punishing offenders is almost certain to fail. It would seem, then, that a better

---

BOX 19.1 **Commonly Self-Reported Types of Academic Dishonesty by Nursing Students**

- Discussing patients in public places or with nonmedical personnel
- Paraphrasing material without appropriate attribution
- Working collaboratively on assignments or tests when it was not allowed
- Obtaining test questions from other students
- Recording vital signs that were not taken or recorded accurately
- Recording patient treatments that were neither performed nor observed
- Recording administration of medications that had not been administered
- Reporting patient responses to treatment that weren't observed
- Attempting procedures without adequate knowledge or asking the instructor for guidance
- Breaking sterile technique without reporting it or replacing contaminated items

approach to dealing with cheating is to inculcate a culture of integrity, rather than focusing on catching perpetrators. As the cheating incident at West Point shows, an honor code can be an important part of a culture of integrity, but isn't enough by itself to ensure academic integrity.

Why Do Students Cheat?

Many researchers have explored the question of why students cheat, and the responses are varied. Running out of the time needed to complete an assignment correctly or to study for an exam adequately is the most common reason students give for cheating (Colorado State University [CSU], 2021). A second reason students give for cheating is not having fully understood the material or assignment at hand. In addition, sloppy note taking leads to unintentional plagiarism, which is often treated just as seriously as intentional plagiarism (Colorado State University, 2021).

Woith and colleagues (2012) found that student participants identified competition among students for grades as fostering an environment conducive to cheating. Buchmann (2014) suggests that competitive pressures placed on children at a very young age carry on with them through high school and college. With so much pressure to stand out as the smartest in a class, some students may give in to the opportunity to succeed at the price of integrity. In fact, there is evidence that the pursuit of "good grades," also known as performance motivation, is associated with a higher propensity to cheating, whereas a mastery motivation, which focuses on learning to acquire knowledge and the desire for achievement, seems to moderate the motivation to cheat (Baran & Jonason, 2020).

Another reason cited by participants as pressures that led to cheating were the time constraints related to acquiring a vast amount of knowledge in the short period offered by nursing programs (typically, approximately 2 years). Krueger (2014) found that participants in her study who worked more than 40 hours per week rated academic dishonesty as more ethical than participants who worked 1 to 10 hours per week. This rationale points up a possible equity issue related to higher education in general, and nursing programs in particular. Do those students who are economically able to attend university without working have an advantage over those students who need to work to support themselves and pay for their schooling? If so, how can we address this inequity?

Institutional apathy has also been identified as a reason why students cheat (Buchmann, 2014). Students may cheat when they do not see the academic environment as one that deserves their honesty. "Just like cheating at Monopoly is easier to justify than tax evasion, if students don't believe their university deserves high standards, then they may see no reason to follow all the rules about grading. Lack of respect for the collegiate institution may also prevent students from reporting instances of dishonesty they see around them" (Buchmann, 2014, para. 8).

Buchmann (2014) suggests that self-interest is also a factor in why people cheat and that this factor appears to encompass all cheating. Students who cheat hope to see a return on their investment of time and resources in college and watching someone else make a better grade can be painful. "With only [themselves] in mind, cheating is hard not to justify when someone can get away with it" (Buchmann, 2014, para. 10). Buchmann's assessment correlates with the research done by Baran and Jonason with 390 Polish university students. Those students who exhibited psychopathy tendencies (meanness, disinhibition, and boldness) had a stronger propensity to cheat: decreased concern about being caught, propensity to exploit other students' work or knowledge reported more frequent academic dishonesty (Baran & Jonason, 2020). See Research Fuels the Controversy 19.1.

Lodhia (2018) agrees, noting that tuition fees and the stress of securing a job mean that some students are fixated on exam results, rather than intellectual development. "For students, the pressure to succeed has never been greater due to the increased cost attached to learning as well as the seeming necessity for students to get jobs as soon as they graduate. Both of these factors have led to an environment where results and grades are more important than scholarship and intellectual development and ultimately undermine the entire purpose of universities" (Lodhia, 2018, para. 2). Baran and Jonason (2020) also concluded that mastery motivation moderated (decreased) perceived pressures to cheat. Reasons that students identify as compelling them to cheat are provided in Box 19.2.

Learning theory also offers insight into the development of a culture of cheating. As Krueger (2014) found in her study, students who witness other students engaging in academically dishonest behavior or who believe their peers are cheating are, themselves, more likely to cheat.

The Woith and team study (2012) had this same observation. This was one of the situational conditions related to cheating that Krueger (2014) identified for her study. The other two were consequences and enforcement of academic dishonesty policies and the students' personal beliefs and values related to cheating and academic honesty. Krueger's study found that students generally perceived that the risk of being caught was high and the consequences severe. Krueger also found a significant negative correlation between a commitment to integrity and the occurrence of dishonest behaviors. In other words, students who valued integrity highly cheated less. These findings suggest some possible approaches to deterring cheating.

Simola (2017) uses the discipline of behavioral ethics to propose several steps to prevent academic dishonesty. In her discussion of students' perceptions of sanctioning

Research Fuels the Controversy 19.1

Why Do Students Cheat?

This study of 390 university students explored the predisposition toward academic dishonesty and which personality traits might discourage cheating as well as potential strategies to decrease cheating.

Source: Baran, L., & Jonason, P. (2020, August 31). Academic dishonesty among university students: The roles of psychopathy, motivation, and self-efficacy. *PLOS One, 15*(8), 1–12.

Study Findings

The researchers found that psychopathy correlated strongly with academic dishonesty. The three traits of psychopathy that were most predictive were disinhibition, meanness, and boldness. Moreover, a student's focus on performance (grades) rather than mastery (competence) was correlated with a predisposition to academic dishonesty. Conversely, an orientation toward mastery and self-efficacy moderated tendencies toward academic dishonesty. The authors concluded by offering teaching strategies that might decrease cheating, as well as suggestions for dealing with known instances of academic dishonesty.

BOX 19.2   **Why Students May Feel Compelled to Cheat**

- Procrastination on assignments and studying
- Time constraints
- Not fully understanding the material or assignment at hand
- Sloppy note taking, leading to unintentional plagiarism
- Competition for grades or success
- Ambiguous attitudes among students about what qualifies as cheating
- Institutional apathy
- Self-interest

Source: Buchmann, B. (2014, February 20). Cheating in college: Where it happens, why students do it and how to stop it. *The Huffington Post.* Retrieved May 28, 2015, from http://www.huffingtonpost.com/uloop/cheating-in-college-where_b_4826136.html; Colorado State University. (2021). *Why do students cheat?* Retrieved November 25, 2020, from https://tilt.colostate.edu/Integrity/FacultyResources/WhyDoStudents

diminished risk of being caught and a resultant lack of fear, both of which mediate, rather than moderate, a propensity to academic dishonesty (Baran & Jonason, 2020).

Student Attitudes Regarding Academic Dishonesty

There seems to be some disagreement among nursing students as to what constitutes academic dishonesty, and even more disagreement as to the seriousness of the conduct described. Most students in McCrink's (2010) study agreed that reporting vital signs that aren't taken are highly or severely unethical. Similarly, falsely reporting medication administration, recording responses to treatment that weren't observed, failure to report an error or incident that involved a patient, and coming to the clinical setting under the influence of alcohol or drugs were all viewed as highly unethical or severely unethical by these same students. However, 21.6% of the participants felt that working with another student when it wasn't allowed wasn't unethical or only slightly unethical. And, 16% of students felt the same way about getting answers from another student.

McCabe (2009) also noted that students tended to engage more readily in behaviors they viewed as less serious. Such a result might be expected, but the question remains as to why students who rate behaviors as very unethical still engage in those behaviors. Similarly, how are we to reconcile the observation that most nursing students in the various studies felt the likelihood of, and penalties for, getting caught cheating were very high with the large number of students who self-report engaging in these behaviors (McCabe, 2009; McCrink, 2010; Woith et al., 2012)? In some cases, students reported that they didn't know that their

systems, or punishment, she makes the observation that the use of punishment or sanctions for academic dishonesty may induce students to use a calculative decision-making process rather than an ethical one. In this model, the student focuses on the probability and cost of getting caught, rather than on the ethical question of whether academic dishonesty is right or wrong (Simola, 2017). This finding is echoed by Baran and Jonason who found that students who exhibit the meanness aspect of psychopathy perceive a

actions constituted unethical conduct or cheating (Beasley, 2014; Bezek, 2014; McCrink, 2010).

> *Consider This* Loschiavo (2017) notes that cheating can "be an intentional, calculated decision in order to get ahead. Often, it is motivated by the path to success that they see around them—people cheating without incurring any real consequences. Students then come to believe that dishonest behavior is rewarded and often do not hesitate to engage in it" (para. 8).

FERTILE GROUND FOR CHEATING?

Nursing school may be a breeding ground for academic dishonesty, despite nursing students' generally wide acceptance that trust, honesty, and fairness are essential to the formation of the therapeutic relationships that are foundational to practice. Although nursing educators and leaders, and even nursing students, may disagree as to whether the factors that promote cheating are actually causes or rationalizations for bad behavior, or just excuses for moral laxity, if we are to deter academic dishonesty we must understand and acknowledge the context within which it occurs. Without question, many of the reasons, cited by students, for cheating exist in nursing programs in abundance: time constraints, a large body of knowledge to assimilate in a short time, significant culture challenge for many students, great pressure for grades, and so on. Moreover, many nursing programs reward collaborative behavior, encouraging nurses to help solve problems. These same students, then, may see little wrong in doing so in situations that call for individual effort. As Adderton notes, the most common kinds of cheating by nursing students are plagiarism and collusion. She also refers to McCabe's work between 2009 and 2015 that found that individual cheating in nursing programs is lower than in other disciplines, but that collaborative cheating is significantly higher (Adderton, 2019).

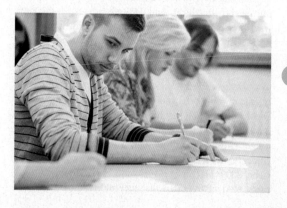

Since the first studies of cheating by nursing students in the mid-1980s, the use of internet-based research and sources, electronic media, electronic submission of papers and exams, online management of courses, complete with quizzes, exams, and various assignments completed online has made the burden of detecting and deterring academic dishonesty even more difficult.

As McCabe (2009) observed, nursing students are exposed to the same influences as students in other disciplines. Opportunities for cheating have certainly increased with the increased use of electronic technologies, but there is little evidence that the actual number of students cheating has increased as a result (McCabe, 2009). The ease with which students can access material is certainly a time-saver, a valuable incentive in nursing programs (McCabe, 2009). In a study by McCabe (2009), more than a third of nursing students reported "copying a few sentences from a web source without citing it." Among the questions raised by this finding is whether students are ignorant of appropriate citation of sources, seduced by the ease of such plagiarism, or whether there is some other explanation for such widespread cheating.

In any case, it is incumbent on nursing educators to work with students to establish a culture of integrity. In 2016, Purdue University's School of Nursing embarked on a continuous quality improvement program to develop strategies to support a culture of honor, ethics, and integrity. The strategies employed include a faculty development program (provided by Generation Z educators), modifications of the academic integrity policies, and more peer-to-peer mentoring as well as standardized, transparent, and consistent communication of expectations regarding academic integrity across the program (Hurn et al., 2020).

Interestingly, student participants in two of the studies (McCrink, 2010; Woith et al., 2012) rejected the neutralization statements (rationales) for academic dishonesty and recognized the correlation between public/patient safety and academic integrity. This finding may offer insight into ways that both faculty and students may cooperate to decrease the incidence of cheating in both the classroom and clinical settings.

WHAT SHOULD BE THE CONSEQUENCES FOR CHEATING?

Both Krueger (2014) and McCabe (2009) report that students who observe their classmates engaging in academic dishonesty are more prone to engage in such activity themselves. Clearly, academic dishonesty must be confronted and addressed so that a culture of cheating is not allowed to exist, much less condoned.

Given that the number of students who admit to cheating has remained constant since it was first measured in 1963, whatever is being done to stop cheating today clearly isn't working (Buchmann, 2014). What, then, should be the consequences of cheating? Clearly, consequences can range from no action to disciplinary expulsion (Box 19.3). Finding an appropriate balance between an excessively punitive culture that allows for no exceptions and an apathetic attitude that actually encourages cheating may be more difficult than one would expect. Moreover, there is often reluctance on the part of faculty to discipline students for academic dishonesty.

Expulsion and formal disciplinary actions clearly affect a student's future as well as career choice. Perhaps even more importantly, and not often addressed, is the fact that students who cheat their way through their education may be missing critical information they need to safely perform in their chosen career path. Certainly, this is the case in nursing, and allowing students who cheat to earn professional degrees clearly places patients at risk.

Discussion Point

Who carries the responsibility for assuring academic integrity in nursing programs, students, or faculty? Support your choice.

HOW CAN ACADEMIC INTEGRITY BE FOSTERED?

Nursing students and faculty, alike, recognize the importance of academic integrity as fostering the kind of ethical behavior essential to nursing care (McCrink, 2010; Woith et al., 2012). Given the positive correlation between academic misconduct in the classroom and unethical behavior in the clinical setting, classroom and clinical faculty as well as nursing leaders must be alert to instances of cheating in both arenas. However, it is important to keep in mind that faculty and students may have different ideas on what constitutes academic dishonesty. As Ok-Hee and Kyung-Hye (2019) found, most students consider academic ethics

| BOX 19.3 | **Common Consequences of Academic Misconduct** |

- No action
- Warning or written reprimand
- General disciplinary probation
- Disciplinary probation with loss of good standing
- Discretionary sanctions such as:
  - Educational programs
  - Restorative justice assignments
- Grading penalties such as:
  - An F on the assignment or exam
  - Failure in the class
  - Reduced grade
  - Academic misconduct or "AM" noted on transcript
- Loss of repeat/delete privilege
- Disciplinary suspension
- Disciplinary expulsion
- Revocation of admission or degree
- Withholding of degree

Source: Colorado State University. (2021). *Why do students cheat?* Retrieved September 20, 2021, from https://tilt .colostate.edu/Integrity/FacultyResources/WhyDoStudents

important, but may not recognize the same behaviors as problematic. Most of the students in their study considered cheating on exams clearly misconduct, but few of them believed that giving overly generous marks to fellow students in peer review or plagiarizing a friend's paper with the friend's consent constituted academic dishonesty (Ok-Hee & Kyung-Hye, 2019).

The approach to fostering academic integrity, however, must not be just reactive (negative sanctions when punishment is discovered). It must be proactive and include establishing an ethical culture, using professional standards as a guide for ethical behavior, establishing clear guidelines and expectations, increasing faculty supervision, fostering self-discipline, implementing honor codes, teaching students about research and appropriate citation, and providing mentoring and support. Given that new nursing students may be ignorant of the rules governing citation formatting, it might be useful for nursing faculty to spend some time early in their students' careers to provide instruction about what constitutes appropriate citation and avoidance of plagiarism (Carter et al., 2019).

The importance of student participation (buy-in) cannot be overemphasized. A study by Robinson and Glanzer (2017) used McCabe and team's model to analyze students' perceptions of academic integrity in general and at their institution. The researchers found that students consistently focused on the negative, punitive aspects of the system and ignored the positive messaging about academic integrity. As a result, they lacked the most important ingredient for an atmosphere that promotes academic integrity: the commitment to values such as mutual trust, respect, and supportiveness (Robinson & Glanzer, 2017).

Establishing an Ethical Culture

Ethical conduct and its role in establishing trustworthiness and a caring, therapeutic relationship among nursing students, nurses, and patients must be a central focus of students, faculty, and professional nurses. The establishment of a culture of ethical behavior and trustworthiness in nursing programs, however, must be a joint endeavor between faculty and students. Without significant participation, "buy-in" by students, faculty efforts to stop cheating are likely to fail. As Krueger (2014) and other researchers point out, if the perceptions among students that they are likely to get caught cheating and the consequences for cheating are quite severe don't deter cheating, a punitive approach alone seems unlikely to solve the problem. Moreover, as Gallant points out, faculty don't want to engage in a technological arms race with students (Gallant, 2020). Nevertheless, faculty, students, and the institution must be resolute that academic dishonesty will not be tolerated.

If the development of a culture of cheating is a result of socialization as Krueger (2014) and Woith and colleagues (2012) suggest, then one avenue toward reversing that course would be to socialize student nurses into a culture of caring, trustworthiness, and accountability. An emphasis on the importance of these attributes to the professional nurse should come early and be repeated often during the course of a student's progression through a nursing program. This socialization would involve teaching and role modeling ethical behavior and integrity as well as clear, consistent communication regarding academic dishonesty. Educators also need to establish the relevance of the work they assign and endeavor to help students manage their time better in order to deal with the increasing complexity and amount of knowledge required of the professional nurse (Woith et al., 2012).

Miron (2016) studied predictors for behaving with academic integrity among nursing students in Canada. She found that attitude, subjective norms, and perceived behavioral control were the strongest predictors for ethical behavior. Her study recommended strategies such as case-based pedagogy, simulation, and instructors finding ways to help students identify and engage in ethical behavior (planned, real-time clinical conferences, for example) as ways to help create an environment of academic integrity. These strategies can promote an atmosphere of mastery-based learning rather than performance-based learning.

Using Professional Standards as a Guide for Ethical Behavior

McCrink (2010), Krueger (2014), and Woith and team (2012) agree that faculty play a central role in helping students incorporate exemplars such as the American Nurses Association (2015) *Code of Ethics* into their interactions with patients. Faculty must also provide clear guidelines and expectations for ethical behavior and model such behavior. In addition, they must help students identify and discuss lapses of ethical conduct they encounter in the clinical setting by both students and professional nurses. Student peer leaders can be helpful in modeling and promoting accountability and trustworthiness (Beasley, 2014; Woith et al., 2012).

The observation of Robinson and Glanzer (2017) that students largely situate responsibility for academic integrity on their teachers and administrators overseeing the system rather than on their student peers seems to support Simola's notion that the more practical approach to achieving academic integrity may lie in actions such as helping students clarify the meaning and types of academic dishonesty, making clear the ethical nature of decisions surrounding academic integrity and its relationship to the ethical norms of nursing, fostering ethical values within courses and classes, and having students sign an honesty pledge before testing, rather than afterward (Simola, 2017). One more suggestion that fits very well with the ethical standards of nursing is that faculty and peers actively encourage and educate students about the importance of seeking help and support early if students are feeling overwhelmed (Simola, 2017).

Indeed, Buchmann (2014) suggests that because cultural ideas may influence the prevalence of cheating, the best long-term solution may be to take a societal approach. Instead of seeing cheating as something that can't be done, students must come to recognize that it should not be done. Faculty have a clear responsibility to model ethical behavior. Not only should clinical standards and expectations regarding original work, allowed collaboration, and so on be crystal clear, but faculty must also be sure to credit sources in lectures, assignments, and so on.

Establishing Clear Guidelines and Expectations

Buchmann (2014) suggests that many students lack understanding of what constitutes cheating because they may not have fully read or comprehended their student rules. This lack of understanding may lead students to cheat by accident or in a way that isn't known to be called cheating. In addition, "ambiguous attitudes among students about what qualifies as cheating may cause more academic dishonesty than intended by students. While most students will call plagiarism cheating, many of them will define plagiarism in a way that allows them to indirectly copy the work of others" (Buchmann, 2014, para. 6).

In addition, faculty should revisit the parameters and expectations of ethical conduct frequently, rather than only at the beginning of the program. Clear delineation of the types of activities that are approved for collaborative work and of those that require individual work would eliminate the rationalization that students didn't realize they weren't to work together. Faculty and students should work together to establish the policies that govern behavior in the academic and clinical settings (Stonecypher & Willson, 2014).

Faculty should also encourage discussions regarding ethical dilemmas associated with academic integrity. This is particularly important in the clinical setting when students may be exposed to unethical conduct by the staff nurses they are working with. Clinical instructors should be clear about their expectations for ethical conduct and the consequences for failing to report errors in an appropriate manner.

Increasing Faculty Supervision

The quality of faculty supervision in test taking can be either a deterrent or a promoter of academic dishonesty. Indeed, Buchmann (2014) suggests that tightening the rules on classroom behavior during exams seems like the most obvious and readily available solution to reducing academic dishonesty. He goes on to detail extensive efforts made by universities to record everything suspicious, efforts made to prevent students from photographing a test, and not allowing students to chew gum because it provides a way to hide that they're talking into a hidden microphone.

Similarly, more faculty are requiring online students to take exams under the supervision of a proctor. Indeed, research demonstrates that students taking online unproctored exams perform better than when they sit for exams before a proctor enforcing the closed-book exam rules (Winneg, 2015). In other words, more students cheat when taking exams unproctored, online at home. However, as noted earlier, in today's world, these strategies often aren't possible. As remote learning becomes more widespread, it is incumbent on faculty to renew their efforts to create engaging learning environments, encourage community among the students, and frequently engage in discussion of honesty and integrity with each assignment and in every environment (Gallant, 2020).

Unfortunately, the internet is filled with strategies students can use to individually or collaboratively cheat, including "the long-sleeved shirt method" (students write important information on their arms for an exam and then roll up their sleeves when instructor is not looking); the "buddy system" (students sit near a student they believe will do well on the test, and that student holds up their exam sheet as if reflecting on their answers so that the other person can copy); "the telephone scam" (students are allowed to use the calculator on their cell phone for exams, but actually use the telephone to text answers to other students or search online); "the distraction method" (one student distracts the instructor so that other students can exchange answers); using crib notes written on Band-Aid, tissues, gum wrappers, and other commonly used innocuous items; and "sign language" (using a series of coughs, Morse code, hand or foot tapping, or other nonverbal cues to let another student know which answer is the correct one), to name just a few.

An attentive instructor may be able to detect some of these strategies, but it is equally clear that the sophistication and skill of academic cheaters are continuing to increase. Using multiple test proctors may be a useful strategy in increasing the degree of faculty supervision.

But new technology is unfolding that includes smartwatches, smart pens, and Google glasses to help students cheat (Vandoorne, 2014). Some new devices are almost impossible to see—such as "invisible" Bluetooth earpieces. They work with a tiny microphone, which is synced to a Bluetooth cell phone and enables questions, whispered from exam rooms, to be answered by someone outside the room. Such wearable technology will only make it more difficult for instructors to spot cheating when it is occurring.

Discussion Point

Can observant teachers detect academic dishonesty or are cheating strategies so sophisticated or well-practiced that being caught is unlikely?

Discussion Point

Is collaborative cheating typically instigated by a few people and others simply follow, or do you believe academic dishonesty is simply more common than most people would like to admit?

Using Test Security or Plagiarism Assessment Tools

Some instructors have begun computerized adaptive testing (CAT) to address cheating concerns. CAT uses an algorithm to choose test items based on the students' strengths and weaknesses (Bleiberg & West, 2013). Every student takes a different test when using CAT, which decreases the number of items tests have in common. Students take the test online, eliminating inappropriately administered testing accommodations and making it difficult for students to share answers.

In addition, plagiarism assessment tools such as Turnitin.com and SafeAssign have become commonplace. These sites have millions of cataloged articles, papers, and webpages to determine what percentage of student papers are original work and what percentage is the work of others.

Instructors are also using webcams to monitor students taking tests offsite and increasingly requiring some type of biometric sign-in to make sure that the student taking the test is the same student taking the course. (The 2008 Higher Education Opportunity Act contains a requirement that schools offering distance learning programs have a system in place to authenticate the identity of their online students.) More computers are being recessed into desktops so that students who attempt to photograph screens are more obvious. In addition, some schools have begun using jamming devices to block the use of cell phones during testing.

Fostering Self-Discipline

A focus on quality improvement rather than a punitive approach to each mistake may encourage students to report errors rather than hiding them. Frank discussion between clinical faculty and students about the problems students observe can help inculcate an attitude of vigilance regarding their own personal practice.

Faculty should also emphasize the findings of the Institute of Medicine's (2004) report linking errors with outcomes in discussions with students regarding academic integrity. Although the evidence that students who cheat become nurses who cheat in the workplace is sketchy, it seems intuitively true, and student respondents in several of the studies cited noted the link (McCabe, 2009; McCrink, 2010; Woith et al., 2012). Instructors should continually discuss with students the importance of the data they're collecting, the procedures they perform, and the dependence of patients' well-being on their honesty and ethical behavior (Krueger, 2014).

Implementing Honor Codes

An academic honor code is a set of rules or expectations that govern an academic community and is based on ideals that define honorable behavior within that community. An honor code's utility depends on the notion that members of the community can be trusted to act with honor. Infractions of the honor code are enforced with various sanctions, including expulsion from the program or institution (Wikipedia, 2020). Honor codes may be quite complex, listing various types of infractions, or they may be quite brief: a

statement that the student who has signed the honor code pledges that all work is their own and that they have received no disallowed assistance.

Woith and team (2012) and Krueger (2014) both noted that earlier researchers had found that schools that had formal honor codes reported fewer instances of student cheating. It may be that the formalization and discussion of these codes not only lay clear guidelines for student behavior but also cause students to actively consider their behavior in the context of the fundamental principles of the nursing profession. Stonecypher and Willson (2014) note that honor codes are effective if students understand the expectations of the code. Honor codes place the responsibility for academic integrity on the student and must be written with clear, easy-to-understand expectations and steps that guide students, faculty, and administrators (Stonecypher & Willson, 2014).

A common feature of honor codes is a "no tolerance" policy that obligates students to report infractions of academic honesty. Others may opt for a policy that allows a student to first confront another student about violations and encourage the accused to self-report before the formal reporting obligation is in force (Wikipedia, 2020). Failure to report a violation is generally considered a violation.

> ### Discussion Point
> Would you report one of your classmates for academic dishonesty? What factors would influence your decision? How does tolerance of academic dishonesty affect the culture of integrity in the nursing program?

Teaching Students About Research and Appropriate Citation

Loschiavo (2017) suggests that one reason students cheat is that they are unprepared for college-level work. He suggests that the reason many students plagiarize is that they were never taught how to write a research paper. He also suggests that students are not being taught how to paraphrase and instead are just expected to cut and paste from the articles they read on the internet.

In addition, Loschiavo (2017) suggests that some students don't have any confidence in their own ideas, so when given the chance to write a paper in which they must share their own thoughts, they simply go to the internet and use others' words or ideas, thinking they are worth more than their own. Or students think that the author's words were so eloquent that they are afraid of their ability to interpret what has been read and to translate it into their own words.

Educators might help students with these deficiencies by requiring the submission of intermediate steps (summaries, rough drafts, etc.) before the deadline for finished papers and assignments. Students might also benefit from a course on research and writing during nursing school. Such a course could also help students learn how to evaluate other research papers and articles in their quest for evidence-based practice.

Providing Mentoring and Support

Loschiavo (2017) suggests that some students cheat because they don't know how to manage their time and thus underestimate how long assignments or studying will take them. They then panic and take shortcuts. In addition, he suggests that some students cheat as a cry for help, subconsciously wishing to be caught so they can share what is going on in their lives with someone they believe may be able to help. He suggests then that faculty should always ask questions about why students made the choices they did.

CONCLUSIONS

Unethical conduct and cheating in both the classroom and the clinical settings are serious concerns for nursing faculty, nursing leaders, and students. Recognition and amelioration of some of the factors in nursing programs that may encourage student dishonesty are critical. Because integrity and trustworthiness are foundations of good nursing practice, faculty must be prepared to help students develop and incorporate these values. As McCabe (2009) put it, "Nursing schools, as the gateway to a profession whose members are assumed to have a strong professional identity that is built on integrity and a desire to serve should assume some responsibility for developing these standards among future members of its profession" (p. 622).

Creating a culture of honesty and accountability is crucial to this end and has been shown to deter cheating. Faculty can also remind students of the importance of integrity, including the effects of a lack of integrity on the well-being of their patients as well as their own self-regard.

Both Stonecypher and Willson (2014) and McCrink (2010) noted that student attitudes toward ethical standards of behavior made the strongest contribution to an ethic of caring and honesty. As one of McCabe's faculty respondents put it, "We have to help students learn that being a student with integrity is a critical part of their socialization into the role of professional health care provider with responsibility for life and death decisions" (McCabe, 2009, p. 620).

For Additional Discussion

1. Which is more important to you—building a culture of integrity in the nursing program and the profession, or loyalty to your classmates or coworkers? How do you handle conflicts between these two values?

2. Do you support the development and use of honor codes in nursing programs?

3. What should an honor code for nursing school look like?

4. Do you believe there is a culture of cheating in your nursing program? What do you do personally to promote academic integrity? What do you think is the relationship between academic integrity and professional integrity? Is a student who cheats in nursing school more likely to cheat in the professional realm? Would you want a nurse who cheated in nursing school caring for someone you cared about?

5. What steps would you recommend to build a culture of strict academic integrity in your nursing program?

References

Adderton, J. (2019, May 2). *Lost integrity: When nursing students cheat.* Retrieved September 20, 2021, from https://allnurses.com/lost-integrity-when-nursing-students-t699207/

American Nurses Association. (2015). *Code of ethics for nurses with interpretive statements (view only for members and non-members).* Retrieved November 25, 2020, from https://www.nursingworld.org/coe-view-only

Bailey, P. A. (2001). Academic misconduct: Responses from deans and nurse educators. *Journal of Nursing Education, 40*(3), 124–131. https://doi.org/10.3928/0148-4834-20010301-07

Baran, L., & Jonason, P. (August 31, 2020). Academic dishonesty among university students: The roles of the psychopathy, motivation, and self-efficacy. *PLOS*

One, 15(8), 1–12. https://doi.org/10.1371/journal
.pone.0238141

Beasley, E. M. (2014). Students reported for cheating explain what they think would have stopped them. *Ethics & Behavior, 24*(3), 229–252. https://doi.org/10.1080/10508422.2013.845533

Bezek, S. M. (2014). *Who is taking care of you? A study of the correlation of academic and professional dishonesty.* Dissertation Abstracts International: Section A. Humanities and Social Sciences, 114. (Publication No. 3630808)

Bleiberg, J., & West, D. (2013, August 20). How technology can stop cheating. *The Huffington Post.* Retrieved September 20, 2021, from http://www.huffingtonpost.com/darrell-west/how-technology-can-stop-c_b_3784392.html

Buchmann, B. (2014, February 20). Cheating in college: Where it happens, why students do it and how to stop it. *The Huffington Post.* Retrieved September 20, 2021, from http://www.huffingtonpost.com/uloop/cheating-in-college-where_b_4826136.html

Carter, H., Hussey, J., & Forehand, J. W. (2019). Plagiarism in nursing education and the ethical implications in practice. *Heliyon, 5*(3), e01350. https://doi.org/10.1016/j.heliyon.2019.e01350

Colorado State University. (2021). *Why do students cheat?* Retrieved November 25, 2020, from https://tilt.colostate.edu/Integrity/FacultyResources/WhyDoStudents

Farkas, K. (2019). *86 Percent of college students say they've cheated. It's easier than ever with mobile devices.* Retrieved September 20, 2021, from https://www.cleveland.com/metro/2017/02/cheating_in_college_has_become.html#:~:text=A%20majority%20of%20college%20students%20in%20a%20recent,have%20cheated%20in%20some%20way%20while%20in%20school

Gaberson, K. B. (1997, July–September). Academic dishonesty among nursing students. *Nursing Forum, 32*(3), 14–20. https://doi.org/10.1111/j.1744-6198.1997.tb00205.x

Gallant, T. (2020, October 23). *Dr. Tricia Bertram Gallant on academic honesty in remote-first instruction.* Retrieved October 31, 2020, from https://unicheck.com/blog/academic-honesty-remote-learning

Gallup. (2020, January 6). *Nurses continue to rate highest in honesty, ethics.* Retrieved November 16, 2020, from https://news.gallup.com/poll/274673/nurses-continue-rate-highest-honesty-ethics.aspx

Glasper, A. (2016, July). Does cheating by students undermine the integrity of the nursing profession? *British Journal of Nursing, 25*(16), 932–933. https://doi.org/10.12968/bjon.2016.25.16.932

Hilbert, G. A. (1985, July–August). Involvement of nursing students in unethical classroom and clinical behaviors. *Journal of Professional Nursing, 1*(4), 230–234. https://doi.org/10.1016/s8755-7223(85)80160-5

Hurn, P., Karagory, P., Sebastian, J., Hagerty, B., & LaFramboise, L. (2020). Upholding the reputation of nurses: Academic integrity. *Nursing Outlook, 68*(4), 383–384. https://doi.org/10.1016/j.outlook.2020.05.003

Institute of Medicine. (2004). *Keeping patients safe: Transforming the work environment of nurses.* National Academic Press.

Krueger, L. (2014, February). Academic dishonesty among nursing students. *Journal of Nursing Education, 53*(2), 77–87. https://doi.org/10.3928/01484834-20140122-06

Lodhia, D. (2018, May 1). More university students are cheating—But it's not because they're lazy. *Guardian News.* Retrieved September 20, 2021, from https://www.theguardian.com/education/2018/may/01/university-students-cheating-tuition-fees-jobs-exams

Loschiavo, C. (2017, June 12). Why do students cheat? Listen to this dean's words. *The Conversation.* Retrieved September 20, 2021, from http://theconversation.com/why-do-students-cheat-listen-to-this-deans-words-40295

McCabe, D. L. (2009, November). Academic dishonesty in nursing schools: An empirical investigation. *Journal of Nursing Education, 48*(11), 614–623. https://doi.org/10.3928/01484834-20090716-07

McCrink, A. (2010). Academic misconduct in nursing students: Behaviors, attitudes, rationalizations, and cultural identity. *Journal of Nursing Education, 49*(11), 653–659. https://doi.org/10.3928/01484834-20100831-03

Miron, J. B. (2016). *Academic integrity and senior nursing undergraduate clinical practice.* Retrieved September 20, 2021, from https://qspace.library.queensu.ca/handle/1974/14708

Morgan, J. (2018, February 14). *How students cheat online, and why stopping them matters.* Inside Higher Ed. Retrieved September 20, 2021, from https://www.insidehighered.com/digital-learning/views/2018/02/14/creative-cheating-online-learning-and-importance-academic

Ok-Hee, C., & Kyung-Hye, H. (2019). Academic ethical awareness among undergraduate nursing students. *Nursing Ethics, 26*(3), 833–844. https://doi.org/10.1177/0969733017727155

Online Degree Programs. (2012, August 9). *7 Most common ways students cheat.* Retrieved September 20, 2021, from http://newsonrelevantscience.blogspot.com/2012/08/7-most-common-ways-students-cheat.html

Robinson, J., & Glanzer, P. (2017, Summer). Building a culture of academic integrity: What students perceive and need. *College Student Journal, 51*(2), 209–221. https://www.ingentaconnect.com/content/prin/cs

Sheer, B. L. (1989). *The relationships among socialization, empathy, autonomy and unethical student behaviors in baccalaureate nursing students* (Unpublished doctoral dissertation). Widener University School of Nursing, Chester, PA.

Shepherd, K. (2020, December 22). More than 70 West Point cadets accused in academy's biggest cheating scandal in decades. *Washington Post.* Retrieved September 20, 2021, from https://www.pressherald.com/2020/12/22/more-than-70-west-point-cadets-accused-in-academys-biggest-cheating-scandal-in-decades/

Simola, S. (2017). Managing for academic integrity in higher education: Insights from behavioral ethics. *Scholarship of Teaching and Learning in Psychology, 3*(1), 43–57. Retrieved October 18, 2021, from https://doi.org/10.1037/stl0000076

Stonecypher, K., & Willson, P. (2014, May). Academic policies and practices to deter cheating in nursing education. *Nursing Education Perspectives, 35*(3), 167–179. https://doi.org/10.5480/12-1028.1

The Conversation. (2018, February 15). *Why students at prestigious high schools still cheat on exams.* Retrieved September 20, 2021, from https://theconversation.com/why-students-at-prestigious-high-schools-still-cheat-on-exams-91041

Vandoorne, S. (2014, June 19). From smartwatch and smartpen... to smartcheat? *CNN.* Retrieved September 20, 2021, from http://www.cnn.com/2014/06/19/business/high-tech-cheating/index.html

Wikipedia, the Free Encyclopedia. (2020, September 4). *Academic honor code.* Retrieved November 25, 2020, from http://en.wikipedia.org/w/index.php?title=Academic_honor_code&oldid=664372276

Winneg, D. (2015, August 1). *Students will cheat—So, deal with it!* [Web log post]. Software Secure. Retrieved September 20, 2021, from https://blog.psionline.com/education/blog/students-will-cheat-deal

Woith, W., Jenkins, S. D., & Kerber, C. (2012, October). Perceptions of academic integrity among nursing students. *Nursing Forum, 47*(4), 253–259. https://doi.org/10.1111/j.1744-6198.2012.00274.x

Assuring Provider Competence Through Licensure, Continuing Education, and Certification

Carol J. Huston

ADDITIONAL RESOURCES

Visit thePoint for additional helpful resources.
• eBook
• Journal Articles
• Web Links

CHAPTER OUTLINE

LEARNING OBJECTIVES

The learner will be able to:

1. Differentiate between competence and continuing competence in a profession.

2. Identify stakeholders who would be affected by a movement to mandate continuing competence in nursing.

3. Identify driving and restraining forces to implementing mandatory reexamination as a prerequisite for license renewal in nursing.

4. Compare support for mandatory reexamination for license renewal in nursing with that of other health professions such as medicine and pharmacy.

5. Identify arguments for and against mandated continuing education for license renewal.

6. Compare continuing education requirements for nurses with those for other health care professionals.

7. Describe personal and professional benefits of professional certification.

8. Delineate the roles and responsibilities assumed by the American Board of Nursing Specialties as the accrediting body for nursing certification.

9. Identify the strengths and weaknesses of using professional certification as an indicator of entry-level competence in advanced practice nursing.

10. Describe how portfolios and self-assessment, as tools for reflective practice, can further the goal of professional competence.

11. Explore the roles and responsibilities of the individual, employers, the state board of nursing, and professional associations in assuring both the initial and the continued competence of health care practitioners.

12. Reflect on beliefs regarding the need for and efficacy of mandating reexamination for licensure, continuing education, and certification for nurses to assure continuing competence.

INTRODUCTION

How can one determine whether a nurse is competent? Does licensure assure competence? Does clinical performance assure competence? Does competence require recency of clinical practice? Is it assured by professional certification? Would nurse residencies increase the competence of the new graduate nurse?

Unfortunately, in many states, a practitioner is determined to be competent when initially licensed and thereafter unless proven otherwise. Yet clearly, passing a licensing examination and continuing to work as a clinician does not assure competence throughout a career. Competence requires continual updates to knowledge and practice, and this is difficult in a health care environment characterized by rapidly emerging new technologies, chaotic change, and perpetual clinical advancements based on new evidence.

For example, the Institute of Medicine (IOM, 2010) report *The Future of Nursing* suggests that nursing graduates need competence in a variety of areas, including continuous improvement of the quality and safety of health care systems, informatics, evidence-based practice, a knowledge of complex systems, skills and methods for leadership and management of continual improvement, and health policy knowledge, skills, and attitudes. One must at least question how many nurses currently in practice would be able to demonstrate competency in all these areas.

In addition, new competencies must be integrated into nursing practice as new science emerges. For example, the Quality, Safety, and Education for Nurses Institute (QSEN, 2020) suggests nurses now need competence for practice in patient-centered care, teamwork and collaboration, evidence-based practice, quality improvement, safety, and informatics.

In addition, the National Human Genome Research Institute (n.d.) suggests nurses also now need competence in incorporating genetic and genomic technologies and information into practice and developing plans of care that incorporate genetic and genomic information. Huston (2018) agrees, noting that genetics is now a requisite competency for nurses, but cautions that it is highly likely that many nurses learned little about what was a newly emerging field of study at the time of their initial nursing education. The result is that some nurses lack both the self-confidence and skills needed to obtain a genetic family history, identify individuals at risk for developing genomic-influenced conditions or drug reactions, and assist consumers in making informed decisions about genetic testing results and therapies.

> *Consider This* Nursing leaders must create practice and curriculum change that establishes genetics as an essential nursing competency. The public's health depends on it and it is nurses who should be the translators of this information (Huston, 2018).

There is little disagreement that the knowledge health care professionals need must be current and appropriate to their area of practice and that their care should be competent at the minimum. The challenge lies, however, in determining how best to assure that competence and in determining who should be responsible for its oversight.

This chapter explores definitions of *competence*, giving particular attention to that of *continuing competence*. Licensure, periodic relicensure, continuing education (CE), and professional certification are examined as potential strategies for assuring provider competence. The chapter also discusses the limitations of each of these strategies for assessing both initial and continuing competence, as well as the difficulties inherent in standardizing continuing competence requirements in a health care system composed of varied stakeholders. Finally, the chapter concludes with an exploration of portfolio development and reflective practice: contemporary strategies that allow health care professionals to carry out a self-assessment of their practice and to develop a personal plan for maintaining competence.

DEFINING COMPETENCE

Competence in nursing can be defined in many ways. Dictionary.com (2021) defines competence as adequacy or the possession of required skill, knowledge, qualification, or capacity. As such, it is tied to experience and context. Hence, professional competence can be defined as the capacity to handle events and challenges effectively.

In 1999, the American Nurses Association (ANA) convened an expert panel that defined three types of competence in nursing: *continuing competence, professional nursing competence,* and *continuing professional nursing competence.* Special attention was given, however, to continuing competence because so many assumptions exist regarding the rights and responsibilities of consumers, individual nurses, and employers to see that such competence is present and promulgated. Indeed, it is continuing competence that is a primary focus of this chapter, given that initial licensure suggests that at least minimum competence levels were met at that time.

In 2007, the ANA released a draft position statement on competence and competency for public review and comment. The purpose of this position paper was to define *competence* ("performing successfully at an expected level") and *competency* ("an expected level of performance that results from an integration of knowledge, skills, abilities, and judgment within the context of current and projected professional directions"). Key excerpts from the final document released in 2008 and reaffirmed in 2014 are provided in Box 20.1.

Clearly, although there is some overlap among these definitions, there is still some lack of consensus around what competence is and how it should be measured. There also appears to be difficulty in relating the continuing competence of providers with the roles they are asked to assume in the clinical setting. For example, some nurses develop high levels of competence in specific areas of nursing practice because of work experience and specialization at the expense of staying current in other areas of practice. Yet, employers who espouse the support of continuing competence often ask registered nurses (RNs) to provide care in areas of practice outside their area of expertise because staffing shortages encourage them to do so. In addition, many current competence assessments focus more on skills than they do on knowledge.

> *Consider This* Nurses are often asked to float to or work in areas where their competence may be in question because their licenses allow them to work in virtually any area of practice.

In addition, professional nursing organizations decline to implement continuing competence mandates because they fear membership repercussions. For example, the American Nurses Credentialing Center (ANCC) continues to offer some certification examinations for RNs without baccalaureate degrees, despite the recognition that such certification suggests advanced rather than basic practice.

BOX 20.1   **Excerpts from the ANA Position Statement on Professional Role Competence (Approved March 28, 2008, and Reaffirmed November 12, 2014)**

The ANA supports the following principles in regard to competence in the nursing profession:
* The public has a right to expect nurses to demonstrate competence throughout their careers.
* Nurses are individually responsible and accountable for maintaining professional competence.
* The nursing profession must shape and guide any process assuring nurse competence.
* Regulatory bodies define minimal standards for regulation of practice to protect the public.
* Employers are responsible and accountable to provide an environment conducive to competent practice.
* Assurance of competence is the shared responsibility of the profession, individual nurses, professional organizations, credentialing and certification entities, regulatory agencies, employers, and other key stakeholders.

Source: American Nurses Association. (2014, November 12). *ANA position statement: Professional role competence.* Retrieved August 27, 2021, from https://www.nursingworld.org/practice-policy/nursing-excellence/official-position-statements/id/professional-role-competence/

The ANA advocates that states defer competence monitoring to the professional association without governmental involvement in the process, partly because of concern about misconduct charges if state regulators are involved and partly because memberships and revenues are likely to increase if the association monitors competence. Clearly, then, stakeholders and politics continue to influence how continuing competence is defined, used, and promulgated.

The issue is also complicated by the fact that there are no national standards for defining, measuring, or requiring continuing competence in nursing. In addition, specialty nursing organizations, state nurses' associations, state boards of nursing, and professional nursing organizations have not reached a consensus about what continuing competence is and how to measure it, although there is little debate that it is needed. The reality is that given the multiplicity and variations of the definition of continuing competence and the number of stakeholders affected by its promulgation, identifying and mandating strategies that assure the continuing competence of health care providers will be difficult.

Consider This   There is no consensus about how to define or objectively measure continuing competence in nursing practice.

PROFESSIONAL LICENSURE

Licensure can be defined as

> *the granting of a permit to perform acts which, without it, would be illegal; The public or governmental regulation of health or other professions for voluntary private-sector programs that attest to the competency of an individual health care practitioner. (The Free Dictionary by Farlex, 2003–2021, para. 1)*

Most health care professionals must be licensed, and this license is assumed to provide at least some assurance that the practitioner was competent in their field at the time of initial licensure.

Licensure Processes in Nursing

One of the most important purposes of the National Council of State Boards of Nursing (NCSBN, 2021b) and its 59 state boards of nursing (one in each of 50 states, two in three states,

one in the District of Columbia, one in each of four U.S. territories, and one with both a board of nursing and a board for advanced practice nurses) is to protect the health, safety, and welfare of the public. This is done by having a regulatory role in the accreditation of nursing education programs, through licensure and by implementing and enforcing the Nurse Practice Act. In addition, the NCSBN has created and disseminated numerous nursing practice and regulation resources on nursing practice and education and maintains a database on nursing disciplinary actions taken across the nation.

It is the licensing examinations for RNs and licensed practical nurses/licensed vocational nurses (LPNs/LVNs), however, that the NCSBN and its state boards of nursing are probably best known. The NCSBN has developed two licensure examinations to test the entry-level nursing competence of candidates for licensure as RNs and as LPNs/LVNs. These examinations, the National Council Licensure Examinations (NCLEX-RN and NCLEX-PN), are administered with the contractual assistance of a national test service (NCSBN, 2021c) and test-integrated nursing content. Passage of the NCLEX suggests that the individual has been deemed by the state to have met minimal competence standards for entry into practice; however, it may not reflect or measure the many higher-level competencies achieved in different types of education programs for nurses.

Despite this flaw, licensure by examination continues to be a highly regarded strategy for assuring competence levels of health care professionals, such as nurses. Indeed, some professional organizations and regulatory bodies suggest that RNs should be required to repeat the NCLEX periodically or that nurses should be required to take examinations similar in scope to the NCLEX for license renewal.

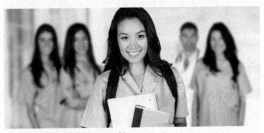

(Rob Marmion/Shutterstock)

Efforts to implement mandatory reexamination as a prerequisite for license renewal in nursing, however, have met with minimal success. This is because there is little agreement about what such an examination should look like, how it would be administered, and how often it should be required. Nonetheless, multiple states have introduced legislation with varying approaches from retesting to requiring a provider to demonstrate competence in the workplace, but resistance is high, and there is little hope that periodic reexaminations to assess competence will be a part of nursing's immediate future.

In addition, the *Nurse Licensure Compact* (NLC), with 33 to 35 participant states as of mid-2021 (two additional states are pending), allows a nurse to have a license in one state and to practice in other states, as long as that nurse is subject to each state's practice laws and discipline (NCSBN, 2021a; Nursing Compact States, 2021; Nursing License Map, 2021). In addition, the NLC was revised in 2015, becoming the enhanced NLC (eNLC). The eNLC allows RNs and LPNs/LVNs in the eNLC member states (Table 20.1) to have one multistate license, which allows them to practice in person or through telehealth in their home state of licensure and other eNLC member states (Nursing License Map, 2021). Having these compacts further reduces the likelihood that a nurse will require NCLEX reexamination during their career, despite crossing state lines where the initial nursing license was obtained.

Licensure Processes in Medicine

In contrast to the NCLEX, U.S. medical licensure examinations are developed using a competence-based process that requires examinees to be cognizant of practice changes, the evidence required for practice, and the knowledge necessary to be competent into the future. In addition, to achieve full authority to practice independently, physicians are required to pass three licensure examinations (U.S. Medical Licensing Examination, 1996–2021). Furthermore, a clinical skills examination was implemented in 2004.

In addition, although periodic reexamination was recommended in 1967 by the Bureau of Health Manpower of the U.S. Department of Health for licensure of physicians as of 1971, the decision regarding whether to do so has been left to the discretion of individual states. In most states, this is simply a matter of completing mandatory CE requirements and having no disciplinary actions filed against their license.

Licensure Processes in Pharmacy

Pharmacists have also been reluctant to embrace the IOM's *To Err Is Human* recommendation that periodic reexamination of key providers is critical to resolving health care

TABLE 20.1	**States That Have Enacted or Have Pending Legislation to Make the Enhanced Nurse Licensure Compact (eNLC) as of August 2021**

1. Alabama
2. Arizona
3. Arkansas
4. Colorado
5. Delaware
6. Florida
7. Georgia
8. Guam (allows nurses who hold active, unencumbered, multistate licenses issued by Nurse Licensure Compact member states to practice in Guam under their multistate licenses)
9. Idaho
10. Indiana
11. Iowa
12. Kansas
13. Kentucky
14. Louisiana (RN and LPN)
15. Maine
16. Maryland
17. Mississippi
18. Missouri
19. Montana
20. Nebraska
21. New Hampshire
22. New Jersey (allows nurses who hold active, unencumbered, multistate licenses issued by Nurse Licensure Compact member states to practice in New Jersey under their multistate licenses)
23. New Mexico
24. North Carolina
25. North Dakota
26. Ohio (law passed and awaiting implementation)
27. Oklahoma
28. Pennsylvania (law passed and awaiting implementation)
29. South Carolina
30. South Dakota
31. Tennessee
32. Texas
33. Utah
34. Virginia
35. West Virginia (RN and LPN)
36. Wisconsin
37. Wyoming

Note: LPN, licensed practical nurse; RN, registered nurse.
Source: Data from *Compact Nursing States List 2021.* (2021). Retrieved August 27, 2021, from https://nurse.org/articles/enhanced-compact-multi-state-license-enlc/

quality problems, especially medical errors. Pharmacists take a licensing examination on graduation, known as the North American Pharmacist Licensure Examination (NAPLEX). The NAPLEX is a computer-adaptive examination that tests general practice knowledge. The NAPLEX is just one component of the licensure process and is used by the boards of pharmacy as part of their assessment of a candidate's competence to practice as a pharmacist (National Association of Boards of Pharmacy [NABP], 2020b).

In addition, 49 boards require a Multistate Pharmacy Jurisprudence Examination (MPJE), which combines federal- and state-specific questions to test the pharmacy jurisprudence knowledge of prospective pharmacists for both initial licensure and license transfer (NABP, 2020a). The five boards that do not utilize the MPJE for their law examinations are Arkansas, California, Idaho, Puerto Rico, and the Virgin Islands. Reciprocity is granted between states by an electronic licensure transfer program. At present, pharmacists are not required to retake the NAPLEX at any point for license renewal.

Discussion Point

Why are professional health care organizations reluctant to support reexamination as a means of ensuring continuing competence? Who are the stakeholders involved? What are some ramifications of adopting such a mandate?

CONTINUING EDUCATION

Instead of requiring health care providers to periodically repeat their initial licensure examinations, many professional associations and states have mandated CE for license renewal. This has been done to promote continued competence and is less controversial than periodic reexamination for licensure.

CE in Nursing

Most of the states in the United States have some kind of requirement for CE for professional nurse license renewal. These requirements typically vary from a few hours to 30 hours, every 2 years (Box 20.2). There is no requirement for CE for RNs in Arizona, Colorado, Connecticut, Indiana, Maine, Maryland (only a refresher course is required), Mississippi, Missouri, Montana, South Dakota, Vermont, and Wisconsin. Every other state has some sort of requirement for RNs (Nursing Continuing Education Requirements by State, 2021).

Some states—Colorado, for example—required CE at one time, but removed that requirement because it felt that CE did not guarantee competence. Similarly, Hawaii

discontinued CE requirements for many professions, including nursing and physical therapy, because of the high costs of these courses to the individual practitioner, considerable costs to the state to administer the legislation, and the inability to demonstrate positive outcomes. Hawaii did reinstitute mandatory CE beginning July 1, 2017, although nurses in that state could also choose to complete a board-approved refresher course, or a minimum of two semester credits of postlicensure academic education related to nursing practice from an accredited nursing program (Nursing Continuing Education Requirements by State, 2021).

Discussion Point

Is the need for CE greater for one type of health care professional than another? When required, should the minimum number of mandated hours be the same for all health care professionals? If not, how many should be required for each health care specialty?

CE in Medicine

Sixty-two boards (46 states plus Guam, Puerto Rico, and the Virgin Islands) require some form of continuing medical education (CME) for relicensure of medical doctors (MDs) and for doctors of osteopathy (DOs), although the requirements frequently differ for the two groups (American College of Physicians, 2021; Medscape Education, 1994–2021).

The number of required hours also varies dramatically by state. For example, as of 2019, Colorado, Indiana, Montana, and South Dakota required no CME hours for either MDs or DOs (Medscape Education, 1994–2021). New York requires only infection control and child abuse content. Illinois requires 150 hours every 3 years, whereas Wisconsin requires only 30 hours every 2 years (must include some content on responsible opioid prescription for physicians holding a drug enforcement agency [DEA] number), and Arkansas requires only 20 hours each year (Medscape Education, 1994–2021). It should be noted, however, that some medical specialty societies, specialty boards, hospital medical staffs, The Joint Commission, and insurance groups require physicians to demonstrate CE, even if the state does not require this for relicensure.

In addition, some states have laws that direct the format of the CME. Required topics often include pain management, AIDS, and domestic violence. Other states require that physicians renewing their licenses must receive instruction on ethics and professional responsibility.

Furthermore, unlike nursing CE, which is typically monitored by the state boards of nursing, there is no central repository of CME. Instead, accredited CME providers are required to keep records of *CE credits* awarded to physicians

---

BOX 20.2   **Sample State CE Requirements for Nurses**

- *Arkansas:* 15 practice-focused contact hours every 2 years, or certification or recertification during the renewal period by a national certifying body or completion of 1 college credit hour course in nursing with a grade C or better during licensure period (Arkansas Department of Health, 2017).
- *California:* 30 hours every 2 years (California Board of Registered Nursing, 2021).
- *Florida:* 16 general hours of CE plus 2 hours on medical error, 2 hours on Florida laws and rules, 2 hours on recognizing impairment in the workplace, 2 hours on human trafficking, 2 hours on domestic violence, and 1 hour of HIV/AIDS every 2 years (Florida Board of Nursing, 2021).
- *Iowa:* 36 hours for a 3-year license (Iowa Board of Nursing, 2020).
- *Michigan:* No less than 25 hours of CE, with at least 2 hours in pain and symptom management every 2 years (Michigan Board of Nursing, 2019).
- *New Jersey:* 30 hours every 2 years (State of New Jersey, 2017).
- *New York:* 3 contact hours of infection control every 4 years and 2 contact hours of child abuse (one time; "New York Board of Nursing State CE Requirements," 2021).
- *North Dakota:* 12 contact hours every 2 years ("North Dakota Board of Nursing State CE Requirements," 2021).
- *Ohio:* 24 hours every 2 years (Ohio Board of Nursing, n.d.).
- *Oklahoma:* (1) RNs must verify 520 hours of employment a year, or (2) complete 24 hours of CE, or (3) verify current certification in a nursing specialty area, or (4) complete a board-approved refresher course, or (5) complete 6 academic semester credits hours of coursework at the current level of licensure or higher (Nursing Continuing Education Requirements by State, 2021).
- *Oregon:* One-time, 7-hour course on pain management. One hour must be a course to be provided by the Oregon Pain Management Commission. The remaining 6 hours can be from a choice of pain management topics. Once this requirement is fulfilled, there are no additional CE requirements for renewal ("Oregon Nursing CE Requirements," 2021).
- *Texas:* 20 hours of CE every 2 years in the nurse's area of practice or the achievement, maintenance, or renewal of a board-approved national nursing certification in the nurse's area of practice. There is also a targeted one-time, 2 contact hours of CE requirement for any RN practicing in an emergency department setting for Forensic Evidence Collection ("Nursing Continuing Education Requirements by State," 2021).

---

who participate in their activities for 6 years, and physicians are responsible for maintaining a record of their CME credits from all sources.

CE in Other Health Care Professions

Almost all states require CE for pharmacists, and most require the CE be from approved sources, such as the American Council on Pharmacy Education. Sometimes carryover of hours or units is allowed, and sometimes the type is proscribed.

In addition, many states require acupuncturists, audiologists, and occupational therapists to have CE for license renewal. Physician assistants must log 100 hours of CME every 2 years and sit for recertification every 10 years to maintain their national certification (U.S. Bureau of Labor Statistics, 2021).

Does Requiring CE Ensure Competence?

The CE approach to continuing competence continues to be very controversial because there is limited research demonstrating correlation between CE, continuing competence,

and improved patient outcomes. In addition, many professional organizations have expressed concern about the quality of mandated CE courses and the lack of courses for experts and specialists. Likewise, there is no agreement on the optimal number of annual credits needed to ensure competence.

Research continues, however, to explore the relationship between CE and continuing competence. A recent retrospective, mixed-method study by Bryant and Posey (2019) of nurses' intent to change practice and actual practice change after completing CE courses found that 88.6% of nurses reported positive intent to change practice and 89.1% reported actual practice change. The researchers concluded that CE can positively influence nursing practice change and lead to broader organizational improvements.

Similarly, Lawrence and Bauer (2020) studied knowledge levels and intent to implement course information by nurses who completed a human trafficking CE course. Postcourse surveys indicated that participants had increased knowledge and desire to implement the course information to identify trafficked individuals, although actual changes in practice outcomes were not measured.

Until consensus can be reached, however, regarding how CE should be provided and how much is needed, and until research findings conclusively demonstrate an empirical link between CE and provider competence, it is difficult to tout CE as a valid and reliable measure of continuing competence. The pros and cons of mandating CE for nurses are summarized in Box 20.3.

Discussion Point

CE is mandated in most states for certified public accountants, optometrists, real estate brokers, nursing home administrators, and insurance brokers. Why are there fewer states mandating CE for health care professionals? What rationale can be given for why these occupations have a greater need for CE than health care professionals?

CERTIFICATION

The Accreditation Board for Specialty Nursing Certification suggests certification "is the formal recognition of the specialized knowledge, skills, and experience demonstrated by the achievement of standards identified by a nursing specialty to promote optimal health outcomes" (American Academy of Ambulatory Care Nursing [AAACN], 2021, para. 1). Certification does not, however, include a legal scope of practice. Instead, it suggests a level of competence in a specific clinical area. Some organizations offering specialty certifications for nurses include the ANCC, the American Association of Critical-Care Nurses, the American Association of Nurse Anesthetists, the

American College of Nurse-Midwives, the Board of Certification for Emergency Nursing, the Oncology Nursing Certification Corporation, and the Rehabilitation Nursing Certification Board.

Becoming Certified

To achieve professional certification, nurses must meet eligibility criteria that may include years and types of work experience, as well as minimum educational levels, active nursing licenses, and successful completion of a nationally administered examination. Certifications normally last 5 years.

The American Board of Nursing Specialties

In addition to the large numbers of certified nurses, there are many different types of nursing certification credentials, and certification programs often have very different standards. This makes it difficult for providers and consumers to determine the value of a specific nursing certification. For this reason, the American Board of Nursing Specialties (ABNS) was created in 1991 to advance knowledge regarding specialty nursing certification through research, support continuing competence as a means for ensuring patient safety, and promote accreditation to recognize quality specialty nursing certification programs. ABNS represents almost 750,000 certified RNs worldwide in a variety of settings (ABNS, 2020).

The ABNS is composed of nurse-certifying organizations from around the world. As the only accrediting body specifically for nursing certification, the Accreditation Council provides a peer-review process for accrediting nursing certification programs that demonstrate compliance with ABNS standards.

BOX 20.3   Pros and Cons of CE Requirements for Nurses

Pros
- Augments knowledge and skills beyond the basic entry-level nursing education
- Provides an opportunity for knowledge and skills updates that reflect best practices
- Provides opportunities to gain new knowledge and skills in a rapidly changing health care environment
- Reflects a professional commitment to continued competence
- Is provided in many forms, allowing individuals the opportunity to learn in a manner that works best for them
- Completing specialty certification and advanced degrees may provide an opportunity for career advancement

Cons
- Participation in learning opportunities does not guarantee learning
- CE content may not be in area of clinical practice/may lack practice relevance
- Can be expensive and time-consuming
- Quality of educational materials and courses is variable
- Just because a course is accredited does not mean that it will be accepted by any state in fulfillment of CE requirements
- Limited empirical data linking mandatory CE to improved practice outcomes

The American Nurses Credentialing Center

The ANA established the ANA Certification Program in 1973 to provide tangible recognition of professional achievement in a defined functional or clinical area of nursing. The ANCC, a subsidiary of the ANA, became its own corporation in 1991, and since then has certified more than a quarter million nurses and approximately 75,000 advanced practice nurses (ANCC, n.d.).

Certification and the Advanced Practice Nurse

Advanced practice nurses were the first nurses to use professional certification as a means of documenting advanced knowledge in practice. In 1946, the American Association of Nurse Anesthetists began certifying nurse anesthetists. The American College of Nurse-Midwives soon followed. Most states now use certification as an indicator of entry-level competence in advanced practice nursing, which includes clinical nurse specialists (CNSs) and nurse practitioners (NPs).

Even the NCSBN, which originally proposed the second licensure for NPs, now recognizes the certification examination as the regulatory mechanism for advanced nursing practice. A master's degree is required to take the certification examinations for advanced practice nurses. Certification, then, in the case of the advanced practice nurse is not voluntary; it is required to ensure public safety and enhance public health.

Discussion Point

The ANCC currently does not allow educational waivers for the CNS- or NP-certifying examination (all applicants must have at least a master's degree). Do you support this decision to not "grandfather in" advanced practice nurses who completed their educations through certifying programs (no master's degree) and who are currently practicing in an advanced role? Why or why not?

The Effect of Professional Certification

A great deal of research has been completed in the past decade regarding the use of certification to ensure competence and its inherent value. Most of these studies suggest that certification does impact both improved patient outcomes and the creation of a positive work environment (Box 20.4).

For example, a recent study by Gigli et al. (2020) found that nursing specialty certification was associated with greater professional identity and higher perceptions of knowledge of and value in evidence-based practices used in the intensive care unit (ICU), whereas education level was not. The researchers concluded that specialty certification could assist with the adoption of evidence-based practices in ICU settings, thereby improving the quality of care (Research Fuels the Controversy 20.1).

Another recent study examined the perceptions of certified registered nurse anesthetists (CRNAs) toward the value of certification in nonsurgical pain management (NSPM) (Ward et al., 2019). Study findings noted perceived benefits of holding the NSPM credential and identified three important constructs: personal satisfaction, professional recognition, and competence. In relation to the construct of competence, study participants reported the specialty certification as validating specialized knowledge, indicating a level of clinical competence, noting the attainment of a practice standard, and enhancing professional credibility.

Certification is also an option for validating the professional competence of academic nurse educators. In a sample of 718 nurse faculty members and administrators from 48 states in the United States, academic nurse educator certification was valued by nurse educators and administrators as representing specialized knowledge, attainment of a professional standard, educator competence, and professional credibility (Poindexter et al., 2019). In addition, the study found that satisfaction with professional accomplishments and professional marketing and recognition subscales reflect National League for Nursing (NLN) nurse educator core competencies and serve to confirm the specialized knowledge and skills expected of nurse educators.

BOX 20.4   Personal Benefits of Professional Certification

- Provides a sense of accomplishment and achievement
- Validation of specialty knowledge and competence to peers and patients
- Increased credibility
- Increased self-confidence
- Promotes greater autonomy of practice
- Provides for increased career opportunities and greater competitiveness in the job market
- May result in salary incentives

Research Fuels the Controversy 20.1

The Association Between Specialty Certification and Nurses' Perceived Knowledge and Value of Evidence-Based Practices

To examine the relationships between critical care nurses' education level and specialty certification, their individual psychosocial beliefs about their place on the ICU team (in relation to three factors: professional identity, self-efficacy, and role clarity), and their perceptions of evidence-based practices used in the ICU, a cross-sectional survey was emailed to nurses in 12 adult ICUs within six hospitals in a single, integrated health care system.

Source: Gigli, K. H., Davis, B. S., Ervin, J., & Kahn, J. M. (2020). Factors associated with nurses' knowledge of and perceived value in evidence-based practices. *American Journal of Critical Care, 29*(1), e1–e8. https://doi.org/10.4037/ajcc2020866

Study Findings

The researchers found a strong association between specialty certification and nurses' perceived knowledge of and value of specific evidence-based practices, supporting the value of nurses with specialty certification, especially among institutions that aim to increase the adoption of evidence-based practices. No significant relationship was found between nurses' education level and perceived knowledge of or perceived value in evidence-based practices. In addition, specialty certification was associated with greater professional identity. The researchers concluded that supporting specialty certification among nurses is a plausible way to assist with the adoption of evidence-based practices to improve ICU quality and should be evaluated further.

Creating Work Environments that Value Certification

It is likely middle- and top-level nurse managers who play the most significant role in creating work environments that value and reward certification. For example, nurse managers can grant tuition reimbursement or salary incentives to workers who seek certification. This is critical because significant barriers to nurses obtaining specialty certification are cost and a fear of failure (Pirschel, 2019). Managers can also show their support for professional certification by giving employees paid time off to take the certification examination and by publicly recognizing employees who have achieved specialty certification.

Managers should also encourage certified nurses to promote their achievements by introducing themselves as certified nurses to patients and wearing their certification pins. In doing so, the certified nurse acts as a role model to other nurses considering specialty certification. Pirschel (2019) agrees, suggesting that nurses should wear their certification like a badge of honor, in demonstrating the qualifications, experience, and expert knowledge they have been able to demonstrate.

Discussion Point

Do most employers value professional certification? Do nurses value it? Does the general public value it? On what criteria do you base your answer?

REFLECTIVE PRACTICE

Reflective practice is defined by the North Carolina Board of Nursing (NCBN, 2021) as a process for the assessment of one's own practice to identify and seek learning opportunities to promote continuing competence. Inherent in the process is the evaluation and incorporation of this learning into one's practice. Such self-assessment is gaining popularity as a tool to promote professional practice and maintain competence. Often, this is done through professional portfolios for competence assessment.

For example, North Carolina now requires RNs to use a reflective practice approach to carry out a self-assessment of their practice and develop a plan for maintaining competence (NCBN, 2021). This assessment is individualized to the licensed nurse's area of practice. RNs seeking license renewal or reinstatement must attest to having completed the learning activities required for continuing competence and be prepared to submit evidence of completion if requested by the board on random audit (NCBN, 2020).

Similarly, the Nurses Association of New Brunswick (NANB, n.d.) developed a mandatory continuing competence program (CCP) for implementation in 2008 (updated in 2018) that requires RNs to demonstrate on an annual basis how they have maintained their competence and enhanced their practice. The CCP requires RNs and NPs to reflect on their nursing practice through self-assessment against their standards of practice, the development and implementation of a learning plan, and then evaluation of the impact of the learning activities on nursing practice (NANB, n.d.). The NANB argues that continuing competence is a necessary component of practice and the public interest is best served when nurses enhance their knowledge, skill, and judgment on an ongoing basis; and reflective practice, or the process of continually assessing one's practice to identify learning needs and opportunities for growth, is the key to continuing competence (NANB, n.d.).

Portfolios and Self-Assessment

Portfolio development is another strategy the individual RN can use to be reflective about their practice and/or to assess or demonstrate competence. The professional portfolio typically contains core components such as biographical information; educational background; certifications achieved; employment history; a resume; a competence record or checklist; personal and professional goals; professional development experiences, presentations, consultations, and publications; professional and community activities; honors and awards; and letters of thanks from patients, families, peers, organizations, and others.

St-Germain and colleagues (2019) add that the purpose of the professional portfolio should not be limited to clinical placements or preparing for admission to higher education in nursing. It can also be used to establish career goals, showcase professional practice and development, illustrate specific areas of expertise, and enhance knowledge and skills.

> **Consider This** All nurses should maintain a portfolio to reflect professional growth throughout their careers.

WHO IS RESPONSIBLE FOR COMPETENCE ASSESSMENT IN NURSING?

Who, then, has the responsibility for competence assessment in nursing? Should it be the individual, the employer, the regulatory board, or the certifying agency? Is it a shared responsibility? If so, are these entities willing to work together to create an integrated and systematic approach to promoting continuing competence in nursing?

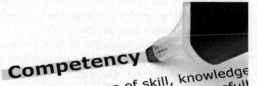

Competency
A specific range of skill, knowledge ability to do something successfully being adequately or well qualified the condition of being capable of to meet demands, requirements

(Ivelin Radkov/Shutterstock)

Certainly, an individual responsibility for maintaining competence is suggested by the *ANA Code of Ethics for Nurses with Interpretive Statements* in its assertion that nurses are obligated to provide adequate and competent nursing care (ANA, 2015). State nurse practice acts also hold nurses accountable for being reasonable and prudent in their practice. Both standards require the nurse to have at least some personal responsibility for continually assessing their professional competence through reflective practice.

> **Consider This** The individual RN has a professional obligation to maintain competence.

The role of the professional association also lacks clarity. Although professional associations develop and promote standards, there is no oversight function of either initial or continuing competence.

Employers also play a role in assuring competence of employees by performing periodic performance appraisals and by carrying out the requirements of the accrediting bodies to ensure the ongoing competencies of employees. Yet, employers are often among the first to argue that "a nurse is a nurse is a nurse" when it comes to meeting mandatory staffing or licensure requirements.

Regulatory boards, such as the state boards of nursing, regulate initial licensure, monitor compliance with requirements for license renewal, and take action when professional standards are breached. Yet, clearly, licensure and relicensure per se do not guarantee competence, particularly in a discipline as broad in scope and practice as nursing.

Finally, certifying organizations do help to identify those individuals who have expertise in a specific area of practice; however, knowledge expertise does not always translate into practice expertise. A lack of professional certification does not necessarily mean that the nurse lacks continuing competence. Recertification does not ensure continued expertise because recertification is usually a product of meeting CE requirements rather than reexamination.

CONCLUSIONS

The challenge in assuring competence in nursing is that nursing practice is dynamic, and thus best practice must be continually redefined because of new discoveries. Licensure, CE, and professional certification can ensure provider competence only if they reflect the latest thinking, research, and clinical practice needs. In addition, each of these three strategies is limited in its effectiveness as a competence assessment strategy.

Clearly, the NCLEX, as it currently exists, assures only minimum entry-level competence for professional nursing practice. Given that NCLEX content derives from a retrospective model and that technologic changes and the rate of knowledge acquisition are increasing exponentially in the 21st century, the knowledge base of the newly licensed nurse has a great likelihood of being dated even before examinations are scored. In addition, as long as a single NCLEX exists and there are multiple levels of educational entry into practice, the examination will continue to have to meet educational content directed at the lowest educational level of entry.

In addition, health care professionals, professional organizations, and regulatory bodies are reluctant to implement mandatory reexamination for licensure. One must at least question whether this is because of the fear that many providers would be unable to demonstrate the continuing competence necessary for relicensure.

CE has similar limitations for assuring provider competence. Some states do not require nurses to complete CE. Those that do demonstrate wide variation in how much CE is required, what content can be included, and how that CE can be provided. In addition, there is no guarantee that completing CE courses results in a change in the provider's knowledge level or practice or even that the content provided in the CE course is current and relevant.

Finally, professional certification does ensure that the nurse has some specialized area of knowledge and practice expertise. The reality, however, is that many nurses perform outside the area of their certification expertise every day in their jobs, particularly if their area of specialty certification expertise is narrow. In addition, Cox and Grus (2019) point out that licensure and initial board certification provide a snapshot of an individual's competence only at a single point in time. To complicate things further, there are multiple certifying bodies and numerous types of certification. Determining the exact value of that certification in terms of improving patient care has not completely been ascertained.

The question of how best to assure provider competence cannot yet be answered. Efforts that address the need to do so are underway, but these efforts have not been coordinated or integrated by the professional associations, regulatory bodies, and stakeholders that are affected. In addition, most professional entities involved in assuring continuing competence are reluctant to mandate interventions for fear of alienating stakeholders. Individual practitioners also seem reluctant to embrace reflective practice or to put thought and effort into creating portfolios that identify continuing competence in concrete and measurable ways. Until the focus rests solely on the need to protect patients and improve the quality of health care, mandated interventions for continuing competence are likely never to occur and provider competence will not be assured.

For Additional Discussion

1. Who should be responsible for the cost of assuring provider competence—the provider, the employer, the patients who are served, or some other entity?

2. How likely is it that states, professional organizations, professional certifying organizations, and employers will be willing to agree on standardized measures for assessing professional competence?

3. Would most RNs support mandatory development of a continuing competence portfolio? Are most RNs actively engaged in reflective practice in an effort to assess their ongoing competence?

4. Why should the entry-level examination for nursing be broad and general in scope, whereas continuing competence is arguably demonstrated by professional certification in specialty areas?

5. Are cost and access deterrents to professional certification? If so, how can these barriers be overcome?

6. Do most nurses view CE coursework as a reliable and valid tool for increasing provider competence?

7. Should nurses be required to complete mandated CE hours in the area of nursing practice in which they work?

8. Are there core competencies all licensed nurses must achieve regardless of the setting in which they practice?

References

American Academy of Ambulatory Care Nursing. (2021). *Nursing certification position statement.* Retrieved August 27, 2021, from https://aaacn.org/certification/nursing-certification-position-statement

American Board of Nursing Specialties. (2020). *About us.* Retrieved August 27, 2021, from https://www.nursingcertification.org/About-ABNS

American College of Physicians. (2021). *State continuing medical education requirements.* Retrieved August 27, 2021, from https://www.acponline.org/cme-moc/cme/state-continuing-medical-education-requirements

American Nurses Association. (2015). *Code of ethics for nurses with interpretive statements.* Author.

American Nurses Credentialing Center. (n.d.). *Our certifications.* Retrieved July 23, 2020, from https://www.nursingworld.org/certification

Arkansas Department of Health. (2017). *ASBN—Continuing education.* Retrieved August 27, 2021, from https://www.healthy.arkansas.gov/programs-services/topics/arsbn-continuing-education

Bryant, T., & Posey, L. (2019, August). Evaluating transfer of continuing education to nursing practice. *Journal of Continuing Education in Nursing, 50*(8), 375–380. https://doi.org/10.3928/00220124-20190717-09

California Board of Registered Nursing. (2021). *Continuing education for license renewal.* Retrieved July 21, 2020, from http://www.rn.ca.gov/licensees/ce-renewal.shtml

Cox, D. R., & Grus, C. L. (2019). From continuing education to continuing competence. *Professional Psychology: Research & Practice, 50*(2), 113–119. https://doi.org/10.1037/pro0000232

Dictionary.com. (2021). *Competence [Definition].* Retrieved August 27, 2021, from http://dictionary.reference.com/browse/competence

Florida Board of Nursing. (2021). *Registered nurse (RN).* Retrieved August 27, 2021, from http://floridasnursing.gov/renewals/registered-nurse-rn

Gigli, K. H., Davis, B. S., Ervin, J., & Kahn, J. M. (2020). Factors associated with nurses' knowledge of and perceived value in evidence-based practices. *American Journal of Critical Care, 29*(1), e1–e8. https://doi.org/10.4037/ajcc2020866

Huston, C. (2018, July 13). *Genomics: Decoding the future of nursing care. Nursing Management. RCNi Learning.* Retrieved September 23, 2021, from https://rcni.com/nursing-management/opinion/comment/genomics-decoding-future-of-nursing-care-136581

Institute of Medicine. (2010, October). *The future of nursing: Leading change, advancing health.* Retrieved August 17, 2020, from http://thefutureofnursing.org/IOM-Report

Iowa Board of Nursing. (2020, January). *CE basic requirements.* Retrieved August 27, 2021, from https://nursing.iowa.gov/continuing-education/continuing-ed-licensees/ce-basic-requirements

Lawrence, M., & Bauer, P. (2020, July). Knowledge base of nurses before and after a human trafficking continuing education course. *Journal of Continuing Education in Nursing, 51*(7), 316–321. https://doi.org/10.3928/00220124-20200611-07

Medscape Education. (1994–2021). *State CME requirements* (last updated Jan. 2019). Retrieved August 27, 2021, from http://www.medscape.org/public/staterequirements

Michigan Board of Nursing. Department of Licensing and Regulatory Affairs. (2019, December). *Continuing education requirements for Michigan nurses.* Retrieved August 27, 2021, from https://www.michigan.gov/documents/lara/LARA_Nursing_Specialty_CE_Brochure_4-11_376430_7.pdf

National Association of Boards of Pharmacy. (2020a). *MPJE—Multistate Pharmacy Jurisprudence Examination. Frequently asked questions.* Retrieved August 27, 2021, from https://nabp.pharmacy/programs/mpje/

National Association of Boards of Pharmacy. (2020b). *NAPLEX: North American Pharmacist Licensure Examination.* Retrieved August 27, 2021, from https://nabp.pharmacy/programs/naplex

National Council State Boards of Nursing. (2021a). *Nurse Licensure Compact (NLC) implementation.* Retrieved August 27, 2021, from https://www.ncsbn.org/enhanced-nlc-implementation.htm

National Council State Boards of Nursing. (2021b). *US members.* Retrieved August 27, 2021, from https://www.ncsbn.org/member-boards.htm

National Council State Boards of Nursing. (2021c). *NCLEX and other exams.* Retrieved August 27, 2021, from https://www.ncsbn.org/nclex.htm

National Human Genome Research Institute. (n.d.). *Competency map.* Retrieved August 27, 2021, from https://genomicseducation.net/competency/nurse

North Carolina Board of Nursing. (2021). *Continuing competence requirements.* Retrieved August 21, 2021, from https://www.ncbon.com/licensure-listing-continuing-competence

New York Board of Nursing State CE requirements. (2021). Retrieved August 27, 2021, from https://www.nurse.com/state-nurse-ce-requirements/new-york

North Dakota Board of Nursing State CE requirements. (2021). Retrieved August 27, 2021, from https://www.nurse.com/state-nurse-ce-requirements/north-dakota

Nurses Association of New Brunswick. (n.d.). *Continuing competence program.* Retrieved August 27, 2021, from http://www.nanb.nb.ca/practice/ccp/requirements

Nursing Compact States. (2021). *Trusted.* Retrieved August 27, 2021, from https://www.trustedhealth.com/compact-states#:~:text=The%20below%2035%20states%20have%20enacted%20the%20nurse,period%20typically%20lasts%20six%20months%20to%20one%20year.%29

Nursing Continuing Education Requirements by State. (2021). Retrieved August 27, 2021, from https://www.aaaceus.com/state_nursing_requirements.asp

Nursing License Map. (2021). *Nursing licensure compact.* Retrieved August 27, 2021, from https://nursinglicensemap.com/resources/nursing-licensure-compact/

Ohio Board of Nursing. (n.d.). *Licensing, certification & continuing education.* Retrieved August 27, 2021, from https://nursing.ohio.gov/licensing-certification-ce/

Oregon Nursing CE requirements. (2021). Retrieved August 27, 2021, from https://www.nurse.com/state-nurse-ce-requirements/oregon

Pirschel, C. (2019). A badge of honor: The value of oncology nurse certification. *ONS Voice, 34*(5), 10–14. Retrieved September 23, 2021, from https://voice.ons.org/news-and-views/the-value-of-oncology-nurse-certification

Poindexter, K., Lindell, D., & Hagler, D. (2019). Measuring the value of academic nurse educator certification: Perceptions of administrators and educators. *Journal of Nursing Education, 58*(9), 502–509. https://doi.org/10.3928/01484834-20190819-02

Quality, Safety, and Education for Nurses Institute. (2020). *Competencies.* Retrieved August 27, 2021, from http://qsen.org/competencies

State of New Jersey. New Jersey Division of Consumer Affairs. (2017). *New Jersey Board of Nursing. Continuing education FAQ.* Retrieved August 27, 2021, from http://www.njconsumeraffairs.gov/nur/Pages/Continuing-Education-FAQ.aspx

St-Germain, D., Cote, V., Gagnon, C., Laurin, A.-C., Bélanger, L., Lambert, A., & Gagné-Sauvé, C. (2019). The INSEPArable research project: A transdisciplinary caring approach to the design of a portfolio for reflexive nursing practices. *International Journal of Caring Sciences, 12*(1), 132–141. Retrieved September 23, 2021, from http://www.internationaljournalofcaringsciences.org/docs/15_st-germain_12_1_1.pdf

The Free Dictionary by Farlex. (2003–2021). *Licensure- [Definition].* Retrieved July 22, 2020, from http://medical-dictionary.thefreedictionary.com/licensure

U.S. Bureau of Labor Statistics. (2021). *Occupational labor handbook. How to become a physician assistant.* Retrieved August 27, 2021, from https://www.bls.gov/ooh/healthcare/physician-assistants.htm#tab-4

U.S. Medical Licensing Examination. (1996–2021). *What is USMLE?* Retrieved August 27, 2021, from https://www.usmle.org/about/

Ward, R. C., Krogh, M. A., Kremer, M. J., Muckle, T. J., & Schoeny, M. E. (2019). The perceived value of certification in nonsurgical pain management. *AANA Journal, 87*(1), 29–36. Retrieved September 23, 2021, from https://pubmed.ncbi.nlm.nih.gov/31587741/

Technology in Health Care

Carol J. Huston

CHAPTER OUTLINE

LEARNING OBJECTIVES

The learner will be able to:

1. Describe emerging applications for biomechatronics in health care.

2. Reflect on the degree to which technologically sophisticated, emotion-sensing, mental service robots will replace professional caregivers in the future.

3. Discuss how biometric technology can increase the likelihood that access to health care information is both targeted and appropriate.

4. Detail how point-of-care barcoding is implemented and the potential benefits and limitations of its use.

5. Explore the effect of computerized physician/ prescriber order entry on the reduction of

medication errors and adverse drug events, as well as barriers to implementation of its use.

6. Identify how clinical decision support systems can both improve existing care processes and provide a means for high-quality clinical decision making.

7. Identify resistance to change and cost barriers to the implementation of electronic health records (EHRs) despite government pressure to develop this technology.

8. Identify how EHRs, telehealth, and point-of-care testing can be used to overcome geography-of-care issues.

9. Analyze how the internet has changed the relationship between providers and patients in terms of the power of information in health care decision making.

10. Describe the perils inherent in having consumers independently seek out and interpret genomic testing without the support of a primary care provider.

11. Engage in futuristic thinking regarding how technology may further alter 21st-century health care and health care provider roles.

12. Identify strategies to optimally integrate the use of technology with the human element as part of the art of nursing.

13. Identify the nurse's role and responsibility in ensuring the ethical use of technology in patient care.

14. Assess personal strengths and weaknesses in terms of technology skill development.

INTRODUCTION

Fisk (2019) notes that the 2020s will be a decade of transformation. Indeed, Fisk suggests there will be more change in the next 10 years than in the last 250 years. Fisk also predicts that technology will fuse with humanity in new ways and there will be few venues where this is more obvious than in health care. Indeed, technology has already dramatically transformed health care, shaping both consumer and provider expectations.

Deloitte (2021) agrees, noting that medicine has undergone a paradigm shift with clinicians now basing their diagnoses and treatment decisions on predictive, preventive, personalized, and participatory medicine, a shift driven by technological and scientific advancements. In addition, technological breakthroughs in artificial intelligence (AI), nanotechnology, quantum computing, and 5G have enabled faster, customized diagnostic pathways and AI-enabled clinical decision tools have helped to deliver hyperpersonalized, evidence-based prevention and treatment interventions (Deloitte, 2021).

With these advances in technology come new opportunities, limitations, and challenges. Technology can cut costs, improve patient outcomes, streamline workflow, and improve information accessibility. It can, however, also be costly, require almost limitless ongoing training, and continually bring about new ethical dilemmas, including the need to ensure the "human element" is not lost in patient care. Determining what technology should be developed and how it should be used in an era of limited resources with increasing vulnerable populations raises multiple ethical questions.

Gabr (n.d.) concurs, suggesting that the ethical consequences associated with technological change must be further examined so that some institutionalization of health ethics can be created. In doing so, new, sensitive, reliable indicators as well as a vigilance system could be developed to monitor inequalities in health care and the abuse or neglect of human rights related to technology use.

> ***Consider This*** Technology is like a rolling freight train—it is difficult to stop it and even more dangerous to get in the way.

This chapter addresses only a few of the technology advances shaping 21st-century health care. Biometrics, point-of-care testing (POCT), and computerized data access/entry are presented as technological approaches for improving documentation and knowledge acquisition. Electronic health records (EHRs) and telehealth are recognized as strategies for overcoming geography-of-care issues, and computerized physician/provider order entry (CPOE) and clinical decision support (CDS) systems are discussed both as strategies for improving existing care processes and promoting high-quality clinical decision making. The internet's effect on both patients and providers is also examined, including the concept of "expert patient" and the resultant need for health care providers trained in consumer health informatics. In addition, genetics and genomics are highlighted as a preventive, diagnostic, and treatment tool for precision medicine, although many ethical issues need further exploration.

Finally, the chapter argues that the "human element" is the art of nursing and that this should not be lost in the quest to develop and use emerging technologies. Huston (2013) asserts that it is nurses who need to be actively involved in determining how best to use technology to supplement, not eliminate, professional nursing care. Questions related to the ethical use of technology should be reviewed by ethics committees prior to technology implementation, but nurses should have a voice in that conversation.

SELECT TECHNOLOGY ADVANCES IN HEALTH CARE
Biomechatronics

Biomechatronics involves technology that replicates or mimics how the body works. This interdisciplinary field, which will continue to increase in prominence in the future, uses biology, neuroscience, mechanics, electronics, and robotics to create devices that interact with the human muscle, skeleton, and nervous systems to establish or restore human motor or nervous system function (Freudenrich, 2021). In addition, applied biomechatronics uses mathematical models that, when applied to engineering principles and techniques in the medical field, can be used in assistive devices that work with body signals.

Future biomechatronics applications are innumerable and will likely include such things as functional stimulation of paralyzed limbs, pancreas pacemakers for people with diabetes, wireless active capsule endoscopy, and mentally controlled electronic muscle stimulators for patients with brain injuries.

Robotics

Surgical Robotics

The use of surgical robotics in health care is becoming commonplace. Indeed, MarketWatch (2021) noted that the robot-assisted surgery market is anticipated to rise considerably between 2021 and 2027. Factors propelling this growth include increased funding for medical robot research, increasing use of surgical robots by ambulatory surgery centers and hospitals, plentiful benefits of robotic-assisted surgery, technological advances, rising prevalence of trauma injuries, a growing need for surgical procedures in the older adult population, and a burgeoning need for accurate laparoscopic surgeries (MarketWatch, 2021).

Robotic surgery, however, is not new. The first robotic-assisted surgery dates to the mid-1980s when a robot was used to place a needle for a brain biopsy using computed tomographic guidance. Robotic-assisted heart bypass surgery followed in the late 1990s, and the first unmanned robotic surgery took place in May 2006 in Italy. Several years later, engineers at Duke University used novel three-dimensional technology and a basic AI program to guide the actions of a rudimentary tabletop robot to perform surgery. The engineers suggested this technology would eventually allow robots to perform surgery on patients in dangerous situations or in remote locations, such as on a battlefield or in space, with minimal or no human guidance.

In addition, similar technology began making certain contemporary medical procedures safer for patients. For example, robots are now performing cataract surgery. With femtosecond laser surgery, a laser can be fired at a target, reducing stress on the retina and other delicate tissues of the eye during cataract extraction. Because this is computer controlled rather than performed with manual surgical tools, greater surgical precision is possible and patient safety is increased (Segre, 2021).

However, surgical robotics is not cheap. A typical surgical robot costs about $2 million (Cedars Sanai, 2021). In addition, the volume of robotic surgery must be large enough to produce a viable financial return within the life of the technology. This is in addition to the ongoing maintenance, special instrumentation, and disposable equipment costs to maintain such a system, not including the annual service contracts of an additional $100,000 to $170,000 (Cedars Sanai, 2021). In addition, each procedure typically costs more than laparoscopic operations because of the need for single-use tools.

Questions have also been raised about whether need is driving surgical robotics or whether the introduction of such robotics is creating a need where one did not exist before. For example, a classic study showed that after Wisconsin hospitals acquired robotic surgery technology, the number of prostate removals doubled within 3 months. In contrast, the number of prostate surgeries stayed the same at hospitals that did not purchase the $2 million technology (Neuner et al., 2011). The researchers questioned whether surgeons at hospitals with robots were recommending this surgery because the outcomes (e.g., potential reductions in incontinence and impotence) were better or whether the new technology was simply more exciting than alternative treatments like radiation or "watchful waiting" (Neuner et al., 2011).

A more recent study by Sheetz et al. (2020) of 169,404 patients in 73 hospitals, found that the use of robotic surgery for all general surgery procedures increased from 1.8% to 15.1% from 2012 to 2018. Hospitals that launched robotic surgery programs had a broad and immediate increase in the use of robotic surgery, which was associated with a decrease in traditional laparoscopic minimally invasive surgery. Sheetz and team (2020) also suggest that their findings highlight a need to continually monitor the adoption of robotic surgery to ensure that enthusiasm for new technology does not outpace the evidence needed to use it in the most effective clinical contexts.

Indeed, Sheetz and colleagues (2020) suggest that there has been rapid growth of robotic surgery in areas with limited evidence to support its use and little theoretical benefit or clinical rationale (e.g., inguinal hernia repair). The findings were similar in a systematic review of the literature completed by Muaddi and team (2021) comparing clinical outcomes (e.g., postoperative complications, survival) after robotic surgery compared to open or laparoscopic surgery. Data demonstrated that robotic-assisted radical prostatectomy offered fewer biochemical recurrences and improvement in quality of recovery and pain scores only up to 6 weeks postoperatively compared to open radical prostatectomy. In addition, robotic surgery for endometrial cancer had fewer conversions to open surgery compared to laparoscopic surgery. Otherwise, robotic surgery outcomes were similar to conventional surgical approaches for other procedures, except for radical hysterectomy where minimally invasive approaches may result in patient harm compared to the open approach (Muaddi et al., 2021).

In contrast, a 2020 study by Pierce et al. showed improved patient outcomes and decreased 90-day episode-of-care costs with robotic arm–assisted total knee arthroplasty (TKA) over manual TKA. No patients in the robotic arm–assisted group required inpatient rehabilitation, whereas 0.90% of the manual TKA patients did. Costs were lower in the robotic arm–assisted TKA patients as well (Research Fuels the Controversy 21.1).

In the end, many argue that robotic surgery has not improved patient outcomes as dramatically as expected, certainly not to the degree that the first wave of minimally invasive surgery did. Additional evidence is needed to determine the efficacy of robotic surgery over traditional minimally invasive surgery for specific procedures.

Robots in Diagnostics

In addition, robots are increasingly being used in diagnostics because their accuracy typically exceeds that of human caregivers. For example, robotics and, more specifically, AI programs like IBM's Watson, can help interpret medical imaging and make more accurate diagnoses than ever before. For example, the Mayo Clinic announced in July 2020 that it would work with Israeli company *Diagnostic Robotics*

to implement its AI-powered patient triage and prediction platform at the Mayo Clinic headquarters in Rochester, Minnesota (NoCamels Team, 2020). These robotics applications will be used to help emergency medicine departments make better informed, quicker decisions about patient care while reducing strain on medical teams, saving on funds, and optimizing emergency room visits. Projections are that the system will cut emergency room wait times (currently 2.5 hours on average in the United States), drastically reduce the burden on physicians, and save health care institutions millions of dollars annually (NoCamels Team, 2020).

In addition, AI is expected to gain ground as health care organizations begin to apply this technology to medical diagnoses and image recognition; however, a drop in demand was seen in 2020 as a result of the COVID-19 pandemic (The Manomet Current, 2021). Adams (2021) notes, however, that hospitals are still expected to increasingly adopt AI-powered tools to streamline workflows, support clinical decision making, diagnose diseases, and generate insights from data. For example, health care AI company *Olive* acquired Empiric Health to introduce new offerings for supply chain and clinical analysis for surgeries and the Mayo Clinic signed a multiyear collaboration with *Pro Medicus* focused on building out and commercializing the health imaging IT provider's AI-powered research platform (Adams, 2021).

Robots as Direct Care Providers

Robots are also being developed to provide direct patient care. In fact, robots are already being used as caregivers,

---

Research Fuels the Controversy 21.1

The Efficacy of Robotic Arm–Assisted Total Knee Arthroplasty

The purpose of this retrospective, longitudinal study examined patient outcomes and costs following

total knee arthroplasty (TKA) in a population under 65 years old.

Source: Pierce, J., Needham, K., Adams, C., Coppolecchia, A., & Lavernia, C. (2020, July). Robotic arm—assisted knee surgery: An economic analysis. *American Journal of Managed Care, 26*(7), e205–e210. https://doi.org/10.37765/ajmc.2020.43763

Study Findings

A total of 357 robotic arm–assisted TKA and 1,785 manual TKA procedures were included in this analysis. Within 90 days of surgery, patients who had robotic arm–assisted TKA were less likely to utilize inpatient services and skilled nursing facilities. No patients in the robotic arm–assisted group went to inpatient rehabilitation, whereas 0.90% of the patients who underwent manual TKA surgery went to an inpatient rehabilitation facility. In addition, patients who underwent surgery using the robot arm and

who worked with home health aides required significantly fewer home health days than their manual surgery counterparts.

In addition, costs associated with overall postoperative expenditures were $1,332 less in the robotics-assisted group ($6,857 vs. $8,189). The 90-day global expenditures (index plus postsurgery) were $4,049 less for those who had robotic surgery and the length of stay after surgery was nearly a day less.

particularly for the older adult population. This is especially true in Japan, which some call the "Robot Kingdom" and where a burgeoning older adult population and a low birth rate have resulted in a severe shortage of caregivers.

Physical Service Robots

Robot caregivers are often divided into two categories: *physical service* and *mental service* robots. Physical service robots are designed to help with basic care tasks such as serving and fetching (already commercially produced) or bathing or carrying people (not yet in commercial production). These robots can serve food and drink from the kitchen and play memory games with those with cognitive deficiencies. They can also remind people to take their pills, track their health, and automatically answer incoming calls from family members and doctors. In addition, robotic walkers can now help users navigate hazardous environments, reducing their risk of falls.

A recent study by Melkas et al. (2020) on the implementation process of the care robot *Zora* in municipal older adult care services in Finland found that the robot's presence stimulated the patients' exercising and interacting. The robots also had the potential for multifaceted rehabilitative functions and became part of the care service with careful systemic planning with a specific focus on orientation.

Clearly, physical service robots, when used appropriately, may improve the effectiveness of care, and provide staff support (Lee et al., 2020). Some providers feel, however, that more attention should be given to defining what the role limitations should be for these robots as well as the impact of reduced human contact for patients (see Research Fuels the Controversy 21.2).

Mental Service Robots

Mental service robots are also being commercially produced and have been in use for some time. Their use, however, is more controversial. One of the best known is *PARO*, a sophisticated, interactive robot designed to help people relax and reduce their stress levels. As of 2021, the robot was in the eighth generation of a design that has been in use since 2003; it is shaped like a baby harp seal and can remember its name and change its behavior depending on how it is treated. It is being used extensively in homes for older adults and with autistic children worldwide. It was also used extensively in Japan after earthquakes and tsunamis to provide emotional support to survivors.

PARO has also been used as a treatment for depression. Indeed, a recent study by Geza et al. (2020) noted that just touching PARO reduced pain perception and salivary oxytocin levels; interacting with PARO induced an increase in

---

Research Fuels the Controversy 21.2

The Use of Bedside Robots

Although robotic systems are used to support health care professionals and to improve the efficiency and quality of nursing, there is a lack of scientific literature on how applied robotic systems can be used to support inpatients. This study used surveys and focus group interviews from a convenience sampling to identify the necessary aspects and functions of bedside robots for hospital inpatients. Ninety health care professionals and 108 inpatients completed a questionnaire, and four physicians and five nurses participated in the focus group interviews.

Source: Lee, H., Piao, M., Lee, J., Byun, A., & Kim, J. (2020). The purpose of bedside robots: Exploring the needs of inpatients and healthcare professionals. *CIN: Computers, Informatics, Nursing, 38*(1), 8–17. https://doi.org/10.1097/CIN.0000000000000558

Study Findings

Health care professionals believed that the most important function of robots was the ability to assist in patient treatment and support safety. They considered that monitoring patient safety and predicting events, such as accidents (i.e., falls) and pressure injuries, which can prolong patients' stays and lead to death or injury, to be important. In addition, the most highly desired functionalities of robotic care were related to patient care and monitoring, including alerting staff, measuring vital signs, and sensing falls.

Nurses and physicians, however, reported different needs for human–robot interaction. Nurses valued robotic functions such as nonverbal expression recognition, automatic movement, content suggestion, and emotional expressions. In addition, the nurses asserted the need for building human–robot rapport so that the robots could provide emotional care and help patients have a positive hospital experience. The need for human–robot interaction was not recognized by the physicians.

The results of the questionnaire's open-ended questions and health care professionals' focus groups indicated that the purpose of the robots should primarily be treatment and nursing. In addition, study participants believed bedside robots could be helpful but had concerns regarding safety and utility. Participants believed direct medical care should primarily be provided by health care professionals.

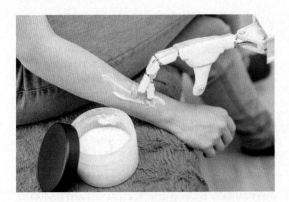

perceived happiness. The researchers concluded that this study revealed a profound effect of human–robot social interaction on pain and emotions; these findings suggest new strategies for pain management and improving well-being.

Many consumers and health care providers have expressed concern, however, about the lack of emotion in robots, suggesting that this is the element of human caregiving that can never be replaced. Indeed, Deloitte Insights (2020) notes that while machine intelligence can currently find patterns in data, it can't interpret whether those patterns have inherent sense since it lacks the ability to recognize and respond to the nuances of human interaction and emotion. Emerging technologies that build on human experience platforms, however, are increasingly able to move beyond the statistical and computational. This will ultimately lead to more capable AI with actual personality (Deloitte Insights, 2020, p. 13).

For example, technology developed in the last decade has resulted in a kind of robot intelligence known as "*kansei*," which means "emotion or feeling." Kansei robots use vision systems to monitor human expressions, gestures, and body language and voice sensors to pick up on intonation and individual words and sentences. When the kansei robot hears a word, it searches through its extensive database to match the results to emotional categories and then to generate an appropriate facial expression in response. In addition, kansei robots can sense human emotion through wearable sensors that monitor pulse rate and perspiration.

Discussion Point

To what degree can health care providers be replaced by technology? Can therapeutic "caring" be demonstrated by robots? Do you feel you could have a therapeutic conversation with a robot?

Kansei robots have been adapted for use with autistic patients. Others have become social robots that can help

individuals in their homes. In Japan, for example, companies are leading the development of a humanoid solution called *Carebots*, which are specifically designed robots for care of older adults (Walker, 2021). In the United States, similar efforts to incentivize researchers are also taking place. Not only does the National Science Foundation invest in the development of service robots but the National Institutes of Health also has been known to fund robotic initiatives to improve health and quality of life—particularly older adult care robotics projects that help increase mobility in older adult patients (Walker, 2021). Similarly, Sardis (2020) provides an overview of three social robots (*ElliQ, iPal, Buddy*) that explicitly state the intention of providing benefits for older adults.

> **Consider This** "Imagine a world in which our senior citizen population is taken care of not by humans, but by fully functional autonomous mobile robots. Imagine these mobile robots, also known as elder care robots, come equipped with state-of-the-art navigation, sensory and perception systems that allows them to complete tasks as simple as picking up a remote control or retrieving a pill box, to actions as complicated as taking a person's temperature or vital signs using sophisticated facial recognition technology. Rest assured, this world in which robotic caregivers are looked upon to help with our world's greying population is very much a reality. It's not a question of if, but when."
>
> —Jason Walker (2021, para. 1), CEO and Founder of WayPoint Robotics

Sharkey and Sharkey (2012) suggest, however, that the increased use of robots in older adult care raises a number of ethical concerns, including a potential reduction in the amount of human contact (opportunities for human social contact can be reduced); an increase in the feelings of objectification and loss of control (robots lack sensitivity to people's feelings and provide care at the convenience of caregivers); a loss of privacy; the loss of personal liberty; deception and infantilization (robots may restrict the behavior of humans); and a lack of clarity regarding the circumstances in which older adults are allowed to control the robots (who is responsible if something goes wrong?).

In addition, as technology continues to advance, robot caregivers have become increasingly lifelike, and the ability to distinguish robot from human caregiver has become more difficult (Huston, 2017). Sharkey and Sharkey (2012) note that this physical embodiment may lead robots to be welcomed in the home and other locations (where, for instance, a surveillance camera would not be accepted) and their personable or animal-like appearance could encourage and mislead people into thinking the robots are capable of more social understanding than they are. Are the older adult and other vulnerable populations at risk for this deception? Can people clearly differentiate between human and machine? Could robots actually further an individual's sense of isolation?

Discussion Point

Do mental health robots improve or further the problem of social isolation in older adults and other vulnerable populations?

Huston (2017) asserts that one of the most significant challenges health care providers face in using technology is finding that balance between maximizing the benefits of technology without devaluing the human element. Nurses need to make sure that the human element is not lost in the race to expand use of technology. This is certainly a potential concern with the use of robots as caregivers.

Robots as Couriers

Another use of robots in health care is as robot couriers for mundane, repetitive jobs such as supply chain automation. Aethon, Inc. has produced mobile robots called *TUGs* that can locate assets as well as transport them, including medications, supplies, equipment, and other goods that rely on scarce, valuable human resources for pushing carts (Aethon, 2018). The TUG, which has algorithms that determine if human intervention is needed, can haul up to 1,400 lb and transport a variety of hospital carts. The hospital worker simply attaches a delivery to the cart, presses a button to select the destination, and pushes the "go" button. The TUG has been programmed to "remember" and navigate the layout of the facility. It automatically travels to its destination, announces that the delivery has arrived, and returns to its home base, where it waits on its charger for the next delivery. In addition, the TUG utilizes the hospital's existing Wi-Fi system to communicate with elevators, automatic doors, and fire alarms as well as the Aethon cloud command center that continuously monitors the TUG.

Biometrics

The health care environment also continues to be rapidly transformed by new technology because of the need to ensure confidentiality and security of patient data and to comply with the Health Insurance Portability and Accountability Act (HIPAA) of 1996. HIPAA calls for a tiered approach to data access in which staff members have access to only the information that they need to know to perform their jobs. New biometric technology ensures that such access being developed is both targeted and appropriate.

Biometrics is the science of identifying people through physical characteristics such as fingerprints, handprints, retinal scans, voice recognition, facial structure, and dynamic signatures. Fingerprint biometrics is still the most common type of biometrics used in health care, primarily because of the ease of use, small size, and affordable price. Detection of facial geometry, however, is also beginning to make inroads. Facial geometry captures facial landmarks such as approach angles, eyebrow and mouth contours, skin texture analysis, and hairstyles, which can then be confirmed by facial recognition software.

Palm vein patterns are also used as biometric identifiers. Using near-infrared light to capture each individual's unique palm vein pattern bypasses the need for quality fingerprints. Right Patient (2021) notes that palm vein biometric patterns are difficult to forge, and because they exist inside of the body, it is practically impossible to recreate someone's biometric template. The palm vein recognition sensor needs the hand and blood flow to register an image. The use of palm veins as a biometric signature is expected to grow at a considerable pace from 2021 to 2026 (22.3%) owing to the growing need for securing confidential information and data in many organizations ("Palm Vein Biometrics Market", 2021).

Smart Cards and Smart Objects

Health care organizations are also increasingly integrating biometrics with "smart cards" to ensure that an individual presenting a secure identification credential really has the right to use that credential. *Smart cards* are credit card–sized devices with a chip, stored memory, and an operating system that records a patient's entire clinical history. The integration of biometrics and smart cards then can eliminate the need for multiple identification requirements.

Smart objects are everyday objects injected with easy-to-use software that give devices some degree of intelligence. For example, "smart hospital rooms" integrate mobile tablets and display technology with cloud-based health care apps (Smith, 2021). This provides caregivers with a real-time patient medical record and instant bedside access to the patient's electronic medical record. Intelligence software monitors patient health as well as ambient room conditions and can alert providers if a patient's condition changes. In addition, patients can view their records and prescriptions, see who is on their care team, and communicate with nurses, doctors, and other hospital staff.

In addition, hospitals are increasingly turning to *smart pumps* for intravenous (IV) therapy infusions. These smart pumps have safety software inside an advanced infusion therapy system that prevents IV medication errors by setting minimum and maximum dose limits as well as preset limits that cannot be overridden at a clinician's discretion. Still, end-user smart pump workarounds and IV-related medication errors are common. This is because health care providers become desensitized to false and repetitive alarms and they lower alarm volumes or simply turn off the alarms to decrease alarm fatigue, placing patient safety at risk. Vanderveen et al. (2020) support this, noting that most smart pumps can be programmed to bypass decision support or opt out of dose error reduction software use. As the primary end users of smart pumps, nurses need to be aware of potential safety issues and play an active role in improving the technology.

> *Consider This*   Smart pumps cannot protect patients from providers who decide to override them or use workarounds.

Point-of-Care Testing

POCT, which has evolved into a multibillion-dollar industry, is another technological advance that is facilitating more timely decision making and treatment, which in turn improves bedside care and promotes more positive outcomes. The College of American Pathologists (CAP) defines POCT as testing that is performed near or at the site of a patient, with the result leading to a possible change in the care of the patient (Allen-Bridson, 2021). In POCT, caregivers gather and test specimens near the patient or at the bedside using handheld analyzers, pulse oximeters, and blood glucose monitoring systems. Then, by networking via the internet and downloading results to a central clinical lab, manual documentation of test results can be eliminated. This allows clinicians to recognize and begin treating life-threatening conditions in real time even when geographic distance is a barrier.

POCT also works for consumer use in the home. Patients can precisely monitor their laboratory values, submit them electronically to the lab, and then have results in minutes. POCT testing represents only a small portion of clinical laboratories' total testing volume, however, and evaluation challenges exist for all POCT programs in terms of accuracy, ease of use, quality control, and accurate data management. Indeed, delivering diagnostic tests at the bedside may be prone to errors because of a failure to follow procedures, inappropriate documentation, improper patient identification, and not performing required quality control tests. More pilot programs are needed to evaluate the use of POCT testing.

Barcode Medication Administration

Barcoding has been developed to help caregivers ensure the right medication in the right dose is given to the right patient at the right time by the right route (the "*five rights*"). Barcoding works by requiring the provider to use a handheld scanner to match their nametag, the barcode on the patient's identification band, and the medication to be given. When one of the five "rights" does not match, an alert is issued, or the medication will not be dispensed from its storage system.

The *Leapfrog Group*, a conglomeration of non–health care Fortune 500 company leaders committed to modernizing the current health care system, has established standards that call for hospitals to implement a barcode medication administration (BCMA) system linked to an electronic medication administration record in 100% of hospital medical-surgical units (adult and pediatric), intensive care units (adult, pediatric, and neonatal), and labor and delivery units; to scan both patient and medication barcodes 95% of the time in units that have implemented BCMA; to have all five elements of decision support that have been identified as best practices by the Leapfrog BCMA Expert Panel; as well as to implement six of the eight best-practice processes and structures to prevent workarounds (Leapfrog Group, 2020b). However, implementation of BCMA is not without problems. Like smart pumps, nurses often develop workarounds that may undermine barcoding's safeguards and thus compromise patient safety.

Computing and Communication

Computerized Physician/Provider Order Entry

CPOE is another rapidly growing technology. Part of this growth has occurred because of its designation as one of three key patient safety initiatives by the Leapfrog Group. In addition, the 1999 Institute of Medicine study, *To Err Is Human*, recommended the use of CPOE to address medical errors. CPOE is a clinical software application designed specifically for providers to write patient orders electronically rather than on paper. With CPOE, providers produce clearly typed orders, reducing medication errors based on inaccurate transcription. Because most medication errors occur during manual ordering and transcribing (handwriting and interpreting the prescription), the use of CPOE systems can help eliminate these types of errors (Leapfrog Group, 2020a).

CPOE also gives providers vital CDS via access to information tools that support a health care provider in decisions related to diagnosis, therapy, and care planning of individual patients. For example, physicians might access evidence-based medicine databases electronically for CDS when writing medication orders. If the provider has ordered a test or treatment that is contraindicated for a specific patient or condition, the CDS will inform that provider of the potential danger at the time the order is entered.

Translating CPOE into action has not, however, been without challenges. Although many health care organizations saw the value in CPOE technology, many did not consider it to be a necessity until government pressure to implement it began and reimbursement incentives were put into place. There may also be cultural obstacles to its implementation; for example, a physician might prefer to write orders by hand instead of using a computer. This may be due to the normal resistance experienced with almost any change or it may reflect a reluctance to take on the increased cognitive workload associated with the use of CPOE.

In addition, cost is a factor. Installation of even "off-the-shelf" CPOE packages requires a significant amount of customization for each hospital and can be expensive, typically more than $2 million. Significant numbers of order sets must be created for CPOE to be put into place, and revisions are ongoing as new evidence emerges about best practice. Providers also need and want some variance within the order sets.

Discussion Point

Should providers have a choice in whether to use CPOE when writing orders?

In addition, the requirements to fully meet Leapfrog's CPOE standards are stringent (Box 21.1). Still, institutional and clinician adoption of CPOE is crucial to helping caregivers reduce medical errors and enhance patient safety, and health care institutions must commit the necessary human and financial resources to make this technological innovation a reality.

CDS Mechanisms and AI

The Centers for Medicare & Medicaid Services (2021) defines a *clinical decision support mechanism* (CDSM) as an interactive, electronic tool for use by clinicians that communicates appropriate use criteria (AUC) information to the user and assists them in making the most appropriate treatment decision for a patient's specific clinical condition. They may be modules within or available through certified EHR technology. Like CPOE, CDSMs will likely be commonplace in the next decade, giving providers the promise of access at the point of care to cutting-edge research, best practices, and decision-making support to improve patient care.

Consider This Technology is never a substitute for clinical judgment or critical thinking. Technology is a tool—an adjunct to nurses' clinical skills—never a replacement.

—Ann Scott Blouin, RN, PhD, FACHE, Executive Vice President of Customer Relations, The Joint Commission (Robert Wood Johnson Foundation [RWJF], 2016a, p. 1)

Electronic Communication

Electronic communication technologies are also expanding at an exponential pace. Computers are increasingly a part of interdisciplinary team communication and care documentation in acute care hospitals, and futurists predict that computers will soon essentially be invisible, replaced with smart objects. Indeed, computerized charting is now the norm. In addition, *personal digital assistants* (PDAs; mobile, handheld devices including smartphones and tablets) give users access to text-based information and the latest computer and cellular applications. With institution-wide documentation systems, everyone uses the same documentation

---

BOX 21.1 **Requirements for Full Compliance with Leapfrog's CPOE Standard**

In order to fully meet the Leapfrog Group's CPOE standard, hospitals must:
1. Ensure that physicians enter at least 85% of inpatient medication orders via a computer system that includes prescribing error prevention software.
2. Demonstrate, via a test, that their inpatient CPOE system can alert physicians to at least 60% of common, serious prescribing errors (applies to adult hospital patients only).

Source: Leapfrog Group. (2020). *Computerized physician order entry*. Retrieved September 10, 2020, from https://ratings.leapfroggroup .org/sites/default/files/inline-files/2021%20CPOE%20Fact%20Sheet_1.pdf

software, and the information is transferred to and retrieved from a central server via "hot syncing" (putting the PDA into a cradle or connecting it via cable to the central server). In addition, the PDA can serve as a reference library, especially for drug information, and as a calculator for computing drug doses.

PDAs, however, are not cheap; in fact, some new smartphones can carry a hefty $1,100-plus price tag. In addition, PDAs can be lost or stolen, posing concerns about patient confidentiality. Finally, some health care providers feel uncomfortable using such technology in front of patients and some feel uncomfortable with the technology itself. However, the quality and number of PDA applications continue to grow, as do their use. Though the use of smartphones continues to grow, however, many health care organizations still limit this specific technology at the point of care.

The use of *wireless local area networking* (WLAN) has also grown exponentially. WLAN uses a spread-spectrum radiofrequency to link two or more computers or devices without using wires. This allows caregivers to access, update, and transmit critical patient and treatment information despite moving between or being located at multiple sites of care. The area of outreach in the network is called the *basic service set*. Similarly, *Bluetooth* technology creates a small wireless network (called a *piconet*) between two pieces of hardware through short-range radio signals. This allows devices such as keyboards to link with personal computers and headsets to link with cell phones.

Electronic Health Records

Even health records have changed because of technology. The EHR is a digital record of a patient's health history that may be made up of records from many locations and/or sources, such as different hospitals, providers, clinics, and public health agencies. For example, an EHR might include immunization status, allergies, demographics, lab test and radiology results, advanced directives, current medications, and current health care appointments. The EHR is available 24 hours a day, 7 days a week and has built in safeguards to ensure patient health information confidentiality and security.

In January 2004, former President George Bush set a goal that most Americans would have their own EHRs by 2014. This goal was later endorsed by former President Barack Obama and supported financially with $30 billion in stimulus funds to support hospital implementation over the next several years. It has not been easy, however, to make such system-wide changes. Cost, debates about ownership of data, and communication across computer systems have posed relentless challenges. Heavy investments are required upfront, with returns that occur only over time, if at all.

Consider This The electronic record is not a single panacea for solving problems related to confidentiality or continuity of medical data access.

Physicians have been especially slow to adopt EHRs because of poor interoperability and difficulty accessing relevant clinical data. EHRs have been shown to increase provider stress and reduce productivity because clinicians must often work longer hours to see the same number of patients (RWJF, 2016b).

In addition, the EHR may interfere with the patient–provider encounter, preventing quality information from being attained. Patients may feel less satisfied if providers focus on their computers instead of them as the face-to-face encounter may feel less personal. In addition, with the de-emphasis on the clinical narrative, the patient's medical record may become a series of "yes" or "no" data points (RWJF, 2016b).

Consider This "As with any recordkeeping system, the value of an EHR is predicated on the amount and quality of information stored there, the way that information is organized, and the ease with which it can be retrieved, analyzed, and shared. EHRs represent a huge advance over paper records on all of these fronts, but they also place new demands on providers" (Charting Nursing's Future, 2016).

Virtual Care/Telehealth

Given declining reimbursement, health care provider shortages, and an increasing shift in care to outpatient settings, health care agencies are increasingly exploring technology-aided options that allow them to avoid the traditional one-to-one health care provider–patient ratio with face-to-face contact. In addition, this technology allows specialists to connect with providers and patients in rural areas where travel is difficult.

Telehealth, also called remote technology, telemedicine, telenursing, telecare, telehomecare, telemanagement, e-health, and telephone care, is a form of virtual care, allowing health care providers to care for patients across a distance, using a combination of telecommunication and multimedia technologies. In more advanced telehealth, providers interact with patients through computer stations hooked up in the patient's home. These stations typically include a video monitor, a movable color video camera, a speakerphone and microphone, and one or more medical peripherals for patient self-monitoring, such as blood pressure and pulse meter, stethoscope, pulse oximeter, scale, and glucometer. Patients record their heart rates, blood pressures, blood glucose levels, and other readings periodically and then transmit these data to a provider with a computer station like theirs. This gives the provider a real-time picture of the patient's health status. In less sophisticated telehealth programs, assessment, intervention, and evaluation may occur by fax, email, telephone, or video chat.

For health care providers, telehealth has meant greater ubiquity; they may now practice across geographic boundaries and be directly involved in patient care even when not directly onsite with patients. It has also typically resulted in improved quality of care and lower costs while providing new strategies for dealing with the health disparities created by geographic location, age, and homebound status. For patients, telehealth has meant increased flexibility and often more personalized care.

Telehealth use grew dramatically in 2020 during the COVID-19 pandemic. Efforts to reduce staff and patient exposure to sick people, preserve personal protective equipment (PPE), and minimize patient surges on health care facilities led to an increased use of telehealth. Indeed, the U.S. Department of Health and Human Services (DHHS, 2020) noted that the meteoric rise of telehealth during the pandemic not only helped limit the spread of the virus but also prompted a new conversation about the future of patient-centered care. DHHS suggests that while in-person patient–provider interactions will always be necessary, the pandemic has accelerated openness to telehealth in ways previously unseen.

Discussion Point

What, if anything, is "lost" when there is no in-person meeting between the health care provider and the patient? Can technology overcome this loss? What does technology offer that face-to-face visits do not?

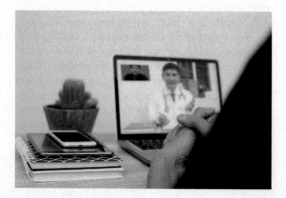

Performance indicators and appropriate measures of quality for telehealth, however, are still evolving. Desired patient outcomes for telehealth include patient satisfaction, increased involvement in health care decision making, reduced travel time and expense, increased time with health care providers, improved health care, improved quality of life, and increased medical record data for clinical decision making. More research is needed, however, to determine what telehealth systems—or a mix of telehealth and in-person visits—add the most value both clinically and financially. Some individuals question what is lost when there is no in-person interaction between the patient and the care provider.

The Internet

The growth of the internet as an information source for all types of information, including health, continues to grow exponentially. Just how significant is this impact? A 2021 report noted that WebMD has 80,000,000 unique monthly visitors, the National Institutes of Health (NIH) website has 55,000,000, and Yahoo Health has 50,500,000 (eBiz, 2021). Clearly, the scope of this use has changed the health care provider–patient relationship.

Historically, providers were recognized as the keepers of medical information. This led them to be the primary health care decision maker, often relegating patients to a somewhat passive and dependent role. The internet, however, has expanded the power and control of health information from providers alone to patients themselves. Indeed, the internet, which is growing faster than any other medium in the world, has enormous potential to improve Americans' health by enhancing communications and improving access to information for care providers, patients, health plan administrators, public health officials, biomedical researchers, and other health professionals.

Indeed, thousands of health information websites currently exist for consumers to explore in attempting to answer their health-related questions, and more are launched daily. The result is that patients have electronic access to medical information on virtually any topic at any time. Many consumers have at least the opportunity to be better informed about their health care problems and needs than in the past. In fact, this increased opportunity for consumers to access information has resulted in the creation of what is known as the *expert patient*—a patient who has the confidence, skills, information, and knowledge to proactively participate in their own health care.

Theoretically, expert patients are better informed and thus better able to be active participants in decision making. Although most providers appreciate well-informed patients who have demonstrated the initiative to learn more about their health care needs and problems, there can be problems with the accuracy and currency of some information on the internet. In addition, some patients do not fully understand the information that is available to them, even when it is accurate. Some providers are concerned that patients will inappropriately self-diagnose, leading them to seek inappropriate treatment or no treatment at all. A smaller number of providers simply do not want to share decision-making power with patients. Students in health care programs must be taught not only to recognize patient expertise but also to actively encourage and support it.

Discussion Point

Empowering patients and involving them in their health care decision making is a socially encouraged value in health care today. Do you believe that most providers truly value and appreciate "expert patients?"

Little research has been done to validate the currency and accuracy of the information available on health care internet sites. In a study of 79 websites from six English-speaking countries, only 43.28% had treatment recommendations for lower back pain that were judged as accurate (Ferreira et al., 2019). The researchers noted that websites from government agencies, consumer organizations, hospitals, nongovernmental organizations, professional associations, and universities demonstrated low credibility standards, provided mostly inaccurate information, and lacked comprehensiveness.

A similar study on websites addressing lower back pain by Costa et al. (2020) found that most websites originated from not-for-profit organizations and that none of the websites provided information on all content areas. At least 55% of the websites reviewed were rated as only poor or fair.

Similarly, a review of websites on the accuracy and quality of medical cannabis use found that 76% of claims made by websites were inaccurate and based on low-quality evidence (Boatwright & Sperry, 2020). Of the medical cannabis claims reviewed, only 10% of websites made appropriate cause-and-effect conclusions. Furthermore, only 3% of the medical cannabis claims were written by health care professionals. Clearly, patients must be savvy about determining which sites yield accurate and timely information and adept at retrieving and deciphering health care information to better empower themselves in health care decision making.

Genetics and Genomics

The National Human Genome Research Institute (2020) defines genomic medicine as "an emerging medical discipline that involves using genomic information about an

individual as part of their clinical care (e.g., for diagnostic or therapeutic decision making) and the health outcomes and policy implications of that clinical use" (para. 1). Ever since the Human Genome Project first began sequencing individual human genomes in 2001, we have learned much about how genetics influences both health and disease. In fact, the day will come soon when a medical checkup consists at least initially of a DNA readout and care will focus on preemptively preventing diseases that patients are at risk for developing rather than retroactively treating illness.

Genetics and genomics will also help us prevent or treat diseases now considered untreatable. For example, in August 2017, the U.S. Food and Drug Administration (FDA) made the first gene therapy available in the United States, ushering in a new approach to the treatment of cancer and other serious and life-threatening diseases (FDA News Release, 2017). Indeed, the FDA anticipates a doubling of new gene therapy applications every year, and Scott Gottlieb, a former FDA commissioner, predicted that by the year 2025, the United States will be approving between 10 and 20 different gene therapies every year (Curran, 2021).

In addition, cellular therapy products include cellular immunotherapies, cancer vaccines, and other types of both autologous and allogeneic cells for certain therapeutic indications, including hematopoietic stem cells and adult and embryonic stem cells (U.S. Food and Drug Administration, 2021, para. 2). With human gene therapy, genetic material is introduced into a person's DNA to replace faulty or missing genetic material, bolstering the immune system to shut down the disease. Because of these new cellular and gene therapy products, futurists suggest that cancer and heart disease deaths could diminish or disappear completely in the coming decade or two.

In the future, organ transplants may no longer be necessary because new organs will be grown from a patient's own tissue, and because organs will be genetically matched to the patient, there will be a much lower chance of rejection. Stem cells will be used to generate replacement cartilage tissue to repair damaged joints, especially for osteoarthritis patients, and total knee and hip replacements may no longer be needed. Dentures will be replaced by stem cell therapies that grow natural teeth. In addition, biologic drugs that can target molecular processes conventional drugs cannot are now available, and they can treat a growing list of diseases including cancer, lupus, Crohn disease, rheumatoid arthritis, multiple sclerosis, kidney failure, asthma, and high cholesterol.

Discussion Point

Do you believe that technology will some day eliminate "disease" as we know it today? If so, what are the implications in terms of life span and the prevalence of chronic disease?

Genetic testing has also created new opportunities for assessing genetic risk for disease so that preventive approaches to care can be taken. Direct-to-consumer companies such as 23andMe and Genos have proven particularly popular, with more than 30 million people around the world having taken a DNA test as of 2020 (Advisory Board, 2020).

How common is genetic testing and how easy is it for a health care consumer to have it done? Provider orders are no longer necessary. In fact, genetic testing is now commonplace, with many commercial DNA sequencing companies charging less than $300 to decode the human genome. All the consumer must do is to send in a saliva sample and a form of payment. Results arrive in a few weeks to a few months.

As patients gain access to information about their personal genetic sequencing, they are increasingly asking their health care providers to help them make informed decisions about what they should do or who they should see with that expertise. Unfortunately, however, many providers have limited knowledge about genetics. Indeed, with the average age of the practicing nurse being in the mid to late 40s, it is highly likely that many nurses learned little about what was a newly emerging field of study when they were undergoing initial nursing education. The result is that many nurses lack both the self-confidence and skills needed to obtain a patient's genetic family history, identify individuals at risk for developing genomic-influenced conditions or drug reactions, and assist consumers in making informed decisions about genetic testing results and therapies (Huston, 2018).

Clearly, having genetic data can ultimately lead to better care and patient empowerment, but there are privacy risks with some genetic testing companies selling user data to outside parties. In addition, consumers and privacy advocates have begun raising concerns about third parties, like tech start-ups and law enforcement, gaining access to their genetic data (Advisory Board, 2020).

In addition, there are ethical dilemmas associated with safeguarding personal genomic information as well as potential emotional consequences for consumers in uncovering unknown medical data without the support of a primary care provider. Also, some genetic tests have limited predictive value or may not be complete, leading patients to consider making decisions with only some of the information they need. Finally, many questions exist regarding whether relatives of someone with a positive predictive genetic test should or must be told about the results.

Consider This Genetic testing poses significant promise for precision medicine as well as significant risk of genetic discrimination and loss of privacy.

IS TECHNOLOGY WORTH THE COST?

The rapid introduction of new technology is a leading cost driver in the U.S. health care system. For example, many of the new biologic drugs, such as T-VEC, (an oncolytic virus agent approved for the treatment of some patients with metastatic melanoma that cannot be surgically removed) cost an average of $65,000 per patient—and that does not come close to topping the list of the most expensive biologic medications.

In addition, because access to technology is often dependent on a person's ability to pay for it, many health care disparities still exist in this regard. Should expensive technologies be available only to those who can pay for them? Huston (2017) agrees, noting that the reality is that emerging diagnostic and treatment technologies are expensive and thus may need to be used selectively. Decisions about who should have access to them and at what cost are at the heart of many ethical debates.

The Markkula Center for Applied Ethics (n.d.) echoes a similar concern in their assertion that the same technologies that offer hope for ever-increasing life expectancy (e.g., promising cancer treatments, surgical procedure and pharmacologic breakthroughs, and advanced genetic research) are also leading to increased demands on the health care system from a growing population of older adults. "Ethicists and health professionals alike are now raising questions about when and from whom treatments should be withheld, as competition for the scarce medical resources of the health care system grows beyond the system's capacity to provide care for everyone. Already, some forms of rationing have been implemented, and more rationing of health care resources may be inevitable" (Markkula Center, n.d., para. 2).

Discussion Point

Should health care technology ever be rationed by age? By ability to pay? By perceived potential contributions to society at large? How were decisions made during the COVID-19 pandemic to ration ventilator use when there weren't enough ventilators for all the patients who needed them?

In addition, some experts argue that technology is not only expensive (both initially and in terms of maintenance and technical support) it needs constant upgrades, and the education needed to truly be competent in the use of all this technology is never ending.

Not all health care providers embrace technology. This may simply represent a resistance to change, or it might be that health care provider input has not historically been used in technology acquisition decisions. Additionally, it is possible that many health care providers have received inadequate orientation to the technology in place.

One must remember that not all technology is worth the cost. Cost must always be weighed against possible benefits, effects on health care provider satisfaction, and projected utilization patterns. Sometimes it is difficult to determine what makes technology worth the cost.

Discussion Point

What makes new technology worth the cost? What criteria should be used in making these potentially value-based decisions (Huston, 2017)?

CONCLUSIONS

Emerging technologies offer great opportunities to improve the quality of patient care, but technology alone is not the answer. Indeed, "in recent years, the pace of technological change has outstripped the ability of many health care providers to fully reap the benefits or mitigate the challenges that come with these advances" (RWJF, 2016a, para. 1). Regardless then of the system that is deployed, health care organizations must consider what technology can best be used in each individual setting and how it should be used. Some pointers to consider in implementing technology are shown in Box 21.2. In addition, successfully adopting and integrating new technology

requires health care providers to understand that technology's limitations as well as its benefits.

Consider This "We need to step back before we adopt new technology and have a conversation about how this will impact care. What do we lose by adding this technology? What will we gain? Nurses on the front lines of care 24/7 are the people to figure this out."

—Carol Huston, as cited in RWJF, 2016c, p. 8

In addition, debates about how best to merge the human element of care (caring) and emerging technology will undoubtedly continue. Historically, machines have been unable to demonstrate caring, though the development of new robotic devices is challenging this long-held belief.

Health care providers also need to overcome their "technophobia" because, clearly, care can be improved with the appropriate use of technology. But far too often, the response of health care providers has been to create "workarounds" to delay a new technology's adoption or worse, mitigate any possible benefits it might bring. It is ironic that it is technology that would likely give nurses more time to do "nursing." Nurses must therefore keep the improvement of patient care first and foremost in their technology development agenda and embrace the use of technology as part of the skill set that will be expected of them in the 21st century.

BOX 21.2   Pointers for Implementing Technology

- Avoid being enticed by technology for its own sake—and be clear on the precise problem the new technology is designed to solve.
- Research the evidence related to new technologies and engage both experts and frontline users in preselection vetting.
- Make sure that nurse leaders are represented on the technology and vendor selection committees and are involved in assessment and design implementation.
- Help establish evaluation criteria and an evaluation process for monitoring the introduction of major technology investments.
- Improve workflow as much as possible before implementation of a new technology so that the new technology enhances workflow rather than impedes it.
- Take part in testing prototypes in real-life scenarios.
- Build in adequate educational resources to ensure a smooth transition.
- Remember that technology is an adjunct to care, not a replacement.

Source: Charting Nursing's Future. (2016). *Boon or bane? Making sure technologies improve (not impede) nursing care* (Issue No. 29). Retrieved September 13, 2020, from https://www.rwjf.org/content/dam/farm/reports/issue_briefs/2016/rwjf433148. Copyright 2016. Robert Wood Johnson Foundation. Used with permission from the Robert Wood Johnson Foundation.

For Additional Discussion

1. Is there a place for technology development in health care even when it does not contribute to the improvement of patient outcomes? In other words, should the technology itself ever be the desired goal?

2. Are nursing schools adequately preparing students with the skill sets and competencies they will need to function successfully in a progressively more technological workplace?

3. How should organizations deal with "technophobic" health care workers? Should health care employers let employees decide what level of expertise they wish to acquire?

4. What safeguards are in place to ensure confidentiality of the EHR?

5. Do you believe confidentiality is greater with electronic or paper records?

6. What technology do you believe has the greatest potential to reduce health care worker shortages? Why?

7. What technologies currently in use would you predict will be obsolete in 10 years?

8. What barriers exist in health care environments that will impede the development of technology in years to come?

9. What safeguards do consumers have that the health information they find on the internet is accurate and appropriate? If such safeguards are not in place, what could the consumers do to reduce their risk of acting on inaccurate information?

References

Adams, K. (2021, July 6). *5 Healthcare AI deals made in 2021. Beckers Health IT.* Retrieved August 31, 2021, from https://www.beckershospitalreview.com/artificial-intelligence/5-healthcare-ai-deals-made-in-2021.html

Advisory Board. (2020, February 20). *Has the consumer DNA test boom gone bust?* Retrieved August 31, 2021, from https://www.advisory.com/daily-briefing/2020/02/20/dna-tests

Aethon. (2018). *Homepage.* Retrieved August 31, 2021, from https://aethon.com/why-aethon/

Allen-Bridson, K. (2021, February 11). *Point of Care Test (POCT) reporting tool for COVID-19. Updates and training post February 4, 2021 release.* Retrieved August 31, 2021, from https://www.cdc.gov/nhsn/pdfs/covid19/ltcf/poc-testing-training-508.pdf

Boatwright, K. D., & Sperry, M. L. (2020). Accuracy of medical marijuana claims made by popular websites. *Journal of Pharmacy Practice, 33*(4), 457–464. https://doi.org/10.1177/0897190018818907

Cedars Sanai Marina del Rey Hospital. (2021). *What is the cost of robotic surgery as compared to other traditional surgery?* Retrieved August 31, 2021, from https://www.marinahospital.com/faq/cost-of-robotic-surgery-as-compared-to-other-traditional-surgery

Centers for Medicare & Medicaid Services. (2021, August 20). *Clinical decision support mechanisms.* Retrieved August 31, 2021, from https://www.cms.gov/Medicare/Quality-Initiatives-Patient-Assessment-Instruments/Appropriate-Use-Criteria-Program/CDSM

Charting Nursing's Future. (2016). *Nursing's role in guiding technological change* (Issue No. 29). Robert Wood Johnson Foundation. Retrieved August 31, 2021, from https://www.rwjf.org/content/dam/farm/reports/issue_briefs/2016/rwjf433148. Copyright 2016. Robert Wood Johnson Foundation. Used with permission from the Robert Wood Johnson Foundation.

Costa, N., Nielsen, M., Jull, G., Claus, A. P., & Hodges, P. W. (2020). Low back pain websites do not meet the needs of consumers: A study of online resources at three time points. *Health Information Management Journal, 49*(2/3), 137–149. https://doi.org/10.1177/1833358319857354

Curran, K. (2021, August 13). *The gene therapy sector is experiencing an acceleration. Rising Tide Biology.* Retrieved August 31, 2021, from https://www.risingtidebio.com/what-is-gene-therapy-uses/

Deloitte. (2021). *Predicting the future of healthcare and life sciences in 2025.* Retrieved August 31, 2021, from https://www2.deloitte.com/ch/en/pages/life-sciences-and-healthcare/articles/predicting-the-future-of-healthcare-and-life-sciences-in-2025.html

Deloitte Insights. (2020). *Tech trends 2020.* Retrieved September 13, 2020, from https://www2.deloitte.com/content/dam/Deloitte/pt/Documents/tech-trends/TechTrends2020.pdf

eBiz. (2021). *Top 15 most popular health websites | March 2021.* Retrieved August 31, 2021, from http://www.ebizmba.com/articles/health-websites

FDA News Release. (2017, August 30). *FDA approval brings first gene therapy to the United States.* Retrieved August 31,

2021, from https://www.fda.gov/NewsEvents/Newsroom/
PressAnnouncements/ucm574058.htm

Ferreira, G., Traeger, A. C., Machado, G., O'Keeffe, M., &
Maher, C. G. (2019, May). Credibility, accuracy, and com-
prehensiveness of internet-based information about low
back pain: A systematic review. *Journal of Medical Internet
Research, 21*(5). https://doi.org/10.2196/13357. Retrieved
August 31, 2021, from https://www.jmir.org/2019/5/e13357/

Fisk, P. (2019, December 23). *Gamechangers*. Retrieved August
31, 2021, from https://www.thegeniusworks.com/2019/12/
the-2020s-will-be-a-decade-of-transformation-power-
redistributed-consumption-reimagined-technology-
enhanced-change-applied/

Freudenrich, C. (2021). *How biomechatronics works. How Stuff
Works*. Retrieved August 31, 2021, from https://science
.howstuffworks.com/biomechatronics.htm

Gabr, M. (n.d.). *Health ethics, equity and human dignity*. Retrieved
August 31, 2021, from http://www.humiliationstudies.org/
documents/GabrHealthEthics.pdf

Geza, N., Uzefovsky, F., & Levy-Tzedek, S. (2020, June 17).
*Touching the social robot PARO reduces pain perception and
salivary oxytocin levels*. Retrieved August 31, 2021, from
https://www.nature.com/articles/s41598-020-66982-y

Huston, C. (2013, May 31). The impact of emerging technology on nursing care: Warp speed ahead. *The Online Journal
of Issues in Nursing, 18*(2), Manuscript 1. Retrieved September 23, 2021, from http://ojin.nursingworld.org/Main
MenuCategories/ANAMarketplace/ANAPeriodicals/OJIN/
TableofContents/Vol-18-2013/No2-May-2013/Impact-of-
Emerging-Technology.html

Huston, C. (2017). Technology in nursing: Emerging ethical
dilemmas. In C. Robichaux (Ed.), *Ethical competence in nursing practice* (Chapter 11, pp. 253–273). Springer Publishing.

Huston, C. (2018, July 13). *Genomics: Decoding the
future of nursing care. Nursing Management. RCNi
Learning*. Retrieved August 31, 2021, from https://
rcni.com/nursing-management/opinion/comment/
genomics-decoding-future-of-nursing-care-136581

Leapfrog Group. (2020a). *Fact sheet. Computerized physician
order entry*. Retrieved August 31, 2021, from https://ratings.
leapfroggroup.org/sites/default/files/2020-08/2020-CPOE-
Fact-Sheet.pdf

Leapfrog Group. (2020b). *Factsheet: Bar code medication
administration*. Retrieved August 31, 2021, from https://
ratings.leapfroggroup.org/sites/default/files/2020-08/2020-
BCMA-Fact-Sheet.pdf

Lee, H., Piao, M., Lee, J., Byun, A., & Kim, J. (2020). The
purpose of bedside robots: Exploring the needs of inpatients and healthcare professionals. *CIN: Computers,
Informatics, Nursing, 38*(1), 8–17. https://doi.org/10.1097/
CIN.0000000000000558

MarketWatch. (2021, July 13). *Robot-assisted surgery system
market size, trend, development analysis 2021 | Covid-19
impact on growth, demand, trends, new technology innovation research report outlook by 2027*. Retrieved August 31,
2021 from https://www.marketwatch.com/press-release/

robot-assisted-surgery-system-market-size-trend-
development-analysis-2021-covid-19-impact-on-growth-
demand-trends-new-technology-innovation-research-
report-outlook-by-2027-2021-07-13

Markkula Center for Applied Ethics. (n.d.). Unhealthy
dilemmas. *Santa Clara University*. Retrieved August 31,
2021, from http://www.scu.edu/ethics/publications/iie/
v3n3/homepage.html

Melkas, H., Hennala, L., Pekkarinen, S., & Kyrki, V. (2020).
Impacts of robot implementation on care personnel and
clients in elderly-care institutions. *International Journal of
Medical Informatics, 134*, N.PAG. https://doi.org/10.1016/j
.ijmedinf.2019.104041

Muaddi H., Hafid, M. E., Choi, W. J., Lillie, E., de Mestral,
C., Nathens, A., Stukel, T. A., & Karanicolas, P. J. (2021,
March 1). Clinical outcomes of robotic surgery compared to conventional surgical approaches (laparoscopic
or open): A systematic overview of reviews. *Annals
of Surgery, 273*(3),467–473. https://doi.org/10.1097/
SLA.0000000000003915. Retrieved August 31, 2021, from
https://pubmed.ncbi.nlm.nih.gov/32398482/

National Human Genome Research Institute. (2020,
December 2). *Genomics and medicine*. Retrieved August
31, 2021, from https://www.genome.gov/27552451/
what-is-genomic-medicine

Neuner, J. M., See, W. A., Pezzin, L. E., Tarima, S., & Nattinger,
A. B. (2011). The association of robotic surgical technology
and hospital prostatectomy volumes: increasing market
share through the adoption of technology. *Cancer, 118*(2),
371–377. https://doi.org/10.1002/cncr.26271

NoCamels Team. (2020, July 5). *Mayo clinic to implement
diagnostic robotics AI patient triage, prediction system*.
Retrieved August 31, 2021, from https://nocamels.
com/2020/07/mayo-clinic-diagnostic-robotics-ai-system/

*Palm vein biometrics market-Growth, trends, COVID-19
impact, and forecasts (2021–2026)*. (2021). Retrieved
August 31, 2021, from https://mordorintelligence.com/
industry-reports/palm-vein-biometrics-market

Pierce, J., Needham, K., Adams, C., Coppolecchia, A., &
Lavernia, C. (2020). Robotic arm—assisted knee surgery:
An economic analysis. *American Journal of Managed
Care, 26*(7), e205–e210. https://doi.org/10.37765/
ajmc.2020.43763

Right Patient. (2021). *RightPatient® palm vein biometrics*.
Retrieved August 31, 2021, from http://www.rightpatient
.com/palm-vein-biometrics-patient-identification

Robert Wood Johnson Foundation. (2016a). Boon or bane?
Making sure technologies improve (not impede) nursing
care. *Charting Nursing's Future*. Issue No. 29. Retrieved
August 31, 2021, from https://www.rwjf.org/content/dam/
farm/reports/issue_briefs/2016/rwjf433148

Robert Wood Johnson Foundation. (2016b). EHRs: Fundamentally changing the nature of care. *Charting Nursing's Future*.
Issue No. 29. Retrieved August 31, 2021, from https://www
.rwjf.org/content/dam/farm/reports/issue_briefs/2016/
rwjf433148

Sardis, B. (2020, July 16). *How can social robots benefit seniors aging in place?* Retrieved August 31, 2021, from https://techforaging.com/social-robots-elderly/

Segre, L. (2021, August). *How much does cataract surgery cost?* Retrieved August 31, 2021, from http://www.allaboutvision.com/conditions/cataract-surgery-cost.htm

Sharkey, A., & Sharkey, N. (2012). Granny and the robots: Ethical issues in robot care for the elderly. *Ethics and Information Technology, 14*, 27–40. https://doi.org/10.1007/s10676-010-9234-6. Retrieved August 31, 2021, from https://bioethics.pitt.edu/sites/default/files/MesserSlides/2020/Sharkey-Sharkey2012_Article_GrannyAndTheRobotsEthicalIssue.pdf

Sheetz, K. H., Claflin, J., & Dimick, J. B. (2020, January 10). Trends in the adoption of robotic surgery for common surgical procedures. *JAMA Network Open, 3*(1):e1918911. https://doi.org/10.1001/jamanetworkopen.2019.18911. Retrieved August 31, 2021, from https://jamanetwork.com/journals/jamanetworkopen/fullarticle/2758472

Smith, T. (2021, April 26). *Smart patient rooms support clinicians and enhance the patient experience.* Retrieved August 31, 2021, from https://insights.samsung.com/2021/04/26/smart-patient-rooms-support-clinicians-and-enhance-the-patient-experience/

The Manomet Current. (2021, August 26). *Global artificial intelligence AI in healthcare market 2021 latest advancements and business outlook-NVIDIA Corporation (NVIDIA) (US) One Up Business Insights.* Retrieved August 31, 2021, from https://manometcurrent.com/global-artificial-intelligence-ai-in-healthcare-market-2021-latest-advancements-and-business-outlook-nvidia-corporation-nvidia-us/

U.S. *Department of Health and Human Services.* (2020, July 28). *HHS issues new report highlighting dramatic trends in Medicare beneficiary telehealth utilization amid COVID-19.* Retrieved August 31, 2021, from https://www.hhs.gov/about/news/2020/07/28/hhs-issues-new-report-highlighting-dramatic-trends-in-medicare-beneficiary-telehealth-utilization-amid-covid-19.html

U.S. *Food and Drug Administration.* (2021, July 9). *Cellular & gene therapy products.* Retrieved August 31, 2021, from https://www.fda.gov/vaccines-blood-biologics/cellular-gene-therapy-products

Vanderveen, O'Neill, and Beard. (2020, February). *How can we tell how "smart" our infusion pumps are?* Retrieved August 31, 2021, from https://www.apsf.org/article/how-can-we-tell-how-smart-our-infusion-pumps-are/

Walker, J. (2021). *Does our future depend on elder care robots? WayPoint Robotics.* Retrieved August 31, 2021, from https://waypointrobotics.com/blog/elder-care-robots/

Health Care Reform in the United States: Is the Affordable Care Act the Answer?

Carol J. Huston

CHAPTER OUTLINE

LEARNING OBJECTIVES

The learner will be able to:

1. Describe key elements contributing to health care costs in the United States and the impact of those costs on the federal budget.

2. Identify driving forces for health care reform in the United States.

3. Describe key components of the *Patient Protection and Affordable Care Act*, more often called the *Affordable Care Act* (ACA) or *Obamacare*.

4. Identify successes as well as flaws of the ACA more than a decade after its implementation.

5. Examine legislative efforts to repeal and replace the ACA as well as revive and bolster it.

6. Debate the degree to which partisanship may continue to be a factor in preserving the ACA.

7. Consider what criteria are most important in a new health care reform bill.

INTRODUCTION

As we entered the second decade of the 21st century, 44 million people in the United States lacked any type of health insurance and an even greater number were underinsured. Of the millions of people unable to afford health insurance, many did not qualify for Medicaid. In addition, small businesses in tough economic times lacked the resources to provide health insurance benefits to all employees. One decade later, 43.4% of American adults ages 19 to 64 were still inadequately insured and 12.5% were uninsured. In addition, 9.5% of adults who were insured, had a gap in coverage in the prior year (Collins et al., 2020). All these factors suggested an ongoing need for health care reform that provides universal health care insurance coverage for all Americans.

Yet, reform efforts to establish such coverage have failed on multiple occasions over the last century, largely due to the opposition of medical–industrial corporate stakeholders. Indeed, comprehensive, systematic efforts to reform a clearly broken health care system achieved no real momentum until late in the first decade of the 21st century. Even then, convergence on proposals for reform in the United States was limited, so the relatively swift passage in 2010 of the *Patient Protection and Affordable Care Act*, more commonly known as the *Affordable Care Act* (ACA) or *Obamacare*, came as a surprise to many. Since its implementation, however, partisan efforts to both repeal and replace it and revise and bolster it have been constant.

Indeed, with the election of Donald Trump (Republican Party) as President of the United States in November 2016, efforts to repeal and replace the ACA became a priority. In fact, on "the very day President Trump was sworn in—January 20, 2017—he signed an executive order instructing administration officials 'to waive, defer, grant exemptions from, or delay' implementing parts of the Affordable Care Act" (Simmons-Duffin, 2019, para. 1).

As a result, a politically contentious 2017 saw significant movement toward incrementally dismantling the ACA as well as a cry for more affordable health care without government mandates. Further, but less significant efforts to repeal and replace the ACA occurred between 2018 and 2020, such as elimination of the individual mandate to have health insurance or face financial penalty (effective January 2019). In addition, the Trump administration cut subsidies to insurers that were in place to encourage them to stay in the ACA insurance exchanges and to help keep premiums down. Formal comprehensive health care reform, however, did not occur during the Trump presidency.

Instead, after a contentious election, Americans chose Joe Biden (Democrat party) to be their new President in November 2020. Biden campaigned on preserving and expanding the ACA and despite the need to divert attention to managing the COVID-19 pandemic, ending the war in Afghanistan, addressing systemic racism in policing and gun violence, and securing passage of a $1.9 trillion American Rescue Plan, progress has been made in reviving and bolstering the ACA during his first 9 months in office.

Important questions, however, should be asked and answered in moving forward with health care reform in the United States. Should desired health care reform be a remake of the ACA with fewer government subsidies, mandates, and regulations? Is there support for a single-payer, universal health care system? If so, what questions must be asked and what form should it take? Is an entirely new model of health care funding indicated, and, if so, is the country prepared to make major shifts in cultural and value expectations about the "right" to health care regardless of the ability to pay? To answer these questions, it may be helpful to first examine why health care reform itself is more necessary than ever in this country.

WHY IS HEALTH CARE REFORM NECESSARY?

Costs Are Uncontrolled

Economics is a leading driver of health care reform in this country, and the U.S. health care system is the most expensive in the world. In fact, the United States spent almost twice as much on health care as a percentage of its economy in 2020 as any other advanced industrialized countries—just over $4 trillion—about 18% of its gross domestic product (Advisory Board, 2020). This equates to a staggering cost of $10,224 per capita in 2021 (Stasha, 2021). In addition, the Centers for Medicare & Medicaid Services (CMS) estimated that prices for medical goods and services will grow at an average annual rate of 2.4% from 2019 to 2028, accounting for 43% of total projected growth in personal health care spending during this time (Advisory Board, 2020).

Much of U.S. health care spending comes out of the coffers of the federal government, now the single largest insurer in this country. The Medicare program provides coverage for items and services for 64 million beneficiaries, approximately 18% of the U.S. population (Kaiser Family Foundation, 2021b). Approximately 86% of enrollees are older adults, 14% are disabled, and fewer than 1% have end-stage renal disease (Kaiser Family Foundation, 2021a). Medicare enrollments are expected to increase dramatically in the coming years as the result of the aging population.

The federal government also heavily subsidizes health care for families below a certain income level through *Medicaid*. Over the past 30 years, Medicaid enrollment increased substantially during two major recessions and again in 2015 with the implementation of the ACA. As a result,

Medicaid provided coverage to about 1 in 5 Americans, or about just over 75.4 million people as of April 2021 (Medicaid.gov, 2021).

In fact, rising health care costs as well as increasing numbers of those using Medicare and Medicaid threaten to consume the entire federal budget in the future. Amadeo and Brock (2021) note that by 2030, spending for Medicare and Medicaid benefits is projected to rise to almost $1.9 trillion. This does not leave much money for Social Security, defense, interest on the national debt, or the rest of the U.S. government.

In addition, for the past 45 years, per capita health care spending has grown much faster than per capita income, resulting in higher out-of-pocket health care costs for most American consumers. Indeed, according to the Bureau of Labor Statistics Consumer Price Index (CPI), in 2019, the cost of medical care rose 4.6% from what consumers were paying in 2018, the largest year-over-year increase since 2007 (Leonhardt, 2020). As a result, medical bankruptcies are a real concern for many Americans. In fact, almost a third of working Americans currently have some type of medical debt; about 28% of those who have an outstanding balance owe $10,000 or more, and more than half of those with medical debt have defaulted on it (Leonhardt, 2020).

Consider This Many adults with medical bill or debt problems report serious financial problems. In a 2020 Commonwealth Fund survey, among those who report any medical bill or debt problem, 37% said they had used up all their savings to pay their bills, 40% had received a lower credit rating as a result of their medical debt, 31% racked up debt on their credit cards, and a quarter were unable to pay for basic necessities such as food, heat, or rent (Collins et al., 2020).

Part of the problem is that out-of-pocket health care costs borne directly by consumers continue to rise dramatically. Much of this increase has come from the transfer of costs (increased *deductibles* and *copayments*) from insurance plans to consumers. Indeed, the share of covered workers enrolled in high-deductible health plans at large employers in the United States reached 51% in 2021, a historic high (Price, 2021). Technologic advances, prescription drugs, and the cost of medical equipment and supplies also contribute to cost increases.

In addition, health care costs are simply higher in the United States. Americans are not consuming significantly more health care than citizens in other industrialized countries, but they are paying more for that care. In the past 20 years, the U.S. CPI, the average change in prices paid by urban consumers for various goods and services, has grown annually at an average of 2.1%, while the CPI for medical care has grown at an average rate of 3.5% per year (Peter G. Peterson Foundation, 2020). Similarly, pharmaceuticals cost far more in the United States because of government-protected "monopoly" rights for drug manufacturers.

Additionally, at least some of the higher costs in the United States have been the result of a historic fee-for-service reimbursement model whereby providers were rewarded for ordering more services rather than taking a more conservative approach. In addition, insurers, until the last couple of decades, primarily paid what was billed, regardless of whether the cost was reasonable for the service provided.

Consider This Fee-for-service reimbursement is like "going to an auto mechanic and agreeing to pay for whatever services he deems necessary, at whatever price he chooses, with no penalties to the provider if the service is poor." —Charles Hugh Smith as cited in Mack, 2019, para. 15

Administrative costs also accounted for about 25% of total health care expenditures in the United States in 2021, a figure about twice that of Canada ("Health Care Costs by Country," 2021). If the United States had cut its administrative spending to match Canadian levels, the country could have saved more than $600 billion in 2017 alone, enough to cover all individuals without insurance, eliminate all the copayments and deductibles, and ramp up home care for older adults and those with disabilities (Abrams, 2020). This inefficiency is only part of the waste that is widely recognized as part of the U.S. health care system.

In fact, in 2021, the United States spent twice as much on health care as comparable Organisation for Economic Co-operation and Development (OECD) countries such as Sweden, Germany, and Austria, all of whom have universal health care ("Health Care Costs by Country," 2021). The country with the second highest expenditure after the United States was Switzerland at $7,317 per capita. Of all these countries, the United States has the highest portion of private insurance.

In addition, there is less price competition in U.S. health care than in other industries, and most people do not pay cash for health care. When consumers do not pay for something out of pocket (because it is being paid by a third party), there are fewer incentives to care about overutilization (a *moral hazard*) or the cost itself, and there is no need to compare costs or shop for the most effective use of resources.

Access Is Unequal

There are also many access problems in the U.S. health care system that suggest a need for health care reform. Geographic access issues to health care providers create disparities for populations living in rural areas. Multiple studies have shown that rural residents are older, have less money, and have fewer physicians to care for them. This inequality is intensified as rural residents are less likely to have employer-provided health care coverage, and even if they are classified as poor, they often are not covered by Medicaid (Rural Health Information Hub, 2002–2021).

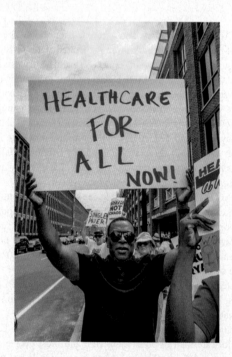

A lack of insurance also creates access barriers. Tolbert et al. (2020) note that people without insurance coverage have worse access to care than do people who are insured. Indeed, 3 in 10 uninsured adults in 2019 went without necessary medical care due to cost. In addition, people without insurance are less likely than those with insurance to receive preventive care and services for major health conditions and chronic diseases (Tolbert et al., 2020). For example, in 2019, non-older adults without insurance were more than three times as likely as younger adults with private coverage to say that they delayed filling or obtaining prescription drugs due to cost (19.8% vs. 6.0%). While insured and uninsured people who are injured or newly diagnosed with chronic conditions receive similar plans for follow-up care, people without health coverage are less likely than those with coverage to obtain all the recommended services (Tolbert et al., 2020).

In addition, with a limited number of primary care providers willing to take on patients without insurance, those without insurance are more likely to be diagnosed with diseases at later stages when treatment is more difficult and outcomes are poorer. Also, when people do not have health care insurance, many seek primary care at the emergency department, raising costs even higher.

Quality Health Care Rankings Are Poor and Medical Errors Permeate the System

Quality concerns are another factor suggesting a need to reform the health care system. Despite having the most expensive health care system in the world, the United States ranked last overall in 2021 compared to 10 other industrialized countries—Australia, Canada, France, Germany, the Netherlands, New Zealand, Norway, Sweden, Switzerland, and the United Kingdom—on comparative health care system performance scores such as access to care, infant mortality rate, and life expectancy (Schneider et al., 2021).

The United States also has the highest chronic disease burden (e.g., diseases like diabetes, hypertension) and an obesity rate that is two times higher than the OECD average (Sousa et al., 2020). The U.S. rate of preventable mortality (177 deaths per 100,000 population) was more than double the best-performing country, Switzerland (83 deaths per 100,000) in 2021 (Schneider et al., 2021).

Finally, medical errors are rampant in the U.S. health care system, though the true number of medical errors is unknown. This is because most medical errors go unreported, and published studies differ widely on exactly how significant the problem is. For example, a 1999 landmark study by the Institute of Medicine suggested 44,000 to 98,000 deaths occur annually in the United States as a result of medical errors, yet a recent meta-analysis of eight studies put the number of preventable deaths at just over 22,000 a year (Hathaway, 2020). Still other frequently cited studies have placed the number of deaths as high as 250,000 deaths per year, which would make medical errors the third leading cause of death behind cancer and cardiovascular disease (Hathaway, 2020). Because medical errors are such a significant problem in the health care system, Chapter 15 has been devoted to this topic. Regardless of what numbers are used to describe the problem, the number of medical errors is significant, and sustained and coordinated efforts will be needed to address the problem as part of health care reform.

THE AFFORDABLE CARE ACT (ACA)

The *ACA* was signed into law in March 2010 by President Barack Obama. It was designed to extend health insurance coverage to millions of uninsured Americans, expand Medicaid eligibility, create the Health Insurance Marketplace, and prevent insurance companies from denying coverage or charging more for preexisting conditions. In addition, *bundled payments, accountable care organizations, value-based purchasing,* and *medical homes* were critical strategies for the achievement of the ACA goals.

With the passage of ACA, approximately 20 million uninsured working-aged adults (aged 18–64 years) gained health insurance coverage (BalancingEverything.com, 2021). The program was especially successful for Black Americans, children, and small business owners. Under the ACA, businesses with more than 50 employees were required to provide health insurance for their employees or pay a fine. More insured small business employees meant fewer bankruptcies, better credit scores, and higher consumer demand. This facilitated individual spending, boosting economic growth.

In addition, the *individual mandate* clause of the ACA required individuals to buy insurance or pay a penalty at tax time unless they qualified for a limited number of exemptions. The penalty for not having insurance in 2018 was $695 per adult or 2.5% of household income exceeding tax-filing thresholds, whichever was higher (ObamaCareFacts .com, 2017). Several exemptions to this penalty, however, were implemented in early 2018, and the mandate was eliminated completely beginning in 2019.

Discussion Point

Should American citizens be required to have health insurance just as they are required to have auto insurance? Is a tax penalty the most appropriate way to finance such a mandate?

Beginning in January 2014, *Health Insurance Marketplaces*, also called *exchanges*, were created as part of the ACA for individuals without access to health insurance through work. Small businesses became eligible to buy affordable and qualified health benefit plans in this competitive insurance marketplace. Every health insurance plan in the marketplace offered comprehensive coverage and could be compared based on price, benefits, and quality, and tax credits were provided to lower the cost of insurance for individuals and families earning below certain levels (Marquis & Huston, 2021). In addition, all exchange plans were required to provide 10 essential health benefits (Box 22.1).

What were the outcomes of the ACA? There were successes (Box 22.2) as well as failures (Box 22.3). Tolbert and colleagues (2020) note that following the ACA, the number of uninsured non-older adult Americans declined by 20 million, dropping to a historic low in 2016. This was especially apparent in some vulnerable populations. For example, Meltzer and Markus (2020) found that the ACA improved access for vulnerable pregnant people who had experienced preterm birth. Although Medicaid continued to provide a final safety net for this population, an additional 4% gained private health insurance and another 4% enrolled in Medicaid due to the ACA (see Research Fuels the Controversy 22.1).

Conversely, when efforts to repeal and replace the ACA began, the number of uninsured Americans increased. In addition, when many of the major coverage provisions of ACA went into effect (e.g., creation of the Health Insurance Marketplace, barring coverage exclusions for preexisting health conditions, expansion of Medicaid, establishment of tax credits, reductions in cost sharing, and other provisions to increase availability and affordability of coverage), the percentage of working-aged adults with health insurance increased.

Under the ACA, reimbursement also increasingly shifted from *volume* to *value*, reducing incentives for redundant and inappropriate care and increasing incentives for quality. The ACA also expanded Medicaid and the Children Health Insurance Program (CHIP). Despite this progress, major opportunities to improve the health care system remained. The ACA itself was shrouded in confusion and misinformation, partly because of partisan politics and partly because of poor public communication starting well before it was signed into law. In fact, 17 million people qualified for subsidies because they did not have insurance from their employer, but only 6.6 million signed up (Amadeo & Brock, 2021).

In addition, negative messages about the ACA in the media outnumbered positive messages and many Americans felt uneasy about what the ACA might mean to them. Some of this discontent came about because of the broken promise that people who were satisfied with their previous coverage could remain on their plan (Wood, 2016). It quickly became apparent this would not be the case, and

BOX 22.1	**The 10 Essential Benefits Guaranteed by Insurance Plans in the Affordable Care Act Health Care Marketplace**

1. Ambulatory patient services (outpatient care)
2. Emergency services
3. Hospitalization
4. Maternity and newborn care
5. Mental health services and substance use disorder services
6. Prescription drugs
7. Rehabilitative services and devices
8. Laboratory services
9. Preventive and wellness services and chronic disease management:
10. Pediatric services

Source: Data from Health for California Insurance Center. (2021). *10 Essential health benefits*. Retrieved September 3, 2021, from https://www.healthforcalifornia.com/affordable-care-act/essential-health-benefits

BOX 22.2	**Successes of the Affordable Care Act (ACA)**

* Between 2010 and 2015, the uninsured rate in the United States fell by over 40%.
* Slowed the rise of health care costs (but did not reduce costs). Indeed, after the ACA was passed, health care prices rose at the slowest rate in 50 years.
* Required all insurance plans to cover 10 essential health benefits including treatment for mental health, addiction, and chronic diseases
* Protected people with preexisting conditions from predatory premiums or denials
* Eliminated lifetime and annual coverage limits (except for grandfathered plans)
* Allowed children to stay on their parents' health insurance plans up to age 26
* Required states to set up insurance exchanges or use the federal government's exchange
* Allowed those earning up to 400% of the poverty level to receive tax credits on their premiums
* Expanded Medicaid to 138% of the federal poverty level and provided this coverage to adults without children for the first time
* Eliminated the Medicare "doughnut hole" gap in coverage by 2020
* Required all qualified health insurance plans to provide free preventive and wellness visits without copays, deductibles, or coinsurance
* Required businesses with more than 50 employees to offer health insurance, though they received tax credits to help with the costs
* Encouraged more small businesses to offer health care benefits
* Altered the 80/20 rule provision so that 80% of premium dollars had to be spent on health care instead of administrative costs
* Created a Payment Advisory Board to set a cap on total health care spending for the nation, which meant regulating health insurance premiums; for individuals, it set limits on maximum annual out-of-pocket costs.

Source: Amadeo & Brock, 2021; Amadeo, K., & Estevez, E. (2021, July 12). *President Donald Trump's economic plans and policies*. Retrieved September 3, 2021, from https://www.thebalance.com/donald-trump-economic-plan-3994106; HealthMarkets.com. (2020, May 23). *The pros and cons of the Affordable Care Act*. Retrieved September 3, 2021, from https://www.healthmarkets.com/resources/health-insurance/affordable-care-act-pros-and-cons; Stasha, S. (2021, August 6). *The state of healthcare industry—Statistics for 2021*. Policy Advice. Retrieved September 3, 2021, from https://policyadvice.net/insurance/insights/healthcare-statistics/; Stasha, S. (2021b, July 18). *27+ Affordable Care Act statistics and facts (2021)*. Policy Advice. Retrieved September 3, 2021, from https://policyadvice.net/insurance/insights/affordable-care-act-statistics/.

BOX 22.3   Failures of the Affordable Care Act (ACA)

- Consumers who were satisfied with their prior insurance plans and providers did not necessarily get to keep them, a promise made to them when the ACA was introduced.
- When businesses found it more cost-effective to pay the penalty and let their employees purchase insurance plans on the exchanges, 3 to 5 million people lost their employment-based health insurance.
- Insurance companies canceled many of the plans for people who never had company plans and relied on private health insurance because their policies did not cover the ACA's 10 essential benefits.
- Many insurance companies made their provider networks smaller to cut costs while implementing ACA requirements. This left customers with fewer providers that were "in-network."
- Increased coverage raised overall health care costs in the short term because many people received preventive care and testing for the first time.
- The ACA taxed those who did not purchase insurance, but many avoided the tax through an ever-expanding list of exemptions.
- Many young people became newly insured because of the ACA provision that children up to the age of 26 years could be covered by their parents' insurance.
- Four million people chose to pay the tax rather than pay for coverage. The Congressional Budget Office estimated they paid $54 billion.
- In 2013, the ACA raised the income tax rate for 1 million individuals with incomes above $200,000. It also raised taxes for 4 million couples filing joint returns on incomes exceeding $250,000.
- Starting in 2013, families could deduct medical expenses that exceeded 10% of income. Before, they could deduct any expenses that exceeded 7.5% of income.
- Pharmaceutical companies paid an extra $84.8 billion in fees between 2013 and 2023 to close the "doughnut hole" in Medicare Part D.
- Three taxes and fees were repealed including the "Cadillac tax" on high-cost group health coverage beginning in 2020; the medical devices excise tax beginning in 2020; and the health insurance providers fee beginning in 2021. A 2018 continuing spending resolution delayed implementation of the Cadillac tax for an additional 2 years until 2022, but a 2019 continuing spending resolution fully repealed the Cadillac tax, beginning with the 2020 taxable year. A 2019 continuing spending resolution fully repealed the health insurance providers fee, beginning with the 2021 calendar year. A 2019 continuing spending resolution fully repealed the medical devices tax beginning in 2020.

Sources: Amadeo & Brock, 2021; Amadeo, K., & Estevez, E. (2021, July 12). *President Donald Trump's economic plans and policies.* Retrieved September 3, 2021, from https://www.thebalance.com/donald-trump-economic-plan-3994106; HealthMarkets.com. (2020, May 23). *The pros and cons of the Affordable Care Act.* Retrieved September 3, 2021, from https://www.healthmarkets.com/resources/health-insurance/affordable-care-act-pros-and-cons; Kamens, J. (2021). *Cadillac tax and other key ACA taxes repealed. Lawley Insurance.* Retrieved September 3, 2021, from https://www.lawleyinsurance.com/affordable-care-act/cadillac-tax/; Stasha, S. (2021, August 6). *The state of healthcare industry—Statistics for 2021. Policy Advice.* Retrieved September 3, 2021, from https://policyadvice.net/insurance/insights/healthcare-statistics/; Stasha, S. (2021b, July 18). *27+ Affordable Care Act statistics and facts (2021). Policy Advice.* Retrieved September 3, 2021, from https://policyadvice.net/insurance/insights/affordable-care-act-statistics/.

government attempts to fix the problem were only partially effective. Other consumers found the rollout of the ACA and the marketplace confusing, and complained that enrollment periods were too limited and the website was too complicated (Wood, 2016).

Consider This Many Americans felt misled by the promise that if they liked their current health care plan, they could keep it under the ACA.

In addition, costs were often prohibitive for both the government and consumers. Indeed, despite the ACA, the cost of health care insurance continued to be unaffordable for many Americans. Many individuals found it difficult to find affordable plans in the Health Insurance Marketplace, often choosing lower cost plans with high deductibles or copayments that they ultimately could not pay (i.e., underinsured). In addition, choice was often limited in the Health Insurance Marketplace, existing coverage was disrupted, and bureaucracy created significant numbers of impeding rules and regulations.

In addition, the costs to implement the ACA as well as marketplace health premiums increased steadily after its implementation, though a decade after its implementation, there is evidence that the ACA has contributed to slower growth U.S. health care spending (Vanderbilt University Medical Center Department of Health Policy, 2020).

Research Fuels the Controversy 22.1

Payer Mix for Preterm Births in the Context of a Post-ACA Insurance Market

The United States has a relatively high preterm birth rate compared with other developed nations. Before the enactment of the ACA in 2010, many pregnant patients at risk for preterm birth were unable to access affordable health insurance or a wide array of preventive and maternity care services. The various health insurance market reforms and coverage expansions contained in the ACA sought in part to address these problems. This analysis describes changes in the patterns of payer mix of preterm births in the context of a post-ACA insurance market, explores possible factors for the observed changes, and discusses some of the implications for the Medicaid program.

Source: Meltzer, R., & Markus, A. R. (2020, July/August). An analysis of payment mix patterns of preterm births in a post-Affordable Care Act insurance market: Implications for the Medicaid program. *Women's Health Issues Paper, 30*(4), 248–259. https://doi.org/10.1016/j.whi.2020.04.003

Study Findings

This study used a repeated cross-sectional study design to explore payment mix patterns of all births and preterm births between 2011 and 2016, using publicly available national vital statistics birth data. Findings revealed a small relative change in payment mix during the study period. Private health insurance (PHI) paid for a higher percentage of all births and this rate increased steadily between 2011 and 2016. Preterm births paid by PHI increased by 1.4 percentage points between 2011 and 2016 and self-pay/uninsured preterm births decreased by 0.3 percentage points over the same time period.

Medicaid had the highest and relatively stable preterm birth coverage percentage (48.9% in 2011, 49.2% in 2014, and 48.9% in 2016). Medicaid was also more likely to pay for preterm births than PHI, but this likelihood decreased by more than half after 2014 (8.2% in 2013 versus 3.8% in 2014).

The researchers concluded that after implementation of the ACA, Medicaid remained a constant source of coverage for vulnerable pregnant people when faced with the high cost of a preterm birth. Nationally, of the 64 million women aged 15 to 44, 4% gained PHI (directly purchased or employer-sponsored) and another 4% Medicaid with a concomitant 8% decrease in uninsured women of reproductive age between 2013 and 2017. The authors recommended further research to conclude with certainty that the reforms worked as intended but noted the undeniable important role of Medicaid as a financial safety net.

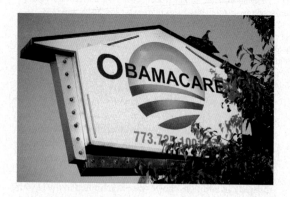

in the health care marketplace or the health exchanges that individual states operate. As much as 80% of the Obamacare-insured population [benefited] from such subsidies" (Wharton, University of Pennsylvania, 2018, para. 5).

> **Consider This** "As long as there are subsidies in place, there will be people who will show up to claim them. That's sort of an iron law of economics."—Mark Pauly, Professor, Health Care Management, Wharton, University of Pennsylvania

Also of great concern were the staggering costs of the federal subsidies to insurers as well as what many perceived to be uneven allocation of their use. Many of the 8.8 million Americans who signed up for coverage via the federal health insurance exchanges in 2018 received subsidies (Wharton, University of Pennsylvania, 2018). "Heavy federal subsidies are designed to offset premium increases by insurers

Tolbert and team (2020) noted, however, that though financial assistance was available to many uninsured individuals under the ACA, not everyone who was uninsured was eligible for free or subsidized coverage. Nearly six in 10 uninsured individuals prior to the COVID-19 pandemic were eligible for financial assistance either through Medicaid or through subsidized marketplace coverage. However, over four in 10 uninsured people were outside the reach of the ACA because their state did not expand Medicaid, their income was too high to qualify for marketplace subsidies, or their immigration status made them ineligible (Tolbert et al., 2020).

In addition, despite claims that the American public would come to like the ACA, public opinion has been largely divided along partisan lines since the law was passed in 2010 (Hamel et al., 2020). Following Republican efforts to repeal the ACA in the summer of 2017, there was a slight uptick in overall favorability toward the law, and since then a somewhat larger share has held a favorable rather than an unfavorable view. A Kaiser Family Foundation tracking poll in December 2020 found that just over half of the public (53%) hold a favorable opinion of the ACA while about one-third (34%) hold a negative opinion of it (Hamel et al., 2020).

Yet, many Americans openly espouse their view that care should be allocated equitably for the common good. Sousa and colleagues (2020) argue that universal health care is in the country's best interests. When people do not have insurance, they are less likely to seek health care, and this increases everyone's risk. In addition, it is the compassionate and moral thing to do. Gerisch (n.d.) agrees, noting that there are rights to which we are entitled, simply by virtue of our humanity, and health care may be the most intersectional and crucial of all of them. Indeed, since universal health care is critical to the ability of the most marginalized segments of any population to live lives of dignity, "the very frailty of our human lives demands that we protect this right as a public good" (Gerisch, n.d., para. 1).

Consider This The right to health care has long been recognized internationally. The origins of this right began in the United States when health care was listed in the Second Bill of Rights drafted by Franklin Delano Roosevelt (FDR). FDR's death kept this Second Bill of Rights from being implemented though Eleanor Roosevelt became the drafting chairperson for the United Nations Universal Declaration of Human Rights (UDHR). Since the adoption of the UDHR, every other industrialized country in the world—and many nonindustrialized countries—have implemented universal health care systems while the United States has not (Gerisch, n.d.).

Yet, Advent Health University (2020) notes that one constant ethical challenge facing health care administrators is how to make capital allocations that strike a balance between patients' medical needs and fiscal responsibility.

Alton (2020) notes that the cost of universal health care could massively increase taxes. If costs remain the same as they are currently, health care could take up nearly the entirety of the federal government's budget and taxes would need to almost double to make up for the shortfall.

In addition, the collective American values of individualism and capitalism often collide with other shared values such as social justice, the right to health care, and utilitarianism when the need for universal health care coverage is discussed. Clearly, there is at least some conflict of values between justice and fairness, and the question about whether health care is a right or a privilege has not been fully answered.

The ACA brought these collective value conflicts to the forefront. Stoltzfus Jost (2017, p. 13) agrees, noting that the ACA "really touched the live wire of political and ethical debates—it attempted to extend public support to low- and moderate-income people of working age who were not obviously among the worthy poor. It also extended government regulation of health insurance and specifically federal government regulation. It thereby came into conflict with a range of conservative values."

Discussion Point

Many Americans oppose some form of universal coverage because they view it as a form of socialism. Do you foresee this public value changing any time soon?

President Trump's Efforts to Dismantle the ACA

President Trump's campaign promises included replacing the ACA with a better health care plan, including the increased use of medical savings accounts, allowing the purchase of health insurance across state lines, weakening Medicaid expansion as offered by the ACA, and allowing consumers to access lower cost imported drugs (The Washington Post, 2021). Only a few of these promises actually resulted in legislation, though active efforts to do so began early in the Trump presidency.

Indeed, multiple bills to repeal and replace the ACA were introduced into either the U.S. House of Representatives or the Senate in 2017, though legislative consensus was not achieved (see Table 22.1). Although the bills were different in some respects, the common theme was a reduction in mandates for individuals and businesses to buy or provide health insurance and a defunding of government subsidies for vulnerable populations like older adults and those living in poverty.

TABLE 22.1	**Congressional Efforts to Repeal and Replace the Affordable Care Act (ACA)**	
March–May 2017	*The American Health Care Act* (passed by the House on May 4, 2017, but failed in the Senate)	Provided a flat tax credit based on age, not income. This subsidy was not based on the cost of plans, so it would have raised costs for many. The Act also included a Patient and State Stability Fund that would help lower premiums by 20% after 2026. The Act would also have allowed states to waive several rules of the ACA under certain conditions. In the states that chose waiver rules, those with chronic diseases would pay much higher rates. The Act also funded Medicare through a fixed block grant and cut funding for Planned Parenthood and ACA taxes.
June–July 2017	*The Better Care Reconciliation Act* (put forth in the Senate but failed to pass)	Allowed states to decide whether to keep all 10 essential health benefits of the ACA. That would have allowed companies to charge more for those with preexisting conditions. The plan penalized those who dropped their insurance and then reapplied for coverage within 63 days. The plan also would have cut Medicaid spending starting in 2020 and reduced ACA tax credits and subsidies. The Act also allowed companies to charge older adults five times more than younger Americans, up from three times as much, and stripped Medicaid and Title X reimbursement for Planned Parenthood health care services for a year. The Act eliminated the tax on the individual insurance mandate and removed the tax on companies that don't provide health insurance. The bill also increased maximum allowable contributions to health savings accounts.
July 2017	"Skinny Repeal" by the Senate (Sen. John McCain, R-Ariz.) cast the deciding vote against the "skinny bill." He disapproved of the process and urged a return to bipartisan lawmaking.	Would have repealed the ACA's mandate that individuals must buy insurance but didn't require companies to provide insurance benefits. It would have repealed the tax on medical device manufacturers as well and defunded Planned Parenthood, the Prevention and Public Health Fund, and the Community Health Center Fund.
September 2017	The Graham-Cassidy Bill (championed by Sens. Lindsey Graham, R-S.C., and Bill Cassidy, R-La). On September 22, 2017, Sen. McCain blocked the Graham-Cassidy Bill. He said there wasn't enough information about how the bill would affect people because it was rushed through to meet Trump's deadline to repeal the ACA by the end of September 2017.	Would have converted the ACA's federal Medicaid funding and insurance subsidies to state block grants. It left it up to the states to design their own health care programs with the funds, benefiting some states and disadvantaging others. The bill also would have allowed states to require that Medicaid recipients have a job unless they were older adults, children, disabled, or pregnant and cut off Medicaid funding by 2027. The bill also sought to eliminate the tax on those who did not buy insurance retroactive to 2016.
December 2017	*The Tax Cuts and Jobs Act* (passed by Congress and signed into law by President Trump in late December 2017)	The bill cut the corporate tax rate to 20% and changed individual tax brackets. It also made significant changes to the ACA, including elimination of the individual mandate to purchase health insurance, or at least reducing the penalty for going uncovered to zero.
February 2018	Expansion of short-term health plans	These regulations made it easier for consumers to obtain coverage through short-term health insurance plans—which did not have to adhere to the ACA's consumer protections—by allowing insurers to sell policies that lasted just under a year.

TABLE 22.1	Congressional Efforts to Repeal and Replace the Affordable Care Act (ACA) (*continued*)	
April 2018	Broadening of the individual mandate exemptions for 2018	The Trump administration announced that those who live in counties with no insurer or with only one choice could apply for a hardship exemption from the individual insurance mandate for 2018. In addition, prolife Americans who could only buy plans that covered abortion could also receive an exemption.
May 2018	President Trump's blueprint for the *American Patients First Plan* to reduce drug prices	This plan attempted to reform the rebates drug companies pay to pharmacy benefit managers (PBMs), who negotiate prices between drug manufacturers, pharmacies, and health insurance companies. The rebates create incentives for PBMs to suggest higher cost drugs. In addition, PBMs can charge insurers more than they charge pharmacies. As a result, everyone pays different prices for drugs. In the first 100 days after the blueprint was presented, numerous actions were taken toward structurally rebuilding drug costs. Full implementation of the blueprint, however, required Congress to amend the act that established Medicare Part D because it prohibits Medicare from negotiating. Although in a July 2021 executive order President Biden said he supports a change in the law, the administration had not outlined a specific process for drug price negotiation as of September 2021 and estimated savings from this proposal were not reflected in the 2022 budget.
August 2018	Expansion of *short-term* health plans as an alternative to plans that meet more stringent standards under the ACA	Short-term plans, which had been limited to no more than 3 months, could now last for up to 1 year, even though short-term plans do not have to meet most standards and consumer protections that apply to regular health insurance.
November 2018	Centers for Medicare & Medicaid Services (CMS) released several "waiver concepts" that invited states to "break away" from federal health care protections and standards—specifically by reviving many of the ideas that were proposed (but failed) during efforts in 2017 to repeal the ACA	This encouraged states to restructure and redirect funding that would otherwise be used for ACA subsidies for low- and moderate-income people.
April 2019	CMS finalized changes to a technical insurance formula that raised premiums for 7.3 million people who purchased subsidized coverage in the ACA marketplace	Analysts predicted the change would cause 70,000 people to drop marketplace coverage and raise limits on total out-of-pocket costs for millions of people, including many with employer coverage.
March 2019	The Department of Justice (DOJ) asked the U.S. Court of Appeals for the Fifth Circuit to invalidate the entire ACA	On January 10, 2020, the DOJ under Biden urged the Supreme Court to delay consideration of the lawsuit in which the Trump administration and 18 states asked the courts to strike down the entire ACA.
June 2020	Proposed increased tax advantages for *health care sharing ministries* and *direct primary care arrangements*, marketed as an alternative to health insurance	Analysts believe that if finalized, these tax incentives would leave more people with coverage gaps and remove them from the protections of the ACA insurance risk pools.

(*continued*)

TABLE 22.1	**Congressional Efforts to Repeal and Replace the Affordable Care Act (ACA)** (*continued*)	
July 2020	President Trump's executive order required health centers to pass any discounts on insulin and epinephrine to their patients. Through participating and enhanced Medicare Part D plans, Americans without access to affordable insulin and injectable epinephrine through commercial insurance or federal programs, such as Medicare and Medicaid, could purchase these pharmaceuticals from a federally qualified health center (FQHC) at a price that aligned with the cost at which the FQHC acquired the medication.	FQHCs receive discounted prices through the 340B Prescription Drug Program on prescription drugs. These steep discounts are now passed through to low-income Americans at the point of sale. A month's supply of insulin became available for a $35 copay.
November 2020	Arguments were heard at the Supreme Court about the constitutionality of the individual mandate to buy insurance under the ACA and to consider if the entire ACA should be thrown out or if a portion of the law was unconstitutional	The Supreme Court issued its final decision in June 2021, concluding that the plaintiffs did not have standing to challenge the constitutionality of the penalty-less individual mandate.
November 2020	The Trump administration announced the *Most Favored Nation* (MFN) Model, to be administered by the CMS beginning January 1, 2021. This order required the U.S. Department of Health & Human Services (HHS) to reduce prices of prescription medications for Medicare Parts B and D by not purchasing medicines at more than most-favored-nation price (price charged in other economically advanced countries). The November 2020 interim final rule established a 7-year nationwide, mandatory MFN Model, under section 1115A of the Social Security Act, with the model performance period beginning on January 1, 2021.	On August 10, 2021, CMS published a proposed rule (86 Fed. Reg 43618) to rescind the "Most Favored Nation Model" interim final rule that was published on November 27, 2020. CMS argues that the nationwide preliminary injunction precluding implementation of the MFN Model on January 1, 2021, findings by multiple courts of procedural issues with the November 2020 interim final rule, and stakeholders' expressions of concern about the model start date, formed an adequate reason to rescind regulations added by the November 2020 interim final rule and to remove the associated regulatory text. CMS is inviting comments on its proposal by October 2021.

Source: Data from Amadeo & Brock 2021; Amadeo, K., & Estevez, E. (2021, July 12). *President Donald Trump's economic plans and policies.* Retrieved September 3, 2021, from https://www.thebalance.com/donald-trump-economic-plan-3994106; Luhby, T. (2018, February 20). *Trump administration unveils alternative to Obamacare. CNN Money.* Retrieved September 3, 2021, from http://money.cnn.com/2018/02/20/news/economy/trump-obamacare-short-term-health-insurance/index.html; Center on Budget and Policy Priorities. (2021, February 2). *Sabotage watch: Tracking efforts to undermine the ACA.* Retrieved September 3, 2021, from https://www.cbpp.org/sabotage-watch-tracking-efforts-to-undermine-the-aca; Simmons-Duffin, S. (2020, November 9). *What Biden's election means for U.S. health care and public health.* Retrieved September 3, 2021, from https://www.npr.org/sections/health-shots/2020/11/09/932071991/what-bidens-election-means-for-u-s-health-care-and-public-health; U.S. Department of Health and Human Services. (2020, November 20). *Trump administration announces prescription drug payment model to put American patients first.* Retrieved September 3, 2021, from https://www.hhs.gov/about/news/2020/11/20/trump-administration-announces-prescription-drug-payment-model-to-put-american-patients-first.html; U.S. Department of Health and Human Services, U.S. Department of the Treasury, U.S. Department of Labor. (n.d.). *Reforming America's healthcare system through choice and competition.* Retrieved September 3, 2021, from https://www.hhs.gov/sites/default/files/Reforming-Americas-Healthcare-System-Through-Choice-and-Competition.pdf; Cubanski, J., Neuman, T., & Freed, M. (2021, July 23). *What's the latest on Medicare drug price negotiations? Kaiser Family Foundation.* Retrieved September 3, 2021, from https://www.kff.org/medicare/issue-brief/whats-the-latest-on-medicare-drug-price-negotiations/; U.S. Department of Health and Human Services. (n.d.). *100 Days of results: President Trump's American Patients First Blueprint.* Retrieved September 3, 2021, from https://www.hhs.gov/sites/default/files/100DaysofResults_AmericanPatientsFirstBlueprint.pdf; Keith, K. (2021a, June 17). *Supreme Court rejects ACA challenge; Law remains fully intact. Health Affairs.* Retrieved August 23, 2021, from https://www.healthaffairs.org/do/10.1377/hblog20210617.665248/full/; Office of Advocacy. (2021, August 13). *CMS proposes to rescind the Most Favored Nation interim final rule and associated regulations.* Retrieved September 3, 2021, from https://advocacy.sba.gov/2021/08/13/cms-proposes-to-rescind-the-most-favored-nation-interim-final-rule-and-associated-regulations/#:~:text=On%20August%2010%2C%202021%2C%20CMS%20published%20a%20proposed,rule%20that%20was%20published%20on%20November%2027%2C%202020.

However, Trump was successful in undermining multiple components of the ACA. The repeal of the individual mandate to purchase health insurance succeeded in late 2017; the penalty for failing to maintain minimum essential health care insurance coverage was reduced to zero in January 2019. In addition, the Trump administration's decision to cut the 2018 open enrollment period to half that of the 2017 enrollment period; to cut advertising by 90%; to reduce navigator funding by 40%; to close the federal marketplace for maintenance several hours each week during open enrollment; and to bar regional office staff members from cooperating in enrollment efforts furthered the undermining of the ACA without repealing it (Stoltzfus Jost, 2017).

In addition, in October 2017, Trump issued an executive order endorsing approaches to siphon healthy individuals from the ACA market (Jost, 2017). The administration also cut off subsidies to insurers that were in place to encourage them to stay in the ACA insurance exchanges and to help keep premiums down. As a result, some health insurance companies left the ACA marketplace (Jost, 2017). The companies that stayed were forced to increase their premiums because of uncertainty around losing subsidies, which would destabilize the marketplace.

Trump also signed executive orders in October 2017 and January 2018 directing the Secretary of Labor to expand access to association health plans (U.S. Department of Health and Human Services, U.S. Department of the Treasury, & U.S. Department of Labor, n.d.). These are policies made available to trade groups, small businesses, and other associations that cross state lines. The order expanded the types of groups that could form associations and prohibited them from refusing coverage or charging more to those with preexisting conditions.

Also in October 2017, Trump requested that the Labor Secretary ease restrictions on short-term health plans; allow employers to use pretax dollars for "health reimbursement arrangements;" find ways to limit consolidation within the insurance and hospital industries; and find additional means to increase competition and choice in health care (Federal Register, 2018). All these plans negatively impacted enrollment in the health care exchanges.

Finally, in late December 2017, *the Tax Cuts and Jobs Act* was passed by Congress, and Trump signed it into law. The bill cut the corporate tax rate to 20% and changed individual tax brackets. It also made significant changes to the ACA, including elimination of the individual mandate to purchase health insurance as of 2019 (Internal Revenue Service, 2021). It did not, however, affect the employer mandate or its related information reporting requirements.

Health care policy remained at the forefront of the 115th Congress from 2018 to 2019 as well, though partisan lines changed. While the Republican Party had a narrow majority in the Senate and a more sizable one in the House of Representatives in early 2018, Democrats took majority control of the House in November 2018 while Republicans maintained majority control over the Senate. As a result, little new legislation made it through Congress, and the ACA continued to be enforced as written while the Trump administration continued to issue regulations and guidance to undermine ACA programs.

In addition, rules were put in place in 2018 to allow states to alter their essential health benefit requirements, reduce transfers among insurers under the risk adjustment program, and diminish required insurer medical loss ratios. The administration also transferred responsibility for marketplace enrollment from the federal marketplace to private web brokers through its enhanced direct enrollment program (Jost, 2018).

The Medicaid program also became a target for reform in 2018 and 2019 since Medicaid expansion was a key part of the ACA and Trump tax cuts increased deficit concerns. Under new legislation, states were encouraged to change the program by allowing for eligibility and enrollment restrictions, restricting benefits, increasing copays, increasing or requiring premiums, (and) implementing work reporting requirements (Simmons-Duffin, 2020).

In addition, Trump made cuts to the *340B Medicare drug discount program* in 2018. The 340B program is a drug price control program that allows qualifying providers, generally hospitals, specialty clinics and their associated outpatient facilities serving uninsured and low-income patients in rural communities, to purchase outpatient drugs from manufacturers at discounted prices (Azalea Health, 2021). In August 2018, the Court of Appeals for the Washington, DC, Circuit upheld the 2018 *Medicare Hospital Outpatient Prospective Payment System* (OPPS) and *Ambulatory Surgical Center Payment System* final rule that cut reimbursement for 340B drugs by 28.5% but later lowered the reimbursement rate cut to 22.5% (Paavola, 2020; Shaw, 2020).

The American Hospital Association, Association of American Medical Colleges and America's Essential Hospitals sued to stop the cuts in December 2018, arguing that the U.S. Department of Health & Human Services (DHHS) exceeded its federal authority to adjust the payment rates (Paavola, 2020). A lower court agreed with the hospital associations. DHHS then appealed the lower court decision in July 2019, and the appellate court reversed the decision, arguing that the lower drug reimbursement rate rested on a reasonable interpretation of the Medicare statute (Paavola, 2020). As a result, DHHS included cuts to the 340B program in its 2019, 2020, and 2021 hospital payment rule.

Discussion Point

Cuts to 340B payments appeared to pit the pharmaceutical industry against 340B hospitals. Because of resultant fiscal losses, many safety net hospitals resorted to patient service cutbacks, with a potential negative impact on the patients they serve. How can we balance the need for hospitals to recover their costs while ensuring vulnerable populations have access to the high-cost drugs they need?

Attacks on the ACA continued in 2020. In April 2020, The Trump administration refused to create a special enrollment period (SEP) to allow people to purchase insurance through the HealthCare.gov website, despite the COVID-19 health and economic crisis (Center on Budget and Policy Priorities, 2021). In July 2020, the Trump administration proposed rules that would make it easier for employers to keep offering pre-ACA plans that were exempt from important consumer protections, giving employers greater leeway to increase deductibles and other cost sharing for workers and their families while maintaining plans' exempt status (Center on Budget and Policy Priorities, 2021).

In November 2020, the Trump administration finalized a regulation weakening important Medicaid managed care plan standards and proposed a regulation that would weaken consumer protections and slash funding for ACA marketplace operations (Center on Budget and Policy Priorities, 2021). In December 2020, the administration finalized rules to make it easier for employers to keep offering pre-ACA plans that were exempt from some consumer protections, giving employers greater leeway to increase deductibles and other cost sharing for workers and their families while maintaining the plans' exempt status (Center on Budget and Policy Priorities, 2021).

The final attempt to dismantle the ACA under the Trump administration occurred in the 10-week transition period between the election and when President Joe Biden took office, with the Republican Party challenging the ACA at the Supreme Court level. The case before the court—*California v. Texas* (known as *Texas v. U.S.* in the lower courts)—addressed the constitutionality of the individual mandate in the ACA to purchase health insurance and questioned whether the ACA could be thrown out entirely if one section of the act was deemed unconstitutional. Earlier courts had ruled that the individual mandate was in fact a tax, not a tax penalty, but because the associated financial penalty no longer "produced at least some revenue" for the federal government, it was considered to be unconstitutional (Tompkins, 2020). Zack (2020) noted that the Trump administration made clear in a June 2020 brief that it was pushing for the invalidation of the entire law, not just the individual mandate.

While Texas's name was on the lawsuit, 20 states including Texas brought the lawsuit. While 17 other states defended the ACA and a handful more states filed briefs in the matter, only Idaho, Wyoming, Oklahoma, and Alaska were not involved in the litigation (Tompkins, 2020). Tompkins (2020) notes that the Court needed to determine whether Texas and the individual plaintiffs had standing to bring the lawsuit to challenge the individual mandate. If so, the Court would need to determine whether the *2017 Tax Cut and Jobs Act* rendered the individual mandate unconstitutional when it reduced the tax for the mandate to zero. After nearly 7 months of review, the Supreme Court, despite a conservative majority on the bench, issued its final decision in June 2021, concluding that the plaintiffs did not have standing to challenge the constitutionality of the now penalty-less individual mandate (Keith, 2021a).

President Biden's Intent to Revive and Bolster the ACA

Simmons-Duffin (2020) notes that while Trump's presidency was marked by scaled-back federal investment and involvement in health care, President Joe Biden pledged to reverse that trend. Indeed, Biden was clear about his intention to double down and invest in the changes the ACA made to the country's health care system. In doing so, he planned to address complaints that ACA premiums are unaffordable and expand subsidies to include people with higher incomes. For example, in the early years of the ACA, the law provided federal premium subsidies only for households that made up to 400% of the federal poverty level, but this cut-off went away as of 2021 (Norris, 2021; Simmons-Duffin, 2020). Biden also stated that he would reverse some ways the Trump administration undercut the exchanges and would restore funding for ACA consumer outreach for help with ACA enrollment.

In addition, Biden's top priorities in preserving and bolstering the ACA included the prohibition of denial of coverage or inflated premiums due to preexisting conditions and annual or lifetime limits on coverage (Bufkin, 2020). Biden also stated he would work to preserve coverage eligibility for adults under 26 to be enrolled in their parents' health insurance.

In addition, to combat the rising cost of prescription drugs, Biden campaigned to repeal the law that stops Medicare from negotiating lower prices with drug corporations.

He also stated he would appoint an independent review board to assess the value of costly specialized drugs, such as cancer drugs, which would then make recommendations on pricing for Medicare and the public coverage option (Bufkin, 2020).

The most significant change Biden proposed to the ACA, however, was the creation of the Medicare-like *public option*, a health insurance program administered by the federal government, that anyone could buy into, that could compete against private insurance plans in the marketplace. This idea was part of the original ACA but did not make it into the final law (Simmons-Duffin, 2020). The public option would also limit price increases of generic drugs to reflect the rate of inflation and impose a tax penalty on companies that did not comply. The plan would also allow consumers to purchase DHHS-certified prescription drugs from other countries, creating more competition in the industry. As of mid-2021, however, the "public option" had fallen off the national radar and will be difficult to revive without a major push by the White House (Sarlin & Kapur, 2021).

Finally, Biden committed to exploring Medicaid expansion. Under the *American Rescue Plan Act of 2021* (ARP), CMS will provide a temporary increase in federal funding to states that newly elect to expand Medicaid coverage to certain low-income adults by offering a temporary 5 percentage-point increase in federal matching funds for certain Medicaid expenditures for a maximum of 2 years (HHS Press Office, 2021). Additionally, these states will qualify for the 90% federal matching funds already available through the ACA for medical services for newly eligible Medicaid-expansion enrollees (HHS Press Office, 2021).

As of August 30, 2021, 39 states, including the District of Columbia, have expanded their Medicaid programs to cover the ACA adult group. Twelve states, however, have yet to expand Medicaid coverage, creating inequalities in coverage for low-income individuals from different communities. Medicaid expansion could reduce these inequalities and bring America closer to ending health disparities—a key priority for this administration and communities across the United States (HHS Press Office, 2021).

CONCLUSIONS

Keith (2021b) notes that as with any complex legislation, the ACA's success has been shaped by how federal officials have interpreted and implemented the law's various requirements and programs. New administrations, each with their own policy preferences, have reached starkly different conclusions about the value of the law and what federal law allows or requires (Keith, 2021b).

While the Trump administration made significant strides to dismantle the ACA, Trump's campaign promise to fully "repeal and replace" the ACA was not realized. President Biden committed to build on the ACA, expand health coverage access, and advance health equity (Centers for Medicare & Medicaid Services, 2021). Thus, the ACA continues to be the organizing framework driving the federal government's current approach to health care.

Yet, the early years of the ACA were not a panacea to health care problems such as limited access and high costs. Indeed, Buerhaus (2020) notes that despite the ACA's success in expanding health insurance coverage to more Americans, the cost of insurance premiums increased for many people, and the cost of government subsidies was staggering. In addition, Warner and colleagues (2020) note that gains in coverage and access notwithstanding, the ACA has been embroiled in political debate since its passage. Its fragmented uptake and implementation, rulings, and administrative actions have hindered the ACA and weakened its impact across the country. Americans, though, are likely to see a further shift in attitude about the ACA in the coming years, and this may be influenced by President Biden's ambitious goal of insuring more than 97% of all Americans by reversing ACA rollbacks, adding in the public option, and increasing the value of certain tax credits (Bufkin, 2020). At the time of writing this chapter in late 2021, however, many unknowns remain.

Warner and colleagues (2020) suggest, however, that future reform efforts should bring the country closer to meaningful health coverage for all U.S. residents. These initiatives must promote a strong, stable health system; adequate provider networks; consumer-focused transparency of costs and coverage benefits; and a health system that is navigable for patients and consumers. In addition, this coverage must facilitate access to the services and treatments needed by patients, including those with unique or complex medical needs, and the patient protections currently in place, including prohibitions on preexisting condition exclusions, annual and lifetime limits, insurance policy rescissions, gender-based pricing, and excessive premiums for older adults, should be maintained (Warner et al., 2020). Given the political stalemate that occurred around the ACA, there is a need to reassess the deeper issues at stake and further ponder the prospects for greatly needed health care reform.

FOR ADDITIONAL DISCUSSION

1. Are current health care reform efforts being driven more by a political or health care agenda?

2. Can traditional market strategies (like competition) be used to increase efficiencies and control rising health care costs in the United States? Why or why not?

3. Did the ACA deliver on its promise to bring universal coverage to vulnerable populations without an increase in taxes or the deficit and with the ability to keep their current insurance plan if desired?

4. What strategies might induce more employers to offer health care insurance as a funded benefit? What keeps them from doing so?

5. Former President Barack Obama suggested that the ACA was likely the most important health care legislation enacted in the United States since the creation of Medicare and Medicaid in 1965. Do you agree or disagree?

6. Do current tax law and regulations discriminate against Americans who do not or cannot get health insurance as part of their employment?

7. Does expanding Medicaid eliminate the problem of American citizens "falling through the cracks" in terms of health care access?

8. What strategies will be needed to address the growing federal deficits related to government-subsidized health care programs like Medicare and Medicaid?

9. Where do the current major health care stakeholders stand on the repeal and replacement of the ACA?

10. How well informed were most Americans about the ACA at the time of its implementation? How much better informed were they 6 years later when efforts began to dismantle it?

11. What should the federal government's role be in ensuring access to care for vulnerable populations?

12. Do Americans consider health care to be a right or a privilege?

13. What might Americans be willing to pay or give up so that all Americans could have affordable, high-quality health care?

References

Abrams, A. (2020, January 6). *The U.S. spends $2,500 per person on health care administrative costs. Canada spends $550. Here's why.* Retrieved September 3, 2021, from https://time.com/5759972/health-care-administrative-costs/

Advent Health University. (2020, May 5). *6 Ethical issues in healthcare in 2020.* Retrieved September 3, 2021, from https://online.ahu.edu/blog/ethical-issues-in-healthcare/

Advisory Board. (2020, April 3). *CMS: US health care spending will reach $4T in 2020.* Retrieved September 3, 2021, from https://www.advisory.com/daily-briefing/2020/04/03/health-spending

Alton, L. (2020, January 8). *Seven big problems with universal health care no one wants to address.* Retrieved September 3, 2021, from https://www.americanthinker.com/articles/2020/01/seven_big_problems_with_universal_health_care_no_one_wants_to_address.html

Amadeo, K., & Brock, T. J. (2021, May 11). *Obamacare facts with the 9 ACA facts that you don't know.* Retrieved September 3, 2021, from https://www.thebalance.com/obamacare-pros-and-cons-3306059

Azalea Health. (2021). *What is the 340b drug pricing program?* Retrieved September 3, 2021, from https://www.azaleahealth.com/blog/340b/#:~:text=The%20federal%20340B%20Program%20is%20a%20drug%20price,prices.%20What%20Is%20The%20340B%20Drug%20Pricing%20Program%3F

BalancingEverything.com. (2021, May 6). *How many Americans are uninsured?* Retrieved August 23, 2021, from https://balancingeverything.com/how-many-americans-are-uninsured/

Buerhaus, P. I. (2020, March/April). Demystifying national healthcare reform proposals: Implications for nurses. *Nursing Economic$, 38*(2), 58–64.

Bufkin, E. (2020, October 30). *Joe Biden vs. Donald Trump on health care in America.* Retrieved September 3, 2021, from https://foxbaltimore.com/news/nation-world/joe-biden-vs-donald-trump-on-health-care-in-america

Center on Budget and Policy Priorities. (2021, February 2). *Sabotage watch: Tracking efforts to undermine the ACA.*

Retrieved September 3, 2021, from https://www.cbpp.org/sabotage-watch-tracking-efforts-to-undermine-the-aca

Centers for Medicare & Medicaid Services. (2021, June 28). *CMS proposed rule to increase Americans' access to health coverage for 2022.* Retrieved September 3, 2021, from https://www.cms.gov/newsroom/press-releases/cms-proposed-rule-increase-americans-access-health-coverage-2022

Collins, S. R., Gunja, M. Z., & Aboulafia, G. N. (2020, August 19). *U.S. health insurance coverage in 2020: A looming crisis in affordability. Findings from the Commonwealth Fund biennial health insurance survey, 2020.* Retrieved September 3, 2021, from https://www.commonwealthfund.org/publications/issue-briefs/2020/aug/looming-crisis-health-coverage-2020-biennial

Federal Register. (2018). *Short-term, limited-duration insurance.* Retrieved September 3, 2021, from https://www.federalregister.gov/documents/2018/08/03/2018-16568/short-term-limited-duration-insurance

Gerisch, M. (n.d.). *Health care as a human right. American Bar Association.* Retrieved September 3, 2021, from https://www.americanbar.org/groups/crsj/publications/human_rights_magazine_home/the-state-of-healthcare-in-the-united-states/health-care-as-a-human-right/

Hamel, L., Kirzinger, A., Muñana, C., Lopes, L., Kearney, A., & Brodie, M. (2020, December 18). *5 Charts about public opinion on the Affordable Care Act and the Supreme Court.* Retrieved September 3, 2021, from https://www.kff.org/health-reform/poll-finding/5-charts-about-public-opinion-on-the-affordable-care-act-and-the-supreme-court/

Hathaway, B. (2020, January 28). *Estimates of preventable hospital deaths are too high, new study shows.* Retrieved September 3, 2021, from https://news.yale.edu/2020/01/28/estimates-preventable-hospital-deaths-are-too-high-new-study-shows

Health care costs by country 2021. (2021). Retrieved September 3, 2021, from https://worldpopulationreview.com/country-rankings/health-care-costs-by-country

HHS Press Office. (2021, August 30). *Biden-Harris administration releases Medicaid and CHIP guidance targeting vaccination and testing for COVID-19.* Retrieved September 3, 2021, from https://www.hhs.gov/about/news/2021/08/30/biden-harris-administration-releases-medicaid-and-chip-guidance-targeting-vaccination-and-testing-for-covid-19.html

Internal Revenue Service. (2021, August 30). *Tax Cuts and Jobs Act: A comparison for businesses.* Retrieved September 3, 2021, from https://www.irs.gov/newsroom/tax-cuts-and-jobs-act-a-comparison-for-businesses

Jost, T. S. (2017, October 12). *Trump executive order expands opportunities for healthier people to exit ACA.* Retrieved September 3, 2021, from https://www.healthaffairs.org/do/10.1377/hblog20171022.762005/full/

Jost, T. S. (2018, August 13). *The Affordable Care Act under the Trump administration.* Retrieved September 3, 2021, from https://www.commonwealthfund.org/blog/2018/affordable-care-act-under-trump-administration

Kaiser Family Foundation. (2021a). *Distribution of Medicare beneficiaries by eligibility category. Timeframe: 2019.* Retrieved September 3, 2021, from https://www.kff.org/medicare/state-indicator/distribution-of-medicare-beneficiaries-by-eligibility-category-2/?currentTimeframe=0&sortModel=%7B%22colId%22:%22Location%22,%22sort%22:%22asc%22%7D

Kaiser Family Foundation. (2021b). *Medicare beneficiaries as a percent of total population. Timeframe: 2018.* Retrieved August 23, 2021, from https://www.kff.org/medicare/state-indicator/medicare-beneficiaries-as-of-total-pop/?currentTimeframe=0&sortModel=%7B%22colId%22:%22Location%22,%22sort%22:%22asc%22%7D

Keith, K. (2021a, June 17). *Supreme Court rejects ACA challenge; Law remains fully intact. Health Affairs.* Retrieved August 23, 2021, from https://www.healthaffairs.org/do/10.1377/hblog20210617.665248/full/

Keith, K. (2021b, May 17). *The Affordable Care Act in the Biden era: Identifying federal priorities for administrative action.* Retrieved September 3, 2021, from https://www.commonwealthfund.org/publications/issue-briefs/2021/may/affordable-care-act-biden-era-federal-priorities

Leonhardt, M. (2020, February 13). *32% of American workers have medical debt—and over half have defaulted on it.* Retrieved September 3, 2021, from https://www.cnbc.com/2020/02/13/one-third-of-american-workers-have-medical-debt-and-most-default.html

Mack, J. (2019, May 20). *7 Reasons U.S. health care is so expensive: Why do we pay more for less? Michigan Live.* Retrieved September 3, 2021, from http://www.mlive.com/news/index.ssf/2017/07/6_reasons_us_health_care_is_so.html

Marquis, B., & Huston, C. (2021). *Leadership roles and management functions in nursing* (10th ed.). Wolters Kluwer.

Medicaid.gov. (2021). *April 2021 Medicaid & CHIP enrollment data highlights.* Retrieved August 23, 2021, from https://www.medicaid.gov/medicaid/program-information/medicaid-and-chip-enrollment-data/report-highlights/index.html

Meltzer, R., & Markus, A. R. (2020, July/August). An analysis of payment mix patterns of preterm births in a post-affordable Care Act insurance market: Implications for the Medicaid program. *Women's Health Issues Paper, 30*(4), 248–259. https://doi.org/10.1016/j.whi.2020.04.003

Norris, L. (2021, August 24). *Will you receive an ACA premium subsidy?* Retrieved September 3, 2021, from https://www.healthinsurance.org/obamacare/will-you-receive-an-aca-premium-subsidy/

Paavola, A. (2020, July 31). *Cuts to 340B payments are legal, appeals court rules.* Retrieved September 3, 2021, from https://www.beckershospitalreview.com/legal-regulatory-issues/cuts-to-340b-payments-are-legal-appeals-court-rules.html

Peter G. Peterson Foundation. (2020, April 20). *Why are Americans paying more for healthcare?* Retrieved September 3, 2021, from https://www.pgpf.org/blog/2020/04/why-are-americans-paying-more-for-healthcare

Price, W. (2021, January 25). *51% of U.S. workforce enrolled in high-deductible health plans, which may leave some underinsured.* Retrieved September 3, 2021, from https://www

.valuepenguin.com/enrollment-changes-to-high-definition-health-insurance-plans#:~:text=51%25%20of%20U.S.%20Workforce%20Enrolled%20in%20High-Deductible%20Health,problems%20for%20many%20consumers.%20Doctor%27s%20office%20waiting%20room

Rural Health Information Hub. (2002–2021). *Rural health disparities.* Retrieved September 3, 2021, from https://www.ruralhealthinfo.org/topics/rural-health-disparities

Sarlin, B., & Kapur, S. (2021, June 5). *The health insurance public option might be fizzling. The left is OK with that.* Retrieved September 3, 2021, from https://www.nbcnews.com/politics/joe-biden/health-insurance-public-option-might-be-fizzling-left-ok-n1269571

Schneider, E. C., Shah, A., Doty, M. M., Tikkanen, R., Fields, K., & Williams II, R. D. (2021, August). *Mirror, mirror 2021. Reflecting poorly: Health care in the U.S. Compared to other high-income countries.* Retrieved September 3, 2021, from https://www.commonwealthfund.org/sites/default/files/2021-08/Schneider_Mirror_Mirror_2021.pdf

Shaw, G. (2020, October 6). *340B health urges Trump administration to eliminate planned Medicare cuts to 340B hospitals.* Pharmacy Practice News. Retrieved September 3, 2021, from https://www.pharmacypracticenews.com/Online-First/Article/10-20/340B-Health-Urges-Trump-Administration-to-Eliminate-Planned-Medicare-Cuts-to-340B-Hospitals/60810

Simmons-Duffin, S. (2019, October 14). *Trump is trying hard to thwart Obamacare. How's that going?* Retrieved September 3, 2021, from https://www.npr.org/sections/health-shots/2019/10/14/768731628/trump-is-trying-hard-to-thwart-obamacare-hows-that-going

Simmons-Duffin, S. (2020, November 9). *What Biden's election means for U.S. health care and public health.* Retrieved September 3, 2021, from https://www.npr.org/sections/health-shots/2020/11/09/932071991/what-bidens-election-means-for-u-s-health-care-and-public-health

Sousa, L. A., Lindblade, V., & Markey, C. (2020, May 13). *Point turning point: The case for universal health care.* Retrieved September 3, 2021, from https://health.usnews.com/health-care/for-better/articles/the-case-for-universal-health-care

Stasha, S. (2021, August 6). *The state of healthcare industry—Statistics for 2021. Policy Advice.* Retrieved September 3, 2021, from https://policyadvice.net/insurance/insights/healthcare-statistics/

Stoltzfus Jost, T. (2017, November). The morality of health care reform: Liberal and conservative views and the space between them. *Hastings Center Report, 47*(6), 9–13. https://doi.org/10.1002/hast.774

The Washington Post. (2021, January 20). *Trump promise tracker.* Retrieved September 3, 2021, from https://www.washingtonpost.com/graphics/politics/trump-promise-tracker/

Tolbert, J., Orgera, K., & Damico, A. (2020, November 6). *Key facts about the uninsured population.* Retrieved September 3, 2021, from https://www.kff.org/uninsured/issue-brief/key-facts-about-the-uninsured-population/

Tompkins, A. (2020, November 9). *Obamacare will be in front of the Supreme Court tomorrow. What you need to know.* Retrieved September 3, 2021, from https://www.poynter.org/reporting-editing/2020/obamacare-will-be-in-front-of-the-supreme-court-tomorrow-what-you-need-to-know/

U.S. Department of Health and Human Services, U.S. Department of the Treasury, U.S. Department of Labor. (n.d.). *Reforming America's healthcare system through choice and competition.* Retrieved September 3, 2021, from https://www.hhs.gov/sites/default/files/Reforming-Americas-Healthcare-System-Through-Choice-and-Competition.pdf

Vanderbilt University Medical Center Department of Health Policy. (2020, March 2). *How the ACA dented the health care cost curve.* Retrieved September 3, 2021, from https://www.vumc.org/health-policy/affordable-care-act-effect-on-health-care-costs

Warner, J. J., Benjamin, I. J., Churchwell, K., Firestone, G., Gardner, T. J., Johnson, J. C., Ng-Osorio, J., Rodriguez, C. J., Todman, L., Yaffe, K., Yancy, C. W., & Harrington, R. A. (2020, February 3). *Advancing healthcare reform: The American Heart Association's 2020 statement of principles for adequate, accessible, and affordable health care: A presidential advisory from the American Heart Association.* Retrieved September 3, 2021, from https://www.ahajournals.org/doi/10.1161/CIR.0000000000000759

Wharton, University of Pennsylvania. (2018, January 5). *Beyond Obamacare: What's ahead for U.S. health care in 2018.* Retrieved September 3, 2021, from http://knowledge.wharton.upenn.edu/article/the-future-of-the-aca

Wood, G. (2016, March 24). *Six broken ObamaCare promises: A retrospective on the ACA's 6th birthday.* Retrieved September 3, 2021, from https://www.heritage.org/health-care-reform/commentary/six-broken-obamacare-promises-retrospective-the-acas-6th-birthday

Zack, E. (2020, November 12). *While the Supreme Court deliberates on the Affordable Care Act, Congress and the White House may act.* Retrieved September 3, 2021, from https://theconversation.com/while-the-supreme-court-deliberates-on-the-affordable-care-act-congress-and-the-white-house-may-act-149891

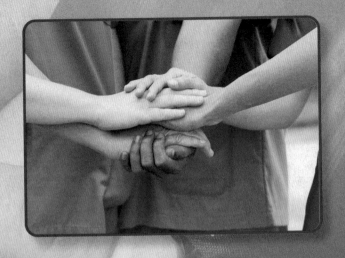

5

PROFESSIONAL POWER

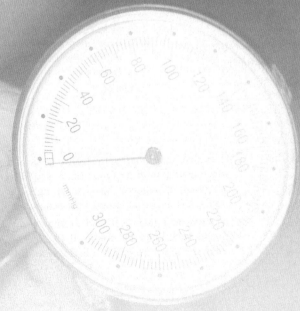

The Nursing Profession's Historic Struggle to Increase Its Power Base

Carol J. Huston

LEARNING OBJECTIVES

The learner will be able to:

1. Explore factors that historically led to nursing's limited power as a profession.

2. Examine characteristics of oppressed groups and analyze whether the nursing profession displays those characteristics.

3. Examine factors that led to the divergence of the nursing profession and feminism in the 1960s and 1970s and subsequently to their convergence in the mid-1980s as part of second-wave feminism.

4. Analyze the influence of gender on how many nurses view policy and politics, the willingness of nurses to work together collectively to achieve

common goals, and the mentoring opportunities available to the profession's future leaders.

5. Identify driving forces in place to increase the nursing profession's power base.

6. Identify potential partners/external stakeholders/alliances that could strengthen the nursing profession's power in national and global policy arenas.

7. Identify nurses currently holding elected office in Congress and state legislatures, as well as the significant committees they serve on or positions they hold.

8. Identify issues currently being debated in the legislature that affect nursing and health care.

9. Explore individual, organizational, and professional responsibilities for succession planning to ensure that an adequate number of highly qualified nursing leaders exists in the future.

10. Reflect on whether the need to be politically competent should be internalized by nurses as a moral and professional obligation.

INTRODUCTION

Power is an elusive concept. The word *power* is derived from the Latin verb *potere*, meaning "to be able." Thus, power may be appropriately defined as that which enables an individual or a group to accomplish goals. Power can also be defined as the capacity to act or the strength and potency to accomplish something (Marquis & Huston, 2021). Having power then gives an individual or a group the potential to change the attitudes and behaviors of others.

How individuals view power, however, varies greatly. Indeed, power may be feared, worshipped, or mistrusted, and it is frequently misunderstood (Marquis & Huston, 2021). Many women (and thus nurses) have historically demonstrated ambivalence toward the concept of power, and some have even eschewed the pursuit of power.

This likely occurred because some women have been culturally socialized to view power negatively, believing that women do not inherently possess power (formal or informal) or authority. In addition, rather than feeling capable of achieving and managing power, some women feel that power manages them. These gender-based perceptions are changing, yet many women still need to learn how to use power as a tool for personal and professional success.

Similarly, the nursing profession has not historically been the powerful force it could have been in dealing with issues directly affecting health care and the profession itself. Indeed, nurses have at times, had limited influence in many areas of the health care system, including health policy, planning, and governance, with some arguing that this focus is far removed from nursing practice and patient care. The Association of Public Health Nurses (APHN) disagrees, noting that nurses spend a lot of time working directly with patients (Regis College,

2021). Thus, they know the specific needs of the communities they serve and can be excellent advocates for public policy development.

> **Consider This** McKeown (2020, p. 1024) suggests that nurses need to reconstruct their professional identity to embrace the positivity of recalcitrant, rebellious, and radical objectives. He also notes that while "we speak a lot about empowerment, of ourselves, of people in receipt of our care, and of communities, we have much less to say about power itself, how this is unfairly distributed, and what to do about this."

Burke (2016, para. 1) agrees, suggesting that to be influential, "nurses must see themselves as professionals with the capacity and responsibility to influence current and future healthcare delivery systems." The general public has said it wants and expects nurses to be more involved in health care policy decision making, and both the American Nurses Association (ANA) *Code of Ethics for Nurses* and the *Social Policy Statement* recognize that influencing public policy is an essential professional expectation for registered nurses (RNs) in every practice setting (Lanier, 2017).

Unfortunately, though, nurses are often thought of as an apolitical group. As a result, nursing has all too often been reactive (rather than proactive) in the policy arena, addressing proposed legislation after its introduction rather than drafting or sponsoring legislation that reflects nursing's agenda. As a result, external forces have often controlled nursing.

These factors have contributed to the nursing profession having a relatively small power base in the political arena and some invisibility as a force in health care decision making. This chapter explores factors that have led to this relative powerlessness as a profession. Driving forces that are in place to increase the nursing's professional power are, however, identified. The chapter concludes with an action plan to increase the nursing's power base so that the profession is recognized as an increasingly significant force in health care decision making in the 21st century.

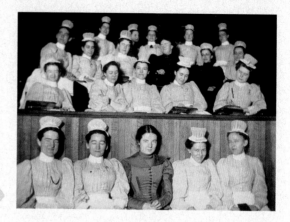

Discussion Point

Why is it that nurses, the largest group of health professionals with perhaps the greatest firsthand knowledge of the health care problems faced by consumers, have not historically been an integral part of health care policy decision making?

FACTORS CONTRIBUTING TO POWERLESSNESS IN NURSING

Many factors have contributed to the nursing profession's relative powerlessness in health care policy setting. Six factors are discussed in this chapter (Box 23.1).

Oppression of Nurses as a Group

The attributes of oppression are unjust treatment, the denial of rights, and the dehumanizing of individuals. As such, it has been suggested that nurses and the nursing profession both work with oppressed groups and are themselves an oppressed group. Indeed, nursing was historically controlled by outside forces with greater prestige, power, and status. Generally, these were patriarchal, male-dominated forces such as medicine and hospital administration. For example, in the early 1900s, physicians attempted to exclude women from the basic sciences. Their refusal to let nurses use new instrumentation sustained women's subordination in nursing, although many nurses continually and actively sought greater scientific knowledge and techniques and incorporated these into their education.

Even at the start of this decade, some physicians openly suggested they should be the only health care professionals qualified to directly treat patients, even though many of the health care professions, including nurses, now hold advanced degrees including doctorates. Indeed, some physicians and their allies continue to push legislative efforts to restrict the right to use the title of "doctor." One must question whether this elitism is more an effort to control money, power, and prestige than it is a concern about whether patients will be confused. Thus, the battle over the title "doctor" is likely a proxy for a larger struggle related to dominance and status.

In addition, some nurse practitioners work with physicians or within physician groups so that they can receive 100% insurance reimbursement for their services. This is called *incident to* billing and indicates that the physician is somehow involved with the care of the nurse practitioner's patients (Nursing Power, 2021). In many U.S. states, however, nurse practitioners have autonomous practice and do not require physician involvement or presence within their practice. In performing identical services, such as a primary care visit for a yearly physical exam, the nurse practitioner typically receives only 75% to 85% compensation from Medicare, Medicaid, and private insurance companies. The Medicare Payment Advisory Commission (MedPAC) examined this payment disparity and determined that there was "no specific analytic foundation" for paying nurse

---

BOX 23.1   Factors Contributing to Powerlessness in Nursing

1. The oppression of nurses as a group
2. Nursing's failure to fully align with the feminist movement
3. Limited collective action by nurses
4. The socialization of women to view power and politics negatively
5. The inadequate recognition of nursing as an educated profession with evidence-based practice
6. The nursing profession's history of being reactive (rather than proactive) in national policy setting

practitioners less than physicians for the same services. This creates nurse practitioner invisibility and decreases nurse practitioner accountability for their own services (Nursing Power, 2021).

When a group is oppressed, it tends to have value confusion and low self-esteem. This occurs because the dominant groups identify their norms and values as the "right ones" and use their initial power to enforce them as the status quo. Oppressed groups accept these norms, at least externally, to gain some power and control. For example, nursing's oppressors have not always held the same values as nursing (i.e., caring, nurturance, and advocacy). This has led to confusion for some nurses and even, at times, contempt for their own profession and what it represents.

> **Consider This** Badmouthing one's own profession may be a sign of oppression and values confusion.

Failure to Align Fully with the Feminist Movement

A second factor contributing to nursing's relative powerlessness is the profession's failure to align fully with the feminist movement. Although both nurses and women have improved their status in the last five decades, nursing has not kept pace with the progress women have made in other areas. This has occurred because, at least in part, nurses have not been fully engaged in the feminist movement.

This occurred for several reasons. One was that many feminists in the 1960s and 1970s were influenced by a more radical feminist perspective and, as a result, spoke out against women becoming nurses because it suggested that female nurses were in subordinate, caregiving roles. In addition, many nurses feared public identification with feminism.

The reality, however, is that nursing continues to be a profession composed of approximately 90% women, and this figure has changed only slowly over time. This is noteworthy, given that there have been major gender shifts in virtually all other traditionally female-dominated professions, such as social workers, librarians, and K-12 teachers since the 1970s.

> **Discussion Point**
>
> Many nursing leaders in the early 1900s were political activists, actively involved in social issues such as women's suffrage and public health. At what point did nursing diverge from a sociopolitical agenda and why?

Although having female dominance in the profession may have some benefits, it also poses some liabilities.

Indeed, some nursing leaders have suggested that nursing will never attain greater status and power until more men join the ranks (see Chapter 9). Others think that adding men to nursing's ranks is not the answer. Instead, nurses need to accept the responsibility for addressing the problems that have historically plagued the profession, and take whatever steps are necessary to proactively build a power base that does not depend on gender.

> **Consider This** Being a female professional in a male-dominated health care system brings to mind the "Ginger Rogers syndrome." Both Ginger Rogers and her dancing partner, Fred Astaire, were known as wonderful dancers, but Fred Astaire's name always came first, and he always received the greater recognition. In reality, "Ginger Rogers danced the same steps as Fred Astaire, but she did them backward and in high heels" (Wikiquote, 2021, para 2). So, who deserved the greater recognition?

In addition, recognition that assertive, independent nurses cannot exist if they have been socialized to be dependent women is growing. Similarly, it is improbable if not impossible for female nurses to implement expanded roles in advanced practice if they are unaware of or unwilling to recognize the social constraints imposed on them because they are women. Clearly, the battles between the American Medical Association (AMA) and advanced practice nurses about the scope of practice, the reimbursement, and the need for medical oversight are likely related as much to gender as they are to competition over patients (see Chapter 4). A reminder of this divide tore through social media just a few years ago when a male anesthesiologist in Florida with ties to a major medical school posted demeaning and inflammatory comments about nurse practitioners:

> Nurse practitioners are not, I repeat, not physicians. They lack the education, IQ and clinical experience. There is no depth of understanding. They are useful but only as minions. (Kalensky, 2017, para. 3)

His comments were posted to Twitter, where many people reacted swiftly, calling for physicians to take a team-based approach and promote unity among health care professionals (Kalensky, 2017). Sociologist Anne Bell suggested, however, that emerging trends in medicine and nursing may lead to a "flattening of the hierarchy" as women move into traditional male roles (Kalensky, 2017). Until then though, women will struggle to establish themselves as equals in health care professions.

Nurses need, then, to continue to examine the progress women have made in other professions and work with them inside and outside of nursing to strengthen power for women everywhere. This holds true for the men in nursing as well because the relative powerlessness of the profession transfers to them too, despite gender differences. Both male and female nurses must solve problems, work to advance the science of nursing, network to increase nursing's knowledge base and power, and provide mutual support.

Limited Collective Representation of Nurses

A third factor limiting the development of the nursing profession's power base is the inadequate collective representation of nurses by groups, such as collective bargaining agents and professional nursing organizations. According to the Bureau of Labor Statistics, as of June 2021, only 20.4% of nurses in the United States belonged to a collective bargaining unit (Burger, 2021). Only about 5% of nurses (approximately 195,884) as of 2017 belonged to the ANA, the nationally recognized professional organization for all RNs, whose mission is to advance and protect the profession (UnionFacts.com, 2021). These relatively small membership numbers directly reflect the money that is available for lobbyists to represent nursing in the political arena. In contrast, the AMA has one of the most powerful lobbying organizations in the United States.

> **Consider This** Nurses must be represented en masse before they will be able to significantly affect the decisions that directly influence their profession.

There are many reasons for the small representation of nurses in the ANA. The dual and often conflicting role of the ANA as both a professional organization for nurses and a collective bargaining agent is certainly one reason. In addition, some nurses think that state nurses' associations have been burdened with the task of collective bargaining under the federation model of the ANA and that other programs have suffered as a result of funds being used for collective bargaining. Other nurses have expressed concerns about the cost of membership in the ANA or argued that the ANA is not responsive enough to the needs of the nurse at the bedside. Other nurses look at nursing as a job and not as a career and have little interest in professional issues outside of their immediate work environment.

Discussion Point

Do you belong to a professional nursing organization? Why or why not? Do contemporary nursing leaders espouse this as a value? Is it encouraged in the workplace and in the academic world?

Whether these issues are valid is almost immaterial. As long as such a small percentage of nurses belong to the ANA, the economic power of the ANA will be limited, as will its ability to significantly influence policy setting and legislation. Perhaps even more importantly, until nurses are willing to work together collectively in some form, they will be unlikely to increase either their personal or their professional power.

> **Consider This** At times, nurses have lacked pride in their collective groups and have viewed alignment with other nurses as alignment with other powerless persons, something that does little to advance an individual's professional power.

Unfortunately, at times, nurses in this country have not acted cohesively, whether at the local level, fighting for wage increases, or at the national level, attempting to influence health policy. Even the various professional nursing organizations to which nurses belong have not historically worked together cooperatively. The reality is that nurses continue to be widely divided on basic issues such as entry into practice, mandatory staffing ratios, and collective bargaining.

> **Consider This** A metaphor for increasing nursing's power base through collective action would be a snowball. Individual snowflakes are fragile, but when they stick together, they become a powerful force.

Socialization of Women to View Power and Politics Negatively

A fourth factor contributing to powerlessness in the nursing profession has been the socialization of women (and thus, the majority of nurses) to view power and politics negatively. Conscious efforts are changing this perception, however. Politics is a part of life. It is also the art of using legitimate power wisely. Therefore, it requires clear decision making, assertiveness, accountability, and the willingness to express one's views (Marquis & Huston, 2021). It also requires being proactive rather than reactive and demands decisiveness.

Unfortunately, nurses' involvement in politics and policymaking has not significantly improved over time according to a recent umbrella literature review completed by Rasheed et al. (2020) (Research Fuels the Controversy 23.1). Rasheed and team (2020) concluded that nursing institutions and regulatory bodies should prepare and encourage nurses to work as policymakers rather than implementers and advocate for the rightful place of nurses at policymaking forums.

Research Fuels the Controversy 23.1

Nurses' Involvement in Politics and Policymaking in the Last Two Decades

The purpose of this literature review was to determine nurses' challenges, extent of involvement, and the impact of involvement in politics and policymaking. Twenty-two articles published from January 2000 to May 2019 were included.

Source: Rasheed, S. P., Younas, A., & Mehdi, F. (2020, July). Challenges, extent of involvement, and the impact of nurses' involvement in politics and policymaking in in last two decades: An integrative review. *Journal of Nursing Scholarship, 52*(4), 446–455. https://doi.org/10.1111/jnu.12567

Study Findings

This review revealed multiple factors and challenges influencing nurses' political participation and role in health and nursing policymaking, and also described the extent and impact of nurses' involvement in policymaking. The researchers noted that major challenges to nurse involvement in politics and policymaking included intra- and interprofessional power dynamics, marginalization of nurses in policymaking, and nursing profession–specific challenges. The extent of involvement was also inadequate and had not improved over time. Nurses mainly worked as policy implementers rather than as policy developers. Those nurses who participated in policy development focused on health promotion to build healthy communities and to empower nurses and the nursing profession.

The researchers concluded that the importance of the nurses' role and involvement in politics and policymaking cannot be overemphasized. They reiterated a need for nurses to participate in policymaking at organizational, system, and national levels and called for adequate preparation of nurses for policymaking.

Clearly, quality nursing care is not separate and distinct from politically informed and engaged professional nursing practice. Nurses, then, become not a group that needs to be controlled and governed, but individuals who must care for themselves before they may care for anyone else.

The International Council of Nurses (ICN, 2014) and the World Health Organization agree, suggesting that nurses can and should be involved in policy development since they are uniquely positioned to provide crucial policy information. Furthermore, health policy often has a direct effect on nurses, and it is in their best interest to be engaged in its formulation. The ICN (2014) argues that a cultural shift must occur within the nursing profession to emphasize the importance of policy and nurses' role in setting and implementing it. In addition, a clear understanding of how policy affects nurses as well as how their unique knowledge regarding patient care is crucial for policy development, must be embedded at the institutional level. This cultural shift must also occur in educational institutions where the integration of policy in practice must be emphasized in nursing classrooms and faculty must be given the proper support to develop and carry out policy research so that policymakers and administrators can draw from the evidence base when developing policy.

Consider This Changing nurses' view of both power and politics is perhaps the most significant key to proactive rather than reactive participation in policy setting.

Nurses, then, must perceive a need not only to be more knowledgeable about power, negotiation, and politics but also to be more involved in broad social and political issues. This requires becoming politically astute. Nurses need to understand what politics means, and they need to become experts in using politics to help nursing achieve both its professional goals and the needs of its patients.

Inadequate Recognition of Nursing as an Educated Profession with Evidence-Based Practice

A fifth factor contributing to the nursing profession's relative powerlessness is the inadequate recognition of nursing as a profession driven by research and the pursuit of higher education. Although nurses should highly value the caring, intuitive, nurturing part of nursing practice, the nursing profession has been negligent about equally emphasizing their extensive scientific knowledge base and the high level of critical thinking and analysis professional nurses use every day in their clinical practice.

Both the art and the science of nursing require highly developed skills and a well-developed knowledge base. The nurse of the 21st century has an extensive knowledge base in the sciences as well as in the arts. In addition, nurses must be expert critical thinkers, as they are required to continually look for and analyze subtle clues in their patient data, make independent nursing diagnoses, and create plans of care. Constant assessment of and adjustment to the plan of care are almost always necessary, so nurses must be highly organized and know how to set priorities. In addition, nurses must have highly refined communication skills, well-developed psychomotor skills, and sophisticated leadership and management skills. This is the image nurses must promote to the public.

Discussion Point

If the public was asked to list five adjectives to describe nursing, what would they be? Would the art or the science of nursing be recognized more? Would nurses themselves use different adjectives?

The Nursing Profession's History of Being Reactive in National Policy Setting

The last factor discussed here as contributing to a relative lack of professional power in nursing is the profession's history of being reactive rather than proactive in national policy setting regarding nursing practice. *Reactive* means waiting until there is a problem and then trying to fix it. *Proactive* is more anticipatory; it means developing appropriate policy before action is taken or a problem occurs.

Unfortunately, the nursing profession has been far from proactive in shaping its own course or that of the health care system. In the 1990s, health care became big business. Managed care proliferated, and gatekeepers, not providers and consumers, began deciding who needed care and how much care was needed. Hospitals lost their place as the center of the health care universe as patient care shifted from inpatient hospital stays to outpatient and ambulatory health care settings. Physicians lost much of their autonomy to practice medicine as they saw fit as insurers increasingly placed restrictions not only on which physicians the patients could see but also on what services the physician was authorized to prescribe.

Patients found themselves with limited choices of providers, longer wait times for care, more rules to follow, and more confusion about what would and would not be a covered expense. At the same time, RNs in record numbers, for the first time in history, were downsized, restructured, and often replaced by a cheaper counterpart to reduce costs.

Many nurses felt both overwhelmed and helpless with this degree of change. However, these changes did not happen overnight. Many of them were incremental and insidious, and the health care system changes occurred with little concerted effort by nurses to stop them.

Senge (1990) wrote about a brief parable in *The Fifth Discipline* that nurses should keep in mind when they think about the need to be proactive, even with incremental change. It is called "The parable of the boiled frog," and it goes like this:

> *If you place a frog in a pot of boiling water, it will immediately try to scramble out. But if you place the frog in room temperature water, and don't scare him, he'll stay put. Now, if the pot sits on a heat source, and if you gradually turn up the temperature, something very interesting happens. As the temperature rises from 70 to 80 degrees Fahrenheit, the frog will do nothing. In fact, he will show every sign of enjoying himself. As the temperature gradually increases, the frog will become groggier and groggier, until he is unable to crawl out of the pot. Though there is nothing restraining him, the frog will sit there and boil. He will boil to death, oblivious to what is happening to him.*

Consider This   Gradual but constant change may be even more dangerous than cataclysmic change because resistance is less organized.

DRIVING FORCES TO INCREASE NURSING'S POWER BASE

So, what is the likelihood that the nursing profession will ever be a powerful force in health care decision making and the political arena? The answer is unclear, although the likelihood of this happening is increasing because of several driving forces in place. This chapter discusses six of these forces (Box 23.2).

The Timing Is Right; Consumers and Providers Want Change

Timing is everything. The political ferment regarding health care reform continues to escalate, and issues of cost and access are paramount in this country. For 2020, the United States was budgeted to spend $2.02 trillion on health care, an amount equal to over 22% of the gross domestic product (Chantrill, 2021). In addition, in mid-2021, President Joe Biden announced his intent to increase health spending by almost 23% to build a new health research agency, eliminate racial and socioeconomic disparities, and beef up the nation's public health preparedness (Baumann et al., 2021). Indeed, since 2000, government health spending has soared by nearly 250% (Matthews, 2021).

In addition, despite spending more than any other industrialized country in the world (two to three times that of most industrialized countries) U.S. rankings in terms of life span, infant mortality, and teenage pregnancy are much lower

---

BOX 23.2   **Driving Forces to Increase Nursing's Power Base**

1. The timing is right
2. The size of the nursing profession and the diversity of nursing practice
3. Nursing's referent power
4. Nursing's increasing knowledge base
5. Nursing's unique perspective
6. The desire for change among consumers and providers

---

than those of many countries that spend significantly less on health care. Matthews (2021) suggests the problem is that more health care spending cannot improve results because it is pushed into health care bureaucracies already struggling to perform unrealistic and ever-expanding missions.

Furthermore, the passage and implementation of the Affordable Care Act (ACA) only escalated public awareness and debate about flaws in publicly funded or subsidized health care in the United States. As a result of publications like *To Err Is Human*, consumers, health care providers, and legislators are more aware than ever of the shortcomings of the current health care system, and the clamor for action has never been louder. Because the flaws of the health care system are no longer secret, nursing can now use its expertise and influence to help create a better health care system for the future.

Size of the Nursing Profession and Diversity of Practice

The second driving force for increasing nursing's professional power base is the size of the profession and the diversity of nursing practice. Numbers are the lifeblood of politics. If nurses do not vote as a block, however, their political voice becomes diluted. The nursing profession's size, then, is perhaps its greatest asset, and its potential for a collective voting block should increasingly be recognized as a force to deal with.

Discussion Point

Collective involvement of only a fraction of the nation's 3.8 million RNs in health care policy would produce a significant voting bloc. Have nurses ever made a concerted effort to vote collectively? What positions have professional organizations such as the ANA taken on recent election issues or candidates for office? Have endorsements by professional nursing organizations influenced how you vote?

Nursing's Referent Power

A third driving force for increasing the power of the profession is the referent power nurses hold. *Referent power* is the power one has when others identify with you or what you symbolize; therefore, you have their admiration or respect (Marquis & Huston, 2021). Nurses have a high degree of referent power because of the trust and credibility given to them by the public.

For 19 consecutive years (2002 to 2021), nurses have been recognized by the public as the most trustworthy of all professions (Gaines, 2021).

> When nurses speak, not only do people listen, but they also believe what is being said. Nurses are seen as selflessly looking after the needs of their patients rather than looking out for more selfish personal interests. In other words, they offer unbiased observations and suggestions that the public believes should be used extensively to shape policy decisions. The public believes nurses should be equal partners with physicians in efforts to address the many problems that challenge the health care system. (Lanier, 2017)

Nursing's Increasing Knowledge Base

A fourth driving force for increasing the power of the profession is nursing's increasing knowledge base. Indeed, the National Academy of Sciences (2021) in *The Future of Nursing 2020-2030* has charged an expert committee to create a vision for the nursing profession into 2030 that empowers the nursing profession to help create a culture of health, reduce health disparities, and improve the health and well-being of the U.S. population in the 21st century. In developing its recommendations for the future, the committee will draw from domestic and global examples of evidence-based models of care that address social determinants of health and help build and sustain a culture of health

To accomplish this vision, more nurses will need to be educated at the master's and doctoral levels than ever before. In 2018, however, only 17.1% of the nation's RNs held a master's degree and 1.9% held a doctoral degree as their highest educational preparation (American Association of Colleges of Nursing [AACN], 2021a). The current demand for master's and doctorally prepared nurses for advanced practice, clinical specialties, teaching, and research roles far outstrips the supply; however, more nurses than ever are achieving advanced degrees. One of the greatest areas of growth is in the number of Doctor of Nursing Practice (DNP) students, with the number of students enrolled in DNP programs increasing from 32,678 in 2018 to 36,069 in 2019 (AACN, 2021b).

Furthermore, leadership, management, and political theory are increasingly a part of baccalaureate nursing education, although most nurses still do not hold baccalaureate degrees. These are learned skills, and, collectively, the nursing profession's knowledge of leadership, politics, negotiation, and finance is increasing. This can only increase the nursing profession's influence outside the field.

Nursing's Unique Perspective

A fifth driving force for increasing the nursing profession's power base is the uniquely philosophical perspective nursing brings to the health care arena. Nursing's perspective is unique because of its blending of art and science—a blending of "caring" and "curing," so to speak. The caring part of the nursing role is better known and better understood by the public. It is what historically has defined nursing. It is important that nurses not forget or underappreciate the unique values nursing represents because these are the values that make the profession different from all the others. These same values will make nursing irreplaceable in the current health care system.

> **Consider This** "The power of nurses' voices and the unique perspective they bring have the potential to be powerful agents for change" (Boerger et al., 2020, p. 257).

The "science" part of nursing, however, is less understood by the public. Nursing has an extensive scientific knowledge base, and the high level of critical thinking and analysis that professional nurses use every day in their clinical practice is enormous. Nursing practice is increasingly becoming *evidence based*, meaning that nursing practice reflects what the literature says is *best practice*. That is, the practice of nursing is research based and scientifically driven (see Chapter 5). Unfortunately, consumers, legislators, and, sometimes even other health care professionals fail to recognize this. Nursing then must do a better job of explaining and emphasizing both the art and the science of its practice.

ACTION PLAN FOR THE FUTURE

Based on these driving forces, an action plan can be created to increase the power of the nursing profession in the 21st century. This chapter identifies seven possible strategies to achieve this goal (Box 23.3).

Place More Nurses in Positions of Influence

Nurses must be a part of decision-making processes in the health care system. This means placing nurses on advisory committees, commissions, and boards where policy decisions are made to advance health systems to improve patient care. Boerger and colleagues (2020) agree, noting that by virtue of their practice, nurses have the inherent skills to plan, organize, and lead. Therefore, the opportunity to include the perspective of a nurse in almost any aspect of community organizations should be encouraged.

Too much can go wrong if decision makers, who do not understand healthcare, are left to make decisions without the input of those who provide professional care 24 hours a day, 365 days a year. Unfortunately, although nurses typically represent the greatest percentage of the workforce in hospitals, too few nurses serve on hospital boards or hold positions of significant power.

Education for board participation, however, is often needed since many nurses lack basic skills in health care

BOX 23.3   Action Plan for Increasing the Power of the Nursing Profession

1. More nurses must be placed in positions of influence.
2. Recognize nursing's potential to make a difference.
3. Nurses must become better informed about all health care policy efforts.
4. Coalition building must occur within and outside of nursing.
5. More research must be done to strengthen evidence-based practice.
6. Nursing leaders must be supported.
7. Attention must be paid to mentoring future nurse leaders and leadership succession.

finance and policy. Cleveland and Harper (2020) concur, noting that many nurse leaders feel unsure about the financial responsibilities and liabilities associated with board involvement, necessitating orientation and continuing education in these areas.

> *Consider This* "No other profession meets people during their most vulnerable experiences and supports them through the health continuum across the thresholds of communities, hospitals, long-term care facilities, and support groups. This position and ability to appreciate and respond to challenges is the unique voice of a nurse" (Cleveland & Harper, 2020, p. 96).

This situation is changing, however, through the work of groups such as the *Nurses on Boards Coalition* (NBC), a coalition founded by the ANA, the American Academy of Nursing, and the American Nurses Foundation (ANF), the charitable and philanthropic arm of the ANA. The coalition, which was first convened in 2014, set a goal to ensure that nurses filled at least 10,000 board seats by 2020 (NBC, 2021). As of September 2021, 10,273 nurses held board seats.

In addition, nurses must be placed in national positions that influence public policy. For example, a significant effort began in 2005 to establish an *Office of the National Nurse* in the United States, who would serve as an assistant to the surgeon general. A National Nursing Network Organization was formed, and legislation has repeatedly been introduced in Congress since 2006 to achieve this goal. Most recently, the National Nurse Act of 2019 ("S.696-116th Congress, 2019-2020") was introduced (Congress.gov, 2019). This bill designated the same individual serving as the Chief Nurse Officer of the Public Health Service as the National Nurse for Public Health. Thus, this bill elevated this nurse into a full-time leadership position to focus on the critical work needed to address national priorities of health promotion and disease prevention and to direct efforts at improving health literacy and decreasing health disparities in the United States. Proponents of the idea suggested that such a position would raise the profile of nursing and assist in a nationwide cultural shift to prevention and health promotion. Opponents suggested that this might not be the best way to effect change both within nursing and in the health care system. The bill was read twice and referred to the Committee on Health, Education, Labor, and Pensions in March 2019 (Congress.gov, 2019).

Not all positions that influence public policy, however, occur at the national level. Indeed, few leaders burst onto the national scene directly. Instead, they assume leadership roles in entities such as medical centers, community hospitals, government agencies, and insurance companies.

Running for and holding elected office is, however, the ultimate in political activism and involvement. Only three nurses were serving in Congress as of fall 2021 (ANA, 2021). Many more nurses hold elected office in state legislatures.

In fact, nurses are uniquely qualified to hold public office because they have the greatest firsthand experience of problems faced by patients in the health care system, as well as an ability to translate the health care experience to the general public. As a result, more nurses must seek out this role. In addition, because the public respects and trusts nurses, nurses who choose to run for public office are often elected. The problem, then, is not that nurses are not being elected but that not enough nurses are running for office.

Recognize Nursing's Potential to Make a Difference

A second part of the action plan to increase the power of the nursing profession in the 21st century is to recognize the nursing profession's potential to make a real difference. It is critical that each nurse never loses sight of this potential.

> **Discussion Point**
>
> Have you ever heard or said "I am just a nurse?" How does this undermine the profession?

In addition, some legislators and employers have argued that "a nurse is a nurse is a nurse." This is wrong. Nurses can be whatever they want to be in nursing, and they can achieve that goal at whatever level of quality they choose. The bottom line, however, is that the profession will only be as smart, as motivated, and as directed as its weakest link. If the nursing profession is to be the powerful force it can be, it needs to be filled with bright, highly motivated people who want to make a difference in the lives of the patients with whom they work, as well as in the health care system itself.

> *Consider This* Individuals may be born average, but staying average is a choice.

Become Better Informed About All Health Care Policy Efforts

The third step of the action plan is that nurses must become better informed about all health care policy efforts—especially those that influence their profession. This is difficult because no one can do this but nurses. This requires grassroots knowledge building and involvement.

Groenwald and Eldridge (2020) suggest that to achieve competence in health policy, nurses will need to obtain knowledge, develop effective communication, collaborate with other health care professionals, and become proactive. They will also need knowledge of the political environment as well as nursing issues because there is a need for both patient and professional advocacy, representing patient outcomes as well as the profession of nursing.

> **Consider This** Nurses who do not understand the legislative process will not be able to influence the policymaking process.

One effort to increase the number of nurses who are well prepared to influence health policy at the local, state, and national levels was the launch of the American Nurses Advocacy Institute (ANAI) in 2009. ANAI fellows complete a year-long mentoring program to strengthen their competence in the political arena. The institute covers content such as the advocacy process, conducting a political environmental scan; bill analysis; preparing and delivering testimony; coalition building; and value of a political action committee (PAC) (Minnesota Organization of Registered Nurses, 2021).

Another program that helps nurses acquire the leadership skills to shape health care locally and nationally is the Robert Wood Johnson Foundation (RWJF) *Future of Nursing Scholars* program. This program creates a diverse cadre of PhD-prepared nurses who are committed to a long-term leadership career; advancing science and discovery through research; strengthening nursing education; and furthering transformational change in nursing and health care (RWJF, 2021).

Not all nurses, however, need to or want to be this involved in politics and policy setting. Determining how directly or indirectly one should be involved is a personal decision. Certainly, being an informed voter should be considered a minimum expectation.

Fortunately, nurses are in the enviable position of having great credibility with legislators and the public. Nurses who choose to be directly involved in politics and policy setting can seek public office or become more involved in lobbying legislators about issues pertinent to health care and nursing. Such lobbying can be done either in person or by writing, and there are many good sources on how to do both. The legislator needs to understand why this is an issue that is critical not only to the nursing profession but also to their constituents. It is important, then, to create a need for the legislator to listen to what is being said.

Nurses can also give freely of their time and money to support nursing's position in the legislative arena. This can be done indirectly by contributing to professional associations such as the ANA, which has lobbyists in the legislative arena

to protect nursing's interests, or by giving money directly to a political campaign. In this case, nurses should try to give early and make as large a contribution as possible. It is the early and significant contributions that are remembered most.

Nurses interested in a more indirect contribution to policy development may work to influence and educate the public about nursing and the nursing agenda to reform health care. Either role is helpful—at least the nurse will have made a conscious decision to be involved.

Finally, nurses must also realize that part of the reason the profession has been invisible or portrayed inappropriately in the media is that nurses have not assumed the spokesperson roles they could have or should have for their profession. More nurses need to gain the skills required to effectively interact with the media about nursing and health care. Other strategies for effecting change through political involvement are noted in Box 23.4.

Build Coalitions Inside and Outside of Nursing

The fourth step of the action plan to increase professional power in the 21st century is for the nursing profession to look within itself as well as beyond its organizations for coalition building. Belonging to professional nursing organizations is one way in which nurses can network for coalition building. Coalitions have been formed within nursing groups as well. The *Tri-Council for Nursing* is an alliance of four autonomous nursing organizations: the AACN, the ANA, the AONE, and the NLN. The Tri-Council focuses on leadership for education, practice, and research.

The Council for the Advancement of Nursing Science (2021) is another example of coalition building among nursing groups. The Council is composed of representatives from the four major regional research societies; Sigma Theta Tau International (STTI); the American Academy of Nursing; the National Institute of Nursing Research (ex officio); the Association of Women's Health, Obstetric and Neonatal Nurses; and the ANF.

Similarly, the National Federation for Specialty Nursing Organizations and the Nursing Organizations Liaison Forum, an entity of the ANA, merged in 2001 to become the *Nursing Organizations Alliance*, also known as The Alliance. The Alliance provides a forum for identification, education, and collaboration building on issues of common interest to advance the nursing profession (The Nursing Organizations Alliance, 2019).

> **Consider This** More collaboration among nursing organizations would increase the power of the nursing profession.

BOX 23.4   **Political Activities to Effect Change**

1. Join professional associations.
2. Be informed about current legislative issues.
3. Know who your current legislators are and how to reach them.
4. Present information and informed opinions to legislators either in writing or face to face.
5. Write letters to newspaper editors.
6. Serve as a media spokesperson.
7. Write political action pieces for professional journals.
8. Contribute to political action committees.
9. Make campaign contributions.
10. Join a campaign and actively participate.
11. Participate in rally days at the capitol.
12. Register to vote and vote.
13. Seek positions of influence on health care and community boards.
14. Attend city council meetings.
15. Use social media to influence a broader audience.
16. Mobilize people to support your causes.

Discussion Point

All too frequently, the AMA and the ANA stand in opposition to each other in the legislative arena. Are there health care issues on which they could partner? Are there issues on which the ANA and the American Hospital Association could partner?

Nurses have not done as well, however, in building political coalitions with other health care professionals with similar challenges. Nor have they done well in building political coalitions with legislators. Most legislators have a great deal of respect for nurses but know little about their qualifications to speak with authority about the health care system. Nurses need to become experts at political networking, making trade-offs, negotiating, and coalition building. They also need to see the bigger picture of health care. This is not to say that nurses should lose sight of patient needs, but that they must do a better job of seeing the bigger picture and of building and strengthening alliances with others before they will be seen as powerful and capable.

Conduct More Research to Strengthen Evidence-Based Practice

Another critical strategy for increasing nursing's power base is to continue to develop and promote evidence-based practice in nursing. Great strides have been made in researching what it is that nurses do that makes a difference in patient outcomes (research on *nursing-sensitive outcomes*), but more needs to be done. Nursing practice must reflect what research has identified as best practices, and a better understanding of the relationship between nursing practice and patient outcomes is still needed.

Consider This Only relatively recently has empirical research been able to prove that patients get better because of nurses, not in spite of them.

Building and sustaining evidence-based practice in nursing will require far greater numbers of highly educated nurse researchers, as well as entry into practice at an educational level similar to that of other professions. Social work, physical therapy, and occupational therapy all now have the master's or doctoral degree as the entry level into practice. Nursing cannot afford to continue debating whether a bachelor's degree is necessary as the minimum entry level into professional practice (see Chapter 1).

Support Nursing Leaders

Another part of the action plan to increase the profession's power is that nurses must support their nursing leaders and recognize the challenges they face as visionary change agents. Nurses have often viewed their leaders as rule breakers, and this has often occurred at a high personal cost to innovators.

In addition, nurses often resist change and new ideas from their leaders, and instead look to leaders in medicine and other health-related disciplines. Some of this occurs because of nurse leaders being discounted, at least in part, because of their female majority, and in part to the low value placed on nursing expertise.

Groenwald and Eldridge (2020) concur, noting that to be able to empower others, including patients, nurses need to feel empowered. Creating an environment where nurses are encouraged and supported to speak out about issues affecting patient care or their profession demonstrates that their expertise and judgment are desired and valued.

It is important to remember that typically, it is not outsiders who divide nursing followers from nursing leaders. Instead, the division of nursing's strength often comes from within. Nursing leaders must be perceived as the profession's best advocates. Differing viewpoints should be not only acknowledged but also encouraged. There is a proper arena for conflict and argument, but the outward force presented must be one of unity and direction.

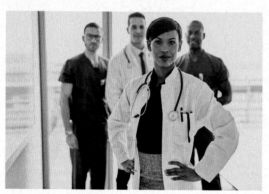

(Flamingo Images/Shutterstock)

Mentor Future Nurse Leaders and Plan for Leadership Succession

Finally, and perhaps most important, before nursing can become a powerful profession, nurses must actively plan for leadership succession and care for younger members by providing mentoring opportunities. It is the future leaders who face the task of increasing nursing's power base in the 21st century.

Some perceive female-dominated professions as having a history of exemplifying what is known as the *queen bee syndrome*. The queen bee is a woman who, after great personal struggle, becomes successful in her career. Her

attitude, however, is that because she had to make it on her own with so little help, other novices should have to do the same. If and when this has been the case, there has been inadequate empowering of young nurse leaders by older, more established nurse leaders. It is the young who hold not only the keys to the present but also the hope for the future. The nursing profession is responsible for ensuring leadership succession and is morally bound to do it with the brightest, most highly qualified individuals.

Discussion Point

Is the nursing profession proactive in planning its leadership succession, or is this a change that occurs by drift?

CONCLUSIONS

Although significant progress has been made, nursing as a female-dominated profession continues to face challenges in having a strong voice in health care policy. Nursing lobbyists in the nation's capital are influencing legislation on quality, access to care, patient and health worker safety, health care restructuring, reimbursement for advanced practice nurses, and funding for nursing education. Representatives of professional nursing organizations regularly attend and provide testimony at government agency meetings to be sure that the "nursing perspective" is heard on health policy issues.

Yet, clearly, nurses, as health care professionals, need to have greater input into and control over how the health care system evolves in this country. We need a health care system that will guarantee basic, affordable health care coverage for all citizens and in which all the members of the multidisciplinary health care teamwork together to create policy and provide care based on what is best for the patient. We also need a health care system that is accountable for its outcomes—that recognizes that individuality, autonomy, quality, and basic human dignity are essential components of health care services and that the bottom line is not always a number.

The nursing profession must be held accountable for being an integral force in shaping such a health care system. Indeed, nursing has a moral and professional obligation to do so.

For Additional Discussion

1. Should the nursing profession target the recruitment of men into nursing in an effort to increase professional power?

2. What partners/external stakeholders should the nursing profession seek in terms of alliances or coalitions to strengthen its position in the policy arena?

3. What are the priority issues the nursing profession should identify in creating a proactive legislative agenda?

4. Will nursing ever be able to increase its power base if it does not increase its educational entry level to a level similar to that of other health care professions?

5. Do nursing schools provide enough content on politics, policy, and leadership for nurses to develop some degree of political competence? If not, what is missing?

6. Do most nurses internalize the need to be politically competent as a moral and professional obligation?

7. What legislative issues being debated have the greatest potential effect on nursing and health care?

References

American Association of Colleges of Nursing. (2021a). *Nursing fact sheet*. Retrieved September 10, 2021, from https://www.aacnnursing.org/News-Information/Fact-Sheets/Nursing-Fact-Sheet

American Association of Colleges of Nursing. (2021b). *DNP fact sheet*. Retrieved September 10, 2021, from https://www.aacnnursing.org/News-Information/Fact-Sheets/DNP-Fact-Sheet

American Nurses Association. (2021). *Nurses serving in Congress*. Retrieved September 10, 2021, from https://www.nursingworld.org/practice-policy/advocacy/federal/nurses-serving-in-congress/

Baumann, J., Lee, J., & Stein, S. (2021, May 28). *Health spending would increase by 23% under Biden budget ask*. Retrieved September 20, 2021, from https://news.bloomberglaw.com/health-law-and-business/health-spending-would-increase-by-23-under-biden-budget-request

Boerger, J., Maisonneuve, V., Nordberg, A., & Judge, K. (2020, June). Illuminating the path, inspiring the future, the power of a nurse's voice. *Nurse Leader, 18*(3), 253–258. https://doi.org/10.1016/j.mnl.2020.03.012

Burger, C. (2021, June 18). *Do unions benefit or harm healthcare & nursing industries?* Retrieved September 10, 2021, from https://www.registerednursing.org/do-unions-benefit-harm-healthcare-nursing/

Burke, S. A. (2016, June 2). *Influence through policy: Nurses have a unique role*. Retrieved September 10, 2021, from https://www.reflectionsonnursingleadership.org/commentary/more-commentary/Vol42_2_nurses-have-a-unique-role

Chantrill, C. (2021). *U.S. Government Spending. Total budgeted government spending expenditure GDP–CHARTS–Deficit debt*. Retrieved September 9, 2021, from http://www.usgovernmentspending.com

Cleveland, K. A., & Harper, K. J. (2020). Prepare and pursue board opportunities: A practical guide for nurse leaders to serve on a board. *Nursing Economic$, 38*(2), 94–97.

Congress.gov. (2019). *S.696—National Nurse Act of 2019. 116th Congress (2019-2020)*. Retrieved September 9, 2021, from https://www.congress.gov/bill/116th-congress/senate-bill/696

Council for the Advancement of Nursing Science. (2021). *Homepage*. American Academy of Nursing. Retrieved September 9, 2021, from http://www.nursingscience.org/home

Gaines, K. (2021, January 19). *Nurses ranked most trusted profession 19 years in a row*. Retrieved September 10, 2021, from https://nurse.org/articles/nursing-ranked-most-honest-profession/

Groenwald, S. L., & Eldridge, C. (2020, January–March). Politics, power, and predictability of nursing care. *Nursing Forum, 55*(1), 16–32. https://doi.org/10.1111/nuf.12377

International Council of Nurses. (2014). Moving towards the greater involvement of nurses in policy development. *International Nursing Review, 61*(1), 1–2. https://doi.org/10.1111/inr.12092

Kalensky, J. (2017, November 3). *More than 'minions': Nurses deserve more respect from doctors*. STAT. Retrieved September 10, 2021, from https://www.statnews.com/2017/11/03/gender-gap-health-care-nurses

Lanier, J. (2017). Feel the power. *Ohio Nurses Review, 92*(2), 6–7. Retrieved September 30, 2021, from https://www.bluetoad.com/publication/?m=&l=1&i=395562&p=6&fbclid=IwAR06VjibOBYswEyZ5GgdAt0bbU1HQDBgJzVVn8-BIJ-SoIykCuD__XuAKa8&ver=html5

Marquis, B., & Huston, C. (2021). *Leadership roles and management functions in nursing* (10th ed.). Wolters Kluwer.

Matthews, B. (2021, August 28). *Health care spending in Biden's budget*. Retrieved September 9, 2021, from https://

townhall.com/columnists/basiamatthews/2021/08/28/
health-care-spending-in-bidens-budget-n2594890

McKeown, M. (2020). Love and resistance: Re-inventing radical nurses in everyday struggles. *Journal of Clinical Nursing, 29*(7/8), 1023–1025. https://doi.org/10.1111/jocn.15084

Minnesota Organization of Registered Nurses. (2021). *The American Nurses Advocacy Institute.* Retrieved September 10, 2021, from https://www.mnorn.org/?SEC=A5968B66-911E-416E-A769-91D0536314AC

National Academy of Sciences. (2021). *The future of nursing 2020-2030.* Retrieved September 10, 2021, from https://nam.edu/publications/the-future-of-nursing-2020-2030/

Nurses on Boards Coalition. (2021). *Homepage.* Retrieved September 10, 2021, from https://www.nursesonboardscoalition.org

Nursing Power. (2021). *Invisibility, just another NP skill?* Posted by DrNurseSally on December 9, 2016. Retrieved July 16, 2020, from http://www.nursingpower.net/nursingpower/invisibility-just-another-np-skill

Rasheed, S. P., Younas, A., & Mehdi, F. (2020, July). Challenges, extent of involvement, and the impact of nurses' involvement in politics and policymaking in in last two decades: An integrative review. *Journal of Nursing Scholarship, 52*(4), 446–455. https://doi.org/10.1111/jnu.12567

Regis College. (2021). *How does nursing influence health care policy?* Retrieved September 9, 2021, from https://online.regiscollege.edu/blog/how-does-nursing-influence-health-care-policy/

Robert Wood Johnson Foundation. (2021). *Future of nursing scholars.* Retrieved September 9, 2021, from http://futureofnursingscholars.org

Senge, P. (1990). *The fifth discipline.* Doubleday/Currency.

The Nursing Organizations Alliance. (2019). *About us.* Retrieved September 9, 2021, from https://www.nursing-alliance.org

UnionFacts.com. (2021, April 8). *American Nurses Association.* Retrieved September 9, 2021, from https://www.unionfacts.com/union/American_Nurses_Association

Wikiquote. (2021, May 13). *Ginger Rogers.* Retrieved September 9, 2021, from https://en.wikiquote.org/wiki/Ginger_Rogers

Professional Identity and Image

Carol J. Huston

CHAPTER OUTLINE

LEARNING OBJECTIVES

The learner will be able to:

1. Explore the roots and prevalence of historic and contemporary nursing stereotypes, including the nurse as angel of mercy, love interest (particularly to physicians), sex bombshell/naughty nurse, handmaiden to the physician, and battle-ax, as well as the stereotype of the male nurse as being gay, effeminate, or sexually predatory.

2. Identify common public portrayals or descriptions of nurses in terms of gender, dress, and role responsibilities.

3. Examine the role that organizations such as the Center for Nursing Advocacy and Truth About Nursing

have assumed in addressing inaccurate or negative portrayals of nursing in the media and the process they use to raise public and professional awareness of the issues surrounding nursing's public image.

4. Analyze the effect of inaccurate nursing stereotypes on the profession's ability to recruit the best and brightest students to nursing, as well as on the collective identity and self-esteem of all nurses.

5. Name well-known fictional nurse characters depicted in contemporary media (television and movies) and identify the nursing stereotypes they best represent.

6. Discuss the challenges inherent in attempting to change deeply ingrained stereotypes about nursing that are likely instilled very early in childhood.

7. Analyze how a lack of uniformity in dress and the way in which nurses introduce themselves to patients may contribute to the public's confusion about who is a nurse.

8. Explore the roles and responsibilities that individual nurses, employers, professional associations, and the media have to ensure that nurses are portrayed accurately and positively to the public.

9. Identify image-building strategies that professional coalitions and corporations have used to promote recruitment and retention in nursing.

10. Reflect on the premise that every nurse controls the image of nursing.

11. Reflect on what image they would like the public to have of the nursing profession.

INTRODUCTION

An *image* can be defined as a reproduction or an imitation of something or as a mental picture or impression of something (*Merriam Webster Online Dictionary*, 2021). In other words, an image is often an unknown reality because it depends on the subjective perception of others. Perhaps that is why the public image of the nursing profession is, at times, one-dimensional and inaccurate.

If asked to describe a nurse, most of the public would use such terms as *nice*, *hardworking*, or *caring*. Indeed, a qualitative descriptive study conducted in 2018 found that from the participants' perspective, a perfect nurse should be *affable* (compassionate, sympathetic, and good-tempered), *responsive* (answering questions, answering requests), *tower of strength* (listening and being patient, understanding, and attentive), and *efficient* (providing careful care, timely care, and proper care) (Valiee et al., 2020). Being well-mannered was also extremely important.

The public would also use the terms *ethical* and *honest* to describe nurses. There is little question that the public trusts and respects nurses. In fact, nurses have ranked number one on every Gallup poll on honesty and ethics for the past 19 years (Gaines, 2021).

Few people, however, would use the terms *highly educated*, *bright*, *powerful*, *professional*, or *independent thinker* to describe a nurse. Even fewer would call the nursing profession *prestigious*. Godsey et al. (2020b) agree, noting that the nursing brand has a long and revered image with various stakeholder groups; however, current public image frequently represents nurses as caring advocates rather than influential leaders who deliver, manage, and administer health care services.

Clearly, public perceptions about the nursing profession are mixed and even contradictory at times. The public trusts and admires nurses, but this does not necessarily equate to respect or prestige. The reality is that much of the public does not understand what nurses really do.

Discussion Point

If the nursing profession is so well thought of, why are many of the brightest students encouraged to look at medicine rather than nursing? Why are there such significant differences in terms of occupational prestige and status between medicine and nursing?

Many people would, however, describe a nurse as a caring young woman, dressed in a white uniform dress, cap, and shoes, altruistically devoted to caring for the ill ("angel of mercy") under the supervision of a physician. Common job functions would be identified as making beds, passing out pills, emptying bedpans, giving shots, and helping doctors. Some people, however, would allude, at least subtly, to a lustier image of sexy young females dressed in provocative attire and seeking sexual gratification from both patients and physicians. Still others might depict stern, aged "battle-ax" females thrusting hypodermic needles into recalcitrant patients and seemingly enjoying the discomfort they cause and the power that they hold.

What do these portrayals have in common? Almost nothing and yet everything. All are part of the convoluted, often conflicting stereotypical images of nurses. In addition, all these images demean the true nature and complexity of nursing, and most are based almost entirely on fiction. Yet these stereotypes are pervasive, and efforts to change them have yielded only limited progress. The result of this public image confusion is that old stereotypes of nurses as overbearing, brainless, sexually promiscuous, and incompetent women are perpetuated, as are images of nurses as caring, hardworking, altruistic, and selfless.

This image conflict is an enduring issue for nursing, and the profession's efforts to address the problem have been fragmented and largely unsuccessful. Indeed, many nurses believe nursing's image to be one of the most important and enduring issues they face as a profession.

This chapter explores common historic and contemporary nursing stereotypes. The effect of these inaccurate stereotypes on recruitment into the profession and the collective self-esteem and identity of nurses is examined. In addition, strategies for improving the public image of nursing are presented, as are the challenges inherent in trying to change stereotypes that are ingrained in the profession's history and even in how nurses view themselves.

NURSING STEREOTYPES

Of the many nursing stereotypes, the most common ones are shown in Box 24.1: the nurse as an angel of mercy; the nurse as a love interest (particularly to physicians); the nurse as a sex bombshell or "naughty nurse;" the nurse as a handmaiden to physicians; the nurse as a battle-ax; and the male nurse as homosexual, effeminate, or sexually predatory. All these stereotypes are profiled in this chapter. In addition, contemporary nursing images as depicted in movies and on television are profiled to better identify what images of nursing are before the public, especially the young people who represent the potential future nursing workforce.

Angel of Mercy

One of the oldest and most common nursing stereotypes is that of the nurse as an angel of mercy. Some individuals suggest that the image of the nurse as an angel with wings comes from the capes nurses historically wore as part of their uniforms. When most people think of nurses as angels of mercy, the image of Florence Nightingale bringing comfort to maimed soldiers during the Crimean War comes to mind. Clearly, Florence Nightingale's legacy of caring is beyond remarkable; however, few individuals outside of nursing would recognize Nightingale as a politically astute, assertive change agent who used her knowledge of epidemiology and statistics to document the effectiveness of nursing interventions. Both images should be equally important parts of her legacy.

The nurse "angel of mercy" stereotype continues to persist today, more than 100 years after Florence Nightingale's death. Indeed, a book published by Harlequin in 2008 titled *Single Dad, Nurse Bride* details the fictional life of an orthopedic doctor, Dr. Dane Hendricks, "who is every nurse's dream—handsome and a take-charge kind of guy when it comes to medicine but also warm and humorous" (Amazon.com, 1996–2021b, para. 2). He is also wealthy. Rikki Johansen is "a conscientious nurse, taking to heart all the lessons she learned in nursing school, ... always puts others before herself and as a result, she must drive a car that doesn't always start right away" (Amazon.com, 1996–2021b, para. 4). "When Dane's brother is diagnosed with cancer and Rikki turns out to be the only bone marrow match, there is never any doubt what her choice will be" (Amazon.com, 1996–2021b, para. 8).

The Center for Nursing Advocacy (2008–2020) has suggested that such images of the nurse as an "angel" or "saint" are generally unhelpful to the profession because they "fail to convey the college-level knowledge base, critical thinking skills, and hard work required to be a nurse. This image also suggests that nurses are supernatural beings who do not require decent working conditions, adequate staffing, or a significant role in health care decision-making or policy" (para. 1).

Some individuals argue that the angel of mercy stereotype is unconsciously promoted by nurses even today—in the Nightingale pledge, for instance (Box 24.2). When one looks closely at the pledge, which originated in 1893 but is still cited frequently in nursing graduation ceremonies, it speaks of nurses forgoing their personal wants and needs

---

BOX 24.1 Common Nursing Stereotypes

1. Angel of mercy
2. Love interest (particularly to physicians)
3. Sex bombshell/naughty nurse
4. Handmaiden to the physician
5. Battle-ax
6. Male nurses as homosexual, effeminate, or sexually predatory

---

BOX 24.2 The Nightingale Pledge

I solemnly pledge myself before God and in the presence of this assembly to pass my life in purity and to practice my profession faithfully. I will abstain from whatever is deleterious and mischievous and will not take or knowingly administer any harmful drug. I will do all in my power to maintain and elevate the standard of my profession and will hold in confidence all personal matters committed to my keeping and all family affairs coming to my knowledge in the practice of my calling. With loyalty will I endeavor to aid the physician, in his work, and devote myself to the welfare of those committed to my care.

Source: Florence Nightingale. (n.d.). *The "Nightingale Pledge."* Retrieved September 9, 2021, from http://www.countryjoe .com/nightingale/pledge.htm

for the good of others. Being giving and caring in nature is a wonderful thing, but to suggest that it should be done to the extent of self-neglect is likely not the desired message.

It is important to remember, however, that being an angel of mercy is not all bad. It does encompass behaviors that many nurses typify, such as caring and dedication. Unfortunately, the angel of mercy image all too often also carries with it the idea that pay is never an issue and that suffering must be a part of the nurse's life if the role is to have value. This intrapersonal conflict between the values of altruism and pay befitting a professional is still experienced by many nurses.

Love Interest (Particularly to Physicians)

Another historic stereotype of nurses is that of a love interest, particularly to physicians. Doctor–nurse romance novels first appeared in the 1930s and 1940s, when becoming a nurse was one of the few career opportunities available to women. Nurses in these novels were generally cast as intelligent, strong women who felt fulfilled in their careers until they met the physicians who would eventually comes their husbands. Then their careers would typically end, and the nurses would live happily ever after, caring for their spouses and children.

Anthony et al. (2019) note these early novels contained nurse characters who were independent thinkers and successful at what they did—caring for patients and saving lives, but the novels glamorized nursing in some ways by including romantic relationships between the nurses and physicians.

With the women's rights movement of the 1970s, women's career opportunities expanded, and fewer books were devoted to women as nurses. In addition, readers' interest in medical romances dwindled. This is not to say that doctor–nurse romance novels do not still exist. They do, but the characters typically are different from what they were in decades past. The female character is now often a determined but compassionate physician or a charge nurse of a critical care unit in a large, urban medical center, who is beautiful. The male character, however, almost always continues to be a physician, coping with a tragedy in his past, who is "brilliant, tall, and muscular" and "with chiseled features, working in emergency medicine" ("Lovesick Doctors," 2007).

Consider This Romantic relationships between nurses and doctors abound on recent television shows as well, such as "Nurse Jackie," "Grey's Anatomy," "Chicago Med," and "The Good Doctor." It could be argued, however, that most of these relationships are not so much love interests as sexual liaisons.

Sex Bombshell/Naughty Nurse

Another common nursing stereotype is that of the nurse as a sex bombshell or "naughty nurse." The depiction of nurses in the sex and pornography industry is even more rampant than the general sexual stereotyping of nurses in the media. In fact, for at least 50 years, nurses have been portrayed as sex objects both on television and in the movies. Indeed, movies for at least six decades have been filled with images of nurses dressed provocatively, who spend most of their time fulfilling sexual fantasies and virtually no time providing care to patients.

Nurses are even depicted as sex objects in television commercials. In 2003, Clairol Herbal Essences shampoo launched a commercial that showed a nurse abandoning her patient to wash her hair in his bathroom and then tossing her hair sensually at the patient as she left the room. Many nurses and nursing organizations condemned the unprofessional stereotype perpetuated in the ad and asked sponsor Procter & Gamble to discontinue it (Clinical Rounds, 2003). Procter & Gamble did issue an apology to nurses and pulled the ad, stating that the company "holds the nursing profession in the highest esteem" (p. 35).

Discussion Point

Do you think that the public truly believes that a nurse would abandon patient care duties to wash her hair in a patient's bathroom and then sensually shake her hair at the patient? If not, does the commercial still cause harm?

Another commercial sexualizing nurses was launched in September 2007 by Cadbury Schweppes Canada for Dentyne gum (Truth About Nursing, 2007). The Cadbury Schweppes ads showed female nurses being lured into bed with male patients the instant the male patients popped Dentyne into their mouths. The tag line for the commercial was "Get Fresh," and the message was that when hospitalized patients used Dentyne products, there would be an instant, erotic reaction from the "always available" bedside nurse.

More than 1,000 protest letters were sent from the website of the Registered Nurses Association of Ontario (RNAO) in response to the Cadbury Schweppes commercial (Truth About Nursing, 2007). Another 500 supporters from the Center for Nursing Advocacy wrote letters to top Cadbury Schweppes executives, leaving long messages explaining that such imagery reinforces a stereotype of workplace sexual availability that contributes to the global nursing crisis. Initially, the company responded that its ads were causing no harm. On October 6, 2007, however, the company told the Center and RNAO that it would pull the ads and consult nurses in creating future U.S. and Canadian ads that involved nurses.

Another more recent example of the perpetuation of the naughty nurse stereotype became apparent when the *Heart Attack Grill*, a theme restaurant in Arizona, began dressing their waitresses in naughty nurse uniforms, which included micro miniskirts, fishnet stockings, and high heels. Because nurses are already a highly sexually fantasized profession, the Center for Nursing Advocacy asked the Heart Attack Grill to reconsider their uniform choice when the restaurant opened in 2006. The Grill's owner, Jon Basso, who calls himself "Dr. Jon" and works in a medical lab coat, refused. In November 2011, a peaceful rally was held in front of the restaurant to protest the image of nursing being presented (Truth About Nursing, 2011). Rally supporters argued that the Heart Attack Grill was reinforcing stereotypes that discouraged practicing and potential nurses (especially men), fostered sexual violence in the workplace, and contributed to a general atmosphere of disrespect that weakened nurses' claims to adequate resources.

In addition, the State Board of Nursing filed a complaint with the Arizona Attorney General's office that Basso was illegally using the term *nurse* in advertising for his restaurant (Arizona Statute A.R.S. 32–1636 states only someone who has a valid nursing license can use the title "nurse"). The Attorney General sent Basso a letter informing him that he was illegally using the word "nurse" at his restaurant and on his website. Basso's response was a refusal to remove the word "nurse" from his website, but he did agree to insert an asterisk next to every nurse reference and to include a disclaimer that none of the women pictured on the website actually had any medical training or provide any real medical services (Truth About Nursing, 2011).

Discussion Point

Do you feel that the uniform policy at Heart Attack Grill is simply good fun, or does it denigrate the nursing profession and sexualize nursing?

Even more recently, in October 2014, Subway launched a television ad that used a naughty nurse costume, among others, to encourage U.S. customers to dine at the sandwich chain (Truth About Nursing, 2014a). In the ad, a young female office worker urged two colleagues not to eat burgers for lunch, but instead to emulate her Subway choices, because Halloween was coming and they had to "stay in shape for all the costumes!" She proceeded to demonstrate, donning a quick series of mostly naughty costumes that she helpfully labeled as "attractive nurse ... spicy Red Riding Hood ... Viking princess warrior ... hot devil ... sassy teacher

... and foxy fullback!" "The nurse outfit wasn't the naughtiest ever, but it was a ridiculously short, flimsy dress" (Truth About Nursing, 2014a, para. 8).

And more recently, a study by McAllister et al. (2018) of the Gothic imaging of nurses in popular culture found that the types of transgressive love nurses expressed to patients ranged from the obsessive and the pornographic to the monstrous. The authors concluded that this illuminates a hidden reality that nursing work that is at once intimate and personal but also hidden, profane, repellent, horrifying, and feared. They also argued that it helps to explain phenomena—including nursing itself—which exist in the shadow of dominant and often stereotyped discourses.

Handmaiden to the Physician

Perhaps the most pervasive stereotype of nurses, however, is that of handmaiden to physicians. In the handmaiden role, the nurse simply serves as an adoring backdrop to the omnipotent physician, demonstrating little, if any, independent thought or action. Certainly, this image is perhaps the most common image perpetuated on contemporary television and movie screens.

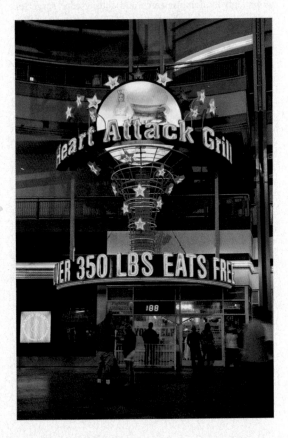

The image, however, is not new. This view of nurses as a handmaiden to physicians was reported in classic research by Philip and Beatrice Kalisch, in the 1970s, a time when nurses generally had no substantial role in television stories and were a part of the hospital background in programs that focused on physician characters. When nurses were the focus of a program, the storyline frequently involved the nurse's personal problems rather than their role as a nurse, and attributes such as obedience, permissiveness, conformity, flexibility, and serenity were emphasized.

Sometimes, though, even health care employers perpetuate this image, even if unintentionally. For example, in 2014, the Baylor Health Care System ran a television ad based on the idea that its employees were faithful "servants" (Truth About Nursing, 2014b). The 1-minute ad featured many apparent nurses in clinical settings, intending to show them in a positive light. But many nurses objected to being presented as "servants." And the nurse scenes in the ad "emphasized what seem to be the most unskilled tasks with which nurses are associated, including hand-holding, mopping brows, wheeling gurneys, changing 'hearts' and sheets, and picking things up off the floor" (para. 13). Meanwhile, apparent physicians in the ad acted as servants by doing research and cutting-edge surgeries and changing minds. Truth About Nursing suggested that "the servanthood theme may hold some appeal as a matter of spirituality or marketing, but it's dangerous to apply to a traditionally female profession that has struggled to overcome the notion that it simply serves physicians and to get respect for its advanced education and skills" (Truth About Nursing, 2014b, para. 13).

> **Consider This** Nursing care is frequently perceived by the public as simple and unskilled.

Many commercial representations of nurses also continue to represent the stereotype of the nurse as a handmaiden. For example, in spring 2008, the Angela Moore jewelry catalog featured "Nurse Nancy" bracelets and necklaces. According to Truth About Nursing (2008), the jewelry was composed of four different types of balls; one ball featured a smiling, rosy-cheeked nurse in white uniform and cap giving a balloon to a girl; the second ball had a ladybug next to a stethoscope; the third ball featured a nurse's cap with a thermometer; and the fourth ball had a stuffed bear holding flowers next to a lollipop. The text in the catalog "asked readers to buy the Nurse Nancy jewelry to celebrate the ladies who give lollipops and band aids a whole new meaning" (Truth About Nursing, 2008, para. 1).

In response to letters of concern from nurses, the jewelry maker did agree to modify the description of the jewelry. According to Truth About Nursing (2008), however, what they changed it to was "Here's a special theme to celebrate the wonderful women who promote health and make us feel so much better. Talented, terrific and leaders to love!" (para. 3). Truth About Nursing (2008) suggested that "while this was probably an improvement over lollipops and band aids" (para. 4), it was still problematic in that it suggested that only women are nurses. In addition, they argued that "statements such as 'makes us feel so much better,' 'leaders to love,' and 'wonderful women' sound like adoration for someone's loving mom who makes them feel so much better by making them soup or tea" (Truth About Nursing, 2008, para. 5), not that nurses are highly trained health care professionals who use both science and art to make a difference in their patients' outcomes.

Even more distressing, however, was the February 24, 2017, suggestion of Nobel Prize winning economist Paul Krugman that nurses were one example of those who perform "menial work dealing with the physical world." When nursing advocacy groups urged Krugman to publicly apologize, he did so, explaining that nursing does deal with the physical work and has "manual" elements, but that it is not "menial" work. This type of uninformed stereotyping in influential media, however, is part of what perpetuates the undervaluation of the profession (Truth About Nursing, 2017c).

Battle-Ax

Few stereotypes in nursing are as dark or demented, however, as that of the nurse as a battle-ax. The battle-ax stereotype often depicts an overbearing, unhappy, mean, senior nurse who intimidates both patients and staff. The movie *One Flew Over the Cuckoo's Nest* (1975) provides a perfect example of the battle-ax. Nurse Ratched, a nurse in a mental hospital, fits the description of a battle-ax in almost every way—craving power and control over others, and forcing her patients to obey her every whim or suffer the repercussions.

Nurse Diesel, in the movie *High Anxiety* (1978), was another stereotypical battle-ax nurse, with the addition of enormous prosthetic breasts. As an overbearing, evil charge nurse, Nurse Diesel continually displayed a dark sneer and a love of domination. Annie Wilkes from the novel and movie *Misery* also gave new meaning to the sociopathic battle-ax nurse as she kidnapped, maimed, and held hostage a writer she admired and wanted to be close to. Similarly, the book *Doctors and Nurses* (Amazon.com, 1996–2021a) depicts Jen, a significantly obese nurse who partners (both sexually and career wise) with her married physician boss to kill their patients. Jen's appetite for food, sex, and violence is whetted when her physician boyfriend happily scams patients and shrugs off lawsuit-worthy mistakes.

Battle-ax stereotypes of nurses have always existed; however, they seemed to hit their peak in the 1970s and 1980s. There are, however, still multiple images of battle-ax nurses available on the internet and even contemporary television. Producer Ryan Murphy and Netflix announced plans to revive the Nurse Ratched character from *One Flew Over the Cuckoo's Nest* for 18 episodes on Netflix (Otterson, 2019).

In addition, a mixed methods study by Stanley et al. (2019) found that 115 of the 485 zombie-focused films produced or coproduced in the United States between 1900 and 2018, were identified with health professionals. Of these, 27 featured nurses, 10 with nurses in the main role. Nurses were portrayed as romantic, sexualized, caring, self-sacrificial, strong, or evil, but the overarching representation of nurses in zombie films was tied to the depravity from which the zombie subculture is based.

It is also of interest that the battle-ax counterpart of male physicians in medicine is viewed less negatively. For example, the television show *House* featured a drug-addicted, rule-breaking, rude, and crude male physician whose bad behavior was excused by his brilliance and ability to often cure patients when all hope was lost.

The Male Nurse: Gay, Effeminate, or Sexually Predatory

Female nurses are not the only ones who are stereotyped. Male nurse stereotypes are at least as prevalent as those for females, which only adds to the difficulty of recruiting men to the profession. Indeed, Lamey (2021) notes that the stigma against men entering nursing is unfair and widespread, and for aspiring male nurses, stereotypes are often a deterrent to pursuing a worthwhile career. Pompilio (2020) agrees, citing a recent study in which 70% of respondents cited stereotypes as a major challenge to recruiting men into nursing.

One stereotype perpetuated for male nurses is being homosexual or effeminate. Indeed, a recent qualitative descriptive study revealed that male graduate nursing students identified two predominant gender scripts: nursing as women's work and male nurses as gay (Jamieson et al., 2019). This resulted in ambivalence or resistance to social context masculinity and active engagement in undoing gender stereotypes. The researchers concluded that the same stereotype-induced barriers to men's engagement in nursing, identified and discussed since the 1960s, remain potent today.

Male nurses may also be stereotyped as being hypersexual and, as a result, the intent of their actions may be questioned as being either sexual in nature or, in some cases, even sexually predatory. Indeed, male nurses may have to address the issue of female patients misinterpreting their actions as sexual assault even when what the nurse has done does not warrant such blame (Nurse Buff, 2020). This makes it difficult for male nurses to demonstrate the caring, therapeutic interactions that are such an important part of nursing.

> *Consider This* Many male nurses fear how their caring actions might be interpreted.

Another popular stereotype for male nurses is that they are nonachievers for going into nursing rather than more traditionally male occupations. This was certainly the case in the 2000 movie *Meet the Parents*. Unfortunately, despite the protestations of Greg Focker, the male registered nurse (RN) in the movie, that he loved nursing and became a nurse by choice, his future in-laws and other relatives constantly questioned his sexual orientation and manliness. They also clearly implied that Greg must have become a nurse because his test scores were not high enough for him to qualify for medical school, which was not the case.

Clearly, men face multiple gender-based barriers in nursing, including lack of history about men in nursing, a lack of male role models, role strain, gender discrimination, and isolation. In addition, finding and staying on the path of nursing presents unique challenges for men. "Men in Nursing" (2020) notes that the recommendations for attracting and recruiting more men to the profession are usually directed at nursing schools, but male nurses can also play a role in improving gender equality in nursing by seeking careers as nurse educators and becoming nurse mentors.

How Ingrained Are Nursing Stereotypes?

Increasingly, researchers are concluding that inaccurate and negative stereotypes of nurses are not only well ingrained but also instilled early in life. Indeed, gender stereotyping about career opportunities begins at an early age. By 3 years, most children already have firmly rooted gender-based ideas about the roles they can and should hold when they grow up.

The reality, then, is that by the end of middle school, most students report having their minds made up about desirable and undesirable careers. An unpublished study by Huston (Research Fuels the Controversy 24.1) suggested that basic beliefs and stereotypes about professions such as nursing may be ingrained at a far younger age, and that waiting until fifth, sixth, or even seventh grade to address inaccurate or negative images of nursing might be too late. Clearly, an early positive image for students is important if this is the population group the profession hopes will solve the current shortage.

Research Fuels the Controversy 24.1

Second-Graders' Image of Nurses

This unpublished study examined stereotypes held by 25 second-graders regarding "important" nursing roles and functions. In an effort to introduce students to nonhospital nursing roles, which students stated they already knew, a 30-minute slide show and discussion were held showing nurses actively engaged in less traditional nursing roles such as cardiac rehabilitation, primary care, flight nursing, education, management, and public health. In addition, nurse practitioners were introduced as primary care providers. Students were shown photos of nurses in all types of garb, except for white uniforms. Efforts were made to ensure ethnic and gender diversity in all presentation materials. At the conclusion of the presentation, students were asked to draw a picture of what they thought was the most exciting role that had been presented for nurses.

Source: Huston, C. (n.d.). Nursing stereotypes ingrained by second grade. Unpublished manuscript.

Study Findings

The caption on the first drawing was "the nurse is doing surgery on a real important disease." In the second, the nurse, with a red cross on her white uniform, was noted to be "rushing" into the hospital. In the third, the nurse, in her white starched cap, was making up a hospital bed. In the fourth drawing, the nurse was giving a hospitalized patient a backrub. In another, a dour nurse, as denoted by a capital N on her starched white cap with a red cross on it, was entering a hospital nursery. In the sixth, a patient in a bed was hooked up to an intravenous line, expressing pain. The smiling nurse was walking away from him.

In the seventh drawing, the nurse was helping the child in the hospital bed, and it included a caption that the "nurse is in a rush." In another drawing, nurses were scurrying to patients in their hospital beds. Rushing, for nurses, was a recurrent theme.

In the eighth drawing, the most exciting role for a nurse was noted as transporting a cot from room to room. Similarly, another student noted that the most important thing a nurse did was to transport people to the operating room, and yet another student noted that transporting patients in wheelchairs to their cars was the most important thing that nurses did.

Several drawings included stern nurses in white uniforms and caps and with red crosses on their chests making patients take medicine that tasted bad. Others depicted nurses working in nurseries or teaching mothers how to care for a crying baby. Another depicted a flight nurse taking an injured patient to the hospital, and yet another showed a nurse, in a white uniform with a red cross on her chest and wearing a cap, taking blood pressures.

All of the nurses in the drawings were female and White. The overwhelming majority wore white uniforms and caps and had red crosses on their chests. All but one drawing depicted nurses in hospital settings. Many associated the nurse with pain or an unpleasant experience. Despite the educational intervention, these second-graders already held deeply ingrained stereotypes about nursing and nursing roles, which were resistant to change. This suggests that if stereotypes are this difficult to modify in second-graders, the challenges in changing the image of nursing with the greater public will likely be very difficult.

Contemporary Nursing Stereotypes on Television

Television medical dramas currently provide the greatest number of visual images of nurses at work. There is little doubt, however, that television medical dramas build on traditional stereotypes of nurses, as well as suggest new ones. One of the best-known medical dramas in the past few decades with strong nurse figures was *ER* (1994–2009). This medical drama focused on the lives and events of the emergency department (ED) staff at County General Hospital in Chicago, a level I trauma center.

The character Carol Hathaway was perhaps the best-known nurse on *ER*. After surviving the September 1994 pilot episode in which she tried to commit suicide, Hathaway became the charge nurse of the ED. She went on to have a sexual relationship with a physician and bore twins out of wedlock. Nurse Hathaway left the show in 1999—to join her physician love interest in another state.

Even with the departure of Nurse Hathaway, *ER* continued to provide influential portrayals of nurses on television. One of the highest profile nurses remaining on the show was Abby Lockhart, an alcoholic and a former obstetric nurse from a family afflicted with bipolar disorder. She started on the show as a medical student, dropped out of medical school, worked as a nurse, and then became a doctor. Abby had sexual relationships with several doctors on the show and eventually married one of them.

In addition, Samantha Taggart, a nurse who joined the staff in 2003, was a tough, free-spirited, single mother of an emotionally troubled child, who almost immediately began a sexual relationship with one of the physicians. In her introductory scene, "Sam" (who had come to the hospital inquiring about employment) grabbed a syringe and leaped to sedate an unruly patient through a central vessel in his neck. This behavior earned her not only a job but also the respect of her soon-to-be coworkers.

Another long-standing TV show to stir nurses to action is *Grey's Anatomy* (2005–present). Physician characters on this show provide all the direct patient care as well as the emotional support of the patient and family. Indeed, in the 2017 lineup of its 15 regular characters, every single one was a surgeon (Truth About Nursing, 2017b). Nurses held only trivial roles.

Similarly, nurses on NBC's show *The Night Shift* (2013–2017) were "mostly there to carry out physician commands. In general, the physicians ran the ED, performed the complex life-saving procedures, and provided the patient advocacy and support. They also did some physician nursing, handling tasks that nurses are more likely to do in real life" (Truth About Nursing, 2017a, para. 1). A similar invisibility of nursing characters exists on the hit series *The Good Doctor* (2017–present).

One of the most alarming contemporary visualizations of a nurse on TV, however, was *Nurse Jackie* (2009–2015). The title character Jackie Peyton was a drug-addicted nurse who worked in the emergency ward at All Saints' Hospital in New York City. Jackie often made unethical and illegal decisions for the "good" of her patients, such as forging organ donor authorizations. In addition, although married, she often had sex with the pharmacist at the hospital in exchange for drugs. In season 2, her drug addiction led her to falsify a magnetic resonance imaging to get a phony prescription and to rip off a local drug dealer who embarked on revenge. Eventually, Jackie's addictions deepened to the point at which she stole drugs from the oncology unit. When her theft was discovered, she was placed on probation by her employer, but a sympathetic colleague in the lab perpetuated her employment by discarding her next contaminated urine drug test. In addition, Jackie was a "world class liar," particularly about her addictions, and alienated almost everyone in her life (Truth About Nursing, 2015).

Perhaps what is most disturbing about *Nurse Jackie* was the attention this utterly dislikable nurse character received solely because of her independent and strong-willed thinking. The reality is that this was a drug-addicted nurse who had little regard for any codes of ethics or the patients she was charged to care for. Her primary mission in life and at work was to attain the drugs she needed to fuel an ever-increasing addiction, and this was often at the expense of patients.

Finally, the May 20, 2014, segment of *Inside Amy Schumer* (Comedy Central), presented four female "RN" characters in patterned scrubs embodying the unskilled physician handmaiden, the naughty nurse/physician gold digger, the backward female serf, and the petty, rule-bound battle-ax (Truth About Nursing, 2018). The first sketch indicated that the practical health advice that nurses deliver is in fact silly or dangerous, since it is delusional for nurses to think they may know more than physicians. The second sketch had the nurse proclaim that although the audience no doubt wanted to hear from physicians, it was going to have to "settle for the unsung heroes who do all the real work. The nurse went on to say that her statement was bogus, because nurses are as far from heroic hard workers as you can get. And the final segment indicated that nurses were helpless to address serious injuries they encountered outside the clinical setting" (Truth About Nursing, 2018).

Yet, there are some positive representations of nurses on contemporary television shows. Shows like *Chicago Med*, *Code Black*, *The Defenders*, *Big Hero 6*, and *Virgin River* offer glimpses of nursing skill, advocacy, and (more rarely) autonomy. In *Code Black*, Latino "senior ER nurse" Jesse Sallander, greeted each new class of physician interns by announcing possessively that he was their "mama" and that they were not "smarter than their mama because you have an MD." He also managed ED logistics, called out vitals, described symptoms, provided psychosocial care, and at times even suggested courses of action and diagnoses (Truth About Nursing, 2017b).

In addition, there are three notable nurse characters on *Chicago Med*, all Black women. All three demonstrate some original thought and risk taking, although the show still spends as much time on their romantic lives and other personal issues as it does on their nursing skill (Truth About Nursing, 2017b). More positive contemporary representations of skilled professional nurses are needed on contemporary television.

The Image of Nursing on the Internet

The internet is also filled with images of nurses, some accurate and some stereotypical. A recent review of nurse images on Google found thousands of inappropriate images of nurses. Many were sexually suggestive as well as demeaning. Some were in caricature, but many were of young women dressed in cleavage-baring uniforms, wearing fishnet stockings, high heels, and garter belts.

Even YouTube includes numerous stereotypical and distorted images. A 2012 study of the most viewed videos for "nurses" and "nursing" on YouTube suggested that nurses were depicted in three main ways—as a skilled knower and doer, as a sexual plaything, and as a witless incompetent (American Association for the Advancement of Science, 2021). The 10 most viewed videos reflected a variety of media, including promotional videos, advertising, excerpts from a TV sitcom, and a cartoon. Some texts dramatized, caricatured, and parodied nurse–patient and interprofessional encounters. Four of the 10 clips, however, were posted by nurses and presented images of them as educated, smart, and technically skilled. They included nurses being interviewed, dancing, and performing a rap song, all of which portrayed nursing as a valuable and rewarding career. The nurses were shown as a distinct professional group working in busy clinical hospitals, where their knowledge and skills counted.

Finally, nurses should recognize that media stereotypes are not limited to nonprofessional sources. Even advertisements in medical and nursing journals often include stereotypical and demeaning nursing images, with frequent depictions of nurses as dependent, passive minor figures on the health care scene. If nurses are not depicted accurately in their own trade publications, how can they expect representation in other types of media to be better?

THE CENTER FOR NURSING ADVOCACY AND TRUTH ABOUT NURSING

Most nurses are upset about their depiction in contemporary media, but their efforts to respond to and change the situation have been fragmented. A more unified voice became possible with the creation of the Center for Nursing Advocacy in 2001. The center was created when Sandy Summers and seven other graduate nursing students at the Johns Hopkins University in Baltimore joined forces to address the media's disrespectful portrayal of nursing.

In 2009, the center was dissolved because of legal wrangling around record keeping and allegations of unpaid taxes. Sandy Summers then set up a new organization, called *Truth About Nursing*, a 501(c)(3) nonprofit organization that seeks to increase public understanding of the central, frontline role nurses play in modern health care, to promote more accurate, balanced, and frequent media portrayals of nurses, and to increase the media's use of nurses as expert sources (Truth About Nursing, 2008–2020). "The Truth About Nursing's ultimate goal is to foster growth in the size and diversity of the nursing profession at a time of critical shortage, strengthen nursing practice, teaching and research, and improve the health care system" (2008-2020, para. 1).

CONSEQUENCES OF INACCURATE OR NEGATIVE IMAGES

Inaccurate or negative public images of nursing have many consequences, particularly because these images influence the attitudes of patients, other health care providers, policy makers, and politicians. They even influence how nurses think about themselves. When someone becomes a nurse, they take on the identity as well as the values and norms of their profession, so inaccurate or undesirable images negatively impact professional self-identity.

Inaccurate or negative images can also influence funding. When decision makers don't understand the value of nursing, they don't fund it. Nursing residencies in the United States receive almost no support compared with physician residency programs. Perhaps even more critical is that negative attitudes about nursing might discourage capable prospective nurses, who will instead choose another career that offers greater appeal in stature, status, and salary.

> **Consider This** Many nurses hold stereotypes about the profession to be true, just as the general public does.

Image-Related Recruitment and Retention Challenges

As with other predominantly female professions, the literature suggests that many patients and their families undervalue nursing and do not understand what it is that nurses do that makes a difference in patient outcomes. Indeed, many nurses will honestly admit that they had little factual basis for what nursing would be like when they chose it as a profession. Instead, what drove them to become nurses were images that emphasized the caring, nurturing, and personal rewards associated with the profession.

Understanding why individuals choose nursing as a career is important. Stereotypical imaging and messaging of the nursing profession shape nurses' expectations and perceptions of nursing as a career, which has implications for both recruitment and retention.

Indeed, a study by Glerean et al. (2019) found that nursing school applicants described using media such as the internet, magazines, and radio and TV series to find information about the nursing profession. However, the media's image of nursing was reported as being negative. This same study found that the historic virtuous caregiver image of the nurse was still prevalent in the applicants' descriptions and that the independence of the nursing profession from medicine was not recognized. Glerean and colleagues (2019) concluded that to prevent misperceptions guiding a career choice in nursing, the nurse image needs to be updated to one that underlines the knowledge, skills, and expertise and recognizes the multiple roles and tasks of the nurse and the independent nature of the profession.

In addition, to recruit young people into the profession, the drug company Johnson & Johnson (J&J) began a series of television advertisements in 2002 as a part of its

Campaign for Nursing's Future. Ads have been released since that time, highlighting different aspects of nursing practice and promotion of diversity in nursing. Recent ads are encompassing and include a website dedicated to promoting men in nursing, with career resources as related reading that emphasize challenges faced by minority male nurses as well as the pride engendered because of being a nurse (Johnson & Johnson, 2021).

CHANGING NURSING'S IMAGE IN THE PUBLIC EYE

Changing nursing's image in the public eye will not be easy, nor will there be a silver bullet. Instead, multiple strategies are needed, including active interaction with the media and restriction of the term *nurse* to licensed nurses. In addition, nurses must increase their efforts to publicly praise and value nursing in addition to emphasizing how nursing uniquely contributes to patients achieving their desired health outcomes. Finally, nurses will need to become even more involved in the political processes that shape their profession.

Accomplishing this will take time and resources, including the time, energy, and funding of coalitions, foundations, and professional nursing organizations. Perhaps most important, it will take a concerted effort by individual nurses that will come only by first recognizing that there is a need to take action and then by doing what is necessary to achieve that goal. Carlson (2017, para. 16) notes that "Florence Nightingale was not a fading Victorian violet who avoided a fight. Rather, she was a disrupter, a change agent, a nurse who used her mind and heart to initiate change in the interest of the health and wellbeing of those she felt called to serve." Nurses today must view the call to change their public image in the same manner.

Indeed, global interest in changing nursing's image is increasing. In February 2018, the Duchess of Cambridge joined nurses and other health leaders across the world in launching a 3-year global campaign (2018–2020) aimed at raising the profile and status of nursing ("Nursing Now Campaign," 2018). This *Nursing Now* campaign recognizes that nurses are at the heart of countries' efforts to provide health for all. The Duchess joined the World Health Organization's chief nursing officer, the president of the International Council of Nurses, health leaders, and nurses from countries around the world calling on governments, health professionals, and service users to value nurses and champion their leadership in providing the best quality of care ("Nursing Now Campaign," 2018).

Similarly, the World Health Organization (WHO) designated 2020 as the *International Year of the Nurse and the Midwife* in recognition of the 200th anniversary of Florence Nightingale's birth and 2021 as the *Covid-19 & International Year of the Health and Care Workers* (International Council of Nurses [ICN], 2021). In addition, WHO (2020) released the *State of the World's Nursing Report* in May 2020 to provide the latest, most up-to-date evidence on and policy options for the global nursing workforce and to present a compelling case for considerable—yet feasible—investment in nursing education, jobs, and leadership. WHO was a partner on the *State of the World's Midwifery 2020 Report*, which was launched around the same time as the State of the *World's Nursing Report* (Swanson, 2020).

Finding a Voice in the Press

One of the most important strategies needed to change nursing's image is to change the image of nursing in the mind of the image makers. That means proactively seeking positive and accurate media exposure of what nursing really is and what nurses really do. Dr. MarySue Heilemann (School of Nursing, University of Wisconsin-Madison, 2017) agrees, noting that while unrealistic nurse characters can misrepresent health care, other relatable nurse characters can be part of innovative and effective interventions with patients. "The media is influential, and inaccurate portrayals of nurses and nursing do a disservice not only to the profession but also to the patients seeking care" (School of Nursing, University of Wisconsin-Madison, 2017, para. 9).

Stephanie Sauvinet, a nurse and published fiction writer, agrees, noting that "Nurses should definitely advocate for realistic representation of their profession. Holding writers and producers accountable for what they put on screen, demanding the use of expert consultants, and encouraging accuracy over drama are just a few ways to do this" (Pirschel, 2018, para. 16).

Finding a voice in the press, however, cannot be left to professional nursing organizations or to the image makers. Nursing's contributions need to be recognized and proclaimed. Unfortunately, many nurses feel ill-prepared or lack the self-confidence to interact with the media. Knowing how to interact with the media is not intuitive for most nurses. Media training should always be provided to give nurses the skills and self-confidence to be effective in this role.

Benjamin (2020), a nursing media expert, agrees, noting that nurses are primed with the knowledge and clinical expertise to deliver important health information using mainstream media, including television, radio, and print, as well as the internet. She suggests, however, that the media puts the audience in a passive role to receive information, which is not how nurses typically communicate with patients and family, so some training is needed. This training prepares nurses to speak succinctly and address important points while being mindful of the Health Insurance Portability and Accountability Act.

> *Consider This* Far too few nurses are both willing and appropriately trained to interact with the media.

Instead of being fearful of the media, nurses should view media as an opportunity to expose the difficulties encountered in the profession as well as more accurate stories about what nurses do and the difference they make in the lives of the populations they serve. Nurses are uniquely qualified to speak with editors, reporters, and media producers on topics related to health care because they have a view from the front lines and can localize national health care issues. Nurses are also well qualified to simplify medical terminology, explain the latest health care research, and identify current trends. Nurses, then, must be taught the basic skills necessary to self-confidently interact with the media. Nurses must also never pass up the opportunity to work with the media and should always view the media as playing a critical role in changing nursing's image.

Salem (2019) agrees, noting that nurses have the chance to "rectify their torn image" by first improving their public involvements and communicating their professionalism over the media. He notes that nurses also need to engage in major public events and discussions that pertain to health matters. Such involvement would convince the public of their professional capabilities and knowledge.

Tips for interacting with the media are shown in Box 24.3.

> *Consider This* Nurses are experts in health care. Their invisibility in the media is likely a result of nurses lacking the basic skills and self-confidence to get involved, not that the media does not want to talk to nurses.

Reclaiming the Title of "Nurse"

Another strategy needed to improve the image of nursing is to ensure that the use of the term *nurse* is limited to licensed nurses. The ICN (2012) reaffirmed in 2012 that the term "nurse" "should be protected by law and applied to and used only by those legally authorized to practice the full scope of nursing" (para. 1). In addition, all state boards of nursing have passed legislation restricting unlicensed personnel from using the title of "nurse." Unfortunately, on a regular basis, nursing aides and attendants either intentionally or unintentionally misrepresent themselves as nurses.

With the increased use of unlicensed assistive personnel and cross-training, a blurring of titles, roles, and responsibilities has occurred among RNs, licensed vocational nurses, and unlicensed support staff. Nametags increasingly recognized all staff as "care partners" or "associates," and some hospitals went so far as to prohibit the listing of RN on a name tag. At the same time, a loss of differentiated uniforms further adds to the public's confusion about who is truly caring for them. In addition, the media frequently perpetuates the inappropriate use of the term "nurse" by referring to all nurse's aides, volunteers who do health-related work, and medical assistants as "nurses."

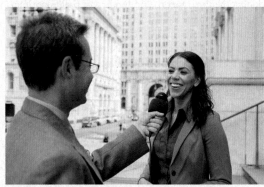

(DW labs Incorporated/Shutterstock)

BOX 24.3   **Tips for Interacting With the Media**

1. Be well informed about the topic.
2. Decide ahead of time what two to three key points you want to make and stay on track with the message.
3. Keep answers short, clear, and concise.
4. Stick to what you know and don't be pressured to answer questions you lack expertise in.
5. Talk in lay terms so that the public you want to reach understands your message.
6. Do not overestimate the reporter's expertise on the topic; be prepared to offer background information if necessary.
7. Remember that nothing is "off the record."
8. Be honest and friendly.
9. Respond immediately to media inquiries for interview since reporters are typically on short deadlines.
10. Be confident that you as a nurse are an expert on many issues consumers need and want to know.

In addition, RNs often contribute to the confusion by how they introduce themselves to patients. Nurses are often very casual when introducing themselves to patients, rarely identifying their specific role as the leader of the health care team. Nor do they explain how the roles of other members of the health care team differ. This may be due in part to typical female role socialization, which encourages women not to promote themselves, or it may be part of a team-building effort. Either way, patients end up confused about who the leader of the team is or how their roles differ.

Jacobs-Summers and Jacobs-Summers (2011) urge nurses to project a professional image in all interactions. They suggest that when nurses meet patients, they introduce themselves as a nurse and include their surname as professionals do. This introduction should not be perceived as cold or formal; instead, it demonstrates respect and pride in the profession.

Jacobs-Summers and Jacobs-Summers (2011) also encourage "nursing out loud." "This means describing more of what you're thinking while you're providing care, consistent with patient confidentiality and sensitivity. If you do, then patients, families, physician colleagues and others will get a better sense of your education and skill" (Jacobs-Summers & Jacobs-Summers, 2011, para. 5).

Dressing as Professionals

Nurses in this country began shedding their white uniforms in the 1960s as part of the anti-conformist movement. As a result, the identity of the RN may be blurred. Whereas nursing caps and white starched uniforms were often impractical in caring for acutely ill patients, 60 years ago, the public knew who the nurse was by the uniform they wore.

Today, many patients are unable to tell the members of the health care team apart, a problem that has become worse as the result of widespread adoption of scrubs as work uniforms. In addition, a study by Pawłowski et al. (2019) found that for hospitalized patients, the nursing dress code affects the level of trust in those who care for them. It also constituted an important element in assessing their professionalism, knowledge, or confidence when performing specific medical interventions. Pawłowski and team (2019) concluded that there is a relationship between the external appearance of nurses and their professional image and the patients' perception of their professional skills as well as the level of their professionalism.

Some nurse leaders have suggested that a return to white uniforms would restore the public's perception of nursing's professionalism. Nurses themselves, however, are split on the issue of whether uniforms are essential to maintaining professionalism in nursing. They argue that comfort and uniformity of dress are equally important and that uniforms

are not a requirement for professional trust and respect. But it is likely naive to believe that how nurses dress does not impact their perceived image or professionalism.

> **Consider This** Is it the white uniform that makes the professional, or is it the actions nurses take that define a nurse's professionalism?

Positive Talk by Nurses About Nursing

Another strategy for improving the image of nursing is to change how nurses talk about nursing to others. Some nurses disparage the profession and discourage young adults from considering nursing as a profession yet go on to bemoan the current nurse shortage. The effect of these comments by nurses on the public should not be underestimated in terms of their effect on the recruitment of young people into the profession.

The reality is that every nurse controls the image of nursing. Nursing, like any other profession, has strengths and weaknesses. It is important, however, that nurses enjoy their work, whatever it might be. Nurses should not stay in jobs that make them unhappy, because it demoralizes everyone around them. Whining and acting like a victim does little to improve the situation.

The bottom line is that nurses must be ambassadors for the profession and tell the public that nursing is an essential service with equal worth to other professions, that it can provide many services more effectively than other health care disciplines, and that nursing is often more cost-effective than other disciplines. The public's demand for nursing likely rests on the demand nursing creates for itself in the public's eye.

Recently published research by Godsey et al. (2020a) concurs, noting that nurses have a unique opportunity to identify the values they wish to convey (and not convey) through their brand image, and to set about purposely developing that brand. Godsey et al. (2020a) also note that most nurses believe they have not put enough effort into creating and maintaining their image, leaving the job to others by default. The researchers concluded that practitioners, educators, administrators, and labor leaders could help shape the image portrayed by the profession in many ways, but nursing needs to take the lead and direct its own future (Research Fuels the Controversy 24.2).

Emphasizing the Uniqueness of Nursing

Another tactic nurses can use to improve nursing's image is not only to emphasize the profession's unique combination of "caring" and "curing" but also to underscore the depth and breadth of the scientific perspective that underlies its

Research Fuels the Controversy 24.2

Nurses' Perceptions of the Brand Image of Nursing

The sample consisted of RN respondents (*n* = 286) from two groups: (a) alumni of a private university in the Midwest who received a bachelor of science (BS) or master of science (MS) degree in nursing (*n* = 152), and (b) a national sample of nursing faculty with graduate degrees (MS or doctoral preparation) from a private Jesuit collegiate network (*n* = 134). Each group was purposely recruited because of their membership as alumni or faculty in this network. Three in-person and webinar focus group sessions were conducted with participants asked to describe their perceptions of the brand image of nursing.

Source: Godsey, J. A., Houghton, D. M., & Hayes, T. (2020, November/December). Registered nurse perceptions of factors contributing to the inconsistent brand image of the nursing profession. *Nursing Outlook, 68*(6), 808–821. https://doi.org/10.1016/j.outlook.2020.06.005

Study Findings

Many respondents expressed concern that the image of nursing portrayed in television shows, in movies, and on the internet contributed to the profession's inconsistent image. The impact of mass media was felt to be far-reaching and had amplified inaccurate perceptions.

Respondents also felt the multiple pathways into the profession had contributed to confusion among those outside of nursing. They noted the lack of a single educational pathway (bachelor of science in nursing [BSN]) prevented their profession from possessing a consistent set of competencies necessary to function as autonomous health care professionals. Respondents also believe that the diluted pathway prevents those with advanced degrees from practicing at the top of their license and fully experiencing the reputational boost that should be associated with their degrees.

In addition, respondents described the nursing profession as "disorganized" and "confused." In order to portray a consistent professional image, respondents suggested that nurses should first agree on the essential role nursing performs in health care and society and the core beliefs or tenets of the profession.

Many respondents also felt the reason nursing has an inconsistent image is because nurses had not put enough effort into creating and maintaining their image. By not prioritizing the image of their profession, nursing may have left the job to others by default. Many nurses responded that their profession simply had not put enough effort into the task of branding itself. Respondents suggested that practitioners, educators, administrators, and labor leaders could help shape the image portrayed by the profession in many ways, but nursing needs to take the lead and direct its own future. As one nurse stated, "Nursing as a profession has not taken command of its profession."

Researchers concluded that nursing has a unique opportunity to identify the values nurses wish to convey (and not convey) through their brand image, and to set about purposely developing that brand. This can build positive associations in the minds of patients, other health care professionals, and administrators, who could further boost nursing's level of responsibility in patient care and involvement in policy and decision making.

practice. Evidence-based practice and the application of best practice principles are an expectation of contemporary professional nursing practice. Nurses, then, must emphasize how clinical research and the use of current best evidence affect their decision making and the care they provide.

> **Consider This** "Competence and caring are interrelated" (Griffin-Stevens, 2018, para. 4).

In addition, newer research on nursing sensitivity and nursing outcomes is able to clarify what it is that nurses do that makes a difference in patient outcomes; there is increasing recognition that patients get better as a result of nursing interventions, not despite them. However, in many cases, the public knows very little about the research base that drives high-quality, evidence-based practice, and it is nurses who are in the best position to tell them about it.

Participating in the Political Arena

The political process can influence nearly everything nurses do and every problem they confront each day. In addition, public opinion is often based on inaccurate images, and nursing is no exception. Participating in the political arena, then, becomes a powerful strategy for changing the public's image of nursing.

The reality, however, is that although the nursing profession has some strong professional organizations, only a small percentage of nurses are members of national nursing organizations. This limits the profession's ability to be a force in the political arena. In addition, many nurses know little about the political process or feel too overwhelmed by the daily demands of their job to become involved in addressing larger professional issues in the political arena. Some nurses just assume that the best interests of the profession are being guarded by some unknown force out there. Legislators wonder whether inactivity means simply not caring or not having an opinion. The result is that nurses are inadequately represented in the political arena, and another opportunity for nurses to be represented as knowledgeable, active participants in the health care system is lost.

Because the underlying causes of the profession's political inactivity are numerous, just as the strategies needed to address this issue are complex, it is discussed only briefly here. Instead, a separate chapter has been dedicated to more fully discuss the issue (see Chapter 22).

CONCLUSIONS

Public identity and image have been a struggle for nurses for at least 200 years in this country. Indeed, Elmorshedy et al. (2020) suggest that negative public perception of the nursing profession is a world-wide problem. From a sociologic perspective, conflicting stereotypes of nursing have not served the nursing profession well, and a disconnect exists between reality and public image. The greater public clearly does not fully understand what professional nursing is about, and the nursing profession has done an inadequate job of correcting long-standing, historically inaccurate stereotypes.

The responsibility for changing nursing's image lies squarely on the shoulders of those who claim nursing as their profession. Until nurses can agree on the desired collective image and are willing to do what is necessary to both tell and show the public what that image is, little will change. Damaging stereotypes are likely to continue to undermine public confidence in and respect for the professional nurse.

For Additional Discussion

1. Historically, images of physicians in the media have been more positive than those of nurses. Why? What factors have led to this difference?

2. Some nurses feel that no longer wearing white uniforms and caps has reduced the professionalism of nursing. Is how nurses dress an important part of public image? Would reverting to more traditional nursing attire improve nursing's public image?

3. Would you want your child to be a nurse? If you have a child, what have you told them about nursing that would either encourage them to enter the profession or discourage them from doing so?

4. Who are the best-known nurses currently depicted in the media (radio, television, movies) you access on a regular basis? Do their characters represent nursing stereotypes that have been discussed in this chapter?

5. What do you believe to be the greatest restraining forces that discourage nurses from interacting with the media? Is media training the answer?

6. The contributions of J&J to improve the image of nursing and increase recruitment into the nursing profession are unparalleled. Why would a corporation such as J&J be interested in this pursuit? Why did such an initiative not originate with a professional nursing organization?

7. Are nurses confused about what shared image they want the public to have of their profession?

References

Amazon.com. (1996–2021a). *Doctors and nurses: A novel (2006) (by L. Ellman)*. Retrieved September 9, 2021, from http://www.amazon.com/dp/1596911026/?tag=reviewsofbooks1-20&link_code=as3&creative=373489&camp=211189

Amazon.com. (1996–2021b). *Single dad, nurse bride (2008) (by Lynn Marshall)* [Reader reviews]. Retrieved September 9, 2021, from http://www.amazon.com/Single-Nurse-Harlequin-Medical-Romance/dp/037319904X

American Association for the Advancement of Science. (2021). *Nurses need to counteract negative stereotypes of the profession in top YouTube hits (July 16, 2012)*. EurekAlert. Retrieved September 9, 2021, from http://www.eurekalert.org/pub_releases/2012-07/w-nnt071612.php

Anthony, M., Turner, J. A., & Novell, M. (2019, May 31). Fiction versus reality: Nursing image as portrayed by nursing career novels. *OJIN: The Online Journal of Issues in Nursing, 24*(2), Manuscript 4. Retrieved September 9, 2021, from https://ojin.nursingworld.org/MainMenuCategories/ANAMarketplace/ANAPeriodicals/OJIN/TableofContents/Vol-24-2019/No2-May-2019/Fiction-vs-Reality-Nursing-Image.html

Benjamin, A. (2020). *This is how I became a media health expert on TV as a nurse.* Retrieved September 9, 2021, from https://nurse.org/articles/nurse-media-health-expert-tv-news-radio/

Carlson, K. (2017, June 7). *Nurses as disrupters and agents of change.* Retrieved September 9, 2021, from https://www.ausmed.com/articles/nurses-as-disrupters-agents-of-change

Center for Nursing Advocacy. (2008–2020). *Are nurses angels of mercy?* Retrieved September 9, 2021, from http://www.truthaboutnursing.org/faq/nf/angels.html

Clinical Rounds. (2003). Procter & Gamble pulls offending ad. *Nursing, 33*(8), 35.

Elmorshedy, H., AlAmrani, A., Hassan, M. H. A., Fayed, A., & Albrecht, S. A. (2020). Contemporary public image of the nursing profession in Saudi Arabia. *BMC Nursing, 19*(1), 1–8. https://doi.org/10.1186/s12912-020-00442-w

Gaines, K. (2021, January 19). *Nurses ranked most trusted profession 19 years in a row.* Retrieved September 9, 2021, from https://nurse.org/articles/nursing-ranked-most-honest-profession/

Glerean, N., Hupli, M., Talman, K., & Haavisto, E. (2019). Perception of nursing profession—Focus group interview among applicants to nursing education. *Scandinavian Journal of Caring Sciences, 33*(2), 390–399. https://doi.org/10.1111/scs.12635

Godsey, J. A., Houghton, D. M., & Hayes, T. (2020a, November/December). Registered nurse perceptions of factors contributing to the inconsistent brand image of the nursing profession. *Nursing Outlook, 68*(6), 808–821. https://doi.org/10.1016/j.outlook.2020.06.005

Godsey, J., Perrott, B., & Hayes, T. (2020b, May). Can brand theory help re-position the brand image of nursing? *Journal of Nursing Management, 28*(4), 968–975. https://doi.org/10.1111/jonm.13003

Griffin-Stevens, D. (2018, May). Impacting the image of nursing. *Georgia Nursing, 78*(2), 14. https://www.thefreelibrary.com/Impacting+the+Image+of+Nursing.-a0624417779

International Council of Nurses. (2012). *Position statement: Protection of the title "nurse."* Retrieved September 9, 2021, from https://www.icn.ch/sites/default/files/inline-files/B06_Protection_Title_Nurse.pdf

International Council of Nurses. (2021). *Covid-19 & International Year of the Health and Care Workers 2021.* Retrieved September 9, 2021, from https://www.2020yearofthenurse.org/

Jacobs-Summers, H., & Jacobs-Summers, S. (2011). *The image of nursing: It's in your hands.* Retrieved September 9, 2021, from http://www.nursingtimes.net/nursing-practice/clinical-specialisms/educators/the-image-of-nursing-its-in-your-hands/5024815.article

Jamieson, I., Harding, T., Withington, J., & Hudson, D. (2019). Men entering nursing: Has anything changed? *Nursing*

Praxis in New Zealand, 35(2), 18–29. https://doi.org/10.36951/NgPxNZ.2019.007

Johnson & Johnson. (2021). *Helpful resources for men in nursing.* Retrieved September 9, 2021, from http://www.discovernursing.com/men-in-nursing

Lamey, K. (2021). *Shattering male nurse stereotypes.* Retrieved September 9, 2021, from https://www.travelnursing.com/news/nurse-news/shattering-male-nurse-stereotypes/

McAllister, M., Brien, D. L., & Piatti-Farnell, L. (2018). Tainted love: Gothic imaging of nurses in popular culture. *Journal of Advanced Nursing, 74*(2), 310–317. https://doi.org/10.1111/jan.13452

Men in Nursing. (2020). Retrieved September 9, 2021, from https://onlinenursingms.com/resources/general/men-in-nursing/

Merriam Webster Online Dictionary. (2021). Image [Definition]. Retrieved September 9, 2021, from http://www.merriam-webster.com/dictionary/image

Nurse Buff. (2020, May 10). *Male nurses: On defying stereotypes.* Retrieved September 9, 2021, from https://www.nursebuff.com/male-nurses-on-defying-stereotypes/

Nurse Ratched's Place. (2007). *Lovesick doctors and lovelorn nurses.* Retrieved September 9, 2021, from http://nurse-ratcheds.blogspot.com/2007/11/lovesick-doctors-and-lovelorn-nurses.html

Nursing Now Campaign Launches. (2018, January). *Reflections on Nursing Leadership, 44*(1), 1–3.

Otterson, J. (2019, January 14). *Sharon Stone, Cynthia Nixon among 10 actors to join Ryan Murphy's 'Ratched' series at Netflix.* Retrieved September 9, 2021, from https://variety.com/2019/tv/news/ryan-murphy-ratched-netflix-cast-1203107796/

Pawłowski, P., Mazurek, P., Zych, M., Zuń, K., & Dobrowolska, B. (2019). Nursing dress code and perception of a nurse by patients. *Nursing in the 21st Century, 18*(1), 60–67. https://doi.org/10.2478/pielxxiw-2019-0008

Pirschel, C. (2018, February 28). *One nurse challenges the profession's stereotypes in fiction.* Retrieved September 9, 2021, from https://voice.ons.org/stories/one-nurse-challenges-the-professions-stereotypes-in-fiction#:~:text=In%20TV%20shows%2C%20movies%2C%20books,depicted%20in%20stereotypically%20inaccurate%20ways.&text=Misrepresenting%20nursing%20goes%20beyond%20a,physicians%2C%20are%20misrepresented%20as%20well

Pompilio, E. (2020, January 14). *Gender roles in nursing.* Retrieved September 9, 2021, from https://www.elitecme.com/resource-center/nursing/gender-roles-in-nursing/

Salem, M. (2019). Public image of nursing. *Advance Practice Nurse, 4*(3). Retrieved September 9, 2021, from https://www.researchgate.net/publication/338998100_Public_Image_Of_Nursing

School of Nursing, University of Wisconsin-Madison. (2017, May 22). *International expert on media portrayal of nurses.* Retrieved October 12, 2021, from nursing.wisc.edu/school-of-nursing-welcomes-international-expert-on-media-portrayal-of-nurses/

Stanley, D., Stanley, K., & Magee, D. (2019, August). Celluloid zombies: A research study of nurses in zombie-focused feature films. *Journal of Advanced Nursing, 75*(8), 1751–1763. https://doi.org/10.1111/jan.14036

Swanson, D. (2020, January 22). *6 Reasons why 2020 is the year of the nurse.* Retrieved September 9, 2021, from https://dailynurse.com/6-reasons-why-2020-is-the-year-of-the-nurse/

Truth About Nursing. (2007, October 6). *Getting fresher.* Retrieved September 9, 2021, from http://www.truthaboutnursing.org/news/2007/oct/06_dentyne.html

Truth About Nursing. (2008). *Let's "celebrate the ladies who give lollipops and band aids" with a Nurse Nancy bracelet!* Retrieved September 9, 2021, from http://www.truthaboutnursing.org/news/2008/mar/18_angela_moore.html

Truth About Nursing. (2008–2020). *Mission statement.* Retrieved September 9, 2021, from http://truthaboutnursing.org/about_us/mission_statement.html

Truth About Nursing. (2011). *November 2011 archives. Heart attack grill: Successful protest in Las Vegas November 12!* Retrieved September 9, 2021, from http://www.truthaboutnursing.org/archives/2011/oct_nov_dec.html#nov

Truth About Nursing. (2014a). *All the costumes.* Retrieved September 9, 2021, from http://blog.truthaboutnursing.org/2014/10/all-the-costumes

Truth About Nursing. (2014b). *Servanthood: Is Baylor ad praising its nurses as "servants" a problem?* Retrieved September 9, 2021, from http://www.truthaboutnursing.org/news/2014/feb/baylor.html

Truth About Nursing. (2015). *Nurse Jackie episode reviews.* Retrieved September 9, 2021, from http://www.truthaboutnursing.org/media/tv/nurse_jackie.html

Truth About Nursing. (2017a). *No nurses. No care. The Night Shift's third season.* Retrieved September 9, 2021, from http://blog.truthaboutnursing.org/2017/10/night-shift-3

Truth About Nursing. (2017b). *The defenders of San Fransokyo.* Retrieved September 9, 2021, from https://blog.truthaboutnursing.org/2017/09/fall-season-preview/#chicago-med

Truth About Nursing. (2017c). *Unskilled. Lowly. Servile.* Retrieved September 9, 2021, from http://blog.truthaboutnursing.org/2017/04/krugman

Truth About Nursing. (2018, May 23). *A comedy of errors. Inside Amy Schumer mocks nurses.* Retrieved September 9, 2021, from https://blog.truthaboutnursing.org/2018/05/amy-schumer

University of Wisconsin-Madison. (2017, May 22). *International expert on media portrayal of nurses—Video available!* Retrieved September 9, 2021, from https://nursing.wisc.edu/school-of-nursing-welcomes-international-expert-on-media-portrayal-of-nurses/

Valiee, S., Nemati, S. M., & Valian, D. (2020). Exploration of service recipients' image of a perfect nurse: A qualitative descriptive study. *Applied Nursing Research, 54.* https://doi.org/10.1016/j.apnr.2020.151272

World Health Organization. (2020, April 6). *State of the world's nursing report—2020.* Retrieved September 9, 2021, from https://www.who.int/publications/i/item/9789240003279

Health and Public Policy: The Influence and Power of Nursing

Sheila A. Burke and Donna M. Nickitas

ADDITIONAL RESOURCES

Visit thePoint for additional helpful resources.
• eBook
• Journal Articles
• Web Links

CHAPTER OUTLINE

LEARNING OBJECTIVES

The learner will be able to:

1. Define the terms public policy, health policy, and politics, and explore their relationship.

2. Differentiate among the problem stream, the political stream, and the policy stream in John Kingdon's three-stream model of policy development.

3. Explore the relationships among social justice, health inequity, and social determinants of health.

4. Describe the role of research in assembling evidence to shape policy change.

5. Identify nursing pioneers who have influenced public and health policy, and describe their contributions in effecting social change.

6. Describe strategies that enhance the integration of health policy into nursing education and practice.

7. Identify the roles that professional membership associations have in shaping policies that address the profession of nursing and societal welfare.

INTRODUCTION

This chapter examines a decade of nursing leadership and influence in advancing and shaping the nation's health. Nursing's contributions to the profession, policy, and politics arise from an underlying belief that nursing is a public good. Nursing has a long history as being the most trusted among all health professions.

Indeed, nurses are well equipped to advance equity, social justice, and antiracism. Through their diverse professional roles, nurses are integrated into every level of society. From nurse executives, parish nurses, school nurses, and occupational and hospital nurses—nurses are present and witness to the health and social challenges across the population. It is incumbent that members of the profession take action in reducing health disparities and improving the health and well-being of the U.S. population. In 2020, nurses again ranked as among the most highly trusted professions in public opinion polls, a position nursing has held for 19 consecutive years (Reinhart, 2020). The evidence supports the public impression that the endorsement of nurses demonstrates a candidate's integrity. Society has also recognized nursing as having a role in advancing the nation's health and well-being (National Academies of Science, Engineering, and Medicine, 2021).

NURSES AS SOCIAL CHANGE AGENTS AND POLITICAL ADVOCATES

Nursing has a long history of social advocacy and action, which includes identifying how to best distribute resources to individuals, families, and populations (Lewenson & Nickitas, 2016). In considering nursing's role in policy development, these activities of advocacy and action toward obtaining and distributing resources align with Lasswell's (1936) classic definition of politics as an activity that determines who gets what, when, and how. Serving in this role, nurses are acting as political agents. Nursing has also been recognized for leading efforts to bring about social change. Early in the 20th century, nurse leaders were involved in passing socially focused legislation that outlawed child labor, supported the suffrage movement, and protected women abandoned by their husbands.

Nursing was also at the forefront of and lent integrity to the civil rights movement. As a result of this movement, poll taxes and literacy tests were made illegal. Also, politicians elected with the aid of newly enfranchised Black citizens passed laws intended to eliminate discrimination based on race.

Nursing was also one of the first professions to eliminate segregation. However, educational opportunities remain out of reach for many students of color, and nursing's responsibility to ensure that the profession reflects the diversity of those entrusted to its care still requires much work. This issue of continued discrimination was dramatically highlighted in May 2020, when, less than 3 months from the beginning of the global COVID-19 pandemic in the United States, the murder of an African American man, George Floyd, by a Minneapolis police officer ignited international protests against racism.

Racism, discrimination, and implicit bias remain deeply rooted in our society and within the nursing profession. However, nurses are acknowledging and addressing the presence of racism within the profession to dismantle structural racism and mitigate the effects of discrimination and implicit bias. For example, in 2021, the American Nurses Association (ANA) launched the National Commission to Address Racism in Nursing. The mission of the group is to include the scope and standard of practice that nurses confront and mitigate systemic racism within the nursing profession and address the impact racism has on nurses and nursing. The ANA uses the *Nursing: Scope and Standards of Practice Fourth Edition* (2021) as a framework to create a roadmap for action, including the goals to:

- Engage in national discussions within the nursing profession to own, amplify, understand, and change how racism negatively affects colleagues, families, and communities and the health care system.

- Develop strategies to actively address racism within nursing education, practice, policy, and research, including issues of leadership and the use of power.

Nurses have a moral and ethical obligation to address all forms of racism and to advocate for policies and laws that promote equity and the delivery of high-quality care to all individuals. This responsibility entails addressing all types of discrimination across sectors such as housing, education, criminal justice, employment, and health care impacting individuals and communities of color. The ANA continues to promote care of the individual, families, groups, communities, and population and strongly encourages the incorporation of advocacy as an important concept within the companion Standards of Professional Performance found in *Nursing: Scope and Standards of Practice, Fourth Edition* (2021).

Indeed, in 1974, the ANA set up a special account to help pass the Equal Rights Amendment to the Constitution. The amendment failed to achieve ratification by a sufficient number of states. The women's movement continued, and nursing and teaching were often used as examples of professions requiring a significant amount of knowledge and skill for which compensation was far below male-dominated jobs requiring similar levels of knowledge and expertise, or "comparable worth." During the 1980s and beyond, nurses in several places went on strike to achieve wages of comparable worth. Nursing's involvement in the women's movement as its interest group, working in coalition with other women's interest groups, strengthened that movement.

> **Consider This** "I am only one, but still I am one. I cannot do everything, but still, I can do something; and because I cannot do everything, I will not refuse to do something that I can do."
>
> —Helen Keller

For nurses to be effective in the creation of intelligent health policy, they must be prepared to use their professional knowledge and intentionally gain access to roles where they can both serve as policymakers and influence policymakers. As nurses work to create improvements in patient care, demanding increased access and pushing for health systems to increase safe, accessible, and cost-effective care, they must face the existing societal and economic factors that shape the health of the populations they serve. The perspective nurses bring to the health care systems makes them valuable leaders and participants in the interprofessional health care, community, and legislative advocacy-preparedness teams (Edmonson et al., 2017).

Nurses have brought essential expertise and a unique perspective to health care settings. They are integral members of the teams responsible for planning, implementing, and evaluating responses to emerging diseases and health care crises. For example, nurses' roles as frontline health care providers became more widely recognized during the COVID-19 pandemic. As the pandemic unfolded throughout 2020, it was clear that nurses had a key role in providing input into policy decisions. For example, nurses were vital contributors to designing systems that addressed the emerging issues related to the disease spread, response, and management. As the cataclysmic arrival of the COVID-19 pandemic created unexpected challenges, nurses across the globe stepped into unknown territory and created new models of care for a population of patients whose needs were just being identified.

Since the outbreak of COVID-19 in early 2020, nurses have garnered attention and moved swiftly to respond to and engage in political and legislative action, calling attention to local, state, and health systems officials to increase nurse staffing, medical supplies, and equipment to all frontline providers who desperately need this support. The social contract between the nursing profession and society authorizes nurses as professionals to meet the needs of those involved in their care as well as society in general. However, the politicization of the pandemic awakened the political will of nurses to do what they know best—leverage nursing science and evidence-based practice to navigate these politics (Nickitas, 2020). Nurses have firsthand knowledge of how COVID-19 has had an inequitable impact on those they serve as well as themselves. It is important to recognize that the pandemic made it clear that nurses are more likely to die than any other health care professional and that nurses of color are far more likely to die (National Academies of Science, Engineering, and Medicine, 2021).

It is time for nurses to use their collective political will to combat the coronavirus and its effects. Nurses took the lead in modeling the way and influencing those around them to follow through on evidence-based policies including screening, social distancing, wearing masks, washing hands, and getting vaccinated. Nurses can use their collective voices and actions to create awareness and political influence to save their own lives and those of others.

The NAM has stated that nursing must be socially and politically engaged in advocacy efforts to address the extensive health inequities exposed by the COVID-19 pandemic. A key to fulfilling nurses' roles in policy now and in the future is to increase the awareness of how nurses should be positioned in the health care system to address the social needs in health care through care coordination and transition management (Hass & Swan, 2020).

An important way for nurses to assume leadership roles is through engaging in the policymaking process (IOM (Institute of Medicine), 2011). Nurses have the accountability to participate in designing health care that is affordable, accessible, and of high quality (IOM, 2011). Because nurses are on the front line of care delivery, they have valuable knowledge that can improve systems and ensure that health care is consistently accessible, equitable, and of high quality. It is important to recognize nurses comprise the largest group of health care providers with more than 20 million nurses worldwide and over 4 million in the United States (National Council of State Boards of Nursing [NCSBN], 2020). Other key nursing facts are given in Box 25.1.

The pace of change in health care has accelerated as technology and science have expanded. These changes have directly added to the complexity of health care and social policy issues. This dynamic environment has expanded opportunities for nurses to be involved in policy development. It is important to recognize that though nurses are recognized as essential health providers and trusted professionals, they have generally not been seen as key players in influencing health care policy decisions. Elevating nurses' participation in policy requires taking steps

---

> **BOX 25.1** **Key Nursing Facts**

- Nurses and midwives account for nearly 50% of the global health workforce.
- There is a global shortage of health workers, in particular nurses and midwives, who represent more than 50% of the current shortage in health workers.
- The WHO estimates that the world needs an additional 9 million nurses and midwives by 2030 for all countries to reach Sustainable Development Goal 3 on health and well-being.
- Nurses play a critical role in health promotion, disease prevention, and delivering primary and community care. They provide care in emergency settings and will be key to the achievement of universal health coverage.
- Achieving health for all will depend on there being sufficient numbers of well-trained and educated, regulated, and well-supported nurses and midwives, who receive pay and recognition commensurate with the services and quality of care they provide.
- Investing in nurses and midwives is a good value for money. The report of the UN High-Level Commission on Health Employment and Economic Growth concluded that investments in education and job creation in the health and social sectors result in a triple return of improved health outcomes, global health security, and inclusive economic growth.

Source: Data from World Health Organization. (2020b). *Nursing and midwifery.* https://www.who.int/news-room/fact-sheets/detail/nursing-and-midwifery

---

to increase recognition of the vital roles nursing should hold in health and social policy issues. The World Health Assembly has stated:

> Nurses and midwives play a vital role in providing health services...are often the first and sometimes the only health professionals that people see and the quality of their initial assessment, care, and treatment is vital. They are also part of their local community, sharing its cultural strengths and vulnerabilities, and shaping and delivering effective interventions to meet the needs of patients and families (World Health Organization [WHO], 2020a, para. 1).

Consider This Professional nurses must work closely with national and international agencies in the governmental, private, and nonprofit sectors to advocate for nursing education, practice, and research to shape legislation, regulation, and standards of care impacting the profession.

For example, the Tri-Council is an alliance of five nursing organizations—the American Association of Colleges of Nursing (AACN), the ANA, the American Organization for Nursing Leadership (AONL, previously known as American Organization of Nurse Executives), the NCSBN, and the National League of Nursing (NLN)—each one has a focus on leadership for nursing education, practice, and research (Tri-Council for Nursing, 2021).

These organizations are linked by common values and regularly collaborate to build consensus as well as provide stewardship within the profession. These organizations represent nursing and collectively speak to the diverse interests of the profession, including the nursing work environment, health care legislation and policy, quality of health care, nursing education, practice, research, and leadership throughout the health care delivery system. In recent years, the Tri-Council established the following policy positions:

1. Increased awareness of incivility by issuing a resolution that spoke to the importance of advancing civility in nursing, within the profession, and in the greater community. The resolution calls upon "all nurses to recognize nursing civility and take steps to systematically eliminate all acts of incivility in their professional practice, workplace environments, and in our communities."

2. Positioned authority and support toward advancing the role of practitioner nurses as a resource for improving health care by releasing a joint statement against the American Medical Association (AMA) Resolution, which has "call[ed] for the creation of a national strategy to oppose legislative efforts that grant independent practice to non-physician practitioners through model legislation and national and state-level campaigns" ("American Nurses Association Responds," 2017, para. 1).

In addition, the American Academy of Nursing (AAN, 2020) argues that patients should have full access to registered nurse (RN) and advanced practice registered nurse (APRN) providers to improve the availability of cost-effective, patient-centered care, consistent with the 2010 Institute of Medicine (now the National Academy of Medicine [NAM]) report, *The Future of Nursing: Leading Change, Advancing Health*, which called for the elimination of regulatory barriers that prevent APRNs from practicing to their full scope. The report outlines several paths by which patient access to care may be expanded, quality preserved or improved, and costs controlled through greater use of APRNs. The report recommended that APRNs should be able to practice to the full extent of their education and training. The *Future of Nursing* report (2011) was revised and expanded, and *The Future of Nursing 2020–2030* report speaks to the path for nursing to advance the health of the nation during the next decade through addressing the disparities in health care that became more evident during and in the wake of the pandemic.

The initiatives presented in the 2011 report and those described in the 2020–2030 report align with the scope of the Tri-Council's role in health care policy, which involves not only the nursing profession but also other professional groups to foster healthy, collaborative work environments that support all clinicians and the patients and communities they serve. In addition to the Tri-Council, the National Forum for State Nursing Workforce Centers, the Health Resources and Services Administration (HRSA), and the National Center for Health Workforce Analysis have provided support with workforce data collection, best practices, and formulation of workforce planning and policy. Additional information about the National Forum for State Nursing Workforce Centers and the Tri-Council are provided in Box 25.2.

POLICY ISSUES AND TRENDS

Today, the nursing profession is expected to be prepared to address myriad health care challenges. Four of these are outlined in Box 25.3. In addition, to promote innovation to scale and sustain health equity, nurses must seek new models of care that eliminate systemic racism that contributes to health inequity; increase early invention screening to reduce the incidence of suicides and depression, particularly in young adults and veterans; and participate in work that combats human trafficking as a social and health issue. It

---

BOX 25.2   Members of the Tri-Council or Nursing

The American Nurses Association (ANA)
The ANA represents the interests of the nation's 4 million RNs through its constituent and state nurses' associations and its specialty nursing and affiliate organizations (ANA, n.d.-a).

The American Association for Colleges of Nursing (AACN)
The AACN is a voice for academic nursing that works to establish quality standards for nursing education, assists schools in implementing those standards, influences the nursing profession to improve health care, and promotes public support for professional nursing education, research, and practice (AACN, 2021).

The National League for Nursing (NLN)
The NLN represents nursing education programs across the spectrum of higher education, health care organizations, and agencies (NLN, 2021). The NLN has created resources for nurses to use in gaining knowledge of policy and policymaking on its Policy Toolkit website at http://www.nln.org/professional-development-programs/teaching-resources/toolkits/advocacy-teaching (NLN 2021).

The National Council of State Boards of Nursing (NCSBN)
The NCSBN is an organization of nursing regulatory bodies of the 50 U.S. states, District of Columbia, and four U.S. territories. The NCSBN works to support these regulatory bodies in their efforts to protect the public. The NCSBN, in collaboration with the Forum of State Nursing Workforce Centers, conducts The National Nursing Workforce Study to provide a national survey of RNs and licensed practical/vocational nurse workforce (NCSBN, 2021a).

The National Forum for State Nursing Workforce Centers
This is a national network of nurse workforce entities that focus on strategies to address the nursing shortage within their states and contribute to the national effort to assure an adequate supply of qualified nurses to meet the health needs of the U.S. population. The Forum of State Nursing Workforce Centers' Minimum Data Sets for Nurse Supply, Demand, and Education is an essential resource to advocates for workforce planning, disaster preparedness, access to care, meeting regional needs of health care professionals, and more (National Forum of State Nursing Workforce Centers, 2012-2021).

BOX 25.3   **Contemporary Health Care Issues Presenting Complex Challenges**

Climate Change

Climate change is a public emergency that threatens the world's health and well-being, most especially children, women, and most vulnerable populations. The WHO estimates that 12.6 million preventable deaths per year can be attributed to environmental factors, all of which are exacerbated by climate change, and an additional 250,000 deaths per year are projected between 2030 and 2050 (Liu et al., 2020).

Gun Violence

For several years now, the AAN on policy has consistently called for action on gun violence (Gonzalez-Guarda et al., 2018). The evidence is clear that gun violence affects the public's health. In fact, the Academy has supported the expansion of background checks as well as increased funding for the National Center for Injury Prevention and Control of the CDC.

Maternal Health and Infant Health

With the recent attention to the causes, consequences, and solutions to address maternal and infant health, specifically increases in rates of maternal mortality and morbidity as well as preterm birth in the United States among Black mothers, nurses have amplified their voices to improve and address the health and racial disparities in maternal and infant health. Black mothers remain the primary group at risk for maternal and infant mortality as well as preterm births. These statistics will only improve significantly when there is better access to quality, equitable health care is achieved.

Patient Protection and Affordable Care Act

On March 23, 2010, President Obama signed H.R. 3590, the Patient Protection and Affordable Care Act (PPACA; hereafter called *The Affordable Care Act*). On March 30, 2010, the House and Senate both approved a package of fixes, H.R. 4872, the Health Care and Education Reconciliation Act of 2010. Chapter 22 contains an exploration of the events surrounding the ACA and discusses the implications in terms of the need for a national health care reform strategy.

---

is incumbent on nurses to work with other health professionals to create and effect policies that result in improved screening and intervention.

Beyond being prepared with knowledge of health care systems and processes, nurses must be willing to engage in policy development and be effective in working with other professions or stakeholders to scale and sustain innovation and interprofessional education that supports access to primary population health care, contains costs, and increases quality improvement initiatives.

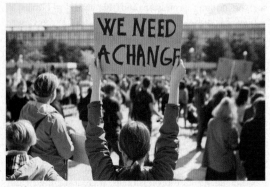

(Halfpoint/Shutterstock)

NURSING AND POLICY

All aspects of the nursing profession are affected by policy issues, including safety and quality, health care standards, educational requirements, and nursing workforce conditions (which include adequate nurse staffing, violence, and workplace incivility). Policy issues also encompass professional protections and requirements for nurses, including whistleblowing, and the management of chemically impaired nurses. Nurses have been active in shaping health care and public policy for over a century. For example, many early nursing leaders and activists, including Florence Nightingale, Lillian Wald, and Lavinia Dock, addressed the social issues of their times from the perspective of the nursing profession. Nurses continue to meet their social responsibility for initiating and supporting action to address the changing health and social needs of the public.

For example, Dr. Bernadette Melnyk and colleagues developed the *COPE* (Creating Opportunities for Personal Empowerment) model for college students and obtained positive outcomes. COPE intervention included assessment and interventions that addressed depression, suicide risk, and anxiety in college students. There are other studies using the COPE model, which indicate the value of early implementation of evidence-based interventions. This is one

Research Fuels the Controversy 25.1

The Global Risks of Poor Physical and Mental Health in the Younger Populations

Many nurse researchers are identifying strategies that can significantly address the dramatic decrease in the health of the younger generations. For the first time in history, the life expectancy for younger population is declining. The rates of obesity and obesity-related conditions, suicide, deaths by other forms of violence, and substance abuse are not only affecting life expectancy; these health issues are going to impact the costs of health care and the lifetime work productivity of the younger generations. Nurse researchers are identifying health promotion and health education strategies that incorporate early intervention and use of nonpharmacological treatments.

Source: Hart Abney, B., Hovermale, R., Lusk, P., & Mazurek Melnyk, B. (2018). Decreasing depression and anxiety in college youth using the Creating Opportunities for Personal Empowerment Program (COPE). *Journal of the American Psychiatric Nurses Association, 25*(2), 89–98. https://doi.org/10.1177/1078390318779205

Study Findings

Multiple nursing led studies in the United States and other countries are defining health education and treatment models that can reduce the risks associated with obesity, depression, and other mental health issues in the younger generation. For example, Dr. Bernadette Melnyk and colleagues developed the COPE (Creating Opportunities for Personal Empowerment) model for college students and obtained positive outcomes. COPE intervention included assessment and interventions that addressed depression, suicide risk, and anxiety in college students. There are other studies using the COPE model, which indicate the value of early implementation of evidence-based interventions. This is one example of how research provides policy opportunities for nursing. Through nurses engaging in policy development, the value of programs such as COPE can be realized. Nurses can educate policymakers and work collaboratively with educational systems so that effective mental and physical health programs become part of the students' experience and can begin to affect the alarming trends toward reduced health quality in younger populations.

example of how research provides policy opportunities for nursing (see Research Fuels the Controversy 25.1).

Similarly, a new statistical brief from the Agency for Healthcare Research and Quality (AHRQ) quantifies potentially avoidable hospital stays in part, through timely and quality primary and preventive care. Indeed, the findings suggest that as many as 3.5 million adult hospital stays are considered potentially preventable, at a cost of nearly $34 billion (McDermott & Jiang, 2020). Heart failure was the most common and most expensive reason for potentially preventable hospital stays among adults.

Discussion Point

What can you do to help ensure nurses can use all their knowledge, skills, and experience to better help patients?

In addition, 8% of approximately 1.3 million pediatric hospital stays were considered potentially preventable, costing nearly $562 million. This finding represented more than 1.1 million hospital stays, with costs totaling $11.2 billion (McDermott & Jiang, 2020).

Indeed, it was professional advocacy and activism that created some of the earliest policy debates within nursing, including the requirements around the "training and education" of nurses. The 2011 IOM and the Robert Wood Johnson Foundation report, The *Future of Nursing, Leading Change, Advancing Health* (IOM, 2011), called for nurses to be better prepared with requisite competencies, such as leadership, health policy, system improvements, research, evidence-based practice, and collaboration, to deliver high-quality care, as well as competency in specific content areas including population and community health, and geriatrics.

The IOM (2011) report represented a turning point for the nursing profession and the need for nurses to achieve higher levels of education and training to ensure the delivery of safe, patient-centered care across health care settings. The report defined the following four key recommendations:

- Nurses should practice to the full extent of their education and training.
- Nurses should achieve higher levels of education and training through an improved education system that promotes seamless academic progression.
- Nurses should be full partners, with physicians and other health care professionals, in redesigning health care in the United States.

- Effective workforce planning and policymaking require better data collection and improved infrastructure (IOM, 2011).

For nurses to practice to the fullest extent of their education and training, the nursing profession must have both regulatory and legislative endorsements for entry into practice, licensure, and scope of practice activities. While there was some progress following the IOM report (2011) and some professional nursing organizations achieved expanded regulatory approval for nurses to practice at the full extent of their training, it was the onset of the COVID-19 pandemic in early 2020 and the subsequent sudden and drastic need to expand the number of practicing nurses that led to multiple states enacting significant policy changes that expanded nursing licensure. Nurses were granted expedited reciprocity, advanced nurse practitioners were permitted to practice without or with less restrictive physician oversight requirements, and nursing graduates who had not yet passed the NCLEX were permitted to accept employment and practice as nurses in a variety of health care settings under a temporary licensure approval.

Discussion Point

What values are reflected in the state nurse practice acts that address the scope of nursing practice for RNs and advanced practice nurses? Do these values promote or restrict nursing practice or nursing licensure, credentialing, and reimbursement for services?

Laws exist today that define the scope of nursing practice and licensure as distinctly separate from medicine and inclusive of responsibilities, independent of medicine (NCSBN, 2021b). The NCSBN is an independent, not-for-profit organization through which boards of nursing confer and develop approaches to address matters of common interest and concern that affect public health, safety, and welfare, including the development of nursing licensure examinations.

Consider This The responsibilities of a licensed nurse include knowledge of, and adherence to, the laws and rules that govern nursing as outlined in the Nurse Practice Act and regulations. Review the nursing laws and rules by locating your state practice act and regulations at https://www.ncsbn.org/npa.htm.

To ensure the public continues to benefit from the care they receive, the NCSBN has conducted research to evaluate safety and quality in nursing practice as well as in educational programs. For example, the NCSBN conducted a landmark, national, multisite, longitudinal study of simulation use in prelicensure nursing programs throughout the country. "The study provided substantial evidence that substituting high-quality simulation experiences (for up to half of the traditional clinical hours) produced comparable end-of-program educational outcomes and new graduates that were ready for clinical practice" (Hayden et al., 2014, p. S3; NCSBN, 2021b). Since the study, multiple state boards of nursing have enacted changes to expand the amount of simulation learning experiences that can be included in prelicensure clinical nursing education. This is one example of how research was used to effect changes in regulatory policies directly affecting nurses' education.

Consider This Nursing's involvement in policy and politics has influenced state Nurse Practice Act that regulates nursing practice for patient safety and public protection.

Another example would be research that examined the relationship between the *Hospital-Acquired Conditions Reduction Program*, patient safety, and Magnet designation in the United States. This research found that Magnet hospitals are more likely to have lower patient safety indicator (PSI) 90 scores but higher catheter-associated urinary tract infection and surgical site infection scores (Hamadi et al., 2020). While the processes, procedures, and educational aspects associated with Magnet recognition seem to improve nursing-sensitive patient safety outcomes, there are still opportunities for improvement, according to researchers who analyzed the association between hospitals' nursing excellence accreditation and patient safety.

Clearly, policy shapes and directs the environment in which nurses provide care and determines the scope of their responsibilities as well as the roles of other health providers and the availability of resources. Nurses must recognize how nursing science and high-quality research can support policy positions for which nurses are advocating and contribute to shaping public policy. This chapter describes nursing's involvement in policy activity and includes contemporary issues being debated in the political arena, such as health care restructuring. Because politics is part of every organization and a part of the government at every level, the chapter describes how becoming politically competent is essential for nurses to act on behalf of their profession and to influence the health care delivery systems where the patients and public will receive care. One way nurses can increase their influence in policy and amplify their voices is by entering into the board rooms of health care organizations. Board service in health care organizations and related entities provides nurses the opportunity to participate in strategic planning and decision making, which can result in improved health care outcomes for the populations being served (Cleveland & Harper, 2020).

Created in 2014, the *Nurses on Boards Coalition* (NOBC) is dedicated to promoting nurse participation on boards to improve the health of communities and the nation. NOBC is a 501(c)(3) independent public charity, championed by over 20 national nursing organization members, 42 strategic partners/sponsors, and seven affiliate members from across the United States. NOBC supports nurses who serve on boards and provides resources to prepare nurses for all types of board positions, including councils, appointments, and commissions (NOBC, 2021).

> *Consider This* In 2020, NOBC was close to achieving its vital strategy of having 10,000 board seats filled by nurses. Its mission of improving the health of our communities and the nation remains strong. It is important to recognize that when nurses are well-prepared to participate in board governance, their actions can be impactful. For example, the experiences of COVID-19 have focused the national spotlight on nurses' value in developing innovative approaches to delivering complex care in dynamic environments. Now, more than ever, nurses must bring the lessons learned in practice to the boardroom. Nurses who serve as board members can shape organizational decisions, influence policy, and resource allocation.

Defining Public and Health Policy

It is essential to describe and differentiate the terms *policy* and *politics* and to clarify the relationship between them. The word *policy* is Greek in origin and is linked to citizenship (Politics, n.d.). In government, policy involves the relationship of citizens to one another in public affairs (Aries, 2016) or is defined as a government plan of action to address an issue (Barbour & Wright, 2017). Government policy and programs often impact organizations and shape the delivery of health care services with the intent to achieve certain outcomes, which have been identified as having value to the population. A broad definition describes a policy as a set of standards that are intended to guide decisions and achieve certain outcomes. It often includes a statement of intent and is implemented as a procedure or protocol. An example of a policy is that all students must be vaccinated against measles, mumps, and rubella before admission into the school system.

Public policy is a term used to describe government actions. The policy is enacted through government systems,

such as in the United States where the three branches of government are the legislative, executive, and judicial systems. These branches have the authoritative capacity to make decisions or influence the actions, behaviors, or choices of others. Each branch of government has a role in the formulation and regulation of health policy.

As licensed health professionals, nurses must be informed and educated about health and public policy, be familiar with their elected government representatives, and be involved with governmental agencies as new laws are developed and enforced. Professional organizations such as the ANA (n.d.-a) have specific departments such as the Department of Governmental Affairs (GOVA) to expand nurses' influence as policies are being created, debated, and implemented. GOVA seeks to foster long-lasting relationships between nurses and their representatives so that nurses are positioned to shape governmental policy. Although policies are often formed in response to societal and health issues, the consistent foundation of nurses' policy work is focused on creating an environment where health services are accessible, of high quality, and sustainable across diverse settings.

Discussion Point

How does health policy connect to how care and treatment are provided at the institutional and governmental levels? What factors must be considered before policy development begins at both levels?

Governmental Policy

At the federal level, the U.S. Congress and the President make policy in three areas: *defense, domestic,* and *foreign.* Health-related policies can be found in all three areas. For example, health-related defense policies include the types of health care the military and their families will receive. *Domestic policy* refers to policies such as the enactment of the 2010 Affordable Care Act (ACA), which originally was planned to be a comprehensive law aimed at protecting consumers, increasing access to care, promoting health, improving the health care delivery system, and controlling costs. Health-related issues are integrated into foreign policy as well. Congress decides whether to assist other nations in preventing HIV/AIDS and providing family planning and nutrition assistance to developing countries. In 2020, the international COVID-19 pandemic prompted policies that included restricting travel to and from the United States as well as multiple policies for health screening and quarantining of travelers.

Consider This Nurses serving in the military are affected by defense policy, nurses working to improve global health in developing countries are affected by foreign policy, and nurses working within the health care system anywhere in the United States are affected by domestic policy. The President and the Congress decide on the allocations of tax dollars to be spent on defense, foreign aid, and domestic health care issues. When more money is spent to fund one policy initiative, less is available for others, unless taxes are increased.

Policies and Values

Policy involves the setting of goals and priorities by a society or an organization and the decisions about how and what resources should be used to achieve those goals. Thus, policies are often expressed as goals, programs, proposals, laws, and regulations that reflect the values and beliefs of those who develop the policies (Milstead, 2016). There are those occasions where policies may develop into moral dilemmas. This is because a policy relates to decisions about how to act toward others. In 2020, the COVID-19 pandemic resulted in policies that created complex ethical situations when family members of frail, older adult residents of nursing homes and assisted living facilities were denied access to their loved ones. There were also ethical issues when nurses and other health care workers were expected to work without proper protective equipment.

Policies developed by nurses have frequently demonstrated a commitment to the value of assisting people to care for themselves despite their illness or disability, and this belief has distinguished nursing from other professions. Caring, whether it is for families, for patients, or the environment, is a value central to nursing. Watson (2008) suggests that to help the current health care system retain its most precious resource—competent, caring professional nurses—a new generation of health professionals must ensure care and healing for the public while learning about the value of serving others. For many years, caring had not been a value that received much attention from institutions and government policymakers. Nurses had some success at the state and federal levels moving such a policy agenda forward; however, results at a national policy level had been limited.

The importance of providing care within a context of caring concerning person- and family-centered care has recently been receiving greater attention. Commonwealth fund research has shown that patient- and family-centered care that incorporates shared decision making can reap potential health care savings of $9 billion over 10 years.

Accordingly, the National Quality Strategy seeks to ensure person- and family-centered care across the health care landscape and has outlined several goals to achieve this aim:

1. Improve patient, family, and caregiver experience of care related to quality, safety, and access across settings.
2. In partnership with patients, families, and caregivers—and using a shared decision-making process—develop culturally sensitive and understandable care plans.
3. Enable patients and their families and caregivers to navigate, coordinate, and manage their care appropriately and effectively (National Quality Forum, 2021a).

POLITICS

Definitions of *politics* stem from the original Greek meaning, which referred to the government of the city-state; the actions of a government, politician, or political party; the process by which communities make decisions and govern; or the managing of a state or government. Politics involves power and influence for key decision making and requires significant investment in social capital. Politics is often defined as the process of who gets to decide how limited resources are allocated and distributed.

In government, politics is an activity that is central to developing the policy that protects the well-being of society. Therefore, nurses must understand how politics drives policy decisions and have the necessary skills and competencies to advocate for societal welfare, regardless of their institution or organizational affiliation. One way nurses can better understand politics is to first assess their political awareness and activity to express their participation in the political process (Box 25.4).

Consider This For nurses to realize their potential to successfully lead change, it is essential to understand the values and political issues at hand. Nurses who are effective advocates will:

1. believe that they have the power and expertise to convince others of the need to change,
2. prepare themselves to handle the broader political value issues, and
3. learn to effectively mobilize their expert power and use strategic planning to influence key stakeholders for the needed change (Robertson & Middaugh, 2016).

1. Are you a registered voter?
2. Are you affiliated with a political party (Republic, Democrat, or Independent)?
3. Did you vote in the last local or state primary election?
4. Did you vote in the most recent presidential election?
5. Did you vote in the last general election—local, state, and national?
6. Can you name your elected city, state, and national representatives?
7. Have you ever contacted any of these elected officials?
8. Have you ever lobbied your elected officials about a personal or professional issue that was important to you?
9. Are you actively monitoring the social media sites related to the policies you want to influence (not necessarily limited to the sites who support the policy as it may be very valuable to be aware of what opponents are doing to contest or dismantle policies you support)?

Politics is a reality of all organized human activity; any group of two or more individuals must establish how to make decisions that require common action and how to resolve conflicts. Kraft and Furlong (2010) suggest that politics involves how conflicts in society are identified and resolved in favor of one set of priorities or values over another. Because resources (money, time, and personnel) are limited or finite, choices must be made regarding their use. There is no perfect process for selecting optimum choices because whenever one valuable option is chosen, usually some other option must be left out. The challenge for effective involvement in policy and political action is to understand how these choices are organized and which ones have the most influence and why. Nurses must consider the implications of how policy initiatives and resources are related in determining priorities and designing strategies for policy development. Consider how policies to support safe patient care require policies for safe work environments and nurses to have adequate equipment and resources.

For nurses to be effective advocates for others and to shape policy (and practice), they must become politically competent and be the active participants in their communities. This includes the ability to understand another's values, motivation, and position and to use that insight to influence others to act. The skills of influence are integral to nursing practice and apply to the arena of political advocacy and action. To be effective in influencing policy at all levels requires specific competencies, which have not traditionally been addressed in many nursing education programs. In 2017, the AACN launched an initiative to increase the amount and depth of education related to preparing all nursing students to be prepared to fulfill their responsibilities in serving as leaders in advocating for and shaping health care. The *Faculty Policy Think Tank* (FPTT)

initiative focused on significantly improving nurses' preparation to impact policy through increasing this area of the educational experience.

Although the *AACN Essentials* had described the expectation for nurses' education at the baccalaureate, masters, and doctoral levels to address that practitioners would participate in policy and improvements to health care, there were wide variations in the degree of curricular content and the approaches to teaching on the subject. The FPTT was created to inform and improve the state of health policy education in undergraduate and graduate nursing programs. The goal of the FPTT was to consider what steps lead to building a generation of future practitioners who understand the elements that impact policy and have the appropriate competencies to bring nursing expertise and insight into the decision-making process and generate change.

CONCEPTUALIZING POLITICS AND POLICY DEVELOPMENT

Although there are many models for conceptualizing politics and policy development, Kingdon's streams of policy development (Sabatier, 1999) provide a broad and comprehensive framework for assessing policy development and a continuum for political engagement.

Kingdon's Three Streams of Policy Development

John Kingdon posited that three streams determine why some problems are chosen over others for policy development (Sabatier, 1999; Box 25.5). The three streams are the *problem stream*, the *policy stream*, and the *political stream*. These three streams often flow endlessly without

BOX 25.5   **John Kingdon's Three Streams**

1. **Problem:** Embodies the process of problem recognition
2. **Policy:** Embodies the formulation and refining of policy proposals as responses to problem recognition
3. **Politics:** Considers the associated benefits and costs to subgroups of the population and the degree of external pressure the legislator feels to take action

converging, but when the streams come together, a window of opportunity opens to move an agenda, to legislate, or to regulate solutions to public problems.

The *problem stream* includes what are defined as problems, indicators of a problem, and the social construction of problems. It also includes how problems come to the attention of policymakers, such as in the form of causal stories or personal experiences. An example of such a problem is the current nursing faculty shortage. According to AACN's report on *2016–2017 Enrollment and Graduations in Baccalaureate and Graduate Programs in Nursing*, U.S. nursing schools turned away 64,067 qualified applicants from baccalaureate and graduate nursing programs in 2016 because of an insufficient number of faculty, clinical sites, classroom space, clinical preceptors, and budget constraints. Most nursing schools responding to the survey pointed to faculty shortages as a reason for not accepting all qualified applicants into baccalaureate programs.

In October 2016, AACN (2019) released a report from its *Special Survey on Vacant Faculty Positions*. The survey achieved an 85.7% response rate from 821 nursing schools and reported a total of 1,567 faculty vacancies from schools with baccalaureate and graduate programs across the country. Besides the vacancies, schools also reported the need to create an additional 133 faculty positions to accommodate student demand. The data show a national nurse faculty vacancy rate of 7.9%. The majority of the vacancies (92.8%) were faculty positions requiring or preferring a doctoral degree.

Strategies to address the shortage have major social relevance as the public's access to quality health care will be affected by a shortage of qualified nurses. Many statewide initiatives are underway to address the shortage of both RNs and nurse educators.

Kingdon's second stream is the *policy stream*. Ideas that are potential policy solutions are considered by their "technical feasibility and value acceptability" (Sabatier, 1999, p. 76). The reality is that policymakers are presented with many problems, and it is impossible to address all of them. Policymakers, then, are expected to set an agenda that reflects the values and issues on which to focus legislation or regulatory action. Because policymakers want to be

successful (for their reelection and job security), most will avoid introducing legislative or regulatory proposals that are unlikely to pass and to be implemented.

For example, since 2013, the increased incidence of mass shootings has caused national and international trauma and concern, with mass shootings in Las Vegas, Nevada (2017); Orlando, Florida (2016); Paris, France (2015); and Parkland, Florida (2018) (Silverstein, 2020). At the same time, nurses have continued to advocate for greater legislative action to reduce gun violence. For decades, the ANA has called on Congress to enact sensible gun control–related legislation. In the wake of the June 2016 Pulse nightclub shooting in Orlando, the ANA, representing the voices of more than 3.6 million RNs, renewed its call to action by urging lawmakers to immediately repeal restrictions prohibiting the Centers for Disease Control and Prevention (CDC) from studying gun violence.

Consider This "The time to unite and take action is now. Together we can halt the growing list of victims. We can stop the madness by forging solutions that address the myriad issues that promote cycles of violence. We must raise our voices to join with members of our communities and at every level of civil society in dialogue and action, to address the underlying issues that result in hate and motivate unspeakable acts of violence."

—ANA President Pamela Cipriano, PhD, RN, NEA-BC, FAAN

When support from the public, professional nursing, consumer, and hospital organizations came together to help fund the Nursing Education Act, it was because of the trust and value the public holds for the profession. In contrast, the ban on assault weapons met with opposition because of the change of national mood, the turnover of Congress and the White House to Republican rule, and opposition from the influential interest group, the National Rifle Association. The issues surrounding gun violence remain unresolved and continued to draw international attention.

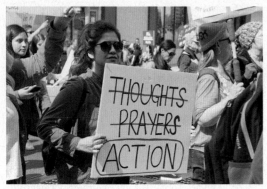

(Sheila Fitzgerald/Shutterstock)

> ***Consider This*** The significance of interest groups as part of the political stream cannot be overestimated. Throughout American history, political and ideologic interest groups have shaped social change and policy decisions. Interest groups provide politicians with one of three resources essential for their success (i.e., reelection), including money, voter mobilization, and image. Image enhancement may be most significant for nurses regarding legislative interest. Having the support of nurses enhances a candidate's image.

Nursing and the professional organizations that represent nursing (interest groups) in the legislature at the state and federal levels must promote policies and vote for candidates that represent their positions. To truly improve health, nursing must be involved in expanding access to quality care across the life span, which includes eliminating racism and improving health equity. Effecting change requires that nursing become involved in the political process. There must be distinct public health policies that remove disparities and enhance the care experience, especially for Black and brown mothers; migrant populations; lesbian, gay, bisexual, transgender, and queer (LGBTQ) individuals; children; older adults; indigenous communities; and other vulnerable populations.

> ***Consider This*** Nursing interest groups have seized upon the public's frustration with rising health care costs and promoted policies that emphasize the cost-effectiveness of advanced practice nurses (stream 1—conditions, plus stream 2—ideas/policies).

Analyzing Policymaking and Professional Nursing

A more traditional approach to analyzing policymaking uses a systems-based model that considers policymaking in sequential stages. It is much like the nursing process: assess, plan, implement, evaluate, and assess again. In a policy system, a problem is identified and placed on the policy agenda and then developed, adopted, implemented, evaluated, and extended, modified, or terminated. The challenge of using a traditional systems model approach is that it fails to consider that the elected government's policy agenda rarely, if ever, reflect a consensus.

For example, leading up to the 2020 election cycle, the country became increasingly more divided along partisan lines, and significant differences were evident in the philosophical perspectives surrounding what role the government should have on health policy. Intense criticism of the ACA and its associated initiatives generated proposals from a variety of stakeholders. By the end of 2020, the nation faced an intensely unsettled political and social environment. The national tension and debates that permeated the politics and policies related to health care coverage escalated as the development and distribution of the COVID vaccines revealed further disparities in health care access and resources. As a new administration was poised to take the lead in 2021, the situation created a new level of opportunity for nurses, as individuals and as members of professional or other stakeholder organizations to step forward and be active in bringing their expertise and influence to support the health care decisions that can provide quality, safety, and social justice.

In Kingdon's model, policy development, adoption and implementation, and politics are inextricably linked, and the political environment in which policy is formed is considered. Nursing has a responsibility to be a participant in all three of Kingdon's policy streams that create windows of opportunity to create and support policy that guarantees high-quality, patient-centered care.

It is a core responsibility of the nursing profession to elevate public awareness about the quality of care or lack of access to care. This includes addressing the social determinants of health. *Social determinants of health* include the issues of age, level of education, socioeconomic status, and access to health care. In addressing the social determinants of health, there is significant potential to improve the health of individuals and communities as well as to reduce the costs of health care. To truly capture the inclusion of social and behavioral determinants of health data, nurses must lobby their legislators and others to ensure that the social determinants of health are effectively addressed within the policies and care delivery systems. These steps can yield significant benefits in increasing the quality and effectiveness of health care (National Quality Forum, 2021b; Sigma Theta Tau International, 2017).

Professional nursing organizations and consumers collectively can develop initiatives and propose policies to solve problems of health care access, health, and safety, or quality of care. Nursing professional organizations and interest groups like the American Association of Retired Persons (AARP) can lobby and engage in political action to influence policy. In all of these examples, nursing is acting as an interest group. The unique thing about nursing as an interest group is that when nurses advocate for nurses and nursing, patients and the public get better care. Political action is a key part of interest group activity. Interest groups do more than support or oppose policies; they help to elect the policymakers by engaging in grassroots campaign activity and raising money for campaigns.

Discussion Point

Nursing has the potential to hold a significant leadership position in policy and politics. At the national level, the profession is represented by the ANA, the AACN, NLN, National Student Nurses Association, and many specialty organizations. What opportunities are available at the local, state, and national levels for you to assume a leadership position?

POLICYMAKING AND POLITICS: THE KEY TO INVOLVEMENT

Nursing's potential to significantly shape health care and be active in policymaking and politics depends on nurses accepting accountability to be change agents. For changes in health care reform to be fully realized, nurses need to see themselves as leaders in the process and engage with others, specifically stakeholders who are committed to health care quality, who will share and support their goals. Political engagement can be viewed along a continuum that extends from no engagement to that of extreme activism, and each individual chooses when and how much political engagement along the continuum they want throughout their lives. For those who choose to enter the nursing profession, there is, however, an expectation that the professional role of the nurse includes accountability to address policy as part of the care environment.

Discussion Point

Political engagement is when individuals make things happen. From where you are in your life today, identify three activities that you can make happen within your school, workplace, and/or your community that can make a difference.

Political Advocacy

Nurses who make things happen fall into three categories: *professionals*, *leaders*, and *political change agents*. All three groups vote in every election and stay informed regarding issues affecting the health care system, and they speak out about working conditions and quality of care. They also participate in professional organizations; know who their local, state, and federal elected officials are; and communicate with them regarding issues of concern. Do not let policy happen "to you"—get involved in the policy committees at work and through state associations.

In addition,

- Seek and enter places where you can use your voice, experience, and expertise to help design and implement care environments and models. No one knows what patients want and need better than nurses do.

- Participate in workforce planning surveys and data collection opportunities. Nurses must measure and broadcast the value of what they do.

- Stay informed about and participate in the activities of a professional association. A few hours of volunteer time can make a big difference; remember there is strength in numbers.

- Embrace and act on the power of nursing expertise and wisdom. Participate in activities that highlight the role nurses have in improving health systems.

Nurses' professional work is linked to and affects policy in the workplace, though nurses often significantly underestimate how much of their work and practice settings are controlled by the government (policy). Across the country, nurses' capacity to influence policy will depend on developing an increased awareness of how government policy decisions impact their practice and then becoming skillful in influencing change. Achieving this level of increased awareness and influence requires that nurses examine their values, use their voices, and take action. It is unrealistic and irresponsible for nurses to sit on the sidelines and say that government policy does not affect them. Health equity, access, and safe, affordable health care requires all nurses to become involved in public and health care policy.

To become engaged in civic participation will require that nurses become and stay informed about health care policy and its impact on their patients and their practice. Find an organization that speaks to your professional and core values. Then investigate the organization's legislative and policy agenda, and learn what legislations impact nurses or nursing. There are several places where information about federal legislation can be located. These are listed in Table 25.1.

To become better informed about current issues affecting nursing and health care, consult additional websites of professional organizations. Other ways for nurses to learn about and increase their influence in politics and health care policy are outlined in Box 25.4. These include becoming involved in electing candidates that nurses want to win. This requires that nurses learn about candidates and their agendas. When nurses support candidates that have a good chance of being elected or with a history of advocating for health care topics nurses support, there is greater opportunity to influence policy.

The nursing profession will benefit from managing its communication to avoid alienating elected officials involved with health care or social policies. One way to avoid eliciting negative responses from elected officials is for nursing (individually and as organizations) to present an evidence-based and objective approach to the issues, focusing on facts and not emotions. Nurses need to be aware that in elections where a candidate is an incumbent, the candidate will still need and value support. Activities nurses can undertake to support such a candidate include working with telephone or in-person outreach, fundraising, sending letters to the media, supporting the candidate in public forums, and either contributing funds personally or through engaging others to support the candidate. Actions that nurses can take to increase their influence in the policy setting are also outlined in Box 25.6.

Shaping policy begins with a nurse selecting and learning about the policy issues that are personally and professionally important enough for that nurse to become an active participant in the policy activities. One way to become engaged is through joining or supporting professional nursing organizations or other relevant organizations that are aligned with professional goals and objectives. Professional membership organizations provide information, education, and opportunities to become active around key professional and societal issues. Most organizations, committees, and task forces provide multiple ways for nurses to learn about organizational structure, function, and governance. Nearly all organizations have a legislative team or political action committee (PAC) focused on addressing policy concerns or issues.

For years, there have been resources for nurses and other members of society to access their legislative representatives. In general, local government representation is available through local offices in nearly all communities. All congressional offices have websites with directories and guidance on how to reach the legislators and their staff. The nurse interested in contacting a legislator, such as a member of the state or national congress, can use the resources available to identify the staff members working with the legislator. Often, the key step to accessing a legislator is to work through the legislator's staff. The district chief of staff is often the only "policy person" in the district. The office in the Capitol deals with legislation and policy issues. Staff members are vital in getting access to a legislator, so the political nurse must be polite and respectful to reach out to these individuals. The entire political system has become invested and engaged in multiple social media platforms, and major policy issues are being addressed in these areas.

Working together, speaking with one strong voice, nurses are a powerful political force. Nurses are, however, quoted only 2% of the time in health news stories (Mason et al., 2018a). Journalists consistently overlook nurses as sources, and when they are cited, they are rarely identified as nurses. Diana J. Mason, principal investigator of *The*

TABLE 25.1 Federal Resources

- Monitored by the Library of Congress
- Wealth of information available about the legislative process, including searches on bill status, public laws. House and Senate roll call votes, current activity in Congress, Senate (www.senate.gov), and House (www.house.gov) websites.
- Information about individual senators and representatives, committees, schedules, and search for legislation.
- Members of Congress can be contacted directly from each of these sites. ANA Government Affairs website http://www.nursingworld.org/MainMenuCategories/Policy-Advocacy
- Contains legislation that has been identified as important to nurses and information about how nurses can contact their legislators to express concern and voice their opinion. National League for Nursing website, the National League for Nursing's Public Policy Action Center (http://capwiz.com/nln/home)

BOX 25.6   **Actions Nurses Can Take to Increase Their Influence in Politics and Policy**

To Influence Politics
- Be knowledgeable and get involved in campaigns (the earlier the better).
- Assist candidates in winning the endorsement of key organizations that you may be involved in, such as nursing organizations, parent–teacher organizations, and neighborhood organizations.

To Influence Policy
- Participate as a member of a nursing organization that influences policy at the local, state, and federal levels.
- Join and work with a group that is addressing a policy you believe is important.
- Educate yourself by subscribing to the social media sites for elected officials who have supported the policies you support and compare their involvement with that of your local representatives.
- Introduce yourself and establish a relationship with your elected officials.
- Participate in the social media sites that your representatives and their staff monitor for feedback.
- Write letters presenting clear and concise information and a request for action on a specific area of policy (e.g., if there is pending legislation or a committee reviewing a particular policy, ask the official to support the position you have presented as benefiting the target population).
- Participate in coalitions of organizations, volunteering to participate in task forces, or to serve as an advocate in the community.

Woodhull Study Revisited (Mason et al., 2018b), affirmed that the most important way to get recognition is by tapping into a variety of media, making nursing voices heard as health care experts.

Consider This To promote a greater understanding of the power, numbers, the impact of nursing, and the nurse's scope of practice, nurses must be ready to engage journalists and use a variety of media to change how nurses are portrayed. Nurses must begin to talk, educate, and engage the public through all forms of print and digital media. They must convey how nurses are improving health care quality and cost savings through evidence-based practice, education, research, and leadership. The full picture of health care will not be portrayed accurately until nurses are included by members of the media who seek nurses as their primary source for stories.

Nurses who want to influence policy should write to their legislative representatives regarding health care issues (Box 25.7). Letters should arrive before any proposed legislation is heard in committee because crucial decisions on proposed legislation are made in committee. Bills that have a financial impact are listened to in a policy committee and a finance committee. Some bills are assigned to two or more committees. This is often a tactic used to defeat the bill before it comes to the floor. If your legislator is not on the committee, write to the Committee Chair at the committee office address. If you write to legislators who do not represent you (you do not reside in their district), however, they are unlikely to respond to your communications because you are not one of their constituents. It is generally more effective to send a copy of the letter with a brief cover letter to your legislator urging their support when the bill comes to the floor. (If bills pass out of committee, they go to the "floor" or the entire house of the legislature.) If your legislator supports your position on legislation, send a thank you note or post your gratitude to the legislator's website or social media site. Thank you notes tell legislators that you are watching what they are doing.

Consider This The ANA was selected to testify at key hearings on national health insurance, amplifying nursing's voice on television to households throughout the country in advocating for comprehensive health coverage, including nursing care in all settings for all Americans.

Finally, nurse political change agents are nurses who use their nursing expertise to lobby elected and appointed officials on issues of concern to the profession, write letters to the editors of professional journals and newspapers, and

Sample Lobbying Letter

[1]Lillian Wald, RN, BSN
Henry Street
New York, New York 00251
[2]The Honorable Harry Nemo
Member, U.S. House of Representatives
House Office Building
Washington, DC 20015
[3]RE: SUPPORT for H.R. 1435
[4]Dear Representative Nemo,
[5]I am an RN, and I have worked in the area of home health care for over 5 years. In the past 2 years, more and more of the older adult patients I care for have had to be readmitted to the hospital shortly after being discharged from the hospital because they are not taking their prescribed medications.
[6]It will save costly hospitalizations to provide needed prescription drugs at affordable costs to seniors. Please support H.R. 1435 and please advise me of your current position on this bill.
Sincerely,
[7]Lillian Wald, RN, BSN

---

[1]Include your address.
[2]Use the proper form of address (most elected and appointed officials are addressed as "the Honorable").
[3]State what the letter is regarding.
[4]Use the office title in the salutation.
[5]State your credentials and experience/belief/position.
[6]Urge support/opposition, and ask for a response with the official's position.
[7]Sign letter. (Please be sure when signing your name to include RN after your name.)

Actions for Media-Savvy Nurses

The following are a few actions to build media competency:
- Compile directories of media-savvy nurses who can speak with journalists at health care organizations, colleges, and universities, and in the community about their clinical and policy expertise.
- Work with your school, workplace, or in your community to develop nurse media competency (how to amplify the voice of nursing).
- Speak with members of the public (friends, family, colleagues in other professions) whenever you can about nurses' contributions and expertise.
- If you spot newsworthy research or work being done by nurses, reach out to your facility's communication professionals and encourage them to share the information with the media.
- Alert journalists about the depth of clinical nursing expertise by writing an op-ed, a letter to the editor, an opinion piece on something you read, or an article that speaks directly to the public.
- Encourage other nurses to develop their own media competencies.

Source: Nickitas, D. M. (2020). Is 2020 the year for increased nurses' visibility in the public sphere through print, television, radio, and social media? *Nursing Economics, 38*(2), 57, 103.

Nursing Political Action Committees

The ANA created the *Nurses Coalition for Action in Politics* (N-CAP; the precursor of the ANA-PAC) to establish political power through the endorsement of candidates and political contributions. The proliferation of nursing specialty organizations and unions all claiming to represent "nursing" may have unintentionally reduced the nursing profession's effectiveness in influencing elected officials because different nursing organizations bring different messages. It can be difficult for elected officials to see how the goals of these organizations are related to each other. Many public officials tend to listen to those who they perceive as best positioned to help elect or reelect them, so the nursing organizations that are most active in political campaigns through contributions and grassroots activity (usually only relevant in an official's first few elections because of the power of incumbency) are the organizations that will be likely to have an impact.

All nurses need to be involved in the organizations that represent nurses, especially those with PACs, because of "money talks." Contributing to candidates that promote nursing's agenda to improve the quality of health care is

ramp up their efforts to get their voices heard in the media (Box 25.8). The work of health and public policy cannot be done in isolation. Nurses must build and participate in coalitions, encourage the participation of other nurses, and mentor future leaders. Most importantly, nurses must use their political muscle to enact and implement policies that enhance access, affordable quality health care, including nursing care; seek appointments or assist other nurses and friends of nursing in securing appointments to governing boards in the public and private sectors; be active members of political parties; query candidates about their positions on health care and assist with fundraising for candidates that support nurses and nursing; seek elected and/or appointed office, and continue to identify themselves as an RN; work on staffs of elected/appointed officials; and extend their policy influence beyond the health system to the community and the globe.

important. The cost of campaigns has grown significantly, and it is a fact that it requires money to buy time in today's expanding media environment and conduct the social research that is now part of any elected official's career.

In 1974, new laws were established, allowing for contributions by PACs. Those laws limited the amount an individual could contribute to a campaign and allowed groups to contribute up to $5,000 per election. Historically, nurses' political contributions have been significantly outpaced in comparison to the contributions of physicians and the hospital political lobbies. Nursing organization's level of political contributions has not approached those from the American Hospital Association. In 2019 to 2020, the AHA-PAC contributed more than $1.1 million to federal candidates (Open Secrets, 2021a). The ANA-PAC in the same period only contributed approximately $260000.00 (Open Secrets, 2021b).

Nursing's future depends on nurses participating in activities that shape policy. Without significant participation, nurses risk having their presence and concerns unrepresented. Nurses can be active members of nursing organizations that take political action; they can take on active roles in a political party and attend political meetings, forums, and rallies; they can help register people to vote; they can contribute and raise money for causes and campaigns through PACs.

Discussion Point

Do all RNs benefit from the contributions made by the ANA members who make monetary contributions to the ANA-PAC and work to elect "nurse-friendly" members of Congress? How would you go about determining the value of the contributions?

NURSES AS POLICY PIONEERS

Nursing has a long history of involvement in politics and policy development. Numerous nursing leaders served as pioneers in public policy formation in the early to mid-1900s. While these nurse change agents had different areas of policy activity, their stories are similar; all of them shared passion, courage, and perseverance. They also shared a commitment to collective strength. These same attributes are recognized by nursing policy activists today.

Lavinia Dock: Organizing Nurses for Social Awareness

At the 1904 ANA convention, Lavinia Dock, a founder of the ANA and the first to donate money to establish the *American Journal of Nursing* that same year, stated that it

was essential that nurses exercise social awareness. As a result, delegates to the ANA convention that year considered social (policy) issues of the time, including child labor, women's suffrage, and sex education.

Lillian Wald: Public Health and Child Welfare

Lillian Wald, one of the founders of the ANA, exemplified involvement in social change, community leadership, and politics. She graduated from nursing school and entered Women's Medical College in New York to become a doctor. During her first year of medical school, she volunteered to teach hygiene to immigrant women attending a school program.

In 1893, she quit medical school with a classmate, Mary Brewster, and moved to New York's Lower East Side neighborhood to provide nursing care in the community. A friend and philanthropist, Jacob Schiff, and Solomon Loeb agreed to fund Wald and Brewster's purchase of a house to support their public health work. This house became the Henry Street Settlement and is considered the founding place for public health nursing.

Martha Minerva Franklin: Segregation and Discrimination

Martha Minerva Franklin was another pioneering public policy nurse in the early 20th century. She founded the National Association of Colored Graduate Nurses (NACGN) in 1908 with the fundraising assistance of Lillian Wald and Lavonia Dock, who mailed letters to more than 1,000 nurses (ANA, n.d.-b). The NACGN was formed because many states barred African American nurses from membership in state nurses' associations. Segregation, discrimination, and racism kept nursing education and hospitals separate.

The NACGN was instrumental, however, in political lobbying efforts to integrate African American nurses into the armed services during World War II. In 1951, the NACGN merged with the ANA (Flanagan, 1976). Today, the National Black Nurses Association exists as one of more than 70 national nursing organizations.

Eddie Bernice Johnson: Legislator

Congresswoman Eddie Bernice Johnson is the highest ranking Texan on the House Transportation and Infrastructure Committee and the first nurse to be elected to the U.S. Congress. She is also the first African American and woman to chair the House Committee on Science, Space, and Technology.

Congresswoman Johnson began her career as the first female African American Chief Psychiatric Nurse at the

VA Hospital in Dallas. In 1972, she was the first nurse ever elected to the Texas State House, and in 1986, she achieved that same distinction when she was elected to the Texas Senate. She has held public office for more than 40 years and has built a reputation for being able to work with both parties to achieve key policies. She has been recognized as one of the most effective legislators in Congress.

During her career, Congresswoman Johnson is credited with authoring and co-authoring more than 177 bills that were passed by the House and Senate and signed into law by the president. She has a long-standing reputation for providing excellent constituent services to the people who elected her. She is the founder of the Diversity and Innovation Caucus, the founder and co-chair of the Congressional Homelessness Caucus, and served as Chair of the Congressional Black Caucus during the 107th Congress. Her initiative, A World of Women for World Peace, has gained national and international recognition (U.S. Representative Eddie Bernice Johnson, n.d.). In October 2020, Congresswoman Johnson was inducted as a fellow into the AAN (U.S. Representative Eddie Bernice Johnson, 2020).

Lauren Underwood: Legislator

Congresswoman Lauren Underwood serves an Illinois Congressional District and was sworn into the U.S. Congress on January 3, 2019. Congresswoman Underwood is the first woman, the first person of color, and the first millennial to represent her community in Congress. She has been a nurse since 2008 and is also the youngest African American woman to serve in the U.S. House of Representatives.

Congresswoman Underwood serves on the House Committee on Education and Labor, the House Committee on Veteran's Affairs, and is the Vice Chair of the House Committee on Homeland Security. Congresswoman Underwood cofounded and co-chairs the Black Maternal Health Caucus, which elevates the African American maternal health crisis within Congress and advances policy solutions to improve maternal health outcomes and end disparities. She also serves on the House Democratic Steering and Policy Committee Representative.

Underwood is also a member of the Future Forum, a group of young Democratic Members of Congress committed to listening to and standing up for the next generation of Americans, the Congressional Black Caucus (CBC), and the LGBTQ Equality Caucus. As a strong supporter of addressing the gun violence epidemic, Congresswoman Underwood is a member of the Gun Violence Prevention Task Force.

She also vowed to preserve and expand access to health care, based on personal experience. "When I was in elementary school, I was diagnosed with a heart condition and had to see my cardiologist quarterly," said Underwood,

who worked as an RN after graduating from the University of Michigan and Johns Hopkins University. "I was inspired by the care that I got from those folks, so that set me on a path toward healthcare." As a career public servant at the U.S. Department of Health and Human Services (HHS), she helped implement the ACA—broadening access for those on Medicare, improving health care quality, and reforming private insurance. Congresswoman Underwood also taught future nurse practitioners through Georgetown University's online master's program. "I love nursing," she added, "because I think you can do anything you want in our profession. We can have several different careers."

Karen Bass: Legislator

U.S. Representative Karen Bass, D-CA, was reelected to her fifth term representing the 37th Congressional District in November 2018. She has served on the House Committee on Foreign Affairs where she was the Chair of the Subcommittee on Africa, Global Health, Global Human Rights and International Organizations. As a member of the House Judiciary Committee, Congressmember Bass also worked to craft sound criminal justice reforms. Congresswoman Bass also served as Chair of the CBC. During her fourth term, Congressmember Bass solidified leadership positions on two issues to which she has personally committed: reforming America's foster care system and strengthening the United States' relationship with Africa (Campaign for Action, 2018).

Bass started her career as a licensed vocational nurse before becoming a physician assistant (PA), and she is the first PA elected to Congress. She has acknowledged that her health professional skills (having a good bedside manner) have helped her to be an effective and diplomatic legislator. Bass serves as a member of the House Judiciary Committee. Her experience as a health care professional working in one of the nation's largest trauma wards in the country is part of what drives her to advocate for legislation that supports the goal of making health care right, not a privilege. With the onset of the 2020 global pandemic, Congressmember Bass continued to advocate for quality, affordable health coverage for all (Representative Karen Bass, 2021).

Bethany Hall-Long, Lieutenant Governor

In November 2016, Dr. Hall-Long was elected lieutenant governor of the State of Delaware. She had previously served 14 years in the General Assembly, where she chaired the Senate Health and Social Services Committee. Dr. Hall-Long is also a professor at the University of Delaware School of Nursing.

During her years in the legislature and as lieutenant governor, Dr. Hall-Long saw the devastating effects the opioid epidemic had on those suffering and their families. She engaged those on the front lines, who were touched by this tragedy, and brought them all together. As the leading voice behind the creation of the Behavioral Health Consortium, her efforts have helped bring substantive and effective change in Delaware to help create a behavioral health system that works for everyone.

CONCLUSIONS

What would Lillian Wald do about health care coverage for children and access to health care? What would Minerva Franklin do about racial health inequalities? What would Florence Nightingale do to elevate nursing in the policy debates? So, the question for today is "What should nursing do to change policies?"

As we entered the second decade of the 20th century, the country passed through a period characterized by intense division along political party lines and expanded and complex political debates occurred about health care access and insurance coverage models. Both had a profound impact on the citizens and residents of the United States regarding their health and well-being.

Nurses must voice their concerns and speak to the public they serve. They are stakeholders in what happens within the delivery of health care (access, insurance coverage, cost, research), in the workplace (quality, staffing levels, safety,

the scope of practice, autonomy, working conditions), in the economy (unemployment's effect on mental and physical health and access to care), and the social environment (addressing environmentally related illnesses and health crises related to social problems such as increased suicides, human trafficking, and opioid abuse).

The health and societal challenges facing the nation provide nurses an opportunity to contribute to a policy framework for more equitable health in the future; a future to improve health and achieve health equity by impacting policy through nursing leadership, innovation, and science. All nurses can influence policies and guide areas ranging from emerging infectious diseases and primary care to military & veterans' health, climate change, and maternal & infant health as well as in the workplace and the community (both public and private). The bottom line is nurses must grasp their responsibility to be active participants and remain involved to address the nation's course of declining health by advocating for better health for all.

Pierce (2004) perhaps said it best:

> As nurses, as voters, and as constituents, we must be a part of the solution. Our elected officials truly want to know what nurses think and it is our obligation as professionals and as citizens to let them know. Our patients and the American public trusts nurses and are counting on us to advocate on their behalf (p. 115).

For Additional Discussion

1. Why are so many nurses reluctant to become active in the political arena? What can be done to engage nurses in political work? The confidence? Do nurses perceive a lack of congruity between professional behavior and politics?

2. Why do you believe nursing was the first profession to eliminate segregation?

3. What are the most significant nursing issues being debated in the policy arena?

4. With the limited membership in the ANA, will nurses ever have a political power base that is representative of the size of their voting block? With the AMA typically being far better represented than the ANA in legislative lobbying, is nursing's risk of being dominated by medicine greater than ever?

5. How well informed are most legislators about contemporary health care and professional nursing issues?

6. What are three major policy issues affecting nursing to be debated in the political arena?

References

American Academy of Nursing. (2020, December 14). *Letter to President-Elect Biden and Vice President-Elect Harris.* Retrieved January 9, 2021, from https://higherlogicdownload.s3.amazonaws.com/AANNET/c8a8da9e-918c-4dae-b0c6-6d630c46007f/UploadedImages/FINAL_Biden_Transition_Letter.pdf

American Association of Colleges of Nursing. (2019, April 1). *Nursing fact sheet.* https://www.aacnnursing.org/news-Information/fact-sheets/nursing-fact-sheet#

American Association of Colleges of Nursing. (2021). *Who we are.* Retrieved October 26, 2021, from https://www.aacnnursing.org/About

American Nurses Association. (2017, November 17). *American Nurses Association responds to Resolution 214 Amendment Presented by the American Medical Association.* Retrieved January 2, 2017, from https://www.nursingworld.org/news/news-releases/2017-news-releases/american-nurses-association-responds-to-resolution-214-amendment-presented-by-the-american-medical-association/

American Nurses Association. (2021). *Nursing: Scope and standards of practice* (4th ed.). American Nurses Association.

American Nurses Association. (n.d.-a). *Federal issues.* Retrieved January 9, 2021, from https://www.nursingworld.org/practice-policy/advocacy/federal/

American Nurses Association. (n.d.-b). *Hall of fame. Martha Minerva Franklin.* Retrieved January 10, 2021, from http://www.nursingworld.org/MarthaMinervaFranklin

Aries, N. (2016). To engage or not engage: Choices confronting nurses and other health professionals. In D. Nickitas, D. Middaugh, & N. Aries (Eds.), *Policy and politics for nurses and other health professionals* (3rd ed., pp. 16–33). Jones & Bartlett.

Barbour, C., & Wright, G. (2017). *Keeping the republic: Power and citizenship in American politics* (8th ed). Sage.

Campaign for Action. (2018). *Nurses (and a nurse champion) win Congressional seats in mid-term election.* Retrieved January 9, 2021, from https://campaignforaction.org/nurses-and-a-nurse-champion-win-congressional-seats-in-mid-term-election/

Cleveland, K., & Harper, K. J. (2020). Prepare and pursue board opportunities: A practical guide for nurse leaders to serve on a board. *Nursing Economic$, 38*(2), 94–97.

Edmonson, C., McCarthy, C., Trent-Adams, S., McCain, C., & Marshall, J. (2017, January 31). Emerging global health issues: A nurse's role. *OJIN: The Online Journal of Issues in Nursing, 22*(1), Manuscript 2. https://doi.org/10.3912/OJIN.Vol22No01Man02

Flanagan, L. (1976). *One strong voice.* American Nurses Association.

Gonzalez-Guarda, R. M., Dowdell, E. B., Marino. A. M., Anderson, J. C., & Laughon, K. (2018). American Academy of Nursing on policy: Recommendations in response to mass shootings. *Nursing Outlook, 66*(3), 333–336. https://doi.org/10.1016/j.outlook.2018.04.003

Hamadi, H., Borkar, S. R., LaRee, M., Tafili, A., Wilkes, J. S., Moreno, F., McCaughey, D., & Spaulding, A. (2020, March 25). Hospital-acquired conditions reduction program, patient safety, and Magnet designation in the United States. *Journal of Patient Safety.* https://doi.org/10.1097/PTS.0000000000000628

Hayden, J. K., Smiley, R. A., Alexander, M., Kardong-Edgren, S., & Jeffries, P. R. (2014). The NCSBN National simulation study: A longitudinal, randomized, controlled study replacing clinical hours with simulation in prelicensure nursing education. *Journal of Nursing Regulation, 5*(2), S1–S44. https://doi.org/10.1016/S2155-8256(15)30062-4

Institute of Medicine. (2011). *The future of nursing: Leading change, advancing health.* National Academy of Sciences.

Kraft, M., & Furlong, S. (2010). *Public policy: Politics, analysis, and alternatives* (3rd ed.). CQ Press.

Lasswell, H. (1936). *Politics: Who gets what, when, how.* Meridian Books.

Lewenson, S. B., & Nickitas, D. M. (2016). Nursing's history of advocacy and action. In D. M. Nickitas, D. J. Middaugh, & N. Aries (Eds.), *Policy and politics for nurses and other health professionals* (2nd ed., pp. 3–13). Jones & Bartlett.

Liu, J., Potter, T., & Zahner, S. (2020, July–August). Policy brief on climate change and mental health/well-being. *Nursing Outlook, 68*(4), 517–522. Published online September 4, 2020. doi: 10.1016/j.outlook.2020.06.003

Mason, D. J., Glickstein, B., Nixon, L., Westphaln. (2018). CPNP-PC original research: Journalists' experiences with using nurses as sources in health news stories. *American Journal of Nursing, 118*(10):42-50. doi: 10.1097/01.NAJ.0000546380.66303.a2

Mason, D. J., Glickstein, B., & Westphaln, K. (2018a). Journalists' experiences with using nurses as sources in health new stories. *American Journal of Nursing, 118*(10), 42–50. https://doi.org/10.1097/01.NAJ.0000546380.66303.a2

McDermott, K. W., & Jiang, H. J. (2020, June). *Characteristics and costs of potentially preventable inpatient stays, 2017* (HCUP Statistical Brief #259). Agency for Healthcare Research and Quality. Retrieved January 9, 2021, from https://www.hcup-us.ahrq.gov/reports/statbriefs/sb259-Potentially-Preventable-Hospitalizations-2017.jsp

Milstead, J. (2016). *Health policy and politics: A nurse's guide* (4th ed.). Jones & Bartlett.

National Academies of Sciences, Engineering, and Medicine. (2021). *The future of nursing 2020-2030: Charting a path to achieve health equity.* The National Academies Press. https://doi.org/10.17226/25982

National Council of State Boards of Nursing. (2020, January). NCSBN's environmental scan. A portrait of nursing and healthcare in 2020 and beyond. *Journal of Nursing Regulation, 10*(4). Supplement. Retrieved October 26, 2021, from https://www.ncsbn.org/2020_JNREnvScan.pdf

National Council of State Boards of Nursing. (2021a). *About NCSBN.* Retrieved January 9, 2021, from https://www.ncsbn.org/about.htm

National Council of State Boards of Nursing. (2021b). *Simulation study.* Retrieved January 9, 2021, from https://www.ncsbn.org/685.htm

National Forum of State Nursing Workforce Centers. (2012–2021). *About us.* Retrieved October 26, 2021, from https://nursingworkforcecenters.org/about-us/

National League of Nursing. (2021). *Advocacy teaching.* Retrieved January 10, 2021, from http://www.nln.org/professional-development-programs/teaching-resources/toolkits/advocacy-teaching

National Quality Forum. (2021a). *Person- and family-centered care.* Retrieved January 10, 2021, from http://www.qualityforum.org/Topics/Person-_and_Family-Centered_Care.aspx

National Quality Forum. (2021b). *NQF and the Aetna Foundation map approach to overcome the health impact of social determinants.* Retrieved January 10, 2021, from https://www.qualityforum.org/Overcoming_the_Health_Impact_of_Social_Determinants.aspx

Nickitas, D. M. (2020). The politics of the COVID-19 pandemic. *Nursing Economic\$, 38*(4), 222–223. https://search.ebscohost.com/login.aspx?direct=true&db=aph&AN=145282247&site=ehost-live

Nurses on Boards Coalition. (2021). *Homepage.* Retrieved January 10, 2021, from https://www.nursesonboardscoalition.org/

Open Secrets. (2021a). *American Hospital Association.* Retrieved January 9, 2021, from https://www.opensecrets.org/political-action-committees-pacs/C00106146/summary/2020

Open Secrets. (2021b). *American Nurses Association.* Retrieved January 9, 2021, from https://www.opensecrets.org/political-action-committees-pacs/C00017525/summary/2020

Pierce, K. M. (2004). Insights and reflections of a congressional nurse detailee. *Policy, Politics & Nursing Practice, 5*(2), 113–115. https://doi.org/10.1177/1527154404264025

Politics. (n.d.). *In online dictionary of social sciences.* Retrieved January 10, 2021, from http://bitbucket.icaap.org/dict.pl?alpha=P

Reinhart, R. J. (2020, January 6). *Nurses continue to rate highest in honesty, ethics.* Retrieved January 9, 2021, from https://news.gallup.com/poll/274673/nurses-continue-rate-highest-honesty-ethics.aspx

Representative Karen Bass. (2021). *Healthcare.* Retrieved January 9, 2021, from https://bass.house.gov/issues/health-care

Robertson, R., & Middaugh, D. (2016). Conclusions: A policy toolkit for healthcare providers and activists. In D. Nickitas, D. Middaugh, & N. Aries (Eds.), *Policy and politics for nurses and other health professionals* (pp. 39–22). Jones & Bartlett.

Sabatier, P. A. (Ed.). (1999). *Theories of the policy process.* Westview.

Sigma Theta Tau International. (2017). *Overcoming the health impact of social determinants.* http://www.sigmanursing.org/connect-engage/our-global-impact/gapfon

Silverstein, J. (2020, January 2). *There were more mass shootings than days in 2019.* Retrieved January 9, 2021, from https://www.cbsnews.com/news/mass-shootings-2019-more-than-days-365/

Swan, B., Hass, S. & Jessie, A. T. (2020). An exploratort descriptive case on care coordination: A consumer perspective. *Nursing Economic\$, 38*(5), 244-251.

Tri-Council for Nursing. (2021). *Homepage.* Retrieved January 10, 2021, from https://tricouncilfornursing.org/#:~:text=The%20Tri-Council%20for%20Nursing%20is%20an%20alliance%20between,consensus%20building%2C%20to%20provide%20stewardship%20within%20the%20

U.S. Representative Eddie Bernice Johnson. (2020, October 29). *Congresswoman Johnson's American Academy of Nursing induction to be streamed live.* Retrieved January 9, 2021, from https://ebjohnson.house.gov/media-center/press-releases/congresswoman-johnson-s-american-academy-of-nursing-induction-to-be

U.S. Representative Eddie Bernice Johnson. (n.d.). *Homepage.* Retrieved January 9, 2021, from https://ebjohnson.house.gov/a-world-of-women-for-world-peace-2019

Watson, J. (2008). Social justice and human caring: A model of caring science as a hopeful paradigm for moral justice and humanity. *Creative Nursing, 14*(2), 54–61. https://doi.org/10.1891/1078-4535.14.2.54

World Health Organization. (2020a). *Year of the nurse and the midwife 2020.* https://www.who.int/campaigns/annual-theme/year-of-the-nurse-and-the-midwife-2020

World Health Organization. (2020b). *Nursing and midwifery.* https://www.who.int/news-room/fact-sheets/detail/nursing-and-midwifery

Professional Nursing Associations

Patricia E. Thompson and Cynthia Vlasich

CHAPTER OUTLINE

LEARNING OBJECTIVES

The learner will be able to:

1. Describe types of nursing associations and their value to members and the profession.

2. Explain the importance of their missions to nursing associations.

3. Examine how nursing associations can strengthen the career-long professional development of their members.

4. Identify data an individual should access and review before selecting an association to join.

5. Identify challenges currently faced by nursing associations and possible solutions.

6. Identify how professional nursing associations respond to health, economic, and environmental crises.

INTRODUCTION

Nurses have many choices to make regarding their careers. Deciding what area and specialty in which they choose to practice, what work setting best suits them, how valuable unique certifications will be to them, the level of education that meets their career goals, and how they balance their careers with their lives are just a few of the key decisions nurses consider on a regular basis. These choices can be relatively easy or quite hard to make, depending on the nurses' specific goals and career aspirations.

Another choice nurses have is which professional associations they will join and, of those they join, how active they will be in each. Every association has a unique mission and vision and offers different benefits to its members. Nursing associations vary in focus from clinical specialty, academic development, scholarship, research, leadership, career advancement, to overall achievement. They also differ in geographic scope, including local or state/provincial, national, and global.

Determining which associations best meet the needs of each nurse at any given time is a personal decision they must make and requires careful consideration, based on that nurse's individual career goals as well as expectations of association membership. However, it is critical for nurses to belong to and engage in professional associations, both to enhance their own development and career potential and to advance the profession.

TYPES OF NURSING ASSOCIATIONS

A nursing association is typically a not-for-profit entity that exists to serve and represent its members, to advance the profession, and to meet the goals of the association based on its specific mission. Most are structured with an individual membership model; however, some organizations are association membership based, such as the International Council of Nurses (ICN), which is a federation model. Other associations may be subsidiaries of a parent organization, such as the Association of Nurse Leaders, which is a subsidiary of the American Hospital Association. Most associations, however, are autonomous. Also, several nursing associations have local/state entities that are part of the greater association.

One of the most important references for members of any association is the association's bylaws. An association's bylaws provide the governance structure through which that organization is led; incorporation laws within the country where the association is established provide the legal framework for the operation of the association.

Other key information about an association can frequently be found on that association's website. This information

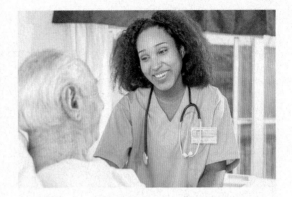

can help prospective members determine what type of nursing association it is, as well as current initiatives, what benefits are offered to members, and other resources that indicate organizational priorities and where the organization invests its resources.

> **Consider This** Bylaws govern an association and provide a list of the association's purposes, but most members never review them.

Nursing associations are usually supported by a governing board of directors, elected officers, and paid and/or volunteer staff. These positions provide opportunities for members to serve in leadership roles on the board and network with stakeholders across the association. No matter how an association is structured, the main goal of every membership-based association should be to support its members and enable their success. Without members, membership associations would not exist. This goal, directly or indirectly, should be reflected in the association's mission, vision, and values, as well as in its programs, events, and services. A membership association exists to serve its members; how well it does so is crucial for prospective members to consider.

MISSION

Each nursing association has an identified mission that sets it apart from other organizations and addresses its main purpose for existence. The association may also have identified a vision and organizational values. The relationship between these is direct: the association mission is what the association does now, the association vision is what it hopes to become/achieve in the future, and the association values are those specific beliefs that, with the mission and vision, guide the governing decisions of the association.

Research Fuels the Controversy 26.1

Program Directors' Perceptions of Student Membership in Professional Organizations

A descriptive national study of program directors of medical imaging and radiation therapy programs was conducted to assess their perceptions of the pros and cons of professional association membership for students. This study also identified possible strategies to increase student involvement in professional associations.

A survey tool was developed by the researchers and pilot tested for validity. A convenience sample of 712 program directors was identified. They were each sent an email and provided consent by completing the survey on the attached link. A reminder email was sent after 2 weeks, and the survey link was active for 3 weeks.

Source: Clark, K. R., & Veale, B. L. (2020). Program directors' perceptions of student membership in professional organizations. *Radiologic Science & Education*, 15–23.

Study Findings

Seven hundred emails were successfully delivered with a 32.7% (N = 229) response rate. There were five incomplete surveys, which were not included in the study. Most of the directors were from community colleges (37.4%) and universities (36.9%). Students were required to belong to professional associations in 39.7% of the educational programs. The top three benefits of belonging to professional associations were "access to educational resources, scholarship opportunities, and professional development." Obstacles preventing students from belonging were "cost of membership, lack of interest in general, and confusion about what the organization represents."

Program directors believed that strategies that would encourage students to belong to associations were "lower costs, offer free access to online resources, and offer free or discounted educational materials." However, when the question was phrased to focus on the most effective perceived strategies, the third response changed to an increase social media presence. Most of the directors believed that professional association membership was important for students and graduates.

For example, the American Nurses Association (ANA), as a voice for nurses in the United States, fosters practice standards and promotes positive work environments to improve health care. The mission of the ANA is to "lead the profession to shape the future of nursing and health care" (ANA, 2021, para. 1). Sigma Theta Tau International (Sigma) is a global nurse member-based association focused on scholarship, leadership, and service. Its mission is "developing nurse leaders anywhere to improve healthcare everywhere" (Sigma Theta Tau International, 2021). The ICN supports nurses globally through a federation model of national nursing associations. Its mission is "to represent nurses worldwide, advance the nursing profession, promote the wellbeing of nurses, and advocate for health in all policies" (ICN, 2021, para. 1).

There are numerous other associations with a focus on practice specialties, education, demographic groups, and administration. Search for detailed information regarding these associations on their websites. Involvement for some nurses begins as a student when they join the National Student Nurses Association to support their professional journey and career.

Meeting the Mission

To effectively support and engage their members, associations must first understand who their members are and why they choose to belong. This process begins with analyzing the organization's member demographics and needs. Age, level of education, place(s) of employment, range of financial income, areas of interest/specialty, certification(s), career goals, motivation to join, and member expectations are examples of demographic data that an association may collect.

In addition, associations should collect data from potential members who have chosen not to join; determining why potential members chose not to join and what their needs are is important in reviewing association benefits. Students are also potential association members, so understanding their motivation for involvement is important. Those who already belong to student professional associations are a key group to engage. Research Fuels the Controversy 26.1 examines program directors' perceptions of the benefits and barriers related to student involvement in professional associations.

Associations must be in compliance with data collection rules, regulations, and policies, however, which limit the data they may collect. For example, the General Data Protection Regulation (GDPR) that went into effect in 2018 has bearing on many associations' ability to gather and utilize data.

Today, most associations have a diverse membership base, with members across multiple age ranges and at different points in their careers. Much has been written about unique characteristics of the various "generations" of people involved in the workplace and who are members of various organizations. Currently, these include the Silent Generation, baby boomers, Generation X, millennials (also referred to as *Generation Y*), Generation Z (Dimock, 2019), and we are now into the birth years of Generation Alpha (born approximately between 2010 and 2025) (Pinsker, 2020).

Data differ on just how diverse the characteristics are between these generations, with some indicating much diversity, and other studies indicating far less than imagined (King et al., 2019).

Associations recognize the differing needs of their members, partly based on generational norms. Their goal is to provide support for members across generations and cultures, with differing career trajectories, with various levels of experience and motivations to join, for the association to meet its mission. Many organizations create a menu of benefit options to address the varied needs of their individual members.

Another way professional membership associations determine member needs is based on the career stages of their members (Rabbitt, 2019). The astute association will provide benefits and opportunities for members within each career stage.

For example, one benefit might be virtual membership options and virtual access to meetings and groups. This might be especially beneficial given the geographic diversity of current and prospective members, as well as public health issues, and trends in virtual education and engagement.

Different interaction modalities are important to meet members' learning preferences and geographic locations, including:

- Face-to-face programs and meetings
- Email, blogs, and communication boards
- Videoconferences, teleconferences, webinars, and other virtual options
- All forms of social media

The need to increase electronic options is more essential during times of public health crises, such as the COVID-19 pandemic. Staying connected with members and addressing their needs is critical to maintaining member engagement and sustaining the association.

Membership associations typically pay attention to the varying characteristics of members in an attempt to meet member needs. However, those associations who are strongest base their offerings on actual member data and recommendations. For example, just because you are a member of a specific generational group, it does not mean that you value or want the same things from organizational membership like everyone else in that same generational grouping; it does, however, mean that you may have had exposure to similar advances in technology, social constructs, and changes in social mores.

As you consider which professional associations to join, it is important that you scrutinize each carefully to determine whether their values align with yours, whether you trust the leadership, whether they communicate and gather in a way that is easy for you to access, whether they offer you education and engagement in ways that are meaningful to you, and most telling: whether you could see yourself now or in the future volunteering your time to support that organization. If not, continue looking.

Discussion Point

What strategies might be used to meet the needs of a geographically diverse membership?

If association data indicate that a key motivator for membership is networking, then ensuring that rich opportunities to network one-on-one and with other members and member groups that have similar interests should become a priority. To be responsive, that association might create networking activities at events and through online communities and opportunities to collaborate on projects and programs that benefit not only the members involved with the actual work but also others in the profession and the profession as a whole. With the shift from face-to-face meetings due to public health concerns, many associations have successfully increased virtual options to meet member needs. With this shift, even after a public health crisis abates, members may continue to expect more virtual options to save time, travel, and costs. However, the importance of face-to-face networking will continue to be valued.

CHOOSING TO BELONG

Nursing is a profession where association membership can provide great personal and professional value. Many of the nurse leaders in our profession today have not only become known within the field of nursing through their involvement in professional associations but also fine-honed their professional and leadership skills and created lifelong relationships with colleagues through such memberships.

Professional membership association benefits vary based on the mission of the association, but they are all important for professional growth across the members' careers. Examples include the following:

- Educational programs providing continuing nursing education on topics related to association mission, with content focused on clinical practice, academic advancement, leadership, scholarship, and so on

- Advocacy for health policy
- Advocacy for political interest
- Networking to connect and collaborate with experts in your area of interest
- Opportunities to identify mentors to assist the member with both short- and long-term goals related to career development
- Association journals and other tools providing current knowledge and updates
- Certification in specialty areas to demonstrate expertise and credibility
- Access to standards of practice
- Awards and recognition such as research grants or travel stipends to present papers at conferences or public recognition for outstanding accomplishments
- Content related to developing knowledge and skills to be a mentor
- Discounts for relevant goods or services per member interest (e.g., malpractice insurance)

Discussion Point

Discuss how mentors/role models in professional associations might advance your professional development, providing specific examples.

Discussion Point

Discuss what information you, as a prospective member, would research regarding each professional association you are considering joining?

We all balance personal and professional demands and need to carefully weigh opportunities and obligations to ensure we maintain the equilibrium needed for a healthy lifestyle and career. Association membership can assist with maintaining that personal/professional balance by providing the benefits listed earlier and many more—all in one place. Instead of seeking out these benefits individually, having the opportunity to find them all through membership in a professional association enhances professional efficiency and convenience.

When considering which association(s) to join, it is important to review the benefits of the association based on a personal cost–benefit ratio. Each nurse must determine what they expect to gain from membership in any given

association or a variety of associations, and in return, what they are willing to give in terms of membership dues and active engagement/participation. Individuals must be able to analyze and determine the value to them of both tangible and intangible benefits. Individuals should research various association options and analyze what each has to offer. In addition to culling through an association's website, they should call the association's membership offices to discuss the benefits of membership, and they should also speak with colleagues about what they recommend.

For example, if a membership association's annual dues are $100 and the benefits include free journal access, free or discounted continuing nursing education, and other tangible benefits, you can calculate a direct cost–benefit ratio based on the expense of these tangible items if purchased separately without the membership benefit. One must then determine and include the value of the intangible benefits, such as networking; the ability to meet and work with professional leaders within the association, to be mentored, to collaborate with others; and free and/or discounted access to events or products. Starting with that analysis, each individual can then also consider how many of the benefits they would actually use to determine what the combined tangible and intangible cost–benefit ratio is, and thus the ultimate value, to them.

Many nursing colleagues choose to participate in two or more associations, gaining different values from each. Frequently, this is a blend of associations with different missions, such as a unique specialty association combined with a more broadly focused national or global organization. Whether interests are focused at the local, state, provincial, national, regional, or global level, and whether they are specifically related to a specialty area or broader in nature, associations exist that can provide individuals with numerous opportunities.

The benefits derived from professional association membership will be directly related to your level of involvement in the association. Many associations have a plethora of opportunities for their members, such as job opportunities and career advice, attending and networking at conferences and seminars, accessing professional journals and continuing education, daily or weekly news briefs/updates, and professional mentoring and networking. In addition, there are opportunities to serve on committees and boards that foster your leadership development and allow you to engage in policy and advocate for patients. Taking advantage of all the opportunities that are of interest to you will be critical to enjoying a full and valuable membership; engagement is key to realize the full benefits of an association. Association membership can provide a wonderfully well-rounded and rich professional experience and greatly enhance one's career.

VALUE TO THE PROFESSION

Nursing associations exist to both support their members and address critical issues and challenges that face the profession and health care. Associations demonstrate support for their members and engage their members effectively through offering various professional education, networking, and mentoring opportunities. Many nursing associations, as a key part of their missions, also have a goal to improve health care, either directly or indirectly. This work may be quite broad or focused in specific educational or clinical practice areas and may be local, regional, provincial, national, and/or global in scope.

Each organization's support of the profession should be mission specific and, depending on the organization, focus on one or more of the following.

Policy, Regulatory, and Legislative Support

Some associations exist to create, enact, and/or monitor compliance with professional practice laws and the standards created by various accrediting bodies. There are legal and voluntary standards that control the profession's work including licensure at all levels of nursing practice. Various accreditation bodies exist to support education, quality, and credentialing regarding practice.

Developing Practice Standards

The mission of many organizations, including those with a specialty focus, is to develop and promote quality and evidence-based practice standards. These professional performance levels are often included or indicated in regulatory statements and used as a benchmark any time a legal question arises regarding professional performance.

Creating Positive Work Environments

Working conditions are often addressed by various accrediting bodies that relate to education and practice settings, as well as associations that may address this topic via research and dissemination of best practices. Addressing safe and healthy work environments is especially critical during a public health crisis as seen with COVID-19 where personal protective equipment (PPE) was limited, or nonexistent in some settings, and health professionals suffered negative consequences from these environments. Also, staff shortages in addition to a lack of needed supplies and equipment to provide care and save lives increased stress and created a negative environment.

Enhancing the Profession

Professional associations are a voice for the profession to consumers and to policymakers. They maintain professional values and standards and support the profession through the opportunities they provide their members to grow and develop. Leadership opportunities to serve on boards, be involved on committees, and take action to move the organization and the profession forward in a positive way are often provided by professional associations.

Advancing Research

Professional associations may also engage in or support conducting research related to professional enhancement in numerous ways, from support for practice standards, positive work environments, impact of performing to scope of practice, to identification of global professional issues and strategies to address them.

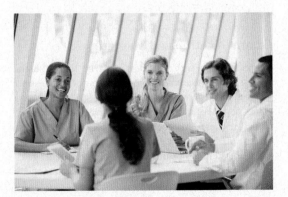

Providing Credentialing

Credentialing is another way professional nursing associations enhance the profession. Credentialing validates nurses' knowledge and expertise in a particular area through assessment against established standards for that area.

> ### Discussion Point
>
> Some of the professional issues nursing associations address include scope of practice, quality and access to care, patient and nurse safety, and legislation that impacts practice. What role do nursing associations play in addressing these issues? What other professional issues do nursing associations address?

PROFESSIONAL ASSOCIATION CHALLENGES

Relevance and Resiliency

Professional associations are charged to remain relevant, resilient, valuable, and significant to all their members. Whether a national, regional, or international organization, the reality is we are a global community with members from diverse cultures. Effectively recognizing and understanding a variety of norms, standards, and protocols, as well as meeting diverse cultural expectations is required for global success.

Associations need to be resilient and flexible to respond to health, economic, and environmental crises. The COVID-19 pandemic is one such example. Strategic planning to position an association's response during times of stress and uncertainty is essential. The plan should include a quick communication system to update staff and members with accurate information. In addition, a strong financial reserve should be in place so the association can continue to support its members and staff, regardless of challenging or unexpected situations.

Global Growth and Diversity

Associations must strategically plan for global expansion, recognizing the implications for the organization and membership. When organizations consider global growth, they must carefully scrutinize their organizational mission, vision for the future, intention, member demographics, and member demand. They must balance these against current and projected organizational resources, to ensure they are positioned not only to initiate global growth but also to achieve sustained, successful, and continued global expansion. Because associations want to design the best multiple strategy approach to reach their members, the strategy must include a variety of modalities to facilitate international participation. Current and prospective members also need to consider whether they would find personal value in being part of an association that is global in scope or one that is planning global expansion.

In addition to generational diversity, today many associations are responding to an increasingly global community because of expansion into multiple countries and regions. This growth broadens the traditional local chapter model to encompass state, province, country, regional, and global models. This global diversity not only impacts how the organization must grow but also brings additional complexity to meeting member needs, far beyond generational issues. Cultural diversity, combined with generational diversity, and the varying values that a rich cultural and generational membership mix provides offer a unique opportunity and challenge for professional associations in meeting their members' needs.

> ### Discussion Point
>
> The practice of nursing differs greatly around the world. How do nursing associations bridge the chasm between diverse cultures, norms, and scopes of practice?

> ### Discussion Point
>
> Discuss the challenges of meeting member needs across generations and options you feel would be effective for associations to reach such diverse membership.

> ### Discussion Point
>
> What are the benefits and challenges to the association and to its members if a country-specific association decides to expand globally?

Communication and Marketing

Communication with members must be fluid, flexible, and varied. For example, some members will prefer communication via phone calls and tangible mailings, whereas others communicate primarily via email, text messages, virtual meetings, and social media. Being aware of their current member preferences regarding communications, communication trends in general, as well as specific guidance to meet legal limitations is vital for the success of any organization.

Members also value timely information about benefit opportunities, as well as how programs, events, products, and services are delivered. For example, an association may have an outstanding program; however, if it is not marketed effectively, and/or delivered in a manner that does not benefit the members, the program is of little value and, indeed, can be detrimental if it leads to a disappointing experience for the members.

To that end, associations need to offer quality programs and market them in such a way so that members recognize the value of the opportunities available for personal and professional growth. From a business construct, positioning the value of the association and its programs based on (a) features, (b) benefits, and (c) member value customized to differing membership audiences may be a highly effective messaging strategy.

Discussion Point

How should communication strategies employed by an association change during a public health crisis?

Discussion Point

Review missions of various professional nursing associations and determine which one(s) best meet your needs.

Discussion Point

Nursing is the most trusted profession according to repeated Gallup poll results (Reinhart, 2020). And yet it is one of the least influential. Discuss how professional associations can develop strategies to change this narrative and increase the *influence of nurses.*

Membership Value and Engagement

A major challenge faced by associations today is increasing their membership when current and potential members are more careful than ever in how they spend their money and time. Associations must develop strategies to demonstrate the actual value received for the dues a member pays and the time they volunteer. Some strategies include allowing payment of dues over time, reduced fees for certain employment levels, discounted fees for multiyear renewals, and so on.

Engaging members can be challenging but is essential for the success of an association. For example, ensuring members are offered opportunities to lead and govern the organization is critical for most associations whose board, committee work, and program content are accomplished through member volunteers. Special emphasis should be placed on engaging new members immediately and often, as well as engaging all members in activities and programs that are meaningful to them; these actions will, in turn, develop long-term loyalty. Providing a diverse variety of rich opportunities for member volunteers can be one of the most powerful strengths of an association.

Leadership Development

Professional associations must have visionary leaders and highly competent staff to thrive. An association may barely survive or fully thrive depending on the knowledge and skill of its paid and volunteer leadership. Advancing the profession and sustaining the association require supporting current nurse leaders, developing future leaders, and encouraging members to grow as leaders.

Associations and their members need to support current nurse leaders who are addressing practice, educational, policy, political, and advocacy change/improvement.

Associations also have a responsibility to help develop the next generation of nurse leaders both for the association and for the profession. They must create an environment to nurture and grow those nurse leaders. Associations have a unique opportunity to encourage and enable members to grow as leaders from the bedside to the boardroom. Providing opportunities and programs to develop leaders to make a difference for both improving health and the profession is essential for our future.

Early identification, development, and mentoring of member and staff leaders, who bring expertise and loyalty to leadership positions within the association, are vital to both current success and long-term sustainability.

Association Collaboration

Although some associations feel a competitive model of work is beneficial, those organizations that have similar missions can benefit in great measure through collaboration with each other. Collaboration can provide a collective voice, a respectful diversity of opinion, experts, and expertise, and strengthen results while minimizing resource outlay.

No one association is as powerful individually as all are collectively. Nursing associations working together provide the foundation for sustaining nursing in the future. The benefit of collaboration has proven to be powerful; it can change practice, establish standards, enact laws, sustain workplace settings in which nurses can best succeed, and support an environment in which our students and new graduates feel welcomed into the profession.

Discussion Point

Collaboration among nursing associations to address key nursing and health care issues conserves resources and strengthens the voice of the profession. What health care issues would best be addressed by a cohesive voice from collaborating nursing associations?

Sustainability

Another strategic decision for associations to make is where to focus their resources and how to prioritize what professional issues to address. There are many nursing and health care issues, and it is easy for the board of an association to enthusiastically slip into a mode of wanting to solve them all. However, it is critical that the association's board of directors ensures all initiatives relate to the mission, so the association stays within its legal parameters. The focus should also support the association's vision and uphold its values.

The association that is nimble, designed to respond quickly and efficiently to new opportunities, able to divest itself of ineffective programs, and provides diverse, meaningful, and impactful programs and opportunities for its members is best poised for long-term success.

Associations that not only meet member needs but surpass member expectations, now and in the future, position themselves for long-term sustainability. And those associations that provide such value so that membership is seen as a necessity, not a choice, will flourish.

As with any organization, associations that thrive in a culture of change are best positioned to succeed. It is essential that organizations are flexible and able to adapt quickly for them to remain relevant. They must not only react to change but also be adept at predicting change. Nowhere is this more apparent than in professional associations. They must be responsive as well as responsible, be able to facilitate change, as well as assist their members in successfully navigating through a changing environment.

The key to sustainability is an infrastructure that includes adequate human and financial resources. Associations need to engage and maintain their members and volunteer leaders, as well as hire expert staff. These are the people who provide the vision, accomplish the work, and maintain the relevance of the organization.

Associations need to develop a multisource revenue base. Relying mainly on dues for revenue will not result in sustainability. Non-dues revenue from programs, products, and services are often used as part of a multisource revenue strategy. However, other options need to be explored. Collaborating with other associations for programming events conserves resources, as well as increases networking opportunities for members and the reach of those programs. In addition, associations that are going to be viable in the future must have a strategy that includes building a reserve fund to access when unexpected situations occur.

RESEARCH OPPORTUNITIES

The focus of professional associations is to meet the needs of members and the nursing profession. Although there are examples and some qualitative data available, there is limited evidence to document the outcomes of association work. Therefore, more research needs to be conducted in this area. Some ideas that can be developed into studies include:

- Survey members in board-level association positions to determine what motivated them to become engaged members. What do they want to achieve as a board member?
- What are the characteristics of associations that will thrive in the future?
- Analyze policy impact/outcomes of those associations with a policy focus.
- Survey association executive officers to assess what actions they are taking to ensure the future success of their association.
- Is there a relationship between early career association membership and nurses in clinical and/or academic leadership roles?
- Does leadership in student nurse associations translate into leadership in professional associations after graduation?
- How can associations address the needs of an increasingly diverse membership?
- What effect will the large number of retiring Baby Boomers have on association viability?
- How do associations plan for and respond to health, economic, and environmental crises?

CONCLUSIONS

Nursing associations seek to elevate the practice of nursing, with the ultimate goal of supporting their members and improving health care and health care outcomes. Every nurse can benefit personally and professionally from active membership in the organization(s) that best meet their needs. With visionary leadership and strong participation, associations advance our profession, locally, regionally, and globally.

For Additional Discussion

1. Determine the cost–benefit ratio for you to join a professional nursing association. Identify both the tangible and intangible benefits.

2. Explain how professional nursing associations enhance the nursing profession.

3. Discuss why effective communication and marketing is key to a professional nursing association's success.

4. Explain how a professional nursing association should make decisions about which professional issues to address.

5. How can professional nursing associations help nursing become more influential?

6. How can collaboration benefit nursing associations and the profession?

7. How can professional nursing associations develop long-term loyalty from their members?

8. Identify key factors necessary for a professional nursing association to thrive.

9. "Resilience" is a popular term and is currently applied to many areas of health care. What does resilience really mean—in the broader framework of health care, as well as in your specific setting? Describe how a professional nursing association can develop and maintain resilience, especially in times of crisis.

10. What professional nursing associations do you know most about? Least about?

11. If you could provide recommendations or advice to any professional nursing association on how best to recruit and retain members, what would those recommendations/that advice be?

12. As you analyze your career goals and direction, which professional nursing associations would be best for you to affiliate with and become a leader of?

13. If you were launching a new professional nursing association, what would its mission be?

14. Of the various types of diversity, for example, culture, gender, age, and socioeconomic status, which do you feel would be most challenging for a professional nursing association to effectively address?

References

American Nurses Association. (2021, September 1). *2020–2023 Strategic plan.* https://www.nursingworld.org/ana/about-ana/anae-strategic-plan-2020–2023/

Dimock, M. (2019, January 17). *Defining generations: Where Millennials end and Generation Z begins.* https://www.pewresearch.org/fact-tank/2019/01/17/where-millennials-end-and-generation-z-begins/

International Council of Nurses. (2021, September 1). *ICN mission, vision and strategic plan.* https://www.icn.ch/who-we-are/icn-mission-vision-and-strategic-plan#:~:text=To%20represent%20nursing%20worldwide%2C%20advance,and%20deliver%20health%20for%20all

King, E., Finkelstein, L., Thomas, C., & Corrington, A. (2019, August 1). *Generational differences at work are small. Thinking they're big affects our behavior.* https://hbr.org/2019/08/

generational-differences-at-work-are-small-thinking-theyre-big-affects-our-behavior

Pinsker, J. (2020, February 21). *Oh no, they've come up with another generation label.* https://www.theatlantic.com/family/archive/2020/02/generation-after-gen-z-named-alpha/606862/

Rabbitt, E. (2019, April 16). *Connect with members across generations.* https://www.asaecenter.org/resources/articles/foundation/2019/connect-with-members-across-generations

Reinhart, R. (2020, January 6). *Nurses continue to rate highest in honesty, ethics.* https://news.gallup.com/poll/274673/nurses-continue-rate-highest-honesty-ethics.aspx

Sigma Theta Tau International. (2021, September 1). *Sigma organizational fact sheet.* https://www.sigmanursing.org/why-sigma/about-sigma/sigma-organizational-fact-sheet

Index

Note: Page numbers followed by b, f and t indicates boxes, figures and tables respectively.

A

AACN. *See* Alliance for Nursing Accreditation
AACN (American Association of Colleges of Nursing), 125
AAMN (American Assembly for Men in Nursing), 128
AAN (American Academy of Nursing), 347, 348
AAP (American Academy of Pediatrics), 112
AARP (American Association of Retired Persons), 383
Abandonment, 176–177, 177b
   employment, 176–177
   patient, 176–177, 177b
ABNS (American Board of Nursing Specialties), 295
Abused drugs, 264–265
ACA. *See* Affordable Care Act of 2010
Academic dishonesty
   student attitudes regarding, 279–280
   types of, 277b
Academic integrity, in nursing education, 275–285
   fostering, 281–285
      clear guidelines and expectations, establishing, 282–283
      ethical behavior, using, 282
      ethical culture, establishing, 282
      faculty supervision, increasing, 283
      honor codes, implementing, 284
      mentoring and support, providing, 285
      self-discipline, fostering, 284
      teaching students about research and appropriate citation, 284–285
      test security or plagiarism assessment tools, using, 283–284
Academic misconduct, consequences of, 281t
Academic-practice-based TPP, 25
Academic-practice gap, in nursing
   changing health care landscape
      health care reform, 19–20
      population aging and sicker, 19

      roles for nurses, 22
      workforce changes, 20–22
   collaborative strategies, 25–26
      academic-practice-based TPP, 25
      dedicated education units, 25
      specialty-specific clinical immersion, 25
      student work-study internships/externships, 25
   curriculum redesign, 26
      California Nursing Schools Pilot Project, 26–27
      Kaiser Foundation School of Nursing, 26
   definition of, 17
   national attention on, 22–23
   practice strategies
      nurse residency programs, 24
   strategies and innovations to bridge gap, 23–26
      active learning/flipped classroom, 24
      competency-based education, 24
      educational strategies, 24
      transition-to-practice program, 19
   understanding, 18–19
Accountable Care Organizations, 323
Accreditation Board for Specialty Nursing Certification, 295
Active learning/flipped classroom, 24
Adaptive leadership, 45
ADEs (adverse drug events), 214
Administration, nursing, 126–128
Administrative leadership, 45
ADN. *See* Associate degree in nursing
Adolescents, social media, 202
Advanced practice nurse certification, 296
Advanced practice nursing (APN), 52–64.
   See also Doctor of Nursing Practice
   clinical nurse specialists in, 53
   Doctor of Nursing Practice in, 60
   history of, 52–53, 55
   nurse practitioners in, 53
Advanced practice registered nurse (APRN), doctor of nursing practice, 57, 60
Adverse drug events (ADEs), 214

Adverse events, definition of, 214
Advocacy
   patient, in whistle-blowing, 253
   political, 383–386
Affordable Care Act of 2010 (ACA), 164, 217, 320, 323–333, 345, 375b, 382
   congressional efforts to replace and repeal, 328–330t
   essential benefits guaranteed by insurance plans, 324b
   failures of, 325b
   successes of, 324b
AFSCME (American Federation of State, County and Municipal Employees), 178
AFT (American Federation of Teachers), 178
Agency for Healthcare Research and Quality (AHRQ), 164
   health care report cards, 221
Aging of nurses, 83
   retention strategies for, 89, 90b
   workplace design for, 89
AHA (American Hospital Association), 387
AHRQ. *See* Agency for Healthcare Research and Quality
Alliance, The. *See* Nursing Organizations Alliance
Alliance for Nursing Accreditation (AACN), 348
   on diversity, 132
Alternative-to-discipline programs, substance use and, 269
American Academy of Nursing (AAN), 347, 348
American Academy of Pediatrics (AAP), 112
American Assembly for Men in Nursing (AAMN), 128
American Association of Colleges of Nursing (AACN), 125
American Association of Community Colleges, 10
American Association of Retired Persons (AARP), 383
American Board of Nursing Specialties (ABNS), 295